HEART
FAILURE

*A Comprehensive Guide to Diagnosis
and Treatment*

Fundamental and Clinical Cardiology

Editor-in-Chief
Samuel Z. Goldhaber, M.D.
Harvard Medical School
and Brigham and Women's Hospital
Boston, Massachusetts

ADDITIONAL VOLUMES IN PREPARATION

Phamacoinvasive Therapy in Acute Myocardial Infarction, *edited by Harold L. Dauerman and Burton E. Sobel*
Clinical, Interventional, and Investigational Thrombocardiology, *edited by Richard Becker and Robert A. Harrington*

HEART
FAILURE

A Comprehensive Guide to Diagnosis and Treatment

Editor

G. William Dec

Massachusetts General Hospital
Boston, Massachusetts, U.S.A.
Harvard Medical School
Cambridge, Massachusetts, U.S.A.

Associate Editors

Thomas DiSalvo, Roger J. Hajjar, and Marc J. Semigran

Harvard Medical School
Cambridge, Massachusetts, U.S.A.

MARCEL DEKKER   NEW YORK

Library of Congress Cataloging-in-Publication Data
A catalog record for this book is available from the Library of Congress.

ISBN: 0-8247-5827-7

This book is printed on acid-free paper.

Headquarters
Marcel Dekker, 270 Madison Avenue, New York, NY 10016, USA
tel: 212-696-9000; fax: 212-685-4540

Distribution and Customer Service
Marcel Dekker, Cimarron Road, Monticello, New York 12701, USA
tel: 800-228-1160; fax: 845-796-1772

World Wide Web
http://www.dekker.com

The publisher offers discounts on this book when ordered in bulk quantities. For more information, write to Special Sales/Professional Marketing at the headquarters address above.

This book is dedicated to
Donna, Sarah, and Jonathan

Preface

Heart failure is a growing world-wide epidemic with a prevalence of more than 5 million cases in the United States and 6.5 million cases in Europe. Epidemiologic data demonstrate a rapid increase in its incidence during the past two decades. This trend is likely to continue as the population ages. It is currently the most common hospital discharge diagnosis for patients over the age of 65 years and accounts for substantial morbidity and high mortality. Fortunately, major advances have occurred in our understanding of the cellular mechanisms, pathophysiological abnormalities, nonpharmacologic therapy and surgical therapeutic options for this syndrome during the past decade. This textbook focuses the most recent developments in the pathogenesis, etiologic considerations, diagnosis, and treatment of heart failure and has been written by internationally recognized physicians and scientists involved on a daily basis in heart failure research and clinical care.

The authors' aim is to provide an up-to-date and comprehensive review of the diagnosis and treatment of heart failure. The text is divided into five sections that concisely summarize fundamental cellular and molecular bases for heart failure, its pathophysiology, current invasive and noninvasive diagnostic techniques, pharmacologic advances and device-based therapy, surgical options, and evolving molecular therapies. The first section focuses on the tremendous advances that have occurred over the last decade in our understanding of the basic mechanisms of heart failure. These discoveries have reshaped our understanding of the basic causes of "the heart failure phenotype" and will allow us to redesign therapeutic strategies for the treatment of this disease. These chapters specifically focus on the genetics of dilated and hypertrophic cardiomyopathy, the role of hypertrophy and apoptosis, beta-adrenergic receptor signaling, and excitation-contraction coupling abnormalities that contribute to ventricular dysfunction. In each of these chapters, the role of new tools, such as microarray analysis, proteomics, and molecular imaging are detailed.

The second section summarizes recent insights into the activation of vasoconstrictor and vasodilator pathways, including a host of crucial neurohormones and cytokines. Ischemic left ventricular remodeling, cardiomyopathies of the adult, and diagnostic and etiologic considerations in diastolic heart failure complete this section.

The third section summarizes current diagnostic methodologies and nonsurgical treatment options. Prognostic markers including brain natriuretic peptides (BNP) are highlighted. Recent pivotal multicenter clinical trials that have evaluated the therapeutic effi-

cacy of beta-adrenergic blockers, angiotensin-receptor antagonists, aldosterone antagonists, and endothelin antagonists are included. Indications and intermediate-term outcomes
for cardiac resynchronization therapy are highlighted. National practice guidelines for
heart failure management from the American Heart Association, American College of
Cardiology and the Heart Failure Society of America are also critically reviewed.

Despite the tremendous success of contemporary pharmacologic treatment, heart
failure remains a progressive disease and the fourth section of the book focuses on the
growing variety of surgical options that are now being adopted for its treatment. The
expanding indications for coronary revascularization and mitral valve repair are summarized. Newer ventricular remodeling procedures, such as the Dor procedure and external
cardiac restraint devices, are reviewed. The contemporary role of cardiac transplantation,
outcome of outpatient left ventricular circulatory support, and the current status of total
artificial heart devices are included.

The next generation of therapies will unquestionably be directed at molecular targets
in the failing myocardium. The last section includes viral-based gene therapies to restore
depressed myocardial contractility, and both stem cell and nonstem cell cellular transplantation techniques designed to repopulate the failing left ventricle. Ongoing advances in
vector and stem cell technology, cardiac cell and gene delivery, and, most importantly,
our understanding of heart failure pathogenesis, encourage consideration of molecular
therapies for heart failure. At the present time, strategies that enhance sarcoplasmic calcium
transport, are supported by substantial evidence in both cardiomyocytes derived from heart
failure patients and animal models. Initial studies evaluating other novel targets appear
promising but have not been as fully evaluated. In ongoing efforts to target cardiac dysfunction, gene and cell transfer provide an important tool to improve our understanding of the
relative contribution of specific pathways. Through such experiments, molecular targets
can be validated for therapeutic intervention whether pharmacologic or genetic. However,
translating these basic investigations into clinical gene therapy for heart failure remains
a formidable challenge. The last section of this book will closely examine the problems
and hope for these novel strategies. Nevertheless, practical advances and our growing
understanding of the molecular pathogenesis of heart failure provide reason for cautious
optimism.

This book will be of particular interest to clinical cardiologists and primary care
specialists involved in the daily care of patients with ventricular dysfunction and symptomatic heart failure. Physician-scientists will also find it useful for integrating mechanistic
laboratory observations with recent clinical advances. Finally, it should appeal to cardiovascular surgeons whose clinical or research interests involve nonpharmacologic treatment
of the failing ventricle. Despite the marked increase in heart failure prevalence, there are
many reasons for optimism that more accurate diagnosis and more individualized, disease-
focused treatment strategies will soon be available. The scientific and clinical approaches
to heart failure management are undergoing dramatic evolution; physicians and surgeons
who care for such patients will benefit from the insights provided into current and future
therapies available in this text.

G. William Dec

Contents

Contents

Contributors

William T. Abraham, MD, FACP, FACC The Davis Heart and Lung Research Institute, The Ohio State University, Columbus, Ohio, USA

Ronen Beeri, MD Cardiac Unit, Massachusetts General Hospital, Boston, Massachusetts, USA

Andrew Clark, MD Department of Cardiology, University of Hull, Hull, UK

John G. F. Cleland, MD Department of Cardiology, University of Hull, Hull, UK

Alison P. Coletta, BSc Department of Cardiology, University of Hull, Hull, UK

G. William Dec, MD Heart Failure and Transplantation Unit, Massachusetts General Hospital, Boston, Massachusetts, USA

Federica del Monte, MD, PhD Cardiovascular Research Center, Massachusetts General Hospital, Boston, Massachusetts, USA

Thomas Disalvo, MD, MPH Massachusetts General Hospital and Harvard Medical School, Boston, Massachusetts, USA

Stefan Engelhardt, MD, PhD Cardiovascular Research Center, Massachusetts General Hospital, Boston, Massachusetts, USA, and DFG-Research Center for Experimental Biomedicine, University of Wuerzburg, Wuerzburg, Germany

Thomas Force, MD Molecular Cardiology Research Institute, Tufts-New England Medical Center, Tufts University School of Medicine, Boston, Massachusetts, USA

William H. Gaasch, MD Department of Cardiovascular Medicine, Lahey Clinic, Burlington, Massachusetts, and the University of Massachusetts Medical School, Worcester, Massachusetts, USA

Justin Ghosh, MBBS   Department of Cardiology, University of Hull, Hull, UK

Roger J. Hajjar, MD   The Program in Cardiovascular Gene Therapy, Cardiovascular Research Center and Cardiology Division, Massachusetts General Hospital, Harvard Medical School, Boston, Massachusetts, USA

Katherine J. Hoercher, RN   George M. and Linda H. Kaufman Center for Heart Failure, Cleveland Clinic Foundation, Cleveland, Ohio, USA

Judy Hung, MD   Cardiac Unit, Massachusetts General Hospital, Boston, Massachusetts, USA

Peter C. Kouretas, MD, PhD   Department of Cardiothoracic Surgery, Stanford University, Stanford, California, USA

Thomas H. Lee, MD, M.Sc.   Partners Community Healthcare, Harvard Medical School, Boston, Massachusetts, USA

Richard Lee, MD   George M. and Linda H. Kaufman Center for Heart Failure, Cleveland Clinic Foundation, Cleveland, Ohio, USA

Robert A. Levine, MD   Cardiac Unit, Massachusetts General Hospital, Boston, Massachusetts, USA

Patrick M. McCarthy, MD   Departments of Cardiovascular and Thoracic Surgery, Northwestern University Medical Center, Chicago, Illinois, USA

Calum A. MacRae, MD   Cardiology Division and Cardiovascular Research Center, Massachusetts General Hospital, Boston, Massachusetts, USA

Dennis M. McNamara, MD   Heart Failure & Transplantation Program, University of Pittsburgh Medical Center, Pittsburgh, Pennsylvania, USA

Anwar Memon, MD   Department of Cardiology, University of Hull, Hull, UK

Philippe Menasché, MD, PhD   Department of Cardiovascular Surgery & INSERM U-633 Hôpital Européen Georges Pompidou, Paris, France

Theo E. Meyer, MD, PhD   Department of Medicine, the University of Massachusetts Memorial Health Center and the University of Massachusetts Medical School, Worcester, Massachusetts, USA

Susan Moffatt-Bruce, MD, PhD   Department of Cardiothoracic Surgery, Stanford University, Stanford, California, USA

Jeffery D. Molkentin, PhD   Department of Pediatrics Division of Molecular Cardiovascular Biology, Children's Hospital Medical Center, Cincinnati, Ohio, USA

Jagat Narula, MD, PhD Division of Cardiology, Hahnemann University Hospital, Philadelphia, Pennsylvania, and The Program in Cardiovascular Gene Therapy, Massachusetts General Hospital, Boston, Massachusetts, USA

Nikolay Nikitin, MD Department of Cardiology, University of Hull, Hull, UK

Bertram Pitt, MD University of Michigan School of Medicine, Ann Arbor, Michigan, USA

Sanjay Rajagopalan, MD University of Michigan School of Medicine, Ann Arbor, Michigan, USA

Kumudha Ramasubbu, MD Baylor College of Medicine and The Methodist DeBakey Heart Center, Houston, Texas, USA

Robert C. Robbins, MD Department of Cardiothoracic Surgery, Stanford University, Stanford, California, USA

Richard Rodeheffer, MD Mayo Clinic School of Medicine, Rochester, Minnesota, USA

Anthony Rosenzweig, MD The Program in Cardiovascular Gene Therapy, Cardiovascular Research Center and Cardiology Division, Massachusetts General Hospital, Harvard Medical School, Boston, Massachusetts, USA

Khurram Shahzad, MD Cardiac Unit, Massachusetts General Hospital, Boston, Massachusetts, USA

Lynne Warner Stevenson, MD Cardiovascular Division, Brigham and Women's Hospital, Boston, Massachusetts, USA

William G. Stevenson, MD Cardiovascular Division, Brigham and Women's Hospital, Boston, Massachusetts, USA

Johan Sundström, MD, PhD National Heart, Lung and Blood Institute's Framingham Heart Study, Framingham, Massachusetts, USA

Usha Tedrow, MD Cardiovascular Division, Brigham and Women's Hospital, Boston, Massachusetts, USA

Guillermo Torre-Amione, MD, PhD The Methodist DeBakey Heart Center, Houston, Texas, USA

Ramachandran S. Vasan, MD National Heart, Lung and Blood Institute's Framingham Heart Study, Framingham, Massachusetts, USA

Cynthia K. Wallace, MSPH Baylor College of Medicine and The Methodist DeBakey Heart Center, Houston, Texas, USA

Clyde W. Yancy, MD Heart Failure/Transplantation, University of Texas Southwestern Medical Center, Dallas, Texas, USA

Paul Zei, MD, PhD Cardiovascular Division, Brigham and Women's Hospital, Boston, Massachusetts, USA

1

The Genetics of Dilated and Hypertrophic Cardiomyopathies

Calum A. MacRae
Cardiology Division and Cardiovascular Research Center
Massachusetts General Hospital
Boston, Massachusetts, USA

The advent of cardiac catheterization and echocardiography changed the landscape of cardiovascular disease. The ability, in routine clinical practice, to objectively assess coronary or ventricular anatomy and to define cardiac physiology led to the reclassification of many conditions [1,2]. Pathological studies had characterized ventricular dilatation and hypertrophy as distinctive adaptive responses of the myocardium to volume or pressure overload, respectively [Figure 1]. These processes were thought of as initial homeostatic responses that led to maladaptive physiology, and ultimately heart failure. The application of new diagnostic tools enabled systematic studies of the natural history of myocardial disease. In many instances there was no evidence of an antecedent valvular lesion or myocardial injury[2,3]. These early descriptions of cardiomyopathy also recognized familial cases, and the concept of primary myocardial disease emerged. Despite these insights, the majority of heart failure cases were still felt to result from occult acquired insults.

The last decade has seen an explosion in the application of genetic approaches to the study of cardiomyopathy. This work was fueled by the promise of identifying the causal genes underlying these primary forms of myocardial dysfunction. Using human and model system genetics, tremendous strides have been made in our understanding of the pathophysiology of both ventricular dilatation and hypertrophy. Although molecular diagnostics have not yet had an impact on day-to-day practice, the interdependence of clinical cardiology and molecular genetics is already evident. This chapter will discuss the relationship between clinical investigation and molecular genetics, emphasizing the role of current knowledge in the diagnosis and management of adult cardiomyopathies.

GENETIC METHODS

In any disease the presence of a major genetic effect has implications, not only for molecular studies of the etiology of the disorder, but also for the design and interpretation of studies of its diagnosis and management. These clinical inferences are often relevant long before the intricacies of the molecular pathways are understood. To place the clinical and

Classic parallel pathways

Dilatation ← Hypertrophy

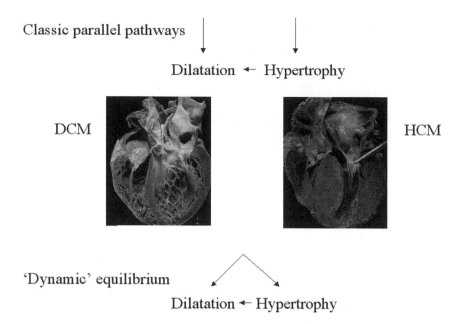

DCM   HCM

'Dynamic' equilibrium

Dilatation ← Hypertrophy

Figure 1   The classic view of HCM and DCM as discrete biological pathways has been challenged by recent molecular genetic studies, although the physiologic profiles are clearly distinct. Hypertrophy is known to progress to dilatation in many situations, including in some familial cardiomyopathies. However, a single mutation in different individuals within the same family may cause hypertrophy or dilatation, as a result, it is presumed, of genetic or environmental modifiers. Understanding the mechanisms favoring the development of hypertrophy or dilatation will help in the dissection of acquired forms of ventricular remodeling.

molecular insights in context, some background on the vocabulary and techniques used in genetic analysis is necessary [see Table 1].

Familial Aggregation

In some instances the genetic nature of cardiomyopathy is obvious, whereas in many cases the symptomatic individuals represent only a subset of those with the underlying trait. Large families with a clear family history of the disease may be the exception rather than the rule, even when a condition is highly heritable. The expression of the phenotype may require additional genetic or environmental factors, or may vary stochastically [Fig 1]. To gain an objective sense of how important genetic factors might be in any given form of heart disease, systematic studies of familial aggregation and lineal transmission are necessary[4]. There are several ways of crudely estimating the degree of heritability, the most common of which is the simple sibling recurrence risk. Detailed assessment of the mode of inheritance and magnitude of any heritable component requires more complex segregation analysis using multiple families. The genetic basis for hypertrophic cardiomyopathy (HCM) was obvious from simple inspection[3,5,6], but these types of analysis first suggested a large heritable contribution to dilated cardiomyopathy (DCM)[7].

Genetic Linkage

Genetics has proven a powerful tool to define causal mechanisms in biology, not because of some unique property of DNA, but rather because of the magnitude of the underlying

Table 1 Basic Genetic Terminology

Allele—Any one of the sequence variants of a particular gene.

Genome—The complete DNA sequence of an organism.

Haplotype—A series of sequence variations that are linked together on a single chromosome.

Introns and exons—Genes are initially transcribed as continuous sequences, but only some segments (the exons) of the resulting messenger RNA molecules contain information that encodes the gene's protein product. The intervening regions between exons (the introns), are excised (or spliced) from the RNA to generate the final RNA from which the protein is translated.

Messenger RNA—Following the initial transcription from a gene of a continuous RNA molecule, this molecule is then processed in a number of ways, including splicing, to generate the final messenger RNA, which is then translated by the cells machinery into a protein.

Mutation—Any variation in sequence from a reference state.

Phenotype—The complete set of characteristics of an organism, including morphology and function.

Proteome—The complete repertoire of proteins encoded by a genome.

Single nucleotide polymorphism (SNP)—Most of the variation in DNA sequence between individual members of a population is the result of changes in single nucleotides. These polymorphisms are known as SNPs.

Transcription—The copying of a gene's DNA into RNA.

Translation—The synthesis of a protein from the information encoded in a messenger RNA.

effect and the segregation of genes through families[8]. In many situations where disease genes have been cloned, the risk to first-degree relatives is several hundred times greater than in the general population. The theory behind proving causality using genetics parallels Koch's postulates in infection–another situation in which an abnormal genome is responsible for disease. If there is a large genetic effect, given the way in which DNA is transmitted to the next generation, it is possible to define a segment of mutated DNA that when inherited is sufficient to cause the phenotype in question. This specific segment of DNA can potentially be isolated, and be shown to be distinct from the normal sequence at that location. Finally, the mutated gene, if introduced into a normal organism, should be capable of causing the disease phenotype. Clearly the literal fulfillment of these criteria is not feasible in humans, but the methods of human molecular genetics allow very similar logic to be applied [see Table 2].

If the DNA of family members can be screened for segments of the genome that are consistently transmitted with the phenotype, then the causative gene can be mapped. The development of panels of informative markers, polymorphic between individuals, made such genetic linkage analyses possible. These anonymous markers allow individual DNA segments to be followed as they pass through a family, defining their relationship (or lack of relationship) with disease. Using a panel of markers that "scans" the entire genome, even in a single large family with a given genetic disease, it is possible to define a minimal location for the disease, and ultimately to identify the causal mutation[9]. The passage, or segregation, of a phenotype through a single lineage is the hallmark of a genetic trait [4]. Segregation also allows other features which track with this phenotype to be identified, informing the investigator about relationships between apparently unrelated clinical findings (Figures 1 and 2) [10].

Clinical Diagnosis and Genetic Mapping

It is impossible to separate human molecular genetics from clinical assessment. A final chromosomal disease interval is defined in terms of recombinants, i.e., individuals whose

Table 2 Criteria for Defining a Causal Mutation-Discrimination from a Polymorphism

I. The "mutation" should segregate perfectly with disease.

The sequence anomaly must be present in all the affected individuals and absent from all the unaffected individuals. Ideally two independent means should be used to confirm that this is the case. The best statistical support for this segregation is a LOD or logarithm of the odds score (also used in anonymous mapping studies), which estimates the likelihood of random cosegregation as a function of the number of informative events.

II. The "mutation" should not be present in a normal population.

Rare polymorphisms may be overrepresented in any given large family. These polymorphisms may have functional significance, yet not be responsible for disease. For example, null alleles have been described for many genes including that encoding the cardiac beta myosin heavy chain, but when present in the heterozygous state may be of no import. It is necessary to screen a large normal population for any putative mutation to ensure that it is not simply an incidental polymorphism.

III. The "mutation" should effect substantial change on the gene sequence.

There should be indirect evidence that the mutation will have a biological effect. This may be obvious for some mutations that disrupt the sense of the entire coding sequence of the gene. Other mutations will have more subtle effects, changing only a single amino-acid residue. The confirmation of these substitutions as disease-causing may require additional studies, such as comparative sequence analyses (with the same gene in other species, or similar genes in the same species, to see if a particular residue is highly conserved), *in vitro* structure function analysis or *in vivo* genetic analyses.

IV. The introduction of the "mutation" should be sufficient to cause disease.

There should be direct evidence that the mutation has a biological effect. The ultimate proof of causality lies in the demonstration that the simple addition of the mutation is sufficient to recapitulate the disease. This is usually done in genetic model organisms, but the specific knock-in of a point mutation (the most common mutations in human disease) is rarely performed. Often a causal role is inferred from transgenic expression of a mutant gene, or from knock-out of the gene. The demonstration of disease in association with a *de novo* mutation in humans is the logical equivalent.

phenotypes and genotypes are discordant due to inferred recombination between the marker and the disease-causing mutation. The definition of recombinant events is, thus, completely dependent on the clinical phenotype[8,9]. Given the central role of the phenotype in mapping and cloning a disease gene, it is conventional to adopt conservative criteria for assigning positive and negative affection status in human molecular genetics. It is better to define an individual as unknown than to attempt molecular studies with the wrong diagnosis. The need to exclude many equivocal family members has restricted positional cloning efforts to very large kindreds with highly penetrant forms of disease. The closer a genetic marker is to the disease-causing mutation the fewer recombinants are evident at that marker, until ultimately the disease-causing mutation itself should segregate perfectly with the phenotype.

Positional Cloning

Once a minimal disease interval has been defined by genetic mapping, the techniques of positional cloning are used to identify all the genes within this interval and to screen these genes for mutations[8]. The ability to grow, in yeast or bacterial artificial chromosomes, long segments of as many as several hundred thousand base pairs of human DNA, allows large stretches of a human chromosome to be cloned in an overlapping set of such segments.

This "contig" of human DNA clones can then be manipulated, and, eventually, sequenced to define the disease gene. Importantly, the cloning of the mutated gene does not require any *a priori* assumptions regarding the mechanism of disease. This lack of dependence on previous hypotheses has resulted in the discovery of truly novel pathways, and is particularly powerful in complicated disorders with multiple manifestations[11]. The recent completion of the Human Genome Project ensures that no matter how large the final disease locus, it is possible to rapidly identify the genes within the final interval[12]. This has expedited the cloning of disease genes, and broadened the scope of positional cloning projects to include progressively smaller families with less penetrant diseases [13].

Genetic Association Studies

Not all phenotypes segregate in large families, so other genetic techniques have been developed that do not use transmission probability, but instead rely on simple association of genotypes with phenotypes within a population[4,14]. These studies are qualitatively different from linkage analyses and have proliferated in recent years[15,16]. Genetic association studies have many limitations[17,18]. By their nature they are biased in favor of small population-wide effects, so that in the face of heterogeneity even major genetic effects might be missed. A second major problem is population stratification, which results in spurious association of a polymorphism with disease, simply because both the disease and the unlinked sequence variant are found in the same population subgroup. This can be partly addressed by replicating the findings in large study cohorts drawn from genetically distinct populations. The prior probability that any observed effect is a result of the specific polymorphism(s) studied is usually extremely low, resulting in an unacceptably high false-positive rate (through Bayesian inference). Importantly, because of the absence of segregation information inherent in these studies, it is also impossible to causally relate specific variants to a phenotype. The phenotype in question may result from variations in linked genes, in so-called dysequilibrium with the tested polymorphism. These issues would, at least in part, be dealt with by using extended haplotypes of markers in large populations. The overall consensus remains that genetic association studies may be extremely difficult to interpret, even when carried out in an exemplary fashion.

Locus and Allelic Heterogeneity

Our ability to distinguish discrete pathologic processes, and to undertake genetic analysis of these phenotypes, is limited by the resolution of current diagnostic techniques. Mutations in many different genes may give rise to very similar phenotypes, a phenomenon known as genetic heterogeneity. This situation is compounded by the fact that inherited cardiac conditions often result in premature mortality, so founder mutations are rare. Virtually every HCM family with mutations in a specific sarcomeric contractile protein has a different mutation (so-called allelic heterogeneity)[11]. This degree of heterogeneity also exists for most other Mendelian cardiac conditions[19]. Importantly, subtle differences between the clinical manifestations of different mutated genes may not be detectable until genetic studies have been completed [19] and "pure" populations studied.

Modifiers of Simple Traits

Any clinician who has cared for families with monogenic forms of cardiomyopathy has been struck by the range of clinical manifestations seen within a single family, in which the primary genetic abnormality is identical in each affected individual. While some of this variable expressivity represents our limited understanding of the phenotype itself, some of the variation is the result of modifier genes or of environmental factors[20]. The discovery of such modifier loci or environmental agents is a major focus of current research. If we cannot discern these modifiers in the context of a simple disease caused by a single major gene, we will have tremendous difficulty understanding those conditions where multiple genes interact[4,14].

USING GENETICS IN CLINICAL PRACTICE

Genotypic information is not yet of any utility in patient management. However, clinical genetic analyses may contribute to patient care long before the genes for all the inherited cardiomyopathies have been cloned. The application of clinical genetic principles in the diagnosis and management of inherited heart disease will be outlined before details of the molecular basis of specific disorders are discussed.

Family-Based Diagnosis

The presence of a definitive diagnosis of HCM or DCM in a first-degree relative dramatically changes the implications of any cardiovascular evaluation. Thus, minor EKG (electrocardiogram) abnormalities are viewed in a different light in the context of a family history of HCM [21]. In some cases, the definitive diagnosis in a particular patient is only clear from the integrated evaluation of multiple individuals within the same family. This is increasingly recognized in families in which several ''discrete'' phenotypes, such as DCM and arrhythmogenic right ventricular cardiomyopathy, cosegregate. Only the complete evaluation of an entire kindred would allow these important features to be detected. The ethical implications of family-based diagnosis remain to be fully explored, but informed consent is critical if the data from multiple individuals are to be collected.

Diagnosis—History

The history often offers evidence that the presenting condition results from an inherited diathesis. Patients with cardiomyopathy may have had subtle evidence of disease from an early age. Functional limitations are often attributed to respiratory illnesses, but it is usually possible to discern other features of the underlying disease. Comparison of exercise capacity at various ages with that of peers is useful in the evaluation of symptoms such as muscle pains or syncope. The presence of other premature medical disorders suggests specific conditions [see Tables 3 and 4].

A comprehensive family history is an integral part of every patient encounter, but is particularly important in the diagnosis and management of adult cardiomyopathies. In addition to defining the basic structure of the family, it is vital to define in as much detail as is possible any cardiac conditions (or even potential cardiac conditions) in first-or second-degree relatives. Probands will often be unaware of subtle distinctions between cardiac diseases, and many affected relatives of patients with cardiomyopathy may have been mislabeled with other cardiac conditions such as valvular heart disease or myocardial infarction. Once the basic family structure is defined and an overview of any inherited traits is obtained, the actual symptoms, ages of onset, specific treatments (e.g., diuretics, pacemakers, ICDs [implantable cardioverter defibrillators] , surgery), and modes of death for every member of the nuclear family should be elicited. Specific enquiry regarding extracardiac phenotypes, including skeletal or other myopathies, peripheral sensory or

Table 3 Adult Dilated Cardiomyopathy Loci

Locus	Mode of inheritance	Disease gene	Specific clinical features	References
1q21 CDDC-1	AD	Lamin A/C	AVB, LGMD, CMT	47
1q31 CMD-1D	AD	Cardiac troponin T		55
2q14–22 CMD-1H	AD	Unknown		79
2q31 CMD-1G	AD	Titin		80
2q35 CMD-1I	AD	Desmin	RCM, Inclusion myopathy	81
3p21 CDDC-2	AD	Unknown	AVB, ARVC	46
4q12	AR	β-sarcoglycan		82
5q33	AD/AR	δ-Sarcoglycan		83
6p24	AR	Desmoplakin	ARVC, Wooly hair	84
6q12-16 CMD-1K	AD	Unknown	Possibly allelic with AFib	85
6q22	AD	Phospholamban		86
6q23 CDDC-3	AD	Unknown	AVB, LGMD	87
6q23-24	AD	Unknown	Sensorineural hearing loss	88
9q13	AD	Unknown		89
10q21-23	AD	Unknown	Possibly allelic with AFib	90
11p15 CMD-1M	AD	Cardiac LIM protein		56
11p11	AD	MYBP-C		91
14q12	AD	β-Cardiac myosin heavy chain (MYH7)		55
15q14	AD	α-cardiac actin	Cosegregating FHC	53
19q13	AD	Myotonin	Anticipation, AVB, arrhythmia	26
Xp21	X-Linked	Dystrophin		48
Xq28	X-Linked	Emery-Dreifuss	AVB, humeroperoneal MD	51

Abbreviations: AD, autosomal dominant; AR, autosomal recessive; AVB, atrioventricular block; MYBP-C, myosin binding protein-C; LGMD, limb girdle muscular dystrophy; CMT, Charcot-Marie-Tooth; RCM, restrictive cardiomyopathy; AFib, atrial fibrillation; FHC, familial hypertrophic cardiomyopathy; MD, muscular dystrophy.

motor neuropathy, and premature diabetes or liver disease is recommended. On many occasions, a family history is not appreciated, simply because the potential connection between different phenotypes is not explicitly considered [22].

It is important to remember that other apparently unrelated disorders or events may represent *formes frustes* of the same primary abnormality [Fig 2]. Thus, for example, atrial fibrillation in a young relative of a patient with cardiomyopathy is likely a manifestation of the same gene defect, and an unexplained motor vehicle accident may represent an undetected sudden death[23]. The family history also allows some sense of the mode of inheritance to be obtained [Figure 2]. A careful family history must also be a prominent

Table 4 Hypertrophic Cardiomyopathy Loci

Locus	Mode of Inheritance	Disease Gene	Specific Clinical Features	References
1q31	AD	Cardiac troponin T	Hypertrophy may be less marked	92
3p	AD/AR	Myosin light chain 3 kinase	Mid-cavity/PAP muscle hypertrophy	70
7q36	AD	PRKAG2	Glycogen storage AVB, WPW	71
9	AR	Frataxin	Ataxia	78
11p15	AD	Muscle LIM protein		93
11p11	AD	MYBP-C	Often later onset disease	94
14q12	AD	MYH7 and MYH 6		66
15q14	AD	α-cardiac actin	Cosegregating DCM	69
15q22	AD	α-Tropomyosin		92
19q13	AD	Cardiac Troponin I	Cosegregating RCM	95
20q13	AD	Myosin light chain kinase	Mid-cavity/PAP muscle hypertrophy	70

Abbreviations: AD, autosomal dominant; AR, autosomal recessive; PRKAG2, adenosine monophosphate activated protein kinase gamma-2 subunit; MYBP-C, myosin binding protein-C; MYH, myosin heavy chain; PAP, papillary; AVB, atrioventricular block; WPW, ventricular preexcitation; DCM, dilated cardiomyopathy; RCM, restrictive cardiomyopathy.

feature in any follow-up visits. Patients will often have gleaned additional family history from interactions with relatives since the initial patient encounter. Indeed, empowering the patient to obtain such information should be a goal of the initial encounter.

Diagnosis–Clinical Evaluation

The physical examination and subsequent clinical investigation of any cardiomyopathy patient are also heavily influenced by the genetic basis of the major syndromes. The examination should look for general morphological abnormalities, such as facial or other

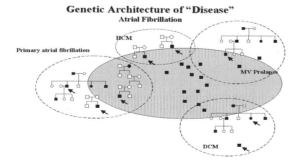

Figure 2 Only the systematic assessment of family members of affected probands reveals the true genetic architecture of a syndrome that may be very homogeneous as in some of the cardiomyopathies, or highly heterogeneous as in this example from a study of atrial fibrillation.

dysmorphism, midline defects, cutaneous anomalies, or the typical features of disorders such as myotonic dystrophy[24]. Several forms of cardiomyopathy are associated with myopathy involving extraocular muscles, the limb girdles, or other muscle groups. The evidence of a skeletal myopathy may be subtle, such as a mild scoliosis or distorted pedal architecture. Finally, it is important to also exclude tendon contractures, ataxia, peripheral neuropathy, or other neurological disorders. Cardiomyopathy is by definition a diagnosis of exclusion, and potentially reversible specific heart muscle diseases, such as coronary artery disease, glycogen storage disorders, hemochromatosis, and dysthyroid heart disease should be formally eliminated[25].

Once appropriate permission has been obtained, objective data from other family members are extremely helpful in the diagnosis and management of adult cardiomyopathies. The direct examination of at-risk family members often will be useful in making a diagnosis in equivocal cases. Pathognomonic components of the phenotype, including extracardiac features, may only be present in a limited subset of the family. Objective phenotypic assignment is especially helpful in inferring the mode of inheritance[24]. Evidence of any mode of inheritance other than an autosomal dominant trait substantially changes the differential diagnosis in any cardiomyopathy [see Tables 3 and 4]. Mitochondrial inheritance is usually seen in the context of left ventricular hypertrophy, X-linked and recessive syndromes are most often seen with DCM, but Friedreich's ataxia is also recessive. Progressive changes in the severity of a phenotype from one generation to the next, known as anticipation or reverse anticipation depending on the direction, are characteristic of triplet repeat expansion disorders such as myotonic dystrophy[26]. The study of extended families offers a unique opportunity to investigate patient cohorts with homogeneous etiologies[27]. In a family with a highly penetrant Mendelian disease, an identical etiology may reasonably be inferred for each affected individual, and the key features of the specific disorder evaluated in exquisite detail. The potential of even a moderate-size family for molecular genetic analysis is changing rapidly, and referral to specialized centers for such studies should be considered[25,28].

Prognosis

The remarkable range of clinical outcomes, even within a single kindred, plagues the clinical management of both DCM and HCM[29–31]. There are families in which multiple members have died suddenly or required transplantation, and others where the disease is little more than an incidental echocardiographic finding. Initial studies of the presentation, natural history, and clinical physiology of the cardiomyopathies were based on highly selected series from large national referral centers. Subsequent series from regional centers have attempted to redress the balance. However, the major biases implicit in inherited disease have not been addressed in most studies. Without knowing the extent to which individuals (particularly phenotypic outliers) are related, or the contributions of specific families to the overall cohort, it is impossible to begin to interpret even simple studies.

The identification of the underlying gene defects led to the hope that molecular diagnostics would revolutionize risk stratification. Preliminary work has suggested that specific mutations may be associated with high rates of adverse outcome, but these studies, by necessity, include multiple members from each family. Contradictory results have emerged from both clinical and molecular studies[32,33]. The extent of genetic heterogeneity, the large size of the genes involved, and the high rates of new mutation have slowed the arrival of genotype-phenotype studies based on serial probands. Understanding the distinctive contributions of the primary mutation, familial modifiers, and therapeutic interventions will require novel statistical methods for extracting information from extended families[20,34].

In the absence of rigorous techniques to attribute risk to specific mutations, the effect of the same mutation in different generations of the same family remains a reasonable (albeit imperfect) index of the likely natural history of the disease, and of the prognosis in an individual patient. Family members share not only the same causative mutation but also much of the genetic background, environment, and experiences. A complete family history and evaluation offers a sense of the range of expressivity of a particular genetic defect. It may be difficult to get an overview of how a condition behaves in a small family, but in larger kindreds clear patterns of natural history sometimes emerge. It is usually possible to assess the penetrance, any major effects of gender, and other features such as anticipation in larger families. At the very least, these data are helpful in genetic counseling of potential parents.

The integration of these imperfect family data with similarly skewed results from heterogeneous clinical cohorts is, unfortunately, the current state of the art. Dogmatic overinterpretation of both types of data is widespread. In most instances, the disparate results seen between studies reflect the underlying etiologic heterogeneity of the study cohorts as much as any true biological differences. Large series of probands are being genotyped by several groups, but the routine clinical use of genotyping will have to await new sequencing methods[35]. The rate of new mutations and the fact that modifiers may significantly affect risk are also stimulating novel approaches to defining prognosis using proteomics or functional assays.

Asymptomatic affected relatives are another group that might benefit from screening[28]. The risk of complications, including death, is not clearly related to symptoms. There are therapies for both DCM and HCM, some of which are proven to reduce mortality. Systematic screening has been recommended for prognostic reasons in "at-risk" asymptomatic relatives of probands with both DCM and HCM[25]. Although there are no objective data to support any form of screening, if undertaken in specialist centers with appropriate counseling, it is reasonable in the context of active research programs.

Management

The management of the cardiomyopathies has also proven difficult to study empirically. Once again the literature contains many equivocal or contradictory studies, and consensus is often lacking. This situation reflects the rarity of many of the conditions, aggregation of heterogeneous populations, and ultimately the failure to deal with familial confounders.

In the face of these uncertainties, clinical decisions must be based on what limited information is available, and, as previously outlined, much of that information is likely to come from the extended family of the patient. Management strategies often must be tailored to the individual family, and their previous experiences with the disease. For example, despite the lack of support from randomized controlled trials, it is difficult not to implant an ICD in an affected young adult whose siblings have died suddenly from HCM. The history of any disease within an extended kindred is usually firmly embedded in the family psyche, and this may also require management approaches that extend far beyond the individual patient. Family meetings and counseling have a role, and involvement with a research group with long-term positive goals can be extremely helpful in engaging individuals who may have withdrawn from dealing with their disease.

SPECIFIC DISORDERS–DILATED CARDIOMYOPATHY
Definitions and Clinical Features

The diagnostic criteria for DCM have evolved little since the earliest definitions of idiopathic cardiomegaly were first proposed as the exclusion of ischemic or valvular causes of heart failure became possible[2]. The most evolved current definition of DCM dates from a NIH (National Institutes of Health) conference, and highlights the lack of positive diagnostic features[36]. Despite being "a diagnosis of exclusion," several key attributes of the syndrome are remarkably consistent across a wide variety of studies. The histological abnormalities seen are almost invariably those of a myocardial dystrophy, with rather patchy myocyte drop-out, inflammatory infiltrates and hypertrophy of remaining myocytes. There are several typical modes of clinical presentation including an acute left ventricular failure syndrome in younger adults, often associated with an upper respiratory prodrome, classic congestive biventricular heart failure, and sudden cardiac death[37]. Increasingly, individuals with asymptomatic left ventricular dysfunction are recognized. Interestingly, the families of probands with overt DCM are enriched not only for DCM, but also for asymptomatic borderline left ventricular enlargement or depression of contractile shortening[38]. These phenotypes are presumed to represent *formes frustes* of DCM in carriers of the mutant gene. There is evidence that these individuals have active myocardial disease, and that some progress to DCM, but the precise relationship to overt DCM remains unclear[39].

The possibility that some subtle phenotypes represent early forms of DCM is particularly attractive in the context of the evidence from randomized controlled trials for the efficacy of several drug regimens in asymptomatic left ventricular dysfunction[40]. These data, combined with the need to identify gene carriers in the genetic analysis of any pedigree, have led to the evolution of less stringent diagnostic criteria for the diagnosis of DCM in the context of a family history[41]. Several extracardiac phenotypes are known to be associated with DCM, and may prove more reliable than subtle cardiac criteria for the diagnosis of gene carriers. It is important to remember that while these criteria may be useful for specialized clinical or molecular studies, they have not been validated formally. Long-term studies of these subclinically affected family members have also described a substantial number of individuals whose echocardiograms revert to normal[42]. The concept is emerging of a genetically determined predisposition to DCM, in the context of a range of common myocardial insults. The variability of progression to overt cardiac disease may be the result of distinctive environmental exposures, modifier genes, or other unknown stochastic factors. In any event, it is clear that the data available at present do not allow easy prognostication from any specific subclinical marker. Hopefully, as our understanding of the etiology of DCM increases, the mechanism for these variations will be uncovered, and it will prove possible to identify those who will develop clinically significant disease, and to institute appropriate preventive measures.

Etiology of DCM

As a consequence of several clinical and pathological features of the disease, a large proportion of DCM was thought to represent the sequelae of previous viral myocarditis[43]. Many cases present with a history of upper respiratory tract symptoms or a vague systemic inflammatory prodrome, and there are often patchy inflammatory infiltrates in myocardial biopsy specimens. Although viral myocarditis undoubtedly may result in persistent ventricular dysfunction, the process is usually associated with reversible abnormalities. Further, there is evidence that even when associated with such an acute prodrome, DCM is the result of a process that has been active for many years, suggesting that this symptom complex is secondary, perhaps to pulmonary or hepatic congestion[44]. Several drugs and other environmental toxins, including alcohol, are known to cause cardiomyopathy through a variety of mechanisms. Similarly, specific nutritional deprivations, such as selenium deficiency or beriberi, occasionally cause heart failure. Autoimmune diseases have been reported to cluster with DCM, and circulating autoantibodies are found in many patients, but primary immunological abnormalities have been difficult to identify[45]. It was in the context of such conflicting hypotheses that genetic studies became attractive.

Clinical Genetics

Even in the earliest descriptions of DCM, an inherited basis was suspected from the occasional observation of extended families. Michels and colleagues studied the role of genetic factors in DCM by systematically evaluating the first-degree relatives of probands with DCM for evidence of the same disease[7]. There was signs of DCM in 25% of at-risk first-degree relatives. Subsequent work from other investigators has confirmed the prevalence of DCM in relatives and demonstrated that when subtle subclinical phenotypes are included up to 40% of DCM probands have affected relatives[38]. These findings, in the context of the successes of positional cloning approaches in HCM and other syndromes, led to an explosion in the number of genetic studies in DCM. Initial anticipation of early etiologic insights in DCM has been tempered by the consistent finding of small kindreds with relatively few definitively affected individuals[30]. Autosomal dominant patterns of inheritance predominate. The large numbers of individuals with subclinical disease have complicated linkage analyses and are one important reason for the high ratio of mapped loci to cloned genes [see Table 3]. The structure of the families seen in DCM likely reflects some real biological attribute of the syndrome, but what this is remains unclear.

Genetic Mapping

Genetic linkage studies have identified at least 20 loci at which DCM is a prominent component of the phenotype. Many loci are represented by only a single published family [see Table 3]. These data suggest a high degree of genetic heterogeneity, as seen in HCM. The detection of any allelic heterogeneity will require the identification of the responsible genes at these loci. This genetic heterogeneity is only partly reflected in clinical or pheno-typic heterogeneity[30,41]. At least two general patterns of disease have been identified, each of which may represent a distinct etiologic pathway. There are several recessive or X-linked muscular dystrophies that are associated with significant cardiomyopathy, often disproportionate to the extent of the skeletal involvement[30,41]. The second phenotypic group is represented by families with autosomal dominant atrioventricular conduction block, intraventricular conduction disease, and DCM. These appear to be manifestations of a syndrome that may also include arrhythmogenic right ventricular cardiomyopathy, or in some cases, limb-girdle muscular dystrophy[30,46,47]. Even these clinical entities are known to be genetically heterogeneous. The vast majority of DCM families are small kindreds with two or three clearly affected individuals in a distribution consistent with autosomal dominant inheritance, with no obvious extracardiac features.

Molecular Genetics and Pathophysiology

The genes responsible for several forms of DCM have been identified, and investigation of the basic mechanisms of disease has been initiated. These genes belong to several different gene families, and at present no unifying theme has emerged.

Dystrophin and Associated Proteins

The cloning of the dystrophin gene responsible for Duchenne and Becker variants of muscular dystrophy, both of which have significant cardiac involvement, suggested this protein and other members of the dystrophin-associated glycoprotein complex (DGC) as potential candidate genes for other forms of DCM. So far occasional families with X-linked DCM have been directly linked to mutations in the dystrophin gene, and other rare recessive cardiomyopathies have been found to result from mutations in the sarcoglycan genes[48,49]. Several screens of multiple affected probands have effectively excluded this protein complex as a common cause of DCM when unselected for mode of inheritance.

Mutations in this pathway are presumed to cause DCM through the role of the large dystroglycan associated glycoprotein complex in the structural integrity of the link between cytoskeleton and extracellular matrix. However, recent work implicating the DGC in membrane cycling, aggregation of signaling molecules into local, functionally important clusters, and in adenoviral pathobiology suggests a much more complicated picture. Abnormalities of smooth muscle, affecting the circulation, have also been implicated in the etiology of skeletal myopathy and cardiomyopathy[50].

Nuclear Membrane Proteins

The discovery of mutations in the lamin A/C gene in families with conduction disease and DCM recently suggested that these nuclear membrane proteins may represent a distinct pathway in cardiomyopathy[47]. These results built on the demonstration of a very similar cardiac phenotype with mutations in emerin, another nuclear membrane protein[51]. It is possible that this pathway results in DCM through defects in the mechanical integrity of the nucleus, however, the biological functions of these genes are only beginning to be understood. Interestingly, lamin A/C is widely expressed, yet the diverse phenotypes associated with mutations in this gene appear tissue-specific. Several other loci exist where the discrete phenotype of conduction disease and DCM cosegregate. The cloning of mutated genes at these loci will add further potential pathway members and may elucidate the mechanisms of disease in this subset[52].

Cytoskeletal and sarcomeric proteins

Given the specialized role of cardiac myocytes, and the adaptation of the cytoskeletal apparatus in the sarcomere, many of these genes became candidates in the search for the causes of DCM[53]. The screening of large numbers of probands for mutations in the cardiac actin gene resulted in the identification of mutations in a very small fraction of these patients. Subsequent screening of series of probands has only confirmed the extreme rarity of actin mutations as causal factors in DCM[54]. Interestingly, mutations in other sarcomeric protein genes, previously implicated in hypertrophic disease, have now been shown to cause DCM infrequently[55,56]. These genes potentially implicate several pathways in the development of DCM, including contractile dysfunction, inefficient energetics, and myocardial sensing of stretch or other stimuli[57,58].

Myotonic Dystrophy

Occasionally myotonic dystrophy will present with DCM or conduction disease as a prominent component, although it is unusual for this to be the case throughout a single pedigree. The mutated gene appears to be a protein kinase, but the mutation, an expanded triplet repeat in the 3' untranslated region of the coding sequence, may also affect transcription of neighboring loci[26]. This triplet repeat is unstable as it is transmitted meiotically, and so disease often will become more severe with each progressive generation, a phenomenon known as anticipation. The mechanism by which the mutation results in cardiomyopathy is unknown, but abnormal levels or localization of the myotonin kinase have been hypothesized.

Disease Models

The identification of the causal human genes in DCM offers a definitive starting point for the generation of true disease models. The production of genetically modified organisms bearing the cognate mutations allows investigators to unravel the mechanisms of cardiomyopathy from the initial insult through to the final phenotype[11]. Insights may also travel in the opposite direction, with model organism phenotypes implicating previously unsuspected genes as candidates for DCM[56]. Importantly, such inferences require confirmation through human molecular work, as null mutants or tissue-specific transgenics may not reflect any naturally occurring human genotype. For example, mouse models of DGC-related DCM confirmed initial hypotheses suggesting that force transmission is somehow disrupted, but importantly have also revealed many other pathways that may be involved in abnormal myocardial function. Clearly, it will be crucial to understand these multiple mechanisms of disease if we are to be able to design specific therapies for primary myocardial disease.

Specific models for other heritable forms of DCM do not yet exist, although there are intense efforts to generate such models, not only in mice but in larger animals, and in the zebrafish[59]. These model systems will enable the detailed pathophysiology of each gene defect to be explored, the causative pathways to be defined, and ultimately allow screening to directly identify modifier loci or novel therapies. The disparate phenotypes already identified in DCM suggest that no single pathway is the sole culprit in this syndrome. The dissection of the fundamental biology of these conditions should illuminate not only such differences, but also the commonalities that may well be shared with acquired forms of heart failure.

HYPERTROPHIC CARDIOMYOPATHY

Definitions and Clinical Features

As recently as the late 1950s, left ventricular hypertrophy (LVH) was believed to always represent an adaptive response to ventricular loading abnormality[2]. Investigators began to describe a syndrome characterized by familial syncope, sudden death, and marked LVH at postmortem[60]. The presence of severe disorganization of muscle cells and myofibrils were originally thought specific to this syndrome, although more recent work suggests this may be a matter of degree. The advent of echocardiography and the study of extended families revealed many asymptomatic, yet obviously affected, individuals[5]. Atypical distributions of left or right ventricular hypertrophy may occur, often with particular patterns seen in a given family. Importantly, as noted earlier, there may be no hypertrophy, and the EKG is reproducibly a more sensitive tool in the context of an extended family[21].

HCM usually presents during, or shortly after, the adolescent growth spurt, unfortunately often as sudden death. The mechanism of premature sudden death is not always certain. Ventricular arrhythmias undoubtedly are a major factor, yet coronary anomalies, pulmonary embolism, or other mechanisms have also been invoked[29]. Nonsustained VT (ventricular tachycardia) is a marker for sudden death risk, but sophisticated assessments of myocardial substrate appear superior[61]. Syncope was a prominent feature of the earliest descriptions of HCM, and a significant cause of confusion with aortic valve disease. Recurrent syncope is one of the most common clinical presentations of HCM, but here too, the precise mechanisms remain obscure[29]. There are documented peripheral vasomotor abnormalities in many of these patients, but these do not correlate perfectly with clinical events[62]. Chest pain is a typical feature, and often quite debilitating. Although ischemia is always invoked, there are few data to support this as a common mechanism[63]. Coronary anomalies should be excluded in those patients with prominent exertional pain. Patchy abnormalities are seen on thallium studies, but other assessments of myocardial blood flow are usually normal[64]. The possibility of primary metabolic mismatch has recently resurfaced in the search for a unifying hypothesis for HCM pathogenesis (see following text)[65]. Less prevalent clinical features include substantial functional subaortic and intra-ventricular obstruction, subaortic membranes, and mitral valve abnormalities. There is progression to ventricular dilatation and congestive heart failure in a proportion of patients. Despite the high heritability of HCM, little is known of the segregation patterns of any of the clinical features other than echocardiographic variables. Two decades of investigation failed to uncover the etiology of HCM, until the molecular genetic basis of the syndrome was revealed by work from the Seidman laboratory[9,66].

Clinical Genetics

Early descriptions of HCM recognized that a large proportion of cases appeared to be familial with autosomal dominant inheritance. Studies based on less extreme echocardio-graphic phenotypes suggested lower rates of familial disease. Systematic family screening now suggests that as many as 90% of cases have evidence of autosomal dominant disease. The remaining, ''sporadic'' cases may represent true *de novo* mutations in the genes that cause Mendelian forms of the disease, or poorly penetrant forms of the underlying trait[5]. A large proportion of the genetic studies, and the majority of all clinical studies, in HCM are dominated by individuals from pedigrees with severe hypertrophic phenotypes or a high incidence of sudden death. Recent attempts to redress this balance have concentrated on nonreferral populations, but virtually every study has failed to assess the potential relatedness of individual subjects from a single center. In a condition dominated by Mende-lian forms, the biases introduced by events or phenotypes in related individuals, genetic founder effects, or other less obvious confounders make many current clinical investiga-tions difficult to interpret. It is not surprising that conflicting data have emerged for the predictive value of most clinical indices[29]. There is an unmet need for proband-based clinical studies (and molecular studies), and the development of segregation-based ap-proaches to the assessment of clinical risk within families.

Clinical genetic studies identified discrete entities within the HCM syndrome several years prior to the use of molecular analyses. Braunwald's initial description of familial HCM noted several large kindreds with evidence of ventricular preexcitation and left ventricular hypertrophy[3] [Figure 3]. In each family, these conditions appeared to cose-gregate tightly, and subsequent work has shown that preexcitation, atrioventricular block, and HCM are linked to a specific locus[22]. Although preexcitation or pseudo-preexcitation are seen with other forms of HCM, spontaneous heart block has not been reported in other autosomal families. Interestingly, preexcitation and atrioventricular block are also seen in HCM due to mitochondrial disease[67]. Families in which both HCM and DCM cosegreg-ate represent a second distinct clinical entity. These kindreds contain multiple individuals with either phenotype, and, importantly, those with DCM do not appear to have progressed from HCM.

Although inbred families with more severe homozygous phenotypes have been re-ported[68], autosomal recessive HCM does not seem common. The most frequent form of recessive ventricular hypertrophy is observed in the context of Friedreich's ataxia, in which there is cardiac involvement in the majority of cases. Other situations in which idiopathic cardiac hypertrophy is seen include Noonan's syndrome, and several of the glycogen storage disorders.

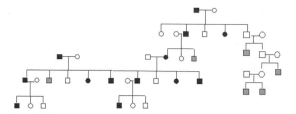

▨ **Hypertrophy**

■ **Sudden Death**

Figure 3 Apparently unrelated phenotypes may be mechanistically related from simple clinical observations in extended families. Here left ventricular hypertrophy and ventricular preexcitation cosegregate in a single pedigree, in a manner consistent with a single autosomal dominant disorder. The study of individual parts of the pedigree, such as the highlighted nuclear family in which hypertrophy is prominent (enlarged symbols), may give a distorted view of the overall nature of the underlying trait.

Molecular Genetics

HCM is caused by mutations in at least 10 genes, the majority of which encode sarcomeric contractile proteins[11]. Many hundreds of genes have been implicated in experimental forms of left ventricular hypertrophy, but only this group of genes appears to cause human hypertrophic disease. Although there is tremendous variation in the expression of HCM even within a single family, some generalizations about the phenotypes seen with specific genes have emerged. Families with cosegregating HCM and DCM seem to have a particular feature of mutations in the cardiac actin gene on chromosome 15[69]. Focal mid-cavity and disproportionate papillary muscle hypertrophy are associated with mutations in the myosin light chains[70]. The syndrome of massive wall thickening, preexcitation, and eventual atrioventricular block has been shown to be a result of activating mutations in the PRKAG2 gene[71]. In this syndrome, the increased wall thickening is due not only to true myocyte hypertrophy, but also to a significant component of inappropriate glycogen storage. Other data have suggested that myosin mutations may be associated with significantly more hypertrophy than troponin mutations[72], and myosin binding protein C mutations may be associated with later onset hypertrophic disease[73,74]. Most recently, mutations in the cardiac troponin I gene have been associated with families exhibiting both HCM and restrictive cardiomyopathy[75].

Disease Models

Murine models of HCM have been generated and recapitulate many of the features of the human disease[11]. There is evidence that the most specific of these models, the Arg403Gln α-cardiac myosin "knock-in" mouse, has significant abnormalities of myocyte calcium handling. The precise pathways involved have not yet been elucidated, but clearly these mice offer the potential to dissect the fundamental mechanisms of hypertrophy most relevant to human disease. The temptation to invoke a single pathway is strong, but evidence of major genetic modifiers, and discrete hypertrophic clinical entities, such as that seen with activating mutations of the AMP-activated protein kinase subunit PRKAG2 suggest otherwise. It is even possible that different mutations in the same gene result in hypertrophy through distinct mechanisms. Inefficient energy utilization may act as an important downstream pathway, and might help reconcile some of the divergent effects of mutations on contractility[76,77]. The disease gene in Friedreich's ataxia is a mitochondrial protein, which appears to be a critical player in oxidative stress pathways[78]. Many other processes, such as sarcomere assembly or cellular transport pathways, might also be perturbed, and the systematic study of genetic models will be vital to unraveling the pathophysiology of primary cardiac hypertrophy.

CONCLUSION

The last few years have seen tremendous advances in the study of the human cardiomyopathies. The major pathways have been identified in HCM, and similar inroads are beginning to be made in DCM. The identification of molecular pathways is the first step in developing a mechanistic understanding of these Mendelian disorders, and also offers the potential for insight into more common types of ventricular remodeling. It is clear that the morphological classification of the cardiomyopathies that has proven so useful for decades will be superceded by a molecular nosology.

There is still much investigation required before molecular diagnostics or prognostics are useful in the management of these disorders. Extremely helpful insights can be gained from simple clinical genetic tools, and these insights may be more immediately applicable than molecular information.

REFERENCES

1. Braunwald E, Bristow MR. Congestive heart failure: fifty years of progress. Circulation, 2000. 102(20 Suppl 4): p. IV14-IV23.
2. Goodwin JF. Congestive and hypertrophic cardiomyopathies. A decade of study. Lancet, 1970. 1(7650): p. 732–9.
3. Frank S, Braunwald E. Idiopathic hypertrophic subaortic stenosis. Clinical analysis of 126 patients with emphasis on the natural history. Circulation, 1968. 37(5): p. 759–88.
4. Risch NJ. Searching for genetic determinants in the new millennium. Nature, 2000. 405(6788): p. 847–56.
5. Maron BJ, Nichols PF 3rd, Pickle LW, Wesley YE, Mulvihill JJ. Patterns of inheritance in hypertrophic cardiomyopathy: assessment by M-mode and two-dimensional echocardiography. Am J Cardiol, 1984. 53(8): p. 1087–94.
6. Greaves SC, Roche AH, Neutz JM, Whitlock RM, Veale AM. Inheritance of hypertrophic cardiomyopathy: a cross sectional and M mode echocardiographic study of 50 families. Br Heart J 1987 58(3): p. 259–66.
7. Michels VV, Moll PP, Miller FA, Tajik AJ, Chu JS, Driscoll DJ, Burnett JC, Rodeheffer RJ, Chesebro JH, Tazelaar HD. The frequency of familial dilated cardiomyopathy in a series of patients with idiopathic dilated cardiomyopathy. N Engl J Med, 1992. 326(2): p. 77–82.
8. Collins FS. Positional cloning: let's not call it reverse anymore. Nat Genet, 1992. 1(1) p. 3–6.
9. Jarcho JA, McKenna W, Pare JA, Solomon SD, Holcombe RF, Dickie S, Levi T, Donis-Keller H, Seidman JG, Seidman CE. Mapping a gene for familial hypertrophic cardiomyopathy to chromosome 14q1. N Engl J Med, 1989. 321(20): p. 1372–8.
10. Freimer N, Sabatti C. The human phenome project. Nat Genet, 2003. 34(1): p. 15–21.
11. Seidman JG, Seidman C. The genetic basis for cardiomyopathy: from mutation identification to mechanistic paradigms. Cell, 2001. 104(4):p. 557–67.
12. Lander ES, Linton LM, Birren B, Nusbaum C, Zody MC, Baldwin J, Devon K, Dewar K, Doyle M, FitzHugh W, Funke R, Gage D, Hartis K, Heaford A, Howland J, Kann L, Lehoczky J, Le Vine R, McEwan P, McKernan K, Meldrim J, Mesirov JP, Miranda C, Morris W, Naylor J, Raymond C, Rosetti M, Santos R, Sheridan A, Sougnez C, Stange-Thomann N, Stojanovic N, Subramanian A, Wyman D, Rogers J, Sulston J, Ainscough R, Beck S, Bentley D, Burton J, Clee C, Carter N, Coulson A, Deadman R, Deloukas P, Dunham A, Dunham I, Durbin R, French L, Grafham D,

Gregory S, Hubbard T, Humphray S, Hunt A, Jones M, Lloyd C, McMurray A, Matthews L, Mercer S, Milne S, Mullikin JC, Mungall A, Plumb R, Ross M, Shownkeen R, Sims S, Waterston RH, Wilson RK, Hillier LW, McPherson JD, Marra MA, Mardis ER, Fulton LA, Chinwalla AT, Pepin KH, Gish WR, Chissoe SL, Wendl MC, Delehaunty KD, Miner TL, Delehaunty A, Kramer JB, Cook LL, Fulton RS, Johnson DL, Minx PJ, Clifton SW, Hawkins T, Branscomb E, Predki P, Richardson P, Wenning S, Slezak T, Doggett N, Cheng JF, Olsen A, Lucas S, Elkin C, Uberbacher E, Frazier M, Gibbs RA, Muzny DM, Scherer SE, Bouck JB, Sodergren EJ, Worley KC, Rives CM, Gorrell JH, Metzker ML, Naylor SL, Kucherlapati RS, Nelson DL, Weinstock GM, Sakaki Y, Fujiyama A, Hattori M, Yada T, Toyoda A, Itoh T, Kawagoe C, Watanabe H, Totoki Y, Taylor T, Weissenbach J, Heilig R, Saurin W, Artiguenave F, Brottier P, Bruls T, Pelletier E, Robert C, Wincker P, Smith DR, Doucette-Stamm L, Rubenfield M, Weinstock K, Lee HM, Dubois J, Rosenthal A, Platzer M, Nyakatura G, Taudien S, Rump A, Yang H, Yu J, Wang J, Huang G, Gu J, Hood L, Rowen L, Madan A, Qin S, Davis RW, Federspiel NA, Abola AP, Proctor MJ, Myers RM, Schmutz J, Dickson M, Grimwood J, Cox DR, Olson MV, Kaul R, Shimizu N, Kawasaki K, Minoshima S, Evans GA, Athanasiou M, Schultz R, Roe BA, Chen F, Pan H, Ramser J, Lehrach H, Reinhardt R, McCombie WR, de la Bastide M, Dedhia N, Blocker H, Hornischer K, Nordsiek G, Agarwala R, Aravind L, Bailey JA, Bateman A, Batzoglou S, Birney E, Bork P, Brown DG, Burge CB, Cerutti L, Chen HC, Church D, Clamp M, Copley RR, Doerks T, Eddy SR, Eichler EE, Furey TS, Galagan J, Gilbert JG, Harmon C, Hayashizaki Y, Haussler D, Hermjakob H, Hokamp K, Jang W, Johnson LS, Jones TA, Kasif S, Kaspryzk A, Kennedy S, Kent WJ, Kitts P, Koonin EV, Korf I, Kulp D, Lancet D, Lowe TM, McLysaght A, Mikkelsen T, Moran JV, Mulder N, Pollara VJ, Ponting CP, Schuler G, Schultz J, Slater G, Smit AF, Stupka E, Szustakowski J, Thierry-Mieg D, Thierry-Mieg J, Wagner L, Wallis J, Wheeler R, Williams A, Wolf YI, Wolfe KH, Yang SP, Yeh RF, Collins F, Guyer MS, Peterson J, Felsenfeld A, Wetterstrand KA, Patrinos A, Morgan MJ, Szustakowki J, de Jong P, Catanese JJ, Osoegawa K, Shizuya H, Choi S, Chen YJ. Initial sequencing and analysis of the human genome. Nature, 2001. 409(6822): p. 860–921.

13. Ellinor PT, Shin JT, Moore RK, Yoerger DM, MacRae CA. A genetic locus for atrial fibrillation maps to Chromosome 6q12-21. Circulation, 2003. 107:2880–2883.

14. Lander ES, Schork NJ. Genetic dissection of complex traits. Science, 1994. 265(5181): 2037–48.

15. Marian AJ, Yu QT, Workman R, Greve G, Roberts R. Angiotensin-converting enzyme polymorphism in hypertrophic cardiomyopathy and sudden cardiac death. Lancet, 1993. 342(8879): 1085–6.

16. Candy GP, Skudicky D, Mueller UK, Woodiwiss AJ, Sliwa K, Luker F, Esser J, Sareli P, Norton GR. Association of left ventricular systolic performance and cavity size with angiotensin-converting enzyme genotype in idiopathic dilated cardiomyopathy. Am J Cardiol,1999. 83(5): p. 740–4.

17. Terwilliger JD, Haghighi F, Hiekkalinna TS, Goring HH. A biased assessment of the use of SNPs in human complex traits. Curr Opin Genet Dev, 2002. 12(6): p. 726–34.

18. Cardon LR, Bell JI. Association study designs for complex diseases. Nat Rev Genet, 2001. 2(2): p. 91–9.

19. Keating MT, Sanguinetti MC. Molecular and cellular mechanisms of cardiac arrhythmias. Cell, 2001. 104(4): p. 569–80.

20. Marian AJ. Modifier genes for hypertrophic cardiomyopathy. Curr Opin Cardiol, 2002. 17(3): p. 242–52.

21. Ryan MP, Cleland JG, French JA, Joshi J, Choudhury L, Chojnowska L, Michalak E, al-Mahdawi S, Nihoyannopoulos P, Oakley CM. The standard electrocardiogram as a screening test for hypertrophic cardiomyopathy. Am J Cardiol 1995; 76(10):689–694.

22. MacRae CA, Ghaisas N, Kass S, Donnelly S, Basson CT, Watkins HC, Anan R, Thierfelder LH, McGarry K, Rowland E, et al. Familial hypertrophic cardiomyopathy with Wolff-Parkinson-White syndrome maps to a locus on chromosome 7q3. J Clin Invest 1995; 96(3): 1216–1220.

23. Gruver EJ, Fatkin D, Dodds GA, Kisslo J, Maron BJ, Seidman JG, Seidman CE. Familial hypertrophic cardiomyopathy and atrial fibrillation caused by Arg663His beta-cardiac myosin heavy chain mutation. Am J Cardiol 1999; 83(12A):13H–18H.

24. McKusick CE. Online Mendelian Inheritance in Man, OMIM (TM). McKusick-Nathans Institute for Genetic Medicine, Johns Hopkins University (Baltimore, MD) and National Center for Biotechnology Information, National Library of Medicine (Bethesda, MD), 2003.

25. Hunt SA, Baker DW, Chin MH, Cinquegrani MP, Feldmanmd AM, Francis GS, Ganiats TG, Goldstein S, Gregoratos G, Jessup ML, Noble RJ, Packer M, Silver MA, Stevenson LW, Gibbons RJ, Antman EM, Alpert JS, Faxon DP, Fuster V, Jacobs AK, Hiratzka LF, Russell RO, Smith SC, Jr. ACC/AHA Guidelines for the Evaluation and Management of Chronic Heart Failure in the Adult: Executive Summary A Report of the American College of Cardiology/American Heart Association Task Force on Practice Guidelines (Committee to Revise the 1995 Guidelines for the Evaluation and Management of Heart Failure): Developed in Collaboration with the International Society for Heart and Lung Transplantation; Endorsed by the Heart Failure Society of America. Circulation 2001; 104(24):2996–3007.

26. Mahadevan M, Tsilfidis C, Sabourin L, Shutler G, Amemiya C, Jansen G, Neville C, Narang M, Barcelo J, O'Hoy K, et al. Myotonic dystrophy mutation: an unstable CTG repeat in the 3' untranslated region of the gene. Science 1992; 255(5049):1253–1255.

27. Leboyer M, Bellivier F, Nosten-Bertrand M, Jouvent R, Pauls D, Mallet J. Psychiatric genetics: search for phenotypes. Trends Neurosci 1998; 21(3):102–105.

28. Crispell KA, Hanson EL, Coates K, Toy W, Hershberger RE. Periodic rescreening is indicated for family members at risk of developing familial dilated cardiomyopathy. J Am Coll Cardiol 2002; 39(9):1503–1507.

29. Spirito P, Seidman CE, McKenna WJ, Maron BJ. The management of hypertrophic cardiomyopathy. N Engl J Med 1997; 336(11):775–785.

30. Grunig E, Tasman JA, Kucherer H, Franz W, Kubler W, Katus HA. Frequency and phenotypes of familial dilated cardiomyopathy. J Am Coll Cardiol 1998; 31(1):186–194.

31. Crispell KA, Wray A, Ni H, Nauman DJ, Hershberger RE. Clinical profiles of four large pedigrees with familial dilated cardiomyopathy: preliminary recommendations for clinical practice. J Am Coll Cardiol 1999; 34(3):837–847.

32. Watkins H, Rosenzweig A, Hwang DS, Levi T, McKenna W, Seidman CE, Seidman JG. Characteristics and prognostic implications of myosin missense mutations in familial hypertrophic cardiomyopathy. N Engl J Med 1992; 326(17):1108–1114.

33. Fananapazir L, Epstein ND. Genotype-phenotype correlations in hypertrophic cardiomyopathy. Insights provided by comparisons of kindreds with distinct and identical beta-myosin heavy chain gene mutations. Circulation 1994; 89(1):22–32.

34. Blair E, Price SJ, Baty CJ, Ostman-Smith I, Watkins H. Mutations in cis can confound genotype-phenotype correlations in hypertrophic cardiomyopathy. J Med Genet 2001; 38(6): 385–388.

35. Richard P, Charron P, Carrier L, Ledeuil C, Cheav T, Pichereau C, Benaiche A, Isnard R, Dubourg O, Burban M, Gueffet JP, Millaire A, Desnos M, Schwartz K, Hainque B, Komajda M. Hypertrophic cardiomyopathy: distribution of disease genes, spectrum of mutations, and implications for a molecular diagnosis strategy. Circulation 2003; 107(17):2227–2232.

36. Manolio TA, Baughman KL, Rodeheffer R, Pearson TA, Bristow JD, Michels VV, Abelmann WH, Harlan WR. Prevalence and etiology of idiopathic dilated cardiomyopathy (summary of a National Heart, Lung, and Blood Institute workshop). Am J Cardiol 1992; 69(17):1458–1466.

37. Braunwald ER. Heart Disease: A Textbook of Cardiovascular Medicine 6th edition. Philadelphia: WB Saunders, 2001.

38. Keeling PJ, Gang Y, Smith G, Seo H, Bent SE, Murday V, Caforio AL, McKenna WJ. Familial dilated cardiomyopathy in the United Kingdom. Br Heart J 1995; 73(5):417–421.

39. McKenna CJ. Abnormal cellularity in asymptomatic relatives of patients with idiopathic dilated cardiomyopathy. J Am Coll Cardiol 2003; 41(4):709; author reply 709.

40. Shekelle PG, Rich MW, Morton SC, Atkinson CS, Tu W, Maglione M, Rhodes S, Barrett M, Fonarow GC, Greenberg B, Heidenreich PA, Knabel T, Konstam MA, Steimle A, Warner Stevenson L. Efficacy of angiotensin-converting enzyme inhibitors and beta-blockers in the management of left ventricular systolic dysfunction according to race, gender, and diabetic status. A meta-analysis of major clinical trials. J Am Coll Cardiol 2003; 41(9):1529–1538.

41. Mestroni L, Rocco C, Gregori D, Sinagra G, Di Lenarda A, Miocic S, Vatta M, Pinamonti B, Muntoni F, Caforio AL, McKenna WJ, Falaschi A, Giacca M, Camerini F. Familial dilated cardiomyopathy: evidence for genetic and phenotypic heterogeneity. Heart Muscle Disease Study Group. J Am Coll Cardiol 1999; 34(1):181–190.

42. Mahon NG, Sharma S, Elliott PM, Baig MK, Norman MW, Barbeyto S, McKenna WJ. Abnormal cardiopulmonary exercise variables in asymptomatic relatives of patients with dilated cardiomyopathy who have left ventricular enlargement. Heart 2000; 83(5):511–517.

43. Kawai C. From myocarditis to cardiomyopathy: mechanisms of inflammation and cell death: learning from the past for the future. Circulation 1999; 99(8):1091–1100.

44. Csanady M, Hogye M, Kallai A, Forster T, Szarazajtai T. Familial dilated cardiomyopathy: a worse prognosis compared with sporadic forms. Br Heart J 1995; 74(2):171–173.

45. Caforio AL, Goldman JH, Haven AJ, Baig KM, McKenna WJ. Evidence for autoimmunity to myosin and other heart-specific autoantigens in patients with dilated cardiomyopathy and their relatives. Int J Cardiol 1996; 54(2):157–163.

46. Olson TM, Keating MT. Mapping a cardiomyopathy locus to chromosome 3p22-p25. J Clin Invest 1996; 97(2):528–532.

47. Fatkin D, MacRae C, Sasaki T, Wolff MR, Porcu M, Frenneaux M, Atherton J, Vidaillet HJ Jr, Spudich S, De Girolami U, Seidman JG, Seidman C, Muntoni F, Muehle G, Johnson W, McDonough B. Missense mutations in the rod domain of the lamin A/C gene as causes of dilated cardiomyopathy and conduction-system disease. N Engl J Med 1999; 341(23):1715–1724.

48. Towbin JA, Hejtmancik JF, Brink P, Gelb B, Zhu XM, Chamberlain JS, McCabe ER, Swift M. X-linked dilated cardiomyopathy. Molecular genetic evidence of linkage to the Duchenne muscular dystrophy (dystrophin) gene at the Xp21 locus. Circulation 1993; 87(6):1854–1865.

49. Melacini P, Fanin M, Duggan DJ, Freda MP, Berardinelli A, Danieli GA, Barchitta A, Hoffman EP, Dalla Volta S, Angelini C. Heart involvement in muscular dystrophies due to sarcoglycan gene mutations. Muscle Nerve 1999; 22(4):473–479.

50. Coral-Vazquez R, Cohn RD, Moore SA, Hill JA, Weiss RM, Davisson RL, Straub V, Barresi R, Bansal D, Hrstka RF, Williamson R, Campbell KP. Disruption of the sarcoglycan-sarcospan complex in vascular smooth muscle: a novel mechanism for cardiomyopathy and muscular dystrophy. Cell 1999; 98(4):465–474.

51. Bione S, Maestrini E, Rivella S, Mancini M, Regis S, Romeo G, Toniolo D. Identification of a novel X-linked gene responsible for Emery-Dreifuss muscular dystrophy. Nat Genet 1994; 8(4):323–327.

52. Hutchison CJ. Lamins: building blocks or regulators of gene expression? Nat Rev Mol Cell Biol 2002; 3(11):848–858.

53. Olson TM, Michels VV, Thibodeau SN, Tai YS, Keating MT. Actin mutations in dilated cardiomyopathy, a heritable form of heart failure. Science 1998; 280(5364):750–752.

54. MacRae CA. Genetics and dilated cardiomyopathy: limitations of candidate gene strategies. Eur Heart J 2000; 21(22):1817–1819.

55. Kamisago M, Sharma SD, DePalma SR, Solomon S, Sharma P, McDonough B, Smoot L, Mullen MP, Woolf PK, Wigle ED, Seidman JG, Seidman CE. Mutations in sarcomere protein genes as a cause of dilated cardiomyopathy. N Engl J Med 2000; 343(23):1688–1696.

56. Knoll R, Hoshijima M, Hoffman HM, Person V, Lorenzen-Schmidt I, Bang ML, Hayashi T, Shiga N, Yasukawa H, Schaper W, McKenna W, Yokoyama M, Schork NJ, Omens JH, McCulloch AD, Kimura A, Gregorio CC, Poller W, Schaper J, Schultheiss HP, Chien KR. The cardiac mechanical stretch sensor machinery involves a Z disc complex that is defective in a subset of human dilated cardiomyopathy. Cell 2002; 111(7):943–955.

57. Towbin JA. The role of cytoskeletal proteins in cardiomyopathies. Curr Opin Cell Biol 1998; 10(1):131–139.

58. Chien KR. Genotype, phenotype: upstairs, downstairs in the family of cardiomyopathies. J Clin Invest 2003; 111(2):175–178.

59. Xu X, Meiler SE, Zhong TP, Mohideen M, Crossley DA, Burggren WW, Fishman MC. Cardiomyopathy in zebra fish due to mutation in an alternatively spliced exon of titin. Nat Genet 2002; 30(2):205–209.

60. Watkins H, Seidman CE, MacRae C, Seidman JG, McKenna W. Progress in familial hypertrophic cardiomyopathy: molecular genetic analyses in the original family studied by Teare. Br Heart J 1992; 67(1):34–38.
61. Saumarez RC, Slade AK, Grace AA, Sadoul N, Camm AJ, McKenna WJ. The significance of paced electrogram fractionation in hypertrophic cardiomyopathy. A prospective study. Circulation 1995; 91(11):2762–2768.
62. Counihan PJ, Frenneaux MP, Webb DJ, McKenna WJ. Abnormal vascular responses to supine exercise in hypertrophic cardiomyopathy. Circulation 1991; 84(2):686–696.
63. Elliott PM, Kaski JC, Prasad K, Seo H, Slade AK, Goldman JH, McKenna WJ. Chest pain during daily life in patients with hypertrophic cardiomyopathy: an ambulatory electrocardiographic study. Eur Heart J 1996; 17(7):1056–1064.
64. Nagata S, Park Y, Minamikawa T, Yutani C, Kamiya T, Nishimura T, Kozuka T, Sakakibara H, Nimura Y. Thallium perfusion and cardiac enzyme abnormalities in patients with familial hypertrophic cardiomyopathy. Am Heart J 1985; 109(6):1317–1322.
65. Ashrafian H, Redwood C, Blair E, Watkins H. Hypertrophic cardiomyopathy: a paradigm for myocardial energy depletion. Trends Genet 2003; 19(5):263–268.
66. Geisterfer-Lowrance AA, Kass S, Tanigawa G, Vosberg HP, McKenna W, Seidman CE, Seidman JG. A molecular basis for familial hypertrophic cardiomyopathy: a beta cardiac myosin heavy chain gene missense mutation. Cell 1990; 62(5):999–1006.
67. Casali C, d'Amati G, Bernucci P, DeBiase L, Autore C, Santorelli FM, Coviello D, Gallo P. Maternally inherited cardiomyopathy: clinical and molecular characterization of a large kindred harboring the A4300G point mutation in mitochondrial deoxyribonucleic acid. J Am Coll Cardiol 1999; 33(6):1584–1589.
68. Ho CY, Lever HM, DeSanctis R, Farver CF, Seidman JG, Seidman CE. Homozygous mutation in cardiac troponin T: implications for hypertrophic cardiomyopathy. Circulation 2000; 102(16):1950–1955.
69. Mogensen J, Klausen IC, Pedersen AK, Egeblad H, Bross P, Kruse TA, Gregersen N, Hansen PS, Baandrup U, Borglum AD. Alpha-cardiac actin is a novel disease gene in familial hypertrophic cardiomyopathy. J Clin Invest 1999; 103(10):R39–R43.
70. Poetter K, Jiang H, Hassanzadeh S, Master SR, Chang A, Dalakas MC, Rayment I, Sellers JR, Fananapazir L, Epstein ND. Mutations in either the essential or regulatory light chains of myosin are associated with a rare myopathy in human heart and skeletal muscle. Nat Genet 1996; 13(1):63–69.
71. Blair E, Redwood C, Ashrafian H, Oliveira M, Broxholme J, Kerr B, Salmon A, Ostman-Smith I, Watkins H. Mutations in the gamma(2) subunit of AMP-activated protein kinase cause familial hypertrophic cardiomyopathy: evidence for the central role of energy compromise in disease pathogenesis. Hum Mol Genet 2001; 10(11):1215–1220.
72. Varnava A, Baboonian C, Davison F, de Cruz L, Elliott PM, Davies MJ, McKenna WJ. A new mutation of the cardiac troponin T gene causing familial hypertrophic cardiomyopathy without left ventricular hypertrophy. Heart 1999; 82(5):621–624.
73. Niimura H, Bachinski LL, Sangwatanaroj S, Watkins H, Chudley AE, McKenna W, Kristinsson A, Roberts R, Sole M, Maron BJ, Seidman JG, Seidman CE. Mutations in the gene for cardiac myosin-binding protein C and late-onset familial hypertrophic cardiomyopathy. N Engl J Med 1998; 338(18):1248–1257.
74. Maron BJ, Niimura H, Casey SA, Soper MK, Wright GB, Seidman JG, Seidman CE. Development of left ventricular hypertrophy in adults in hypertrophic cardiomyopathy caused by cardiac myosin-binding protein C gene mutations. J Am Coll Cardiol 2001; 38(2):315–321.
75. Mogensen J, Kubo T, Duque M, Uribe W, Shaw A, Murphy R, Gimeno JR, Elliott P, McKenna WJ. Idiopathic restrictive cardiomyopathy is part of the clinical expression of cardiac troponin I mutations. J Clin Invest 2003; 111(2):209–216.
76. Witt CC, Gerull B, Davies MJ, Centner T, Linke WA, Thierfelder L. Hypercontractile properties of cardiac muscle fibers in a knock-in mouse model of cardiac myosin-binding protein-C. J Biol Chem 2001; 276(7):5353–5359.
77. Mukherjea P, Tong L, Seidman JG, Seidman CE, Hitchcock-DeGregori SE. Altered regulatory function of two familial hypertrophic cardiomyopathy troponin T mutants. Biochemistry 1999; 38(40):13296–13301.

78. Campuzano V, Montermini L, Molto MD, Pianese L, Cossee M, Cavalcanti F, Monros E, Rodius F, Duclos F, Monticelli A, et al. Friedreich's ataxia: autosomal recessive disease caused by an intronic GAA triplet repeat expansion. Science 1996; 271(5254):1423–1427.

79. Jung M, Poepping I, Perrot A, Ellmer AE, Wienker TF, Dietz R, Reis A, Osterziel KJ. Investigation of a family with autosomal dominant dilated cardiomyopathy defines a novel locus on chromosome 2q14-q22. Am J Hum Genet 1999; 65(4):1068–1077.

80. Gerull B, Gramlich M, Atherton J, McNabb M, Trombitas K, Sasse-Klaassen S, Seidman JG, Seidman C, Granzier H, Labeit S, Frenneaux M, Thierfelder L. Mutations of TTN, encoding the giant muscle filament titin, cause familial dilated cardiomyopathy. Nat Genet 2002; 30(2): 201–204.

81. Li D, Tapscoft T, Gonzalez O, Burch PE, Quinones MA, Zoghbi WA, Hill R, Bachinski LL, Mann DL, Roberts R. Desmin mutation responsible for idiopathic dilated cardiomyopathy. Circulation 1999; 100(5):461–464.

82. Barresi R, Di Blasi C, Negri T, Brugnoni R, Vitali A, Felisari G, Salandi A, Daniel S, Cornelio F, Morandi L, Mora M. Disruption of heart sarcoglycan complex and severe cardiomyopathy caused by beta sarcoglycan mutations. J Med Genet 2000; 37(2):102–107.

83. Tsubata S, Bowles KR, Vatta M, Zintz C, Titus J, Muhonen L, Bowles NE, Towbin JA. Mutations in the human delta-sarcoglycan gene in familial and sporadic dilated cardiomyopathy. J Clin Invest 2000; 106(5):655–662.

84. Norgett EE, Hatsell SJ, Carvajal-Huerta L, Cabezas JC, Common J, Purkis PE, Whittock N, Leigh IM, Stevens HP, Kelsell DP. Recessive mutation in desmoplakin disrupts desmoplakin-intermediate filament interactions and causes dilated cardiomyopathy, woolly hair and keratoderma. Hum Mol Genet 2000; 9(18):2761–2766.

85. Sylvius N, Tesson F, Gayet C, Charon P, Benaiche A, Peuchmaurd M, Duboscq-Bidot L, Feingold J, Beckmann JS, Bouchier C, Komajda M. A new locus for autosomal dominant dilated cardiomyopathy identified on chromosome 6q12-q16. Am J Hum Genet 2001; 68(1): 241–246.

86. Schmitt JP, Kamisago M, Asahi M, Li GH, Ahmad F, Mende U, Kranias EG, MacLennan DH, Seidman JG, Seidman CE. Dilated cardiomyopathy and heart failure caused by a mutation in phospholamban. Science 2003; 299(5611):1410–1413.

87. Messina DN, Speer MC, Pericak-Vance MA, McNally EM. Linkage of familial dilated cardiomyopathy with conduction defect and muscular dystrophy to chromosome 6q23. Am J Hum Genet 1997; 61(4):909–917.

88. Schonberger J, Levy H, Grunig E, Sangwatanaroj S, Fatkin D, MacRae C, Stacker H, Halpin C, Eavey R, Philbin EF, Katus H, Seidman JG, Seidman CE. Dilated cardiomyopathy and sensorineural hearing loss: a heritable syndrome that maps to 6q23-24. Circulation 2000; 101(15):1812–1818.

89. Krajinovic M, Pinamonti B, Sinagra G, Vatta M, Severini GM, Milasin J, Falaschi A, Camerini F, Giacca M, Mestroni L. Linkage of familial dilated cardiomyopathy to chromosome 9. Heart Muscle Disease Study Group. Am J Hum Genet 1995; 57(4):846–852.

90. Bowles KR, Gajarski R, Porter P, Goytia V, Bachinski L, Roberts R, Pignatelli R, Towbin JA. Gene mapping of familial autosomal dominant dilated cardiomyopathy to chromosome 10q21-23. J Clin Invest 1996; 98(6):1355–1360.

91. Daehmlow S, Erdmann J, Knueppel T, Gille C, Froemmel C, Hummel M, Hetzer R, Regitz-Zagrosek V. Novel mutations in sarcomeric protein genes in dilated cardiomyopathy. Biochem Biophys Res Commun 2002; 298(1):116–120.

92. Thierfelder L, Watkins H, MacRae C, et al. Alpha-tropomyosin and cardiac troponin T mutations cause familial hypertrophic cardiomyopathy: a disease of the sarcomere. Cell 1994; 77(5): 701–712.

93. Geier C, Perrot A, Ozcelik C, et al. Mutations in the human muscle LIM protein gene in families with hypertrophic cardiomyopathy. Circulation 2003; 107(10):1390–1395.

94. Watkins H, Conner D, Thierfelder L, et al. Mutations in the cardiac myosin binding protein-C gene on chromosome 11 cause familial hypertrophic cardiomyopathy. Nat Genet 1995; 11(4):434–437.

95. Kimura A, Harada H, Park JE, et al. Mutations in the cardiac troponin I gene associated with hypertrophic cardiomyopathy. Nat Genet 1997; 16(4):379–382.

2

Molecular Signaling Networks Underlying Cardiac Hypertrophy and Failure

Jeffery D. Molkentin
Department of Pediatrics Division of Molecular Cardiovascular Biology,
Children's Hospital Medical Center
Cincinnati, Ohio, USA

Thomas Force
Molecular Cardiology Research Institute, Tufts-New England Medical Center,
Tufts University School of Medicine
Boston, Massachusetts, USA

INTRODUCTION

Physiological hypertrophy is a normal part of the growth response of cells, including cardiomyocytes, which are terminally differentiated and cannot undergo hyperplastic growth. This form of hypertrophy is described as both concentric (characterized by addition of sarcomeres in parallel, leading to increased width of the myocyte) and eccentric (characterized by the addition of sarcomeres in series, leading to increased length). Concentric cardiac hypertrophy can also develop as a response to stressors, in most cases an excess load placed on the heart; for example, with uncorrected hypertension or valvular disease, or post-MI (myocardial infarction) when the remote noninfarcted myocardium hypertrophies. Hypertrophy is initially believed to be adaptive, normalizing systolic wall stress, though this concept has been challenged recently and it is not clear that hypertrophy is really necessary to maintain systolic function in the face of moderately elevated afterloads. Eccentric hypertrophy results most often from volume loads such as those seen with valvular insufficiency.

If the load placed on the heart is not normalized, the heart may continue to hypertrophy, eventually leading to elevated filling pressures and "so-called" diastolic heart failure. The hypertrophied heart may also begin to decompensate, leading to progressive dilatation, systolic dysfunction, and heart failure on that basis. Not surprisingly, cardiac hypertrophy is a significant risk factor for the development of heart failure and, in addition, for sudden death [1,2]. Given this predisposition, investigators have begun to dissect the molecular determinants that underlie the cardiac hypertrophic response in an attempt to identify novel pharmacologic targets of potential clinical relevance. The focus of these investigations has been on the cell surface receptors for agonists that trigger the hypertrophic response, including receptors for angiotensin II, endothelin-1, and α- and β-adrenergic agents. However, given the vast number of agents that have been reported to induce hypertrophy (see following text), and the increasing evidence that hypertrophy is multifactorial in origin, more recent investigations have begun to focus on intracellular signaling pathways, with the hope of identifying one or a few final common pathways necessary for the hypertrophic response, irrespective of the inciting stimuli. With the rapid advances in the development of small molecule inhibitors of components of these pathways that can be used in vivo, we are rapidly approaching the point of being able to readily manipulate these pathways in patients. Therefore, it is essential to understand the signaling networks that regulate hypertrophic growth.

Irrespective of the type of hypertrophy, the processes of growth and hypertrophy require a dramatic reprogramming of gene expression to upregulate gene products necessary for growth of the cardiomyocyte (including genes encoding contractile elements and proteins of the basic transcriptional and translational machinery that allow new protein production), and genes that encode proteins that remodel the extracellular matrix, allowing growth to proceed. This process of reprogramming gene expression occurs in response to specific growth signals that are generated from a multitude of sources and include soluble factors (growth factors, neurohormonal mediators), or biomechanical forces (stretch of the myocyte induced, for example, by an acute MI or an acute pressure load)(reviewed in [3,4]). To reprogram gene expression, however, these signals must be sensed at the cardiomyocyte membrane, and transmitted into the interior of the cell, and eventually into the nucleus, by a process called signal transduction. It is the purpose of this chapter to provide an introduction into the field of signal transduction, specifically as it applies to hypertrophy of the heart, and in so doing to help the reader understand how gene expression becomes reprogrammed. The complexity of the field, including the large number of growth factors that have been reported to induce growth of cardiomyocytes, and the even larger number of signaling molecules that have been reported to mediate growth, makes it impossible to cover all pathways that have been implicated. Rather than a laundry list of pathways and molecules, we will focus on two major arms for which strong evidence exists implicating components of the pathway in the hypertrophic response: (a) the calcineurin pathway, and (b) the phosphoinositide 3-kinase (PI3-kinase)/Akt pathway and its interactions with the mammalian target of rapamycin (mTOR)—a pathway that has been implicated in growth of species from Drosophila to human [5]. In addition, we will explore how the role of these pathways are evaluated in mouse models of human disease, allowing the reader to understand this rapidly growing field from which crucial discoveries leading to therapeutic benefits will likely come. It is possible that after reading this chapter, the reader may be overwhelmed with the complexity of these pathways and wonder how, or even whether, they all fit together in some coherent manner. This view is shared by many in the field, and one must realize that this is simply a reflection of the complexity of the entire process itself and the large number of factors that must be recruited to allow the coordinated end-result, hypertrophic growth. Finally, we will explore dysregulation of these pathways in the hearts of patients with advanced heart failure, discuss how this dysregulated signaling is altered when hemodynamic stresses are reduced, and speculate about potential targets for the treatment of heart failure.

THE SIGNAL AT THE CELL MEMBRANE

There are two types of stimuli that are believed to trigger the hypertrophic response-mechanical deformation of the membrane (cell stretch) and growth-promoting ligands binding to their cognate receptors in the myocyte cell membrane, though as will be demonstrated, mechanical deformation activates ligand/receptor interactions as well.

Mechanical Deformation

Stretch of cardiomyocytes in culture leads to gene transcription and protein synthesis in a pattern that closely resembles the load-induced hypertrophic response in vivo [6]. Stretch triggers responses both via the direct activation of signaling molecules and by inducing the release of humoral factors that appear to be of paramount importance in the maintenance of the response. Although the identity of the stretch "sensor" remains unknown, stretch results in the direct recruitment of integrin signaling and stretch-activated ion channels, both of which could be true sensors of membrane deformation [7–11]. Heterotrimeric G proteins (Gq and Gi), which clearly play a role in transducing signals from prohypertrophic factors released following stretch, and possibly small G proteins, appear to be activated so early after stretch that it is possible that these are also directly activated [12]. One critical consequence of activation of these proximal mediators of the stretch response is an increase in cytosolic calcium, which plays a role in activating several signaling pathways including calcineurin, as will be discussed in detail in the following text. Until the sensors are identified and fully characterized, however, the precise mechanisms by which cytosolic signaling pathways are activated by stretch will remain speculative. One potential shortcoming of the stretch-sensing hypothesis is that in most biological response pathways, a stretch signal gradually accommodates so that the response is lost unless a new or greater stimulus is applied. In this manner, it is uncertain how an acute stretch stimulation mediates long-term hypertrophic growth (and maintains it).

Humoral Factors

One of the central features of hypertrophic signaling is that membrane deformation induces the release of growth factors that act in an autocrine or paracrine fashion to amplify hypertrophic responses. In a seminal paper in 1993, Sadoshima, Izumo, and co-workers first reported that autocrine release of angiotensin II (Ang II) was, at least in part, responsible for the hypertrophic response of cardiomyocytes in culture to cell stretch [13,14]. Ang II activates a number of prohypertrophic signaling pathways via at least two mechanisms, one triggered directly by the receptor and its associated heterotrimeric G protein, Gq (see following text), and the other triggered by transactivation of growth factor receptors with intrinsic tyrosine kinase activity, most notably the epidermal growth factor (EGF) receptor. Transactivation of the EGF receptor was originally noted by Ullrich and co-workers in 1996 [15]. The current model involves calcium transient-induced (and possibly oxidant stress-induced [16]) activation of a metalloprotease that releases heparin-binding EGF-like growth factor, which then binds to the receptor, activating additional signaling pathways not directly activated by the Ang II receptor [17,18]. A second group of factors released by mechanical stretch are the IL-6 family of cytokines, including cardiotrophin-1 (CT-1), which act via receptors specific to the cytokine and via the common receptor, gp130 [19–21].

A wealth of data implicates the insulin-like growth factor-1 (IGF-1) axis, including growth hormone, which acts in large part via inducing production of IGF-1, as the dominant regulator of normal postnatal growth of the mammalian heart [22–24]. In pathological states, IGF-1 signaling is activated by a variety of stimuli that induce remodeling including pressure overload and following myocardial infarction [25]. IGF-1 signaling is also activated in the remodeled hearts of patients with advanced heart failure [26].

Many of the prohypertrophic peptides, including Ang II, endothelin-1 (ET-1), and α-adrenergic agents bind to receptors that are linked to heterotrimeric G proteins of the Gq family. These G proteins convert receptor activation into mobilization of intracellular signaling pathways, and are the initial trigger for downstream events. Heterotrimeric G proteins of the Gq family clearly play a major role in ventricular adaptation to pressure overload. Overexpression, specifically in the heart of the α subunit of Gq or of an activated mutant of αq, led to cardiac hypertrophy [27–30]. Later, in a landmark study, Ahkter and colleagues demonstrated that expressing a peptide that inhibited Gq-dependent signaling significantly limited the hypertrophic response to pressure overload in vivo [31]. More recently, conditional inactivation of the gene encoding the α subunit of Gq (and the related G_{11}) was shown to blunt the hypertrophic response [32]. These studies, taken together, confirm a critical role for Gq in hypertrophic signaling and in the hypertrophic response to pressure overload.

SIGNALING WITHIN THE CELL

There are two essential features of hypertrophic growth-reprogramming of gene expression and protein synthesis. Each is regulated by a series of intracellular pathways that are activated by events occurring at the membrane as previously described. We will consider each of these components separately, though they are inextricably intertwined.

Reprogramming of Gene Expression

In order to mount a hypertrophic response, the cardiomyocyte must upregulate the expression of a number of genes, including genes encoding components of the sarcomere and more specific growth-related and stress-induced genes. Other genes are downregulated as part of the response. Characteristic of the response is a reestablishment of a gene program that is often described as ''embryonic'' or ''fetal'' because several of the reexpressed genes are normally expressed in utero, but expression declines rapidly after birth. The genes induced by the hypertrophic response are often divided into three groups based on their time of expression—immediate early, intermediate, and late [33]. Immediate-early genes include the neurohormonal mediator, brain natriuretic peptide (BNP), as well as several stress-induced genes or genes involved in growth control, including c-fos, c-jun, c-myc, egr-1, and heat shock protein 70 (HSP70). Intermediate-response genes include atrial natriuretic peptide (ANP) and angiotensinogen as well as several sarcomeric components, -myosin heavy chain (β-MHC) (and corresponding downregulation of α-MHC), myosin light chain-2, and skeletal α-actin (replacing cardiac α-actin). Late-response genes include angiotensin converting enzyme and the Na/Ca exchanger.

Signal transmission from the cell membrane, where the initiating stimulus is generated, to the nucleus is essential for this reprogramming. This is generally accomplished by linear cascades of proteins, most commonly protein kinases (but also the protein phosphatase calcineurin [see following text]), phosphorylating and activating one another in sequence, culminating in the phosphorylation and activation of one or more transcription factors (Fig. 1). The transcription factors then bind to promoter elements, specific DNA sequences, usually of ~6 to 12 base pairs in length, within the promoters of genes. Thus, each transcription factor will usually target several genes. The net result of the activation of the entire set of genes is the hypertrophic response.

As noted, a host of different pathways have been implicated in regulating the hypertrophic response [4]. However, many of these studies have relied exclusively on overexpression of specific signaling molecules either in cardiomyocytes in culture or in the heart in vivo (transgenic models with genes expressed downstream of a cardiac-specific promoter, such as the α-MHC promoter). One must be very cautious in drawing conclusions based on these findings alone, however, since the level of expression of the transgene is often many-fold higher than the level of the endogenous protein, producing nonphysio-

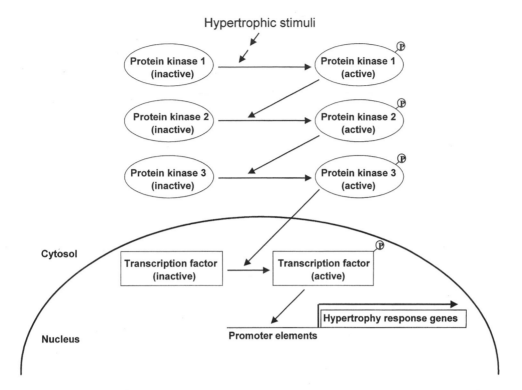

Figure 1   Schematic representation of a signal transduction pathway linking the cell surface receptor to nuclear events. Hypertrophic stimuli sensed at the membrane lead via a variety of signal transducers (e.g., Gq) to the activation of a protein kinase at the the top of a multitiered cascade of protein kinases. This kinase phosphorylates kinase 2 in the cascade that in turn phosphorylates kinase 3 in the cascade. Kinase 3 then phosphorylates one or more transcription factors that bind to promoter elements in the regulatory regions of various "hypertrophic response genes" and activate gene expression. This multitiered cascade serves to both amplify the signal (one kinase molecule at each level activates many molecules at the next level) and prevent the need for kinase 1 to translocate to the nucleus each time it is activated.

logical levels of activation of normal downstream targets. In addition, gross overexpression of a transgene leads to "cross talk" with other signaling pathways that are not normally regulated by that transgene [34]. That said, many signaling pathways have fairly striking fidelity so that cross talk is often minimal and valuable information can certainly be obtained using an overexpression approach. The optimal approach is that in addition to demonstrating that a specific molecule is sufficient to induce the hypertrophic response using a gain-of-function approach, it is also important to demonstrate that the molecule is necessary for the response (e.g. the complementary studies of the role of Gq in hypertrophic growth previously discussed). This is a much more difficult task because it requires deleting or "knocking out" a gene, whereas sufficiency can be suggested with a transgenic model.

In-Depth Evaluation of Calcineurin–Nuclear Factor of Activated T-Cell Signaling

Herein, we will focus on one pathway that has consistently been shown, in a number of different models, to regulate hypertrophic growth—the calcineurin pathway (Fig. 2).

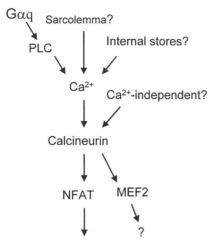

Hypertrophic gene expression

Figure 2   Schematic representation of the calcineurin/NFAT pathway. Diagram shows the possible sources of Ca^{2+} necessary for the activation of calcineurin as well as the possible contribution of Ca^{2+}-independent inputs into calcineurin activation. See text for more details.

Calcineurin (also known as protein phosphatase 2B, PP2B) is a calcium-calmodulin-activated protein phosphatase. Calcineurin specifically dephosphorylates proteins previously phosphorylated on serine or threonine residues. It is uniquely activated by sustained elevations in intracellular calcium [35–37]. Calcineurin comprises a 59–63 kDa catalytic subunit referred to as calcineurin A, a 19 kDa calcium binding protein referred to as calcineurin B, and the calcium binding protein calmodulin [35,36]. Three mammalian calcineurin A catalytic genes have been identified (α,β,γ) that are highly homologous to one another. The calcineurin Aα and Aβ gene products are expressed in a ubiquitous pattern throughout the body, whereas calcineurin Aγ expression is more restricted [38–41].

Calcineurin catalytic activity is inhibited by the immunosuppressive drugs cyclosporine A (CsA) and FK506 through complexes with immunophilin protein [35,36]. The identification of calcineurin as a target for CsA and FK506 suggested a critical role for this phosphatase in the regulation of T-cell reactivity and cytokine gene expression. Once activated, calcineurin directly dephosphorylates members of the nuclear factor of activated T-cells (NFAT) transcription factor family in the cytoplasm, promoting their translocation into the nucleus. Once in the nucleus, NFAT family members participate in the transcriptional induction of various immune response genes [42,43].

More recently, calcineurin was identified as a hypertrophic signaling factor in the heart suggesting a conservation in the function of calcineurin as a reactive signaling factor in multiple cell-types. For example, overexpression of an activated form of calcineurin in the hearts of transgenic mice induced a profound hypertrophic response (two- to threefold increase in heart size) that rapidly progressed to dilated heart failure within 2 to 3 months [44]. Such data implicated calcineurin as a sufficient inducer of the hypertrophic response and as a potential causative factor associated with the transition to decompensation and heart failure. More recent investigation has focused on an evaluation of calcineurin's requirement as a hypertrophic mediator. Treatment of cultured neonatal cardiomyocytes with the calcineurin inhibitory agent CsA attenuated agonist-induced hypertrophy in vitro [44]. This initial observation suggested that calcineurin is likely activated in cultured cardiomyocytes in response to agonist stimulation. Indeed, agonist stimulation (e.g. phen-ylephrine, angiotensin II) significantly increased calcineurin enzymatic activity in cultured cardiomyocytes, which was associated with an increase in both calcineurin Aβ mRNA and protein levels [45]. Endothelin-1-stimulated hypertrophy of cultured cardiomyocytes also induced a significant (three-fold) increase in calcineurin activity [46]. Calcineurin enzymatic activity and protein levels were each significantly upregulated in hearts from juvenile tropomodulin transgenic mice, a model of dilated heart failure [47,48]. Similarly, a number of groups have reported increased cardiac calcineurin activity in aortic-banded rats, exercise-induced cardiac hypertrophy, or salt-sensitive hypertension-induced hyper-trophy [49–51]. A few studies have also examined the activity of calcineurin in failed or hypertrophic human heart samples. Analysis of human hypertrophic or failed heart tissue due to ischemic and idiopathic cardiomyopathy, revealed a significant increase in cal-cineurin activity [26,52]. These results were recently extended in patients with hypertrophic obstructive cardiomyopathy and aortic stenosis-induced pressure overload, who showed a significant increase in cardiac calcineurin activity that was associated with a differentially processed form of the calcineurin catalytic subunit in the heart, presumably due to partial proteolysis [53]. Collectively, the observations previously discussed have demonstrated a linkage between cardiac hypertrophy and failure and the activation of a pivotal reactive signaling molecule in the heart.

Use of CsA and FK506 in Animal Models of Cardiac Hypertrophy

Although CsA can attenuate agonist-induced cardiomyocyte hypertrophy in vitro [44,54], its effectiveness in vivo is somewhat more controversial. CsA and FK506 each prevented the phenotypic manifestations of hypertrophic and dilated cardiomyopathy in three separate transgenic mouse models of intrinsic heart disease [47]. In the same report, CsA administra-tion to aortic-banded rats over 6 days prevented the induction of cardiac hypertrophy [47]. However, four subsequent studies concluded that calcineurin inhibitors did not signifi-cantly block pressure overload hypertrophy in either aortic-banded mice or rats, suggesting that CsA and FK506 might not be effective antihypertrophic agents [55–58]. In addition, a more recent study concluded that CsA was detrimental to disease progression in α-MHC 403 mutant mice [59]. Although the studies previously discussed have concluded a somewhat negative correlation between calcineurin and cardiac disease states, such evidence should be weighed against the large number of positive accounts. To date, approx-imately 20 individual reports have shown that inhibition of calcineurin with either CsA or FK506 can antagonize cardiac hypertrophy and/or disease progression in pleiotropic rodent models [47–51,60–74]. While the overwhelming majority of pharmacologic animal studies support a role for calcineurin in the hypertrophic response, the few negative ac-counts may reflect factors such as drug dosage, differences in the surgical preparations, sex, age, or type of animal model.

Targeted Inhibition of Calcineurin Attenuates Hypertrophy

Another aspect of the controversy surrounding CsA and FK506 studies in animal models of hypertrophy pertains to drug specificity. To address the issue of specificity, the noncom-petitive calcineurin inhibitory domains from the calcineurin interacting proteins Cain/Cabin-1 and AKAP79 were recently employed [75–77]. Adenovirus expressing the inhibi-tory domains of Cain or AKAP blocked calcineurin activity and attenuated phenylephrine- and angiotensin II-induced hypertrophy in cultured cardiomyocytes [45]. The inhibition of hypertrophy by Cain and AKAP adenoviral infection was similar to the inhibition observed with CsA and FK506, suggesting calcineurin as the determinative factor [45]. More recently, transgenic mice were generated that express the calcineurin inhibitory domains of Cain or AKAP [78]. Cain and AKAP transgenic mice demonstrated a significant reduction in pressure overload (aortic banding) and agonist-induced (isoproterenol infusion) cardiac hypertrophy [78]. Calcineurin activity is also negatively regulated by the muscle-enriched calcineurin inhibitory proteins MCIP1 and MCIP2 (DSCR1 and ZAKI-4), which are each highly expressed in the heart and skeletal muscle [79,80]. Transgenic mice expressing the calcineurin inhibitory domain from MCIP1 have also been recently characterized and shown to have reduced cardiac hypertrophy in response to stress stimulation or pressure overload [81,82]. Lastly, transgenic mice expressing a dominant negative mutant of calcineurin within the heart also demonstrated reduced cardiac hypertrophy to stress stimuli (aortic banding) [83]. More recently, *calcineurinAβ* gene targeted mice were generated as a further means of evaluating the necessary function of this phosphatase in the heart. *CalcineurinAβ* null mice were viable, fertile, and had reduced cardiac calcineurin activity that was associated with an impaired hypertrophic response to Angiotensin II infusion, isoproterenol infusion, or abdominal aortic constriction [84]. These data not only extend the transgenic approaches previously discussed, but they more specifically implicate the *calcineurinAβ* gene in regulating the hypertrophic response.

Calcineurin Targets Regulating the Hypertrophic Response

The downstream transcriptional mechanisms whereby calcineurin might function in vivo remain largely uncharacterised. However, both NFAT and MEF2 transcriptional regulators are regulated by calcineurin (Fig. 2), suggesting obvious candidates for genetic analysis in the heart. The NFAT family consists of five members, four of which (NFATc1-c4) are partitioned between the cytoplasm and nucleus so that calcineurin activation sends them to the nucleus where they activate gene expression [42]. Analysis of mRNA levels suggests that multiple NFAT factors are expressed in the heart [85], although the lack of good antibodies and the relatively low abundance of NFAT proteins has made it difficult to identify the most prominent NFAT member expressed in the heart. To potentially identify the downstream effectors of calcineurin in mediating the hypertrophic response both *NFATc3* and *NFATc4* null mice were evaluated. Remarkably, *NFATc3* null mice, but not *NFATc4* null, were determined to have impaired hypertrophy induced by activated calcineurin, abdominal aortic constriction, or angiotensin II infusion [86]. These data suggest that NFATc3 functions as a necessary transducer of calcineurin signaling in mediating the cardiac hypertrophic response. Collectively, analysis of multiple genetically modified mouse models with altered calcineurin-NFAT signaling leaves little doubt that calcineurin is an important regulator of the cardiac hypertrophic response. The data obtained with these animal models also suggest that CsA and FK506 attenuate cardiac hypertrophy through a calcineurin-dependent mechanism. However, enthusiasm for calcineurin inhibitory agents in treating human heart disease should be considered within the framework of drug toxicity and lack of clinical data (see following text).

Clinical Use of CsA and FK506

Although calcineurin inhibitory drugs can attenuate cardiac hypertrophy and/or failure in most rodent models of induced heart disease, their potential usefulness in humans is uncertain. Both CsA and FK506 have a number of side-effects in humans, including nephrogenic and neurogenic toxicity and immunosuppression [87]. Indeed, chronic CsA therapy in human transplant patients induces renal toxicity leading to hypertension and potentially secondary cardiac hypertrophy [88]. Although this observation suggests that CsA might be associated with cardiac hypertrophy in humans (albeit secondary), drug dosage is an important consideration. The dosage of CsA or FK506 that is required to attenuate cardiac hypertrophy in animal models is five- to 10-fold higher than the dosage used for immuno-suppression [49,89]. In this respect, lower dosages of CsA used for immunosuppressive purposes would not effectively inhibit cardiac calcineurin activity and, therefore, might not act as an antihypertrophic agent. The reason for the differing sensitivity to CsA likely relates to a higher calcineurin protein content in cardiomyocytes relative to T- and B-cells, or to differences in tissue accessibility.

Despite the concerns listed, there is still a general lack of convincing clinical data regarding the affects of CsA on human cardiac hypertrophy, which further complicates assessment of calcineurin as a therapeutic target. However, a large number of patients receiving CsA for its immunosuppressant qualities fail to demonstrate significant cardiac side-effects, at least suggesting that cyclosporine is innocuous to the heart (in contrast to the suggestion of Fatkin and colleagues [59]). Indeed, one small clinical study of heart transplant patients, which employed a cocktail of immunosuppressants that included CsA, even demonstrated smaller left ventricular masses indexed to body surface area at 3, 6, 9, and 12 months posttransplantation [90]. This study is provocative, however, more defini-tive data is needed before such a paradigm can be extended from animal models to humans. In addition, novel approaches to selectively inhibit calcineurin within the heart would be advantageous given the known side-affects of CsA and FK506.

In summary, the calcineurin/NFAT pathway illustrates the paradigm of how a signal, increased cytosolic [Ca^{2+}], generated in response to either deformation of the membrane or to hypertrophic agonist binding to its receptor, activates one signaling factor (cal-cineurin), which then dephosphorylates and activates a transcription factor (NFATc3) that, in turn, translocates to the nucleus, reprogramming gene expression.

Regulation of Protein Synthesis

The second critical component of hypertrophic growth is the ability to dramatically upregu-late protein synthetic capabilities. This is regulated by two very complex and interacting pathways. One is the mammalian target of rapamycin (mTOR) pathway [91]. The other is the PI3-kinase pathway that, in addition to its role in regulating protein synthesis, also plays a major role in reprogramming gene expression. These pathways are essential in determination of cell, organ, and body size (i.e., normal growth) in species as diverse as *Drosophila* and man [5,92–95]. The pathways are also recruited in, and regulate the response to, pathologic stress-induced hypertrophic growth [96–98]. A schematic of these interacting pathways is shown in Figure 3. Both the mTOR and PI3-K pathways regulate protein synthesis by modulating the activity of various translation factors, either initiating factors (which initiate the translation of mRNAs into proteins) or elongation factors (which are responsible for elongation of the polypeptide chain) (reviewed in [99,100]).

Evaluation of mTOR

mTOR is a protein kinase whose importance is illustrated by its conservation throughout evolution, from yeast to human. The critical importance of mTOR in regulating hypertro-phic growth in vivo was recently demonstrated when its inhibitor, rapamycin, was found to attenuate the hypertrophic response to pressure overload in mice [98]. Although it is abundantly clear that mTOR is absolutely critical in the regulation of protein synthesis, and studies employing rapamycin have identified specific targets of mTOR that regulate

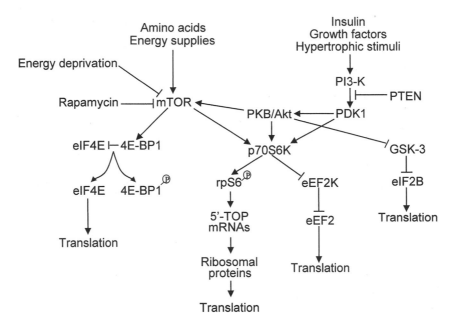

Figure 3 Schematic representation of the PI3-K and mTOR pathways. See text for details. Other abbreviations/notes: rpS6, S6 ribosomal protein; eEF2K, the eukaryotic elongation factor 2 kinase that phosphorylates and inactivates eEF2 (eEF2K is inhibited by p70S6K) [99].

synthesis, the mechanisms regulating mTOR activity remain something of a mystery. In brief, mTOR is activated when amino acids and energy supplies are plentiful (Fig. 3). In addition, growth factors, including those leading to cardiac growth, such as insulin and IGF-1, also activate mTOR probably via activation of PI3-K signaling. Teleologically this makes sense because protein translation is an enormous consumer of energy in the cell, and, therefore, one would not want translation proceeding at times of amino acid or energy deprivation.

One of mTOR's major targets is a protein, 4E-binding protein 1 (4E-BP1), which binds to and inactivates the eukaryotic initiation factor 4E (eIF4E), preventing the initiation of translation [100–102]. When activated, mTOR leads to the phosphorylation 4E-BP1, causing it to dissociate from eIF4E, thus allowing translation to proceed (Fig. 3). A second target activated by mTOR, in cooperation with the PI3-K pathway, is the p70S6 kinase that phosphorylates the S6 protein of the small ribosomal subunit [5]. The p70S6K may regulate the translation of a specific set of mRNAs, the so-called 5'-TOP (tract of pyrimidines) mRNAs that encode ribosomal proteins. In addition, it may regulate one of the elongation factors, eEF2 [99]. The importance of p70S6K in cell and organ growth is illustrated by the marked reduction in cell, organ, and body size in mice deleted for even one of the two p70S6K genes [93]. Furthermore, p70S6K is activated by pressure overload, and it is possible that the ability of rapamycin to block pressure overload hypertrophy is due, to the inhibition of p70S6K activation by rapamycin [98].

The PI3-K Pathway

This highly conserved pathway (Fig. 3) is remarkable in the fact that virtually every component of the pathway has been shown in animal models in vivo to regulate cell and organ growth, including growth of the heart, thus presenting a consistent message concerning the importance of the pathway [96–98,103–112]. The pathway is activated by most (if not all) of the agonists implicated in inducing cardiac hypertrophy, including pressure overload. When activated, the PI3-K phosphorylates the integral membrane phosholipid, phosphatidylinositol, at the 3′ position of the inositol ring. This leads to the recritment of the protein kinase, Akt (also known as protein kinase B, PKB) to the cell membrane via interactions of a specific domain of PKB/Akt (the plekstrin homology [PH] domain) with the phosphorylated lipid [113]. This brings PKB/Akt into proximity to its activator, the 3-phosphoinositide-dependent protein kinase-1 (PDK1), which phosphorylates and activates PKB/Akt (in addition to the p70S6K previously discussed). PKB/Akt then plays a role in activating mTOR and, consequently, p70S6K and the protein translation machinery [114]. Given this, it is probably not surprising that PI3-K, PDK1, and PKB/Akt have all been shown to regulate cell and organ size, including size of the heart. Indeed, one of the more striking cardiac-specific transgenic models is the mouse overexpressing PKB/Akt that has a markedly enlarged heart [108,111]. Although it is likely that activation of the translational machinery is an important mechanism driving the increased heart size in these mice, PKB/Akt has transcriptional targets that also likely play a role in reprogramming gene expression in response to hypertrophic stress, however these remain to be clearly identified [115].

PKB/Akt has another target, glycogen synthase kinase-3 (GSK-3), which also plays a role in regulating normal and pathologic stress-induced growth of the heart [103,105,106,116,117]. GSK-3 (β and likely GSK-3α as well) is a negative regulator of cardiac growth. Transgenic animals expressing GSK-3β have dramatic reductions in normal cardiac growth and also have a markedly reduced hypertrophic response to pressure overload [103,118]. Furthermore, inhibition of GSK-3β is necessary for the hypertrophic response to a number of agonists, likely mediated via several mechanisms. For example, GSK-3β negatively regulates activity of the initiation factor, eIF2B [119], and reviewed in [120]. Thus inhibition of GSK-3β may be important for upregulating protein translation. However, GSK-3β also inhibits the activity of a number of targets that function as transcription factors. Since several of them have been implicated in cardiac growth, GSK-3β may be particularly important in the reprogramming of gene expression and relatively less important in regulating protein translation. This might make GSK-3β an attractive target for therapeutic intervention because therapies targeting the translation machinery can be expected to have significant toxicity when used long-term. The GSK-3β targets include the NFATs, and thus, GSK-3β acts in opposition to the calcineurin pathway [105,121,122]. Phosphorylation of NFATs by GSK-3β leads to exclusion of NFATs from the nucleus, thus preventing access to target genes. In fact, when the GSK-3β transgenic was bred with the calcineurin transgenic, hypertrophy was markedly reduced [103]. Other known growth regulators negatively regulated by GSK-3β include c-Myc, GATA-4, β-catenin, and c-Jun (reviewed in [123,124]).

The PI3-kinase pathway is negatively regulated by a phosphatase that dephosphorylates 3-phosphorylated phosphoinositides at the 3′ position called PTEN (phosphatase and tensin homolog) (Fig. 3) [125]. Overexpression of a catalytically inactive mutant of PTEN in cultured cardiomyocytes led to cardiomyocyte hypertrophy [110]. Furthermore, conditional inactivation of the PTEN gene in the heart also led to hypertrophy, further supporting a critical role for the PI3-K pathway in regulating cardiomyocyte growth [96].

Other Pathways Involved in Growth Regulation

As suggested in the introduction, a large number of signaling pathways have been implicated in the regulation of cardiomyocyte growth. However, either there are insufficient data at this point to support a claim, or the data are too conflicting to make definitive statements concerning their role. This is probably most apparent when one examines the literature on the role of stress-activated mitogen-activated protein (MAP) kinases in the hypertrophic response (Fig 4). These kinases, the c-Jun N-terminal kinases (JNKs) and the p38-MAP kinases, have been exhaustively studied but there remains no consensus on their role. This is, in large part, due to the models that have, out of necessity, been employed and, until very recently, the lack of adequate pharmacologic inhibitors that can be used in vivo. Both of these kinases are members of multigene families so that gene-targeting experiments have been complicated by functional redundancy and embryonic lethality. This has forced a variety of approaches, none of which are ideal, and include studying transgenics or conditional transgenics (with problems inherent to overexpression), knock-outs of upstream activators, or utilizing adenovirus-mediated gene transfer of dominant inhibitory mutants [126–130]. Given the central role of these kinases in very basic responses of all cells to a wide range of cellular stressors (oxidant stress, ionizing radiation, cytokine stimulation, osmolar stress, heat shock, etc.) compensatory adaptations are likely to be profound in these models. It is likely that a definitive conclusion on the role of these kinases in hypertrophic growth will have to await the commerical availability of truly specific inhibitors of these kinases, or better yet, inhibitors of specific isoforms of these kinases, because there is evidence that different isoforms (and even different splice variants) may serve different functions within the cell. Alternatively, tissue-specific gene targeting experiments, or controlled dominant negative transgenic studies, may provide additional insight. However, assessment of the present data suggests that the JNKs and p38-MAP kinases may be more involved in the progression of heart failure, including remodeling of the matrix, and may play much less of a role in hypertrophic growth. If confirmed, they may be very attractive drug targets in the failing heart.

The ERK family (extracellular signal-regulated kinases) of MAP kinases (Fig. 4) are also potently activated by hypertrophic stimuli. For studies of the role of the ERKs

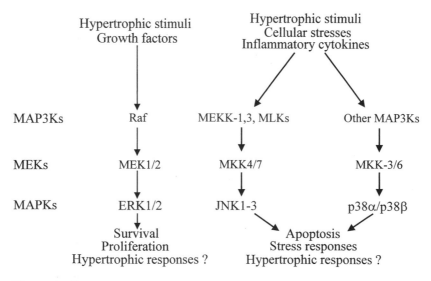

Figure 4 Schematic representation of the major mitogen-activated protein kinase (MAPK) pathways. The three-tiered kinase cascade consists of a MAP kinase kinase kinase (MAP3K), that phosphorylates and activates a MAP kinase kinase (also known as MAPK and ERK kinase, MEK), that, in turn, phosphorylates the MAP kinases (MAPK), either the ERKs, JNKs, or p38–MAPKs.

in hypertrophy, relatively specific inhibitors of the MEKs (MAPK and ERK kinases), kinases immediately upstream of the ERKs are available and, in general, studies have found them to inhibit at least part of the hypertrophic response of cardiomyocytes in culture (reviewed in [33]). Interestingly, cardiac-specific overexpression of MEK1 (one of the immediate upstream activators of the ERKs) produced concentric cardiac hypertrophy, but unlike most other models, such as the calcineurin transgenic, the MEK1 transgenic animals did not progress to contractile failure [131]. These data raised the concept of ''beneficial'' hypertrophy vs ''detrimental'' hypertrophy by clearly demonstrating that hypertrophy per se need not inexorably progress to heart failure. This may have to do with the fact that the ERKs (in contrast to many other prohypertrophic signaling molecules including calcineurin, the JNKs, and the p38-MAP kinases) are in many circumstances, cytoprotective. Of note, hypertrophy induced by overexpression of PI3-K also leads to hypertrophy without heart failure, and the PI3-K pathway, like the ERK pathway, is also cytoprotective [97]. These data suggest a potential approach to the treatment of patients with heart failure wherein pathways promoting progression of heart failure are inhibited while those prohypertrophic pathways that are also cytoprotective are stimulated.

In summary, the PI3-K and mTOR pathways are critical regulators of cell and organ growth via effects on the general protein synthesis machinery as well as via effects on the activity of several transcription factors regulating expression of hypertrophic response genes. Calcineurin is another important regulator that appears to act largely via effects on the NFAT family of transcription factors. Many other pathways have been implicated, however, the data supporting an important role for these other pathways in physiological or pathological hypertrophy are not, at least at this time, nearly as convincing. Thus, it seems likely as drugs become available for the treatment of hypertrophic disorders, the focus, at least initially, will likely be on components of the calcineurin and PI3-K/mTOR pathways. It remains to be determined whether these pathways, with their known roles in the most basic of cellular responses of many (or all) cells in the body, will be able to be inhibited for prolonged periods of time without inducing toxicity. Alternative approaches, such as gene therapy, which can be delivered in an organ-specific (and even cell type-specific) manner, or organ-specific drug delivery may be necessary to target these pathways safely.

ALTERATIONS IN SIGNALING IN THE DISEASED HUMAN HEART

We have discussed the signaling profile of the hearts of experimental animals exposed to pressure overload. These data raise two questions: (a) How do the signaling alterations seen in the heart of these animals compare to signaling alterations in the hearts of patients with hypertrophy or heart failure? and (b) Is there any evidence that abnormalities seen in these clinical scenarios are a cause of heart failure (as opposed to a consequence of the heart failure) and, therefore, will manipulating their activity alter the progression of disease?

One study has examined the signaling profile of hypertrophied hearts [26]. In this study, patients were scheduled to be transplant donors but for a variety of reasons were not considered to be appropriate. Several of these patients were found to have significant cardiac hypertrophy, allowing a comparison of the signaling profiles in those hearts vs. normal hearts, that were also rejected as donors. Of the signaling factors examined (calcineurin, ERK1/2, JNK, p38-MAP kinase, Akt, and GSK-3), the only factor consistently found to be activated in the hypertrophied hearts was calcineurin [26]. Of note, although some of these patients clearly had hypertension, they were not suspected of having any cardiac disorder and, in all cases, systolic function was not depressed. Therefore, clinically, they would be described as "compensated" hypertrophy. These data raised calcineurin as one potential therapeutic target, inhibition of which might be able to regress hypertrophy, at least in this phase of the disease.

In contrast to the paucity of data on hypertrophied hearts, several studies have examined the signaling profile of hearts explanted from patients with advanced failure either going to transplant or undergoing left ventricular assist device (LVAD) placement prior to transplant [26,52,132–137]. The following signaling factors were examined in at least one of the studies: calcineurin, ERK1/2, JNKs, p38-MAP kinases, ERK5, the MAP kinase phosphatases (which inactivate the MAP kinsaes), Akt, GSK-3, and a signaling pathway activated by Ang II and cytokines, the Janus kinase (Jak)/signal transducer and activator of transcription (STAT) pathway. Where examined, calcineurin expression and activity were increased, though not to the same degree as seen in the hypertrophied hearts previously discussed [26,52]. Unfortunately, no clear consensus has emerged from the studies examining the MAP kinase pathways despite the fact that the patient populations studied appear to be similar. The most consistent results are probably in relation to p38-MAP kinase activity. Three studies have reported activation of p38-MAP kinases in ischemic cardiomyopathy [26,133,136], with only one reporting inhibition [135]. In contrast, in idiopathic cardiomyopathy, p38-MAPK activity has generally been reported to be decreased or unchanged, with only one reporting activation, although the magnitude of activation was very low in that study [26]. No consistent results have been reported for the JNKs and ERKs. Single reports have examined the other factors. In these, ERK5 has been reported to be inhibited [137] and the MAP kinase phosphatases were activated [132]. Akt was also found to be activated, irrespective of the etiology of the heart failure, and accordingly, its downstream target, GSK-3, was inhibited [26]. This profile suggested to the authors that the heart may be attempting to mount a hypertrophic response in the face of severe contractile dysfunction [26]. Differences between the studies could be accounted for by a number of factors, including different medical therapies, device therapies, status of the patient, and, maybe most importantly, methods of preserving the tissue because suboptimal harvest and storage techniques can lead to the rapid dephosphorylation and inactivation of protein kinases.

To summarize, not only can one not define a signaling profile of the failing heart at this point, it is also entirely unclear whether any signaling alterations are causal or simply a consequence of the heart failure. As a result, it is unclear what if any effect manipulating these pathways would have on the progression of disease. Interestingly, hearts that have been mechanically unloaded with LVAD support do show changes in activity of MAP kinases, with ERK 1/2 and JNK activity decreasing and p38-MAP kinase activity increasing, concomitant with a decrease in cardiomyocyte size (i.e., regression of hypertrophy) and a decline in the rate of myocyte apoptosis [134]. Again, however, it is unclear if the regression of hypertrophy and reduction in apoptosis is due to the changes in activity of these MAP kinases.

Finally, the complexity of the heart failure signaling abnormalities and the changing activities of various pathways at various times in the progression of disease (as evidenced by the differences in signaling in the hypertrophied vs. failing hearts) creates a "moving target" and leads to significant challenges for translational research in this area. The patients with compensated hypertrophy vs. advanced heart failure were obviously at different ends of the pathophysiological spectrum of heart failure, and in between these points, including the transition to and early progression of heart failure, we have very little data on what pathways might be reasonable targets. It is very likely, however, that interventions at different points in the progression of heart failure will have to be aimed at very different targets, and it is not clear that these interventions will be equally or uniformly successful. Given the aggressive pursuit of inhibitors of these pathways by the pharmaceutical/biotech industry, we should, in a very short time, have the tools to be able to address these questions.

REFERENCES

1. Levy D, Garrison RJ, Savage DD, Kannel WB, Castelli WP. Prognostic implications of echocardiographically determined left ventricular mass in the Framingham heart study. N Engl J Med 1990; 322:1561–1566.
2. Ho KK, Levy D, Kannel WB, Pinsky JL. The epidemiology of heart failure: the Framingham study. J Am Coll Cardiol 1993; 22:6–13.
3. Force T, Michael A, Kilter H, Haq S. Stretch-actvated pathways and left ventricular remodeling. J Card Fail 2002; 8:S351–S358.
4. Molkentin JD, Dorn GW. Cytoplasmic signaling pathways that regulate cardiac hypertrophy. Annu Rev Physiol 2001; 63:391–426.
5. Fingar DC, Salama S, Tsou C, Harlow E, Blenis J. Mammalian cell size is controlled by mTOR and its downstream targets S6K1 and 4EBP1/eIF4E. Genes Dev 2002; 16:1472–1487.
6. Ruwhof C, van der Laarse A. Mechanical stress-induced cardiac hypertrophy: mechanisms and signal transduction pathways. Cardiovasc Res 2000; 47:23–37.
7. Hu H, Sachs F. Stretch-activated ion channels in the heart. J Mol Cell Cardiol 1997; 29:1511–1523.
8. Keller RS, Shai SY, Babbitt CJ, Pham CG, Solaro RJ, Valencik ML, Loftus JC, Ross RS. Disruption of integrin function in the murine myocardium leads to perinatal lethality, fibrosis, and abnormal cardiac performance. Am J Pathol 2001; 158:1079–1090.
9. MacKenna DA, Dolfi F, Vuori K, Ruoslahti E. ERK and JNK activation by mechanical stretch is integrin-dependent and matrix-specific in rat cardiac fibroblasts. J Clin Invest 1998; 101:301–310.
10. Pham CG, Harpf AE, Keller RS, Vu HT, Shai SY, Loftus JC, Ross RS. Striated muscle-specific β 1D-integrin and FAK are involved in cardiac myocyte hypertrophic response pathway. Am J Physiol 2000; 279:H2916–H2926.
11. Ross RS, Pham CG, Shai SY, Fenczik C, Glembotski CC, Ginsberg MH, Loftus JC. β1 integrins participate in the hypertrophic response of rat ventricular myocytes. Circ Res 1998; 82:1160–1172.
12. Gudi SRP, Lee AA, Clark CB, Frangos JA. Equibiaxial strain and strain rate stimulate early activation of G proteins in cardiac fibroblasts. Am J Physiol 1998; 274:C1424–C1428.
13. Sadoshima J, Izumo S. Mechanical stretch rapidly activates multiple signal transduction pathways in cardiac myocytes: potential involvement of an autocrine/paracrine mechanism. EMBO J 1993; 12:1681–1692.
14. Sadoshima J, Xu Y, Slayter HS, Izumo S. Autocrine release of angiotensin II mediates stretch-induced hypertrophy of cardiac myocytes in vitro. Cell 1993; 75:977–984.
15. Daub H, Weiss FU, Wallasch C, Ullrich A. Role of transactivation of the EGF receptor in signaling by G-protein-coupled receptors. Nature 1996; 379:557–560.
16. Ushio-Fukai M, Griendling KK, Becker PL, Hilenski L, Halleran S, Alexander RW. Epidermal growth factor receptor transactivation by angiotensin II requires reactive oxygen species in vascular smooth muscle cells. Arteriocler Thromb Vasc Biol 2001; 21:489–495.
17. Eguchi S, Dempsey PJ, Frank GD, Motley ED, Inagami T. Activation of MAPKs by angiotensin II in vascular smooth muscle cells. J Biol Chem 2001; 276:7957–7962.
18. Prenzel N, Zwick E, Daub H, Leserer M, Abraham R, Wallasch C, Ullrich A. EGF receptor transactivation by G-protein-coupled receptors requires metalloproteinase cleavage of proHB-EGF. Nature 1999; 402:884–888.

19. Kunisada K, Tone E, Fujio E, Matsui H, Yamauchi-Takihara K, Kishimoto T. Activation of gp130 transduces hypertrophic signals via STAT3 in cardiac myocytes. Circulation 1998; 98:346–352.

20. Murata M, Fukuda K, Ishida H, Miyoshi S, Koura T, Kodama H, Nakazawa HK, Ogawa S. Leukemia inhibitory factor, a potent cardiac hypertorphic cytokine, enhances L-type Ca^{2+} current and $[Ca^{2+}]i$ transient in cardiomyocytes. J Mol Cell Cardiol 1999; 31:237–245.

21. Oh H, Fujio Y, Kunisada K, Hirota H, Matsui H, Kishimoto T, Yamauchi-Takihara K. Activation of phosphatidylinositol 3-kinase through gp130 induces protein kinase B and p70 S6 kinase phosphorylation in cardiac myocytes. J Biol Chem 1998; 273:9703–9710.

22. Lupu F, Terwilliger JD, Lee K, Segre GV, Efstratiadis A. Roles of growth hormone and IGF-1 in mouse postnatal growth. Dev Biol 2001; 229:141–162.

23. Pete G, Fuller CR, Oldham JM, Smith DR, Ercole AJ, Kahn CR, Lunk PK. Postnatal growth responses to insulin-like growth factor I in insulin receptor substrate-1-deficient mice. Endocrinology 1999; 140:5478–5487.

24. Tamemoto H, Kadowaki T, Tobe K, Yagi T, Sakura H, Hayakawa T, Terauchi Y, Ueki K, Kaburagi Y, Satoh S. Insulin resistance and growth retardation in mice lacking IRS-1. Nature 1994; 372:182–186.

25. Ren J, Samson WK, Sowers JR. IGF-1 as a cardiac hormone: physiological and pathophysiological implications in heart disease. J Mol Cell Cardiol 1999; 31:2049–2061.

26. Haq S, Choukroun G, Lim HW, Tymitz KM, del Monte F, Gwathmey J, Grazette L, Michael A, Hajjar R, Force T, Molkentin JD. Differential activation of signal transduction pathways in human hearts with hypertrophy versus advanced heart failure. Circulation 2001; 103: 670–677.

27. Adams JW, Sakata Y, Davis MG, Sah VP, Wang Y, Liggett SB, Chien KR, Brown JH, Dorn GW. Enhanced Gαq signaling: a common pathway mediates cardiac hypertrophy and apoptotic heart failure. Proc Natl Acad Sci 1998; 95:10140–10145.

28. D'Angelo DD, Sakata Y, Lorenz JH, Boivin GP, Walsh RA, Liggett SB, Dorn GW. Transgenic Gαq overexpression induced cardiac contractile failure in mice. Proc Natl Acad Sci 1997; 94:8121–8126.

29. Mende U, Kagen A, Cohen A, Aramburu J, Schoen FJ, Neer EJ. Transient cardiac expression of constitutively active Gαq leads to hypertrophy and dilated cardiomyopathy by calcineurin-dependent and independent pathways. Proc Natl Acad Sci 1998; 95:13893–13898.

30. Sakata Y, Hoit BD, Liggett SB, Walsh RA, Dorn GW. Decompensation of pressure-overload hypertrophy in Gαq-overexpressing mice. Circulation 1998; 97:1488–1495.

31. Ahkter SA, Luttrell LM, Rockman HA, Iaccarino G, Lefkowitz RJ, Koch WJ. Targeting the receptor-Gq interface to inhibit in vivo pressure overload myocardial hypertrophy. Science 1998; 280:574–577.

32. Wettschureck N, Rutten H, Zywietz A, Gehring D, Wilkie TM, Chen J, Chien KR, Offermans S. Absence of pressure overload induced myocardial hypertrophy after conditional inactivation of Gαq/G α11 in cardiomyocytes. Nature Med 2001; 7:1236–1240.

33. Vlahos CJ, McDowell SA, Clerk A. Kinases as therapeutic targets for heart failure. Nat Rev Drug Disc 2003; 2:99–113.

34. Kyriakis JM, Avruch J. Sounding the alarm: protein kinase cascades activated by stress and inflammation. J Biol Chem 1996; 271:24313–24316.

35. Klee CB, Ren H, Wang X. Regulation of the calmodulin-stimulated protein phosphatase, calcineurin. J Biol Chem 1998; 273:13367–13370.

36. Crabtree GR. Generic signals and specific outcomes: signaling through Ca2 +, calcineurin, and NF-AT. Cell 1999; 96:611–614.

37. Dolmetsch RE, Lewis RS, Goodnow CC, Healy JI. Differential activation of transcription factors induced by Ca2 + response amplitude and duration. Nature 1997; 386:855–858.

38. Takaishi T, Saito N, Kuno T, Tanaka C. Differential distribution of the mRNA encoding two isoforms of the catalytic subunit of calcineurin in the rat brain. Biochem Biophys Res Commun 1991; 174:393–398.

39. Muramatsu T, Giri PR, Higuchi S, Kincaid RL. Molecular cloning of a calmodulin-dependent phosphatase from murine testis: identification of a developmentally expressed nonneural isoenzyme. Proc Natl Acad Sci U S A 1992; 89:529–533.

40. Buttini M, Limonta S, Luyten M, Boddeke H. Distribution of calcineurin A isoenzyme mRNAs in rat thymus and kidney. Histochem J 1995; 27:291–299.

41. Jiang H, Xiong F, Kong S, Ogawa T, Kobayashi M, Liu JO. Distinct tissue and cellular distribution of two major isoforms of calcineurin. Mol Immuno 1997; 34:663–669.

42. Rao A, Luo C, Hogan PG. Transcription factors of the NFAT family: regulation and function. Annu Rev Immunol 1997; 15:707–747.

43. Lopéz-Rodríguez C, Aramburu J, Rakeman AS, Rao A. NFAT5, a constitutively nuclear NFAT protein that does not cooperate with Fos and Jun. Proc Natl Acad Sci USA 1999; 96: 7214–7219.

44. Molkentin JD, Lu JR, Antos CL, Markham B, Richardson J, Robbins J, Grant SR, Olson EN. A calcineurin-dependent transcriptional pathway for cardiac hypertrophy. Cell 1998; 93: 215–228.

45. Taigen T, De Windt LJ, Lim HW, Molkentin JD. Targeted inhibition of calcineurin prevents agonist-induced cardiomyocyte hypertrophy. Proc Natl Acad Sci USA 2000; 97:1196–1201.

46. Zhu W, Zou Y, Shiojima I, Kudoh S, Aikawa R, Hayashi D, Mizukami M, Toko H, Shibasaki F, Yazaki Y, Nagai R, Komuro I. Ca2 + /calmodulin-dependent kinase II and calcineurin play critical roles in endothelin-1-induced cardiomyocyte hypertrophy. J Biol Chem 2000; 275:15239–15245.

47. Sussman MA, Lim HW, Gude N, Taigen T, Olson EN, Robbins J, Colbert MC, Gualberto A, Wieczorek DF, Molkentin JD. Prevention of cardiac hypertrophy in mice by calcineurin inhibition. Science 1998; 281:1690–1693.

48. Lim HW, De Windt LJ, Mante J, Kimball TR, Witt SA, Sussman MA, Molkentin JD. Reversal of cardiac hypertrophy in transgenic disease models by calcineurin inhibition. J Mol Cell Cardiol 2000; 32:697–709.

49. Lim HW, De Windt LJ, Steinberg L, Taigen T, Witt SA, Kimball TR, Molkentin JD. Calcineurin expression, activation, and function in cardiac pressure-overload hypertrophy. Circulation 2000; 101:2431–2437.

50. Eto Y, Yonekura K, Sonoda M, Arai N, Sata M, Sugiura S, Takenaka K, Gualberto A, Hixon ML, Wagner MW, Aoyagi T. Calcineurin is activated in rat hearts with physiological left ventricular hypertrophy induced by veluntary exercise training. Circulation 2000; 101: 2134–2137.

51. Shimoyama M, Hayashi D, Zou Y, Takimoto E, Mizukami M, Monzen K, Yazaki Y, Nagai R, Komuro I. Calcineurin inhibitor attenuates the development and induces the regression of cardiac hypertrophy in rats with salt-sensitive hypertension. J Cardiol 2001; 37:114–118.

52. Lim HW, Molkentin JD. Calcineurin and human heart failure. Nat Med 1999; 5:246–247.

53. Ritter O, Hack S, Schuh K, Rothlein N, Perrot A, Osterziel KJ, Schulte HD, Neyses L. Calcineurin in human heart hypertrophy. Circulation 2002; 105:2265–2269.

54. Xia Y, McMillin JB, Lewis A, Moore M, Zhu WG, Williams RS, Kellems RE. Electrical stimulation of neonatal cardiac myocytes activates the NFAT3 and GATA4 pathways and up-regulates the adenylosuccinate synthetase 1 gene. J Biol Chem 2000; 275:1855–1863.

55. Luo Z, Shyu KG, Gualberto A, Walsh K. Calcineurin and cardiac hypertrophy. Nat Med 1998; 10:1092–1093.

56. Mäller JG, Nemoto S, Laser M, Carabello BA, Menick DR. Calcineurin inhibition and cardiac hypertrophy. (letter to editor) Science 1998; 282:1007.

57. Ding B, Price RL, Borg TK, Weinberg EO, Halloran PF, Lorell BH. Pressure overload induces severe hypertrophy in mice treated with cyclosporine, an inhibitor of calcineurin. Circ Res 1999; 84:729–734.

58. Zhang W, Kowal RC, Rusnak F, Sikkink RA, Olson EN, Victor RG. Failure of calcineurin inhibitors to prevent pressure-overload left ventricular hypertrophy in rats. Circ Res 1999; 84:722–728.

59. Fatkin D, McConnell BK, Mudd JO, Semsarian C, Moskowitz IG, Schoen FJ, Giewat M, Seidman CE, Seidman JG. An abnormal Ca(2 +) response in mutant sarcomere protein-mediated familial hypertrophic cardiomyopathy. J Clin Invest 2000; 106:1351–1359.

60. Meguro T, Hong C, Asai K, Takagi G, McKinsey TA, Olson EN, Vatner SF. Cyclosporine attenuates pressure-overload hypertrophy in mice while enhancing susceptibility to decompensation and heart failure. Circ Res 1999; 84:735–740.

61. Shimoyama M, Hayashi D, Takimoto E, Zou Y, Oka T, Uozumi H, Kudoh S, Shibasaki F, Yazaki Y, Nagai R, Komuro I. Calcineurin plays a critical role in pressure overload-induced cardiac hypertrophy. Circulation 1999; 100:2449–2454.

62. Hill JA, Karimi M, Kutschke W, Davisson RL, Zimmerman K, Wang Z, Kerber RE, Weiss RM. Cardiac hypertrophy is not a required compensatory response to short-term pressure overload. Circulation 2000; 101:2863–2869.

63. Sakata Y, Masuyama T, Yamamoto K, Nishikawa N, Yamamoto H, Kondo H, Ono K, Otsu K, Kuzuya T, Miwa T, Takeda H, Miyamoto E, Hori M. Calcineurin inhibitor attenuates left ventricular hypertrophy, leading to prevention of heart failure in hypertensive rats. Circulation 2000; 102:2269–2275.

64. Shimoyama M, Hayashi D, Zou Y, Takimoto E, Mizukami M, Monzen K, Kudoh S, Hiroi Y, Yazaki Y, Nagai R, Komuro I. Calcineurin inhibitor attenuates the development and induces the regression of cardiac hypertrophy in rats with salt-sensitive hypertension. Circulation 2000; 102:1996–2004.

65. Murat A, Pellieux C, Brunner HR, Pedrazzini T. Calcineurin blockade prevents cardiac mitogen-activated protein kinase activation and hypertrophy in renovascular hypertension. J Biol Chem 2000; 275:40867–40873.

66. Mervaala E, Muller DN, Park JK, Dechend R, Schmidt F, Fiebeler A, Bieringer M, Breu V, Ganten D, Haller H, Luft FC. Cyclosporin A protects against angiotensin II-induced end-organ damage in double transgenic rats harboring human renin and angiotensinogen genes. Hypertension 2000; 35:360–366.

67. Øie EB, Reidar OPF, Clausen H. Attramadal. Cyclosporin A inhibits cardiac hypertrophy and enhances cardiac dysfunction during postinfarction failure in rats. Am J Physiol Heart Circ Physiol 2000; 278:2115–2123.

68. Wang Z, Nolan B, Kutschke W, Hill JA. Na+-Ca2+ exchanger remodeling in pressure overload cardiac hypertrophy. J Biol Chem 2001; 276:17706–17711.

69. Wang Z, Kutschke W, Richardson KE, Karimi M, Hill JA. Electrical remodeling in pressure-overload cardiac hypertrophy: role of calcineurin. Circulation 2001; 104:1657–1663.

70. Goldspink PH, McKinney RD, Kimball VA, Geenen DL, Buttrick PM. Angiotensin II induced cardiac hypertrophy in vivo is inhibited by cyclosporin A in adult rats. Mol Cell Biochem 2001; 226:83–88.

71. Deng L, Huang B, Qin D, Ganguly K, El-Sherif N. Calcineurin inhibition ameliorates structural, contractile, and electrophysiologic consequences of postinfarction remodeling. J Cardiovasc Electrophysiol 2001; 12:1055–1061.

72. Yang G, Meguro T, Hong C, Asai K, Takagi G, Karoor VL, Sadoshima J, Vatner DE, Bishop SP, Vatner SF. Cyclosporine reduces left ventricular mass with chronic aortic banding in mice, which could be due to apoptosis and fibrosis. J Mol Cell Cardiol 2001; 33:1505–1514.

73. Youn TJ, Piao H, Kwon JS, Choi SY, Kim HS, Park DG, Kim DW, Kim YG, Cho MC. Effects of the calcineurin dependent signaling pathway inhibition by cyclosporin A on early and late cardiac remodeling following myocardial infarction. Eur J Heart Fail 2002; 4: 713–718.

74. Takeda Y, Yoneda T, Demura M, Usukura M, Mabuchi H. Calcineurin inhibition attenuates mineralocorticoid-induced cardiac hypertrophy. Circulation 2002; 105:677–679.

75. Sun L, Youn HD, Loh C, Stolow M, He W, Liu JO. Cabin 1, a negative regulator for calcineurin signaling in T lymphocytes. Immunity 1998; 8:703–711.

76. Lai MM, Burnett PE, Wolosker H, Blackshaw S, Snyder SH. Cain, a novel physiologic protein inhibitor of calcineurin. J Biol Chem 1998; 273:18325–18331.

77. Coghlan VM, Perrino BA, Howard M, Langeberg LK, Hicks JB, Gallatin WM, Scott JD. Association of protein kinase A and protein phosphatase 2B with a common anchoring protein. Science 1995; 267:108–111.

78. De Windt LJ, Lim HW, Bueno OF, Liang Q, Delling U, Braz JC, Glascock BJ, Kimball TF, del Monte F, Hajjar RJ, Molkentin JD. Targeted inhibition of calcineurin attenuates cardiac hypertrophy in vivo. Proc Natl Acad Sci U S A 2001; 98:3322–3327.

79. Rothermel B, Vega RB, Yang J, Wu H, Bassel-Duby R, Williams RS. A protein encoded within the Down syndrome critical region is enriched in striated muscles and inhibits calcineurin signaling. J Biol Chem 2000; 275:8719–8725.

80. Fuentes JJ, Genesca L, Kingsbury TJ, Cunningham KW, Perez-Riba M, Estivill X, de la Luna S. DSCR1, overexpressed in Down syndrome, is an inhibitor of calcineurin-mediated signaling pathways. Hum Mol Gen 2000; 9:1681–1690.

81. Rothermel BA, McKinsey TA, Vega RB, Nicol RL, Mammen P, Yang J, Antos CL, Shelton JM, Bassel-Duby R, Olson EN, Williams RS. Myocyte-enriched calcineurin-interacting protein, MCIP1, inhibits cardiac hypertrophy in vivo. Proc Natl Acad Sci U S A 2001; 98: 3328–3333.

82. Hill JA, Rothermel B, Yoo KD, Cabuay B, Demetroulis E, Weiss RM, Kutschke W, Bassel-Duby R, Williams RS. Targeted inhibition of calcineurin in pressure-overload cardiac hypertrophy. Preservation of systolic function. J Biol Chem 2002; 277:10251–10255.

83. Zou Y, Hiroi Y, Uozumi H, Takimoto E, Toko H, Zhu W, Kudoh S, Mizukami M, Shimoyama M, Shibasaki F, Nagai R, Yazaki Y, Komuro I. Calcineurin plays a critical role in the development of pressure overload-induced cardiac hypertrophy. Circulation 2001; 104: 97–101.

84. Bueno OF, Wilkins BJ, De Windt LJ, Molkentin JD. Impairment of cardiac hypertrophy in CnAβ-deficient mice. Proc Natl Acad Sci U S A 2002; 99:9398–9403.

85. Hoey T, Sun YL, Williamson K, Xu X. Isolation of two new members of the NF–AT gene family and functional characterization of the NF-AT proteins. Immunity 1995; 2:461–472.

86. Wilkins BJ, De Windt LJ, Bueno OF, Braz JC, Glascock BJ, Kimball TF, Molkentin JD. Targeted disruption of NFATc3, but not NFATc4, reveals an intrinsic defect in calcineurin-mediated cardiac hypertrophic growth. Mol Cell Biol 2002; 22:7603–7613.

87. Haverich A, Costard-Jackle A, Cremer J, Herrmann G, Simon R. Cyclosporin A and transplant coronary disease after heart transplantation: facts and fiction. Transplant Proc 1994; 26: 2713–2715.

88. Ventura HO, Malik FS, Mehra MR, Stapelton DD, Smart FW. Mechanisms of hypertension in cardiac transplantation and the role of cyclosporine. Curr Opin Cardiol 1997; 12:375–381.

89. Batiuk TD, Urmson J, Vincent D, Yatscoff RW, Halloran PF. Quantitating immunosuppression. Transplantation 1996; 61:1618–1624.

90. Leenen FH, Holliwell DL, Cardella CJ. Blood pressure and left ventricular anatomy and function after heart transplantation. Am Heart J 1991; 122:1087–1094.

91. Schmelzle T, Hall MN. TOR, a central controller of cell growth. Cell 2000; 103:253–262.

92. Montagne J, Stewart MJ, Stocker H, Hafen E, Kozma SC, Thomas G. Drosophila SK kinase: a regulator of cell size. Science 1999; 285:2126–2129.

93. Shima H, Pende M, Chen Y, Fumagalli S, Thomas G, Kozma SC. Disruption of the p70(s6k)/ p85(s6k) gene reveals a small mouse phenotype and a new functional S6 kinase. EMBO J 1998; 17:6649–6659.

94. Stocker H, Hafen E. Genetic control of cell size. Curr Opin Genet Dev 2000; 10:529–535.

95. Weinkove D, Leevers SJ. The genetic control of organ growth: insights from Drosophila. Curr Opin Genet Dev 2000; 10:75–80.

96. Crackower MA, Oudit GY, Kozieradzki I, Sarao R, Sun H, Sasaki T, Hirsch E, Suzuki A, Shioi T, Irie-Sasaki J, Sah R, Cheng HY, Rybin VO, Lembo G, Fratta L, Oliveirados-Santos AJ, Benovic JL, Kahn CR, Izumo S, Steinberg SF, Wymann MP, Backx PH, Penninger JM. Regulation of myocardial contractility and cell size by distinct PI3K-PTEN signaling pathways. Cell 2002; 110:737–749.

97. Shioi T, Kang PM, Douglas PS, Hampe J, Yballe CM, Lawitts J, Cantley LC, Izumo S. The conserved phosphoinositide 3-kinase pathway determines heart size in mice. EMBO J 2000; 19:2537–2548.

98. Shioi T, McMullen JR, Tarnavski O, Converso K, Sherwood MC, Manning WJ, Izumo S. Rapamycin attenuates load-induced hypertrophy in mice. Circulation 2003; 107:1664–1670.

99. Browne GJ, Proud CG. Regulation of peptide-chain elongation in mammalian cells. Eur J Biochem 2002; 269:5360–5368.

100. Proud CG. Regulation of mammalian translation factors by nutrients. Eur J Biochem 2002; 269:5338–5349.

101. Dennis PB, Jaeschke A, Saitoh M, Fowler B, Kozma SC, Thomas G. Mammalian TOR: a homeostatic ATP sensor. Science 2001; 294:1102–1105.

102. Rohde J, Heitman J, Cardenas ME. The TOR kinases link nutrient sensing to cell growth. J Biol Chem 2001; 276:9583–9586.

103. Antos CL, McKinsey TA, Frey N, Kutschke W, McAnally J, Shelton JM, Richardson JA, Hill JA, Olson EN. Activated glycogen synthase kinase-3 suppresses cardiac hypertrophy in vivo. Proc Nat Acad Sci 2002; 99:907–912.

104. Chen WS, Xu PZ, Gottlob K, Chen ML, Sokol K, Shiyanova T, Roninson I, Weng W, Suzuki R, Tobe K, Kadowaki T, Hay N. Growth retardation and increased apoptosis in mice with homozygous deletion of the Akt1 gene. Genes Dev 2001; 15:2203–2208.

105. Haq S, Choukroun G, Kang ZB, Lee K-H, Ranu H, Matsui T, Rosenzweig A, Alessandrini A, Molkentin JD, Woodgett J, Hajjar R, Michael A, Force T. Glycogen synthase kinase-3 is a negative regulator of cardiomyocyte hypertrophy. J Cell Biol 2000; 151:117–129.

106. Haq S, Michael A, Andreucci M, Bhattacharya K, Dotto P, Walters B, Woodgett JR, Kilter H, Force T. Stabilization of -catenin by a Wnt-independent mechanism regulates cardiomyocyte growth. Proc Nat Acad Sci 2003; 100:4610–4515.

107. Lawlor MA, Mora A, Ashby PR, WIlliams MR, Murray-Tait V, Malone L, Prescott AR, Lucocq JM, Alessi DR. Essential role of PDK1 in regulating cell size and development in mice. EMBO J 2002; 21:3728–3738.

108. Matsui T, Li L, Wu JC, Cook SA, Nagoshi T, Picard MH, Liao R, Rosenzweig A. Phenotypic spectrum caused by transgenic overexpression of activated Akt in the heart. J Biol Chem 2002; 277:22896–22901.

109. Scanga SE, Ruel L, Binari RC, Snow B, Stambolic V, Bouchard D, Peter M, Calvieri B, Mak TW, Woodgett JR, Manoukian AS. The conserved PI3′K/PTEN/Akt signaling pathway regulates both cells size and survival in Drosophila. Oncogene 2000; 19:3971–3977.

110. Schwartzbauer G, Robbins J. The tumor suppressor gene PTEN can regulate cardiac hypertrophy and survival. J Biol Chem 2001; 276:35786–35793.

111. Shioi T, McMullen JR, Kang PM, Douglas PS, Obata T, Franke T, Cantley LC, Izumo S. Akt/Protein kinase B promotes organ growth in transgenic mice. Mol Cell Biol 2002; 22: 2799–2809.

112. Shiojima I, Yefremashvili M, Luo Z, Kureishi Y, Takahashi A, Tao J, Rosenzweig A, Kahn CR, Abel ED, Walsh K. Akt signaling mediates postnatal heart growth in response to insulin and nutritional status. J Biol Chem 2002; 277:37670–37677.

113. Yang J, Cron P, Thompson V, Good VM, Hess D, Hemmings BA, Barford D. Molecular mechanism for the regulation of protein kinase B/Akt by hydrophobic motif phosphorylation. Molec Cell 2002; 9:1227–1240.

114. McManus EJ, Alessi DR. TSC2: a complex tale of PKB-mediated S6K regulation. Nature Cell Biol 2002; 4:E214–E216.

115. Cook SA, Matsui T, Li L, Rosenzweig A. Transcriptional effects of chronic Akt activation in the heart. J Biol Chem 2002; 277:22528–22533.

116. Morisco C, Seta K, Hardt SE, Lee Y, Vatner SF, Sadoshima J. Glycogen synthase kinase 3 regulates GATA4 in cardiac myocytes. J Biol Chem 2001; 276:28586–28597.

117. Morisco C, Zebrowski D, Condorelli G, Tsichlis P, Vatner SF, Sadoshima J. The Akt-glycogen synthase kinase-3 pathway regulates transcription of atrial natriuretic factor induced by β-adrenergic receptor stimulation in cardiac myocytes. J Biol Chem 2000; 275:14466–14475.

118. Michael A, Haq S, Kilter H, Chen X, Walters B, Battacharya K, Cui L, Liao R, Patten RD, Molkentin JD, Force T. Cardiac-specific expression of glycogen synthase kinase-3 impairs cardiac growth and calcium handling, leading to systolic and diastolic dysfunction and heart failure. 2003, Submitted.

119. Pap M, Cooper GM. Role of translation initiation factor 2B in control of cell survival by the phosphatidylinositol 3-kinse/Akt/glycogen synthase kinase-3beta signaling pathway. Mol Cell Biol 2002; 22:578–586.

120. Frame S, Cohen P. GSK3 takes centre stage more than 20 years after its discovery. Biochem J 2001; 359:1–16.

121. Beals CR, Sheridan CM, Turck CW, Gardner P, Crabtree GR. Nuclear export of NF-ATc enhanced by glycogen synthase kinase-3. Science 1997; 275:1930–1934.

122. Graef IA, Mermelstein PG, Stankunas K, Neilson JR, Deisseroth K, Tsien RW, Crabtree GR. L-type calcium channels and GSK-3 regulate the activity of NF-ATc4 in hippocampal neurons. Nature 1999; 401:703–708.

123. Cohen P, Frame S. The renaissance of GSK-3. Nat Rev Mol Cell Biol 2001; 10:769–776.

124. Woodgett JR. Judging a protein by more than its name: GSK-3. Sci STKE 2001; 100:RE12.

125. Cantley LC, Neel BG. New insights into tumor suppression: PTEN suppresses tumor formation by restraining the phosphoinositide 3-kinase/Akt pathway. Proc Natl Acad Sci 1999; 96: 4240–4245.

126. Choukroun G, Hajjar R, Fry S, del Monte F, Haq S, Guerrero JL, Picard M, Rosenzweig A, Force T. Regulation of cardiac hypertrophy in vivo by the stress-activated protein kinases/ c-Jun NH_2-terminal kinases. J Clin Invest 1999; 104:391–398.

127. Liao P, Georgakopoulos D, Kovacs A, Zheng M, Lerner D, Pu H, Saffitz J, Chien KR, Xiao R-P, Kass DA, Wang Y. The in vivo role of p38 MAP kinses in cardiac remodeling and restrictive cardiomyopathy. Proc Nat Acad Sci 2001; 98:12283–12288.

128. Minamino T, Yujiri T, Terada N, Taffet GE, Michael LH, Johnson GL, Schneider MD. MEKK1 is essential for cardiac hypertrophy and dysfunction induced by Gq. Proc Nat Acad Sci 2002; 99:3866–3871.

129. Petrich BG, Molkentin JD, Wang Y. Temporal activation of c-Jun N-terminal kinase in adult transgenic heart via cre-loxP-mediated DNA recombination. FASEB J 2003; 17:749–751.

130. Sadoshima J, Montagne O, Wang Q, Yang G, Warden J, Liu J, Takagi G, Karoor V, Hong C, Johnson GL, Vatner DE, Vatner SF. The MEKK1-JNK pathway plays a protective role in pressure overload but does not mediate cardiac hypertrophy. J Clin Invest 2002; 110: 271–279.

131. Bueno OF, De Windt LJ, Tymitz KM, Witt SA, Kimball TR, LKlevitsky R, Hewett TE, Jones SP, Lefer DJ, Peng CF, Kitsis RN, Molkentin JD. The MEK1-ERK1/2 signaling pathway promotes compensated cardiac hypertrophy in transgenic mice. EMBO J 2000; 19: 6341–6350.

132. Communal C, Colucci WS, Remondino A, Sawyer DB, Port JD, Wichman SE, Bristow MR, Singh K. Reciprocal modulation of mitogen-activated protein kinases and mitogen-activated protein kinase phosphatase 1 and 2 in failing human myocardium. J Card Fail 2002; 8:86–91.

133. Cook SA, Sugden PH, Clerk A. Activation of c-Jun N-terminal kinases and p38-mitogen-activated protein kinases in human heart failure secondary to ischaemic heart disease. J Mol Cell Cardiol 1999; 31:1429–1431.

134. Flesch M, Margulies KB, Mochmann HC, Engel D, Sivasubramanian N, Mann DL. Differential regulation of mitogen-activated protein kinases in the failing human heart in response to mechanical unloading. Circulation 2001; 104:2273–2276.

135. Lemke LE, Bloem LJ, Fouts R, Esterman M, Sandusky G, Vlahos CJ. Decreased p38 MAPK activity in end-stage failing human myocardium: p38 MAPK alpha is the predominant isoform expressed in human heart. J Mol Cell Cardiol 2001; 33:1527–1534.

136. Ng DC, Court NW, dos Remedios CG, Bogoyevitch MA. Activation of signal transducer and activator of transcription (STAT) pathways in failing human hearts. Cardiovasc Res 2003; 57:333–338.

137. Takeishi Y, Huang Q, Abe J, Che W, Lee JD, Kawakatsu H, Hoit BD, Berk BC, Walsh RA. Activation of mitogen-activated protein kinases and p90 ribosomal S6 kinase in failing human hearts with dilated cardiomyopathy. Cardiovasc Res 2002; 53:131–136.

3

Mechanisms of Cell Death in Heart Failure

Jagat Narula and Anthony Rosenzweig
Division of Cardiology, Hahnemann University Hospital, Philadelphia, Pennsylvania
The Program in Cardiovascular Gene Therapy,
Massachusetts General Hospital
Boston, Massachusetts, USA

A progressive, often self-perpetuating process of myocardial remodeling is an important determinant of HF (heart failure) and myocardial cell loss by any mechanism is an important component in the genesis of remodeling. Although necrosis has been regarded as the predominant mode of myocardial cell death, there is increasing evidence that cells die through a variety of programmed and nonprogrammed mechanisms of cell death. In addition to necrosis, cardiac cells may be lost through apoptosis, and also autophagy associated with ubiquitinated protein accumulation (Fig. 1) [1–3]. Apart from mechanistic insights, understanding of mechanisms of cell survival and death may offer novel therapeutic approaches.

MORPHOLOGIC FEATURES OF CELL DEATH

The distinct types of cell death in heart failure have been traditionally defined based on cell morphology [4]. The morphological distinctions are reinforced when reproducible mechanisms are found to underlie the different types of cell death. There is severe disruption of cell membrane in necrosis that is associated with loss of cell contents. On the other hand, apoptosis involves a genetically programmed cell death that takes place within a preserved cell boundary and is characterized by negligible inflammatory response [2,5]. It has recently been demonstrated that ubiquitinated protein aggregates may also mediate cell death in heart failure at a rate comparable to necrotic and apoptotic mechanisms of death. The proportion of cells dying through each mechanism may differ at various stages in the natural history of HF and therapeutic interventions may radically alter the proportions of cells dying of apoptosis, autophagy, and necrosis [6]. ACE inhibitors and beta-blockers inhibit apoptotic, and to a lesser extent necrotic, cell death, and may make autophagy more prominent. This becomes an important issue because one of the goals is to interdict the natural history of heart failure.

45

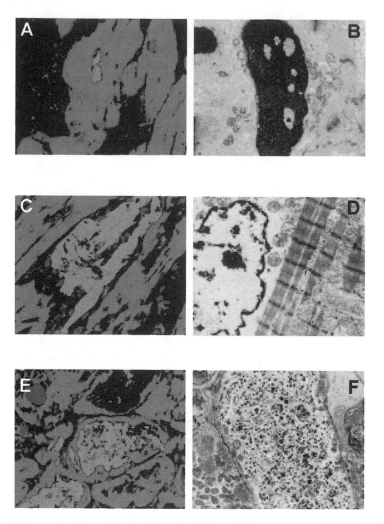

Figure 1 *Morphologic characteristics of different types of cell death.* A, C, E are confocal and B, D, F are electron micrographs. *A and B, Apoptotic cell death.* (**A**) Nuclei with DNA fragmentation. (**B**) Nuclei show condensed chromatin. *C and D, Oncotic cell death.* (**C**) Single cell oncosis labeled with complement 9. (**D**) Nuclei are electron-lucent with clumped chromatin, mitochondria are damaged with flocculent densities. *E and F, Autophagic cell death.* (**E**) Ubiquitin deposition and loss of nuclei (**F**) Ultrastructural appearance with numerous autophagic vacuoles. (From Ref. 1; modified.)

CELL DEATH BY NECROSIS IN HEART FAILURE

The causes of necrotic cell death in heart failure are multiple. Ongoing ischemia is the commonest cause and infringes on aerobic oxidative respiration [7,8]. Infective agents, postinfective immune processes, hypersensitivity phenomenon, and autoimmune diseases result in predominantly inflammatory injury. In addition, chemical insults, including alcohol and doxorubicin toxicity, are infrequent causes of myocardial damage. Regardless of the inciting agent, several common biochemical pathways mediate cell necrosis (Fig. 2), the most important of which is ATP (adenosine triphosphate) depletion that occurs com-

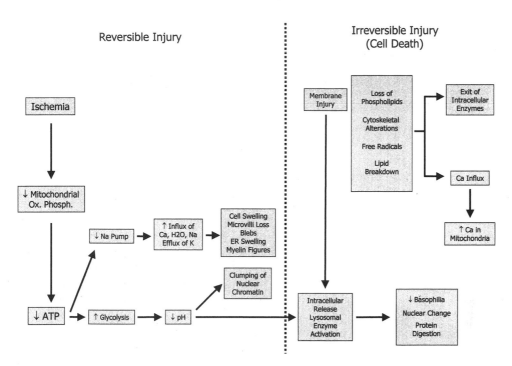

Figure 2 *Mechanisms of necrotic cell death.* Necrosis is mediated by downregulation of aerobic oxidative respiration, ATP depletion, production of partially reduced reactive oxygen forms, and a distinct increase in intercellular calcium (with loss of calcium homeostasis). This is accompanied by activation of deleterious enzymes, such as phospholipases, proteases, ATPase, and endonucleases, and mitochondrial damage by formation of mitochondrial permeability transition pores. Although reversible in its early stages, the nonselective pores become permanent upon persistence of inciting stimuli. The biochemical alterations, including mitochondrial damage, lead to loss of integrity of cell membrane, which is the hallmark of necrotic cell death. (From Ref. 7; modified.)

monly during hypoxia and ischemia. Partially reduced reactive oxygen species, produced during oxidative phosphorylation, are exaggerated during reperfusion injury and lead to cellular damage. In addition to ATP depletion and oxidative stress, an increase in intracellular calcium activates potentially deleterious enzymes, such as phospholipases, proteases, ATPase, and endonucleases. These biochemical events contribute to mitochondrial and cell membrane damage. Formation of a permeability transition pore in the mitochondrial membrane leads to loss of mitochondrial membrane potential, which is otherwise critical for oxidative phosphorylation. On the other hand, the loss of integrity of the cell membrane, which is the hallmark of necrotic cell death, leads to cell swelling, extrusion of intracellular content, and induction of inflammation [9].

Morphologically, the scattered necrotic cells in heart failure may demonstrate increased eosinophilia with loss of striations and nuclei, with and without interstitial inflammatory cells. Ultrastructurally, necrotic cells are characterized by overt breach in the plasma membrane, dilation of mitochondria with large amorphous densities and intracytoplasmic myelin figures or accumulation of fluffy material representing denatured protein. Nuclear changes occur due to nonspecific breakdown of DNA and may present as karyolysis (loss of chromatin), pyknosis (nuclear/DNA shrinkage), or karyorrhexis (fragmentation of pyknotic nuclei) [7]. Most necrotic cells and their debris are removed by a combined process of digestion and fragmentation, with phagocytosis of particulate debris. If not destroyed and removed, they attract calcium salts and other minerals and develop dystrophic calcification.

The prevalence and importance of myocyte necrosis in heart failure cannot be estimated histologically and has been best demonstrated by noninvasive radionuclide imaging with antimyosin antibody [10–12] (Fig. 3). This antibody binds specifically to myocardial cells that have lost their sarcolemmal integrity, allowing either the presence of myosin on the cell surface or the penetration of antimyosin antibody into the cell. Because myocardial necrosis is an obligatory component of myocarditis, scintigraphic evidence of abnormal antimyosin antibody scans was initially considered to represent myocarditis in the setting of dilated cardiomyopathy [13,14]. However, a large number of patients test positive for the disease by antimyosin scintigraphy but test negative by biopsy. This may reflect myocyte degeneration that is responsible for their clinical presentation as acute onset or worsening of heart failure without accompanying mononuclear cell infiltration [11,12].

In our study of 50 such consecutive patients with LV systolic dysfunction (left ventricular ejection fraction [LVEF] <45%), right ventricular endomyocardial biopsy and noninvasive cardiac imaging with Indium-111 – labeled antimyosin antibodies were performed [11]. Endomyocardial biopsy uncovered myocarditis in 10 patients. A comparison of the histopathological findings was performed for the remaining 40 patients with apparent nonmyocarditic dilated cardiomyopathy (mean LVEF, 27% ± 11%). Of these 40 patients with dilated cardiomyopathy, 25 showed left ventricular antimyosin uptake establishing the presence of myocyte necrosis. However, biopsy evidence of myocyte necrosis was observed in only one patient; instead myofibrillarlysis (Fig. 3) was observed on the endomyocardial biopsy specimen in 22 of these 25 (88%) patients with positive findings on scans. In addition to myofibrillarlysis, four (16%) patients had evidence of interstitial lymphocyte infiltration not sufficient for the diagnosis of myocarditis. Evidence of focal interstitial fibrosis and variable degrees of myocyte hypertrophy were observed in two-thirds of patients. Myofibrillarlysis was closely related to antimyosin antibody uptake and was the only significant independent predictor of antimyosin positivity. Myofibrillarlytic cells in the biopsy specimens were sparsely distributed.

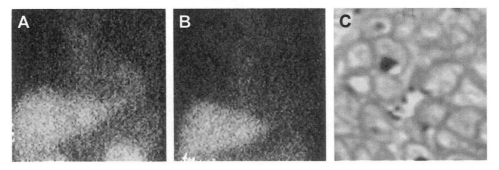

Figure 3 *Antimyosin antibody imaging for the detection of myocyte necrosis.* (**A**) Scintigraphy with Indium-111 antimyosin antibody in a patient with heart failure and left ventricular ejection fraction of 20%. He initially had positive scan (arrows) (**B**). The follow-up scan showed clearly reduced uptake of antibody compared with the initial study. Patients ejection fraction had increased to 65%. The right ventricular endomyocardial biopsy demonstrated an evidence of myofibrillarlysis. The cells reveal cytoplasmic clearance and loss of contractile proteins. (From Refs. 11 and 12; modified.)

Improvement in ventricular function assessed as change in resting LVEF (ΔEF) from the time of antimyosin scan (EF1) to 6 months later (EF2) in these patients divulged interesting results. Stepwise multiple regression analysis revealed that multiplicative interaction of antimyosin scan and myofibrillarlysis was the only significant predictor of improvement in ventricular function as assessed by ΔEF. Initial ejection fraction and the interaction of myofibrillarlysis with myocyte hypertrophy (MH) made a slightly negative contribution to the predictive value. These factors yielded the following regression equation: ΔEF = 19 ($\pm$15) + 20 ($\pm$6) AMS $\times$ Mfl $-$ 0.6 ($\pm$0.2) EF1 $-$ 12 ($\pm$6) Mfl $\times$ MH where AMS, Mfl and MH and binary variables (0 = negative, 1 = positive) and EFI (the initial ejection fraction) is expressed as a percentage. Thus, a positive antimyosin scan and the presence of myofibrillarlysis predicted an eventual additional improvement in ejection fraction of 20% ($\pm$6.5%) above those patients who had negative antimyosin scan results or the absence of myofibrillarlysis in a given clinical situation where all other histological variables were kept constant. For example, a patient with initial ejection fraction of 40% had ΔEF of -5% (an eventual loss in ejection fraction) in case of lack of antimyosin uptake or myofibrillarlysis (or both). However, a patient with positive antimyosin scan results and biopsy evidence of myofibrillarlysis had ΔEF of 15% (an eventual gain in ejection fraction). This example assumes that myocardial hypertrophy was not observed in the endomyocardial biopsy samples. Spontaneous improvement of LVEF greater than 10% was observed in 10 of 22 (45%) patients with positive antimyosin uptake and evidence of myofibrillarlysis on biopsy specimens. Only three of the 18 patients lacking one or both of these markers had a comparable improvement. The mean ejection fraction of the 22 patients with positive results on antimyosin scans and positive myofibrillarlysis rose from 27% $\pm$ 10% to 41% $\pm$ 17% (ΔEF = 12% $\pm$ 20%). The mean ejection fraction of the other 18 patients remained unchanged (EF1, 24% $\pm$ 10% and EF2, 25% $\pm$ 12%).

Scintigraphic evidence of necrosis predicting resolution of ventricular dysfunction appears to be counterintuitive. Although the precise relationship between myofibrillarlysis observed in this study and myocardial uptake of antimyosin antibody is not clear, their concurrence offers some explanation. It suggests that myocyte damage in chronic myocardial diseases may retain a potential of reversibility to an extent, a concept that is better vindicated in energy-hungry forms of cell death (see following text). It can be presumed that the myofibrillarlytic myocyte population is expected to be a mixture of cells at various stages of injury and can comprise a wide spectrum between reversibly and irreversibly damaged myocytes on the basis of integrity of the sarcolemma. Necrotic myocytes in the myofibrillarlytic myocyte population are postulated as the source of antimyosin uptake. Although myocyte necrosis was not identified by light microscopy, the antimyosin positivity provided scintigraphic evidence of early myocyte necrosis. Myocytes permitting sarcolemmal entry to small Fab fragments of antimyosin antibody require very small pores that may only permit exchange of small soluble molecules, ions, and water resulting in gradual osmotic lysis but may escape detection by standard light microscopy. In addition to the likelihood of reversibility, myocyte necrosis detected by antimyosin scintigraphy may also be a marker of a larger population of reconstitutible myofibrillarlytic myocytes with intact sarcolemma.

CELL DEATH BY APOPTOSIS IN THE FAILING MYOCARDIUM

The initial hemodynamic compensation in various cardiovascular substrates that result in heart failure is accomplished by neurohormonal and cytokine activation. The hypertrophic response is also associated with the reappearance of fetal gene expression within the myocytes for entry into cell cycle. However, since cardiac myocytes are terminally differentiated such that DNA synthesis is generally undetectable in these cells, a hyperplastic response may become associated with apoptosis. Hypertrophy of myocardium in various experimental models [15–17], such as with activation of some hypertrophic genes (such as c-myc, c-fos and TGF-β) may also promote apoptosis [18]. Experimental evidence for a continuum between the growth and apoptotic responses in cardiomyocytes can be observed by forced expression of a transcription factor E2F1, which results in DNA synthesis followed by apoptosis [19].

Apoptosis is markedly different from necrosis. It is a genetically programmed and energy-requiring series of events that permits the cell to die without inducing an inflammatory response [4]. The classic changes of apoptosis include cell shrinkage and formation of apoptotic bodies [8]. The activation of DNAses results in cleavage of chromatin into multimers of oligonucleosomal-length DNA fragments, evident on agarose gel electrophoresis. Chromatin marginalizes as the nucleus becomes segmented. Sarcolemmal integrity is preserved but progressive convolution of membrane breaks up the cell into clusters of membrane-bound subcellular organelles referred to as apoptotic bodies. Unlike necrosis, because cell swelling and sarcolemmal disintegration do not occur, cytoplasmic contents are not released and inflammation not provoked. Apoptotic bodies are phagocytosed and removed. Identification of such cells is feasible by histochemical characterization of upstream signaling (such as caspase activation) or DNA fragmentation.

Two distinct, but not mutually exclusive, pathways of apoptotic cell death have been well desribed. Both involve activation of highly specific proteolytic enzymes referred to as caspases [20] (Fig. 4). In the *extrinsic* pathway, soluble or cell surface death ligands, such as TNF-α and Fas ligand, bind to the corresponding death receptors inducing activation of upstream caspases, such as -8, followed by activation of downstream executionary caspases, such as -3, -6, and -7. In the second, *intrinsic* pathway, cytochrome c from mitochondria is released in to the cytoplasm [21], often initiated by stress stimuli, such as ischemia, oxidative stress, genotoxic stress, and calcium excess. Cytoplasmic cytochrome c in presence of dATP/ATP binds Apaf-1 to activate caspase-9 and subsequently downstream effector caspases. Once activated, the executionary caspases fragment intracellular proteins resulting in the orderly destruction of the cell. The effector caspases also activate DNAses and lead to fragmentation of nuclear DNA [22]. The death receptor and mitochondrial pathways are linked by Bid, which can be cleaved by caspase-8 to truncated Bid (tBid) following death receptor activation [23], and translocates to the mitochondria where it stimulates cytochrome c release through interactions with the proapoptotic Bcl-family members, Bax and/or Bak. The anti-apoptotic Bcl-family members, Bcl-2 and Bcl-xL also reside in the outer mitochondrial membrane and inhibit cell death by competing with Bax and Bak for tBid as well as possibly through direct interactions with Bax and Bak [24]. These death pathways are inhibited by several other prosurvival pathways, which include ARC or FLIP (inhibitors of caspase-8), and XIAP or related proteins (inhibitors of caspases-3 and -9) [25]. When apoptosis is induced, in addition to cytochrome c, SMAC is also released from the mitochondria that binds to XIAP precluding its inhibition of caspases.

Apoptosis in human heart failure was initially demonstrated by Narula and colleagues. [2] based on the histochemical demonstration of DNA fragmentation; apoptosis occurred both in ischemic and dilated cardiomyopathy (Fig. 5). They proposed that slow ongoing apoptotic loss of myocytes may contribute to inexorable progression of CHF (chronic heart failure). Their ultrastructural studies in explanted hearts demonstrated cytochrome c release from mitochondria to cytoplasm in failing hearts [26]. In contrast, cyto-

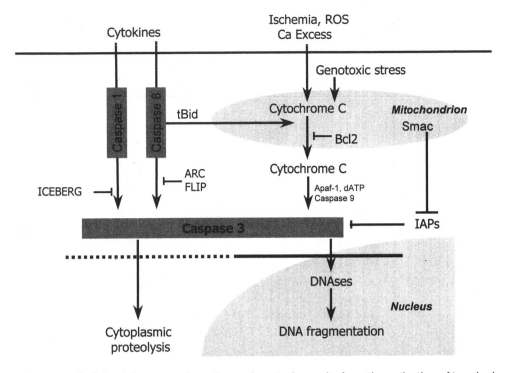

Figure 4 *Cell death by apoptotic pathway.* Apoptosis results from the activation of terminal caspases (such as caspase-3), which fragment various cytoplasmic proteins and nuclear DNA. The activation of caspase-3 occurs either by mitochondrial stress (such as ischemia, calcium excess, or oxidative stress in cardiomyopathic disorders) that leads to release of cytochrome c and processing of caspase-9, or cytokine-based inducers of death receptors and upstream caspases (such as caspase-1 and -8). The two pathways, however, may not be mutually exclusive, and caspase 8 leads to amplification of caspase 3 activation via mitochondrial release of cytochrome c. In cardiomyopathic hearts, caspase-8 is activated due to Flip downregulation, leads to Bid truncation, cytochrome c release from mitochondria, and caspase-3 activation. Upregulation of IAPs with decreased Smac-L restricts active caspase-3. Residual active caspase-3 leads to contractile protein cleavage but fails to induce DNA fragmentation due to complete abolition of DNA fragmentation factors (DFF). Although interrupted apoptotic cascade allows myocyte to survive, loss of cytochrome c and contractile proteins lead to systolic dysfunction. (From Ref. 3; modified.)

chrome c is exclusively localized to the mitochondria in normal hearts. (Fig. 5) Downstream to cytochrome c release, caspase 3 was found to be activated in the cardiomyopathic hearts. Unprocessed caspase-3 was also upregulated, whereas only minimal inactive caspase 3 was observed in normal myocardium. A systematic destruction of cytoplasmic proteins is expected after the activation of caspase-3. A conceptual proof of this has been offered by Communal and co-workers [27], who demonstrated caspase-3 mediated fragmentation of myofibrillar proteins and consequent loss of contractile function of cultured cardiomyocytes (Fig. 6). A 4-hour exposure to active caspase-3 resulted in the cleavage of α-actin and α-actinin. Treatment with the caspase-3-specific and polycaspase inhibitors abolished the cleavage. Myofilaments isolated from adult rat ventricular myocytes after induction of apoptotic pathway by beta-adrenergic stimulation, displayed a similar pattern of contractile protein cleavage. Further, exposure of skinned fiber to caspase-3

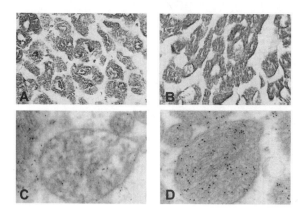

Figure 5 *Apoptosis of myocytes in heart failure.* Simultaneous staining for apoptosis (TUNEL, black) and myocytes (actin) was performed. (**A**) Few myocytes are apoptotic with stained nuclei in a myocardial sample from dilated cardiomyopathy patient. Other myocytes have clear nuclear areas as in control myocardial sample (**B**). (**C, D**) Ultrastructural magnification of normal myocardial specimen from a donor heart (*D*) and cardiomyopathic heart (*C*) demonstrate striking difference in cytochrome-c immunoreactivity. Localization of cytochrome-c is represented by (black) gold particles. The cytochrome-c is predominantly localized in mitochondria in normal hearts (*D*). On the other hand, cytochrome-c is substantially reduced in mitochondria (*C*) in cardiomyopathic heart and is spilled in the cytoplasmic compartment. The cytochrome c was predominantly seen distributed either over Z-bands or near intercalated disc (*data not shown*). Of note, the sarcolemma was intact and nucleus not affected in most of the cells showing cytochrome c release. (From Refs. 2 and 26; modified.)

decreased maximal Ca^{+2} activated force and myofibrillar ATPase activity. In cardiomyopathic hearts, although the majority of myocytes demonstrate ultrastructural evidence of cytochrome c release and there is variable loss of cytoplasmic proteins, the nuclei in all these cells remain essentially normal. Intactness of nuclei ensures the viability of cardiomyocytes.

We have observed that although there is continuous evidence of mitochondrial cytochrome c release, myocytes inhibit activation of caspase-3, and lose DNAses to preserve nuclear integrity [28] (Fig. 4). Such a phenomenon represents an interrupted apoptotic cascade in CHF and possible altered myocardial state of cell survival [29]. In our recent study of activation of death receptor pathways, release of mitochondrial activators of caspase 3, inhibitors of caspase 8 and active caspase 3, and DNA fragmentation factors (DFF-35,40,45) in end-stage ischemic and dilated cardiomyopathic hearts, we observed that activated caspase-8 remained uninhibited due to Flip-L downregulation, and led to Bid truncation, cytochrome c release from mitochondria, and caspase-3 activation. Upregulation of XIAP with decreased Smac-L, restricted active caspase-3. Residual active caspase-3 led to contractile protein cleavage but fails to induce DNA fragmentation due to complete abolition of DNAses.

The ability of caspase-8 to induce cardiomyopathy and heart failure has been demonstrated in transgenic animals, using myocardium-specific expression of a ligand-activatable caspase-8 construct [30]. The catalytic domain of caspase-8 was coupled with the FK506 binding site to engineer the transgenic mouse wherein FK1012 administration allowed dimerization and activation of caspase-8, with subsequent activation of caspase 3 and aggressive myocardial apoptosis, and evolution of dilated cardiomyopathy.

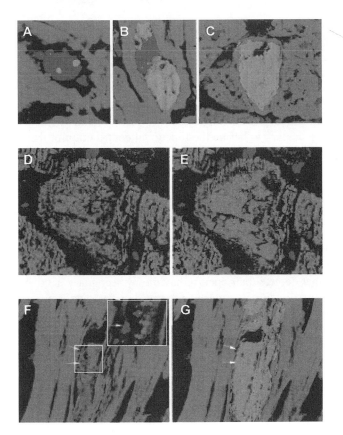

Figure 6 *Ubiquitin-accumulations in myocytes in heart failure.* (**A**), Only two small dots of ubiquitin in a myocyte nucleus. (nucleus). (**B**) Massive cytoplasmic ubiquitin labeling in myocyte. (**C**) Massive deposition of ubiquitin in a myocyte without a nucleus. (**D, E**) Double labeling for ubiquitin and myosin showing colocalization of these proteins and that ubiquitinated myosin lacks a typical cross-striated pattern. (**F, G**) Double labeling for ubiquitin (green) with autophagic vacuoles. Shown with arrows in *F* are the autophagic vacuoles. Inset, Enlarged view of the box area and shows monodansylcadaverine (arrows). (**G**) Double labeling for ubiquitin and monodansylcadaverine showing colocalization of these two signals. (From Ref. 1; modified.)

Cardiomyopathy could be prevented by simultaneous administration of a broad-spectrum caspase inhibitor. These studies demonstrate that caspase activation and apoptotic loss of myocytes are sufficient to induce cardiomyopathy. Whether activation of caspases in general or caspase-8 in particular is *necessary* for the development of more routine forms of heart failure, remains unclear. However, recent studies from our group have provided evidence of the functional significance of death receptor signaling and caspase-8 activation in hypoxia-induced cardiomyocyte apoptosis [31]. Using adenoviral expression of wild-type and dominant negative forms of the adaptor molecule, FADD, that links death receptors to caspase-8 activation, we found, not surprisingly, that expression of FADD in cardiomyocytes was sufficient to induce cardiomyocyte apoptosis. However, expression of dominant negative FADD (DN-FADD) was remarkably effective at inhibiting cardiomyocyte apoptosis in response to serum and oxygen deprivation. A detailed analysis revealed that in this context FADD inhibition blocked activation of caspase-8, -9, and -3, thereby abrogating the apoptotic response [31]. These studies suggest that in hypoxic cardiomyocytes both the intrinsic and extrinsic pathways play a role, but that the intrinsic, mitochondrial pathway is activated downstream of death receptor signaling. More recent in vivo studies by Lee and colleagues demonstrated that mice harboring a mutation in Fas have smaller infarcts after ischemia reperfusion injury [32]. Thus, inhibition of death receptor signaling may prove a productive avenue for future efforts to reduce myocardial injury. Future studies will be necessary to define the functional contribution of these apoptotic signaling pathways in models of heart failure.

From the previous discussion, it is clear that the apoptotic process is initiated in failing cardiomyocytes but damage to the nucleus does not occur and appears to be different from that seen in the classic apoptosis. It is likely that terminally differentiated cells resist nuclear fragmentation despite continued activation of upstream cascade of apoptosis [33]; low levels of cytoplasmic damage may continue to occur. It is likely that a very small number of cells undergo complete apoptosis in a smoldering and slowly progressive disease state. However, because apoptosis in an energy-requiring process, it is also conceivable that a tiny fraction of these cells that deplete their energy may die by secondary necrosis [34,35]. Therefore, a myocyte that maintains its nuclear integrity but has compromised its respiratory chain and oxidative phosphorylation, and allows variable destruction of its contractile proteins, should contribute to systolic dysfunction of the cell [29]. Also, such cells with intact nuclei may be amenable to recovery.

ROLE OF UBIQUITIN-PROTEOSOME PATHWAY IN MYOCYTE DEATH IN HEART FAILURE

Involvement of the ubiquitin pathway has recently been suggested in cardiac myocytes from failing hearts [1]. The evolutionarily highly conserved ubiquitin system labels substrate proteins with a ubiquitin molecule on lysine residues enroute to degradation by the 26S proteosome [36]. Interestingly, although four or more ubiquitin molecules condemn a protein to destruction [37], shorter chains may regulate survival functions, including gene transcription and DNA repair. Ubiquitination is a reversible process; a number of deubiquitinating enzymes remove ubiquitin molecules from discarded proteins and can enhance protein survival. Similar to apoptosis, ubiquitination intersects with death decisions in a large way in the failing myocardium.

Ubiquitinated protein aggregates have been observed in cardiomyocytes. Many aggregates are observed in cells showing marked structural changes, including autophagic vacuoles [1] (Fig. 6). This is accompanied by increased tissue ubiquitin mRNA, polyubiquitinated proteins, increase in of E2 UBC, but no change in E3 ubiquitin ligase, and reduction in some deubiquitinating enzymes. The authors postulate that defects in this pathway may lead to increased ubiquitylation, protein aggregates, and cell death by autophagy. The hypothesis is similar to observations in neurons susceptible to death after cerebral ischemia, wherein ubiquitylated protein aggregates were commonly found and correlated with dying cells; such deposits were rarely seen in cells destined to live [38]. Thus, a high density of ubiquitylated protein aggregates in myocytes may be a marker of cells destined to die. In an accompanying editorial to this report, we had proposed that the cells, at least those with mild ubiquitylation, were invoking protective responses to avoid cell death and may die when such responses are overwhelmed. Evidence is accumulating that cells exposed to death signals actively try to protect themselves through a number of mechanisms. There is a fascinating link between endoplasmic reticulum (ER) stress, ubiquitylation, and cell survival or death. Various ER stress stimuli, such as ischemia, altered redox status or calcium homeostasis (which are all prevalent in the failing myocardium), invoke a series of protective responses called the unfolded protein response (UPR) or the endoplasmic overload response (EOR). Such mechanisms help the cells survive by reducing the entry of new proteins into the ER, and increasing protein translocation out of it. Retrotranslocated proteins need to be rapidly marked for degradation, or else they accumulate in the cell as toxic protein aggregates. The increased degradation of ER-translocated proteins in the proteosome through the ubiquitin pathway reduces ER stress [39], which has been demonstrated in ischemic cardiomyopathy [40]. Prolonged ER stress can lead to protein aggregates, and apoptotic or necrotic cell death [39]. Protein aggregates can turn off synthesis of many important proteins, including those in the UPP, to mediate necrotic cell death [18] or increase apoptotic signaling to mediate apoptotic death [39,41]. In the study by Kostis and Colleagues [1], myocytes accumulated ubiquitinated proteins in the presence of normal proteosome activity that could imply large amount of misfolded protein translocation to ER-associated degradation (ERAD) from stressed ER. Therefore, cell death could reflect a prolonged UPR and overwhelmed ERAD pathway (Fig. 7) rather than a primary defect in the ubiquitin/deubiquitination system.

CROSS-TALK IN DEATH PATHWAYS

It is becoming clearer that various forms of death may be a part of the same spectrum [2,8], and multiple morphologies of cell death may coexist in the same microscopic field, sometimes even in adjacent cells [1]. The predominant form of death may depend upon highly modifiable intracellular and extracellular conditions. For instance, a low intensity stress, such as a short period of ischemia or interruption of ischemia by reperfusion, may lead to apoptotic death, while a longer period of ischemia may bring on necrotic death [42]. Similarly, the degree of ATP depletion [43], amount of PARP cleavage [44], or rate of MPT formation [45] could drive a cell toward apoptosis or necrosis [46] depending on when substrate changes occur. Further, cells sometimes die with a hybrid morphology that is intermediate between apoptosis and necrosis [47]. It has been demonstrated that inhibiting one pathway of death may simply switch it to die by another pathway. For example, caspase-9, mediates a nonapoptotic cell death when apoptosis is inhibited by zVAD.fmk [48]. Also during some developmental process of interdigital resorption (which is mediated by apoptotic) digits still mature after inhibiting apoptosis by inducing necrosis [49]. Furthermore, ubiquitination can modulate apoptosis by ubiquitination or deubiquitination of apoptotic proteins (like caspases) or its regulators (Bcl2, p53, NF-kb); ubiquitin-mediated modulation of p53 and proapoptotic and antiapoptotic p53 family members can regulate apoptosis depending on the circumstances [50]. Also, the endogenous antiapoptotic proteins (IAPs), which have ubiquitylation activity, inhibit apoptosis by ubiquitylating caspases [51].

However, the cross-talk between modes of cell death and their intimate connection to myocyte function suggests that it may be possible to identify points of intervention based on common signaling pathways modulating all of these phenomena that would mediate meaningful rescue. Some studies suggest that this may, in fact, be the case in cardiomyocytes. For example, we found that activation of the kinases, PI 3-kinase and its downstream effector, Akt, are sufficient to block apoptosis in cardiomyocytes in vitro [52] without apparent induction of alternative modes of cell death. Moreover, adenoviral gene transfer of activated Akt to the heart in vivo mediated a dramatic reduction in cardiomyocyte apoptosis as well as infarct size after IRI [53]. More importantly, Akt activation

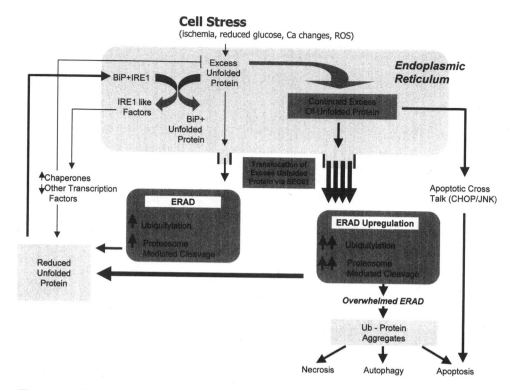

Figure 7 *Cell death by ubiquitin pathway*. Multiple stimuli can stress the ER and result in an accumulation of unfolded proteins in the ER. The normal response (*left half of the figure*) to clear this involves (a) BiP mediated release of IRE1 like factors, which then increase chaperone protein production (which will improve protein folding) and suppression of non-chaperone related protein transcription (which reduced protein load coming into the ER), and (b) increased translocation of unfolded protein via the ER channel SEC61. Continued unfolded protein excess in the ER increases protein retrotranslocation that is matched by an upregulated ERAD—this normalizes the amount of unfolded protein and allows the cell to recover from ER stress. When ERAD is overwhelmed (*right panel in the figure*) by either continued excess of unfolded protein coming from the ER or if proteosome function "reserve" is exhausted, unfolded proteins accumulate in the cell and can form insoluble ubiquitylated protein aggregates (Ub-protein aggregates), which are cytotoxic. (From Ref. 3; modified.)

substantially improved regional and overall cardiac function, likely related to its ability to simultaneously block block apoptosis, reduce necrosis, and preserved function (contraction, Ca^{++}-handling) in the surviving cells [53].

Based on the discussion above, the following assumptions can be made [3]. First, multiple death signals are active at any given time within the failing myocardium. Second, cells likely to die invoke multiple protective mechanisms [29]. Finally, doomed cells, once compensatory mechanisms are overwhelmed, may succumb to death pathways, cross over to other morphologic variety or die of a hybrid form of death [54,55]. One could speculate that cross talk in death pathways might be dependent on a number of associated factors such as the energy state of cell and intensity of damage. Preserved energy states and lower intensity stimuli can drive a cell towards "energy hungry" death pathways like apoptosis and possibly UPPathways. On the other hand, exhaustion of energy during these (energy-requiring processes) and exaggeration of severity of inducing stimuli may upset calcium homeostasis and mediate necrosis. Repletion of the cytosolic ATP pool before irreversible damage may redirect the death program towards energy-dependent death pathways [3,56].

CONCLUSIONS

Death by any or many mechanisms is a loss of contractile heart muscle mass that is predominantly irreplaceable. The adaptation of myocytes particularly in heart failure associated with upregulation of protective factors (or downregulation of death factors) renders the cells into a dysfunctional yet metastable state. Such adaptive processes significantly retard the rate of loss of muscle mass and allow reversibility of contractile function to an extent.

REFERENCES

1.   Kostin S, Pool L, Elsasser A, Hein S, Drexler HC, Arnon E, Hayakawa Y, Zimmermann R, Bauer E, Klovekorn WP, Schaper J. Myocytes die by multiple mechanisms in failing human hearts. Circ Res 2003; 92:715–724.

2.   Narula J, Haider N, Virmani R, DiSalvo T, Hajjar RJ, Kolodgie F, Schmidt U, Semigran MJ, Dec GW, Khaw BA. Apoptosis in cardiomyocytes in end-stage heart failure. N Engl J Med 1996; 335:1182–1189.

3.   Chandrashekhar Y, Narula J. Death hath a thousand doors to let out life ⋯. Circ Res 2003; 92:710–714.

4.   Majno G, Joris I. Apoptosis, oncosis, and necrosis. An overview of cell death. Am J Pathol 1995; 146:3–15.

5.   Schaper J, Elsässer A, Kostin S. The role of cell death in heart failure. Circulation 1999; 85: 867–869.

6.   Yue TL, Ma XL, Wang X, Romanic AM, Liu GL, Louden C, Gu JL, Kumar S, Poste G, Ruffolo RR, Feuerstein GZ. Possible involvement of stress-activated protein kinase signaling pathway and Fas receptor expression in prevention of ischemia/reperfusion-induced cardiomyocyte apoptosis by carvedilol. Circ Res 1998; 82:166–174.

7.   Cellular pathology I: cell injury and cell death: In Cotran RS , Kumar V , Collins T, Eds. Robins Pathologic Basis of Disease. 6th ed.. Philadelphia: WB Saunders, year:8.

8.   Narula J, Hofstra L. Imaging myocardial necrosis and apoptosis. In Braunwald E, Dilsizian V, Narula J, Eds. Atlas of Nuclear Cardiology, Philadelphia: Current Medicine, 2003:197–216.

9.   Narula J, Zaret BL. Noninvasive detection of cell death: from tracking epitaphs to counting coffins. J Nucl Cardiol 2002; 9:554–60.

10. Narula J, Khaw BA, Dec GW, Palacios IF, Southern JF, Fallon JT, Strauss HW, Haber E, Yasuda T. Recognition of myocarditis masquerading as acute myocardial infarction. N Engl J Med 1993; 328:100–104.

11. Narula J, Southern JF, Dec GW, Palacios IF, Fallon JT, Strauss HW, Khaw BA, Yasuda T. Antimyosin uptake and myofibrillarlysis in dilated cardiomyopathy. J Nucl Cardiol 1995; 2: 470–477.

12. Narula J, Khaw BA, Dec GW, Newell JB, Palacios IF, Southern JF, Fallon JT, Strauss HW, Haber E, Yasuda T. Evaluation of diagnostic accuracy of antimyosin scintigraphy for the detection of myocarditis. J Nucl Cardiol 1996; 3:371–381.

13. Yasuda T, Palacios IF, Dec GW, Fallon JT, Gold HK, Leinbach RC, Strauss HW, Khaw BA, Haber E. Indium 111-monoclonal antimyosin antibody imaging in the diagnosis of acute myocarditis. Circulation 1987; 76:306–311.

14. Dec GW, Palacios I, Yasuda T, Fallon JT, Khaw BA, Strauss HW, Haber E. Antimyosin antibody cardiac imaging: its role in the diagnosis of myocarditis. J Am Coll Cardiol 1990; 16:97–104.

15. Teiger E, Dam TV, Richard L, Wisnewsby C, Tea BS, Gaboury L, Tremblay J, Schwartz K, Hamet P. Apoptosis in pressure overload induced heart hypertrophy in the rat. J Clin Invest 1996; 97:2891–2897.

16. Li Z, Bing OH, Long X, Robinson KG, Lakatta EG. Increased cardiomyocyte apoptosis during the transition to heart failure in the spontaneously hypertensive rat. Am J Physiol 1997; 272: H2313–H2319.

17. Cheng W, Kajstura J, Nitahara JA, et al. Programmed myocyte cell death affects the viable myocardium after infarction in rats. Exper Cell Res 1996; 226:316–327.

18. Katz AM. The cardiomyopathy of overload: an unnatural growth response in the hypertrophied heart. Ann Inter Med 1994; 121:363–371.

19. Agah R, Kirshenbaum LA, Abdellatiff M, Truong LD, Chakraborty S, Michael LH, Schneider MD. Adenoviral delivery of E2F-1 directs cell cycle reentry and p 53-independent apoptosis in post mitotic adult myocardium in vitro. J Clin Invest. 1997; 100:2722–8.

20. Green DR. Apoptotic pathways: the roads to ruin. Cell 1998; 94:695–698.

21. Zamzami N, Kroemer G. The mitochondrion in apoptosis: how Pandora's box opens. Nat Rev Mol Cell Biol 2001; 2:67–71.

22. Green DR. Apoptotic pathways: paper wraps stone blunts scissors. Cell 2000; 102:1–4.

23. Gross A, Yin XM, Wang K, Wei MC, Jockel J, Milliman C, et al. Caspase cleaved BID targets mitochondria and is required for cytochrome c release, while BCL-XL prevents this release but not tumor necrosis factor-R1/Fas death. J Biol Chem 1999; 274:1156–1163.

24. Gross A, McDonnell JM, Korsmeyer SJ. BCL-2 family members and the mitochondria in apoptosis. Genes Dev 1999; 13:1899–1911.

25. Salvesen GS, Duckett CS. Apoptosis: IAP proteins: blocking the road to death's door. Nat Rev Mol Cell Biol 2002; 3:401–410.

26. Narula J, Pandey P, Arbustini E, Haider N, Narula N, Kolodgie FD, Dal Bello B, Semigran MJ, Bielsa-Masdeu A, Dec GW, Israels S, Ballester M, Virmani R, Saxena S, Kharbanda S. Apoptosis in heart failure: release of cytochrome c from mitochondria and activation of caspase-3 in human cardiomyopathy. Proc Natl Acad Sci USA 1999; 96:8144–8149.

27. Communal C, Narula J, Solaro J, Hajjar RJ. Functional consequences of caspase activation in cardiac myocytes. Proc Natl Acad Sci USA 2002; 99:6252–6256.

28. Haider N, Narula N, Narula J. Apoptosis in heart failure represents programmed cell survival, not death, of cardiomyocytes and likelihood of reverse remodeling. J Card Fail 2002; 8: S512–S517.

29. Narula J, Arbustini E, Chandrashekhar Y, Schwaiger M. Apoptosis and systolic dysfunction in congestive heart failure. Cardio Clin 2001; 19:113–126.

30. Weneker D, Nguyen KT, Khine CC, Chandra M, Carantziotis S, Ng K, Factor SM, Shirani J, Kitsis RN. Myocyte apoptosis is sufficient to cause dilated cardiomyopathy. Circulation 1999; 100:1–17.

31. Chao W, Shen Y, Li L, Rosenzweig A. Importance of FADD signaling in serum-deprivation- and hypoxia-induced cardiomyocyte apoptosis. J Biol Chem 2002; 277:31639–31645.

32. Lee P, Sata M, Lefer DJ, Factor SM, Walsh K, Kitsis RN. Fas pathway is a critical mediator of cardiac myocyte death and MI during ischemia-reperfusion in vivo. Am J Physiol Heart Circ Physiol 2003; 284:H456–H463.

33. Reed JC, Paternostro G. Postmitochondrial regulation of apoptosis during heart failure. Proc Natl Acad Sci USA 1999; 996:7614–7616.

34. Leist M, Single B, Castoldi AF, Kuhnle S, Nicotera P. Intracellular adenosine triphosphate (ATP) concentration: a switch in the decision between apoptosis and necrosis. J Exp Med 1997; 185:1481–1486.

35. Eguchi Y, Shimizu S, Tsujimoto Y. Intracellular ATP levels determine cell death fate by apoptosis or necrosis. Canter Res 1997; 57:1835–1840.

36. Glickman MH, Ciechanover A. The ubiquitin-proteasome proteolytic pathway: destruction for the sake of construction. Physiol Rev 2002; 82:373–428.

37. Thrower JS, Hoffman L, Rechsteiner M, Pickart CM. Recognition of the polyubiquitin proteolytic signal. EMBO J 2000; 19:94–102.

38. Hu BR, Janelidze S, Ginsberg MD, Busto R, Perez-Pinzon M, Sick TJ, Siesjo BK, Liu CL. Protein aggregation after focal brain ischemia and reperfusion. J Cereb Blood Flow Metab 2001; 21:865–875.

39. Kaufman RJ. Orchestrating the unfolded protein response in health and disease. J Clin Invest 2002; 110:1389–1398.

40. Chandrashekhar Y, Gupta S, Erickson M. Chaperone proteins are reduced in the nonischemic remote myocardium in rats with heart failure following an anterior wall myocardial infarction. Circulation 1998; 98:1–840 (abstract).

41. Häcki J, Egger L, Monney L, Conus S, Rosse T, Fellay I, Borner C. Apoptotic crosstalk between the endoplasmic reticulum and mitochondria controlled by Bcl-2. Oncogene 2000; 19:2286–2295.

42. Fischer S, Maclean AA, Liu M, et al. Dynamic changes in apoptotic and necrotic cell death correlate with severity of ischemia-reperfusion injury in lung transplantation. Am J Respir Crit Care Med 2000; 162:1932–1939.

43. Lieberthal W, Menza SA, Levine JS. Graded ATP depletion can cause necrosis or apoptosis of cultured mouse proximal tubular cells. Am J Physiol Renal Physiol 1998; 274:F315–F327.

44. Los M, Mozoluk M, Ferrari D, Stepczynska A, Stroh C, Renz A, Herceg Z, Wang ZQ, Schulze-Osthoff K. Activation and caspase-mediated inhibition of PARP: a molecular switch between fibroblast necrosis and apoptosis in death receptor signaling. Mol Biol Cell 2002; 13:978–988.

45. Lemasters JJV. Necrapoptosis and the mitochondrial permeability transition: shared pathways to necrosis and apoptosis. Am J Physiol Gastrointest Liver Physiol 1999; 276:G1–G6.

46. Dong Z, Saikumar P, Weinberg JM. Internucleosomal DNA cleavage triggered by plasma membrane damage during necrotic cell death. Involvement of serine but not cysteine proteases. Am J Pathol 1997; 151:1205–1213.

47. Vercammen D, Brouckaert G, Denecker G, Van de Craen M, Declercq W, Fiers W, Vandenabeele P. Dual signaling of the Fas receptor: initiation of both apoptotic and necrotic cell death pathways. J Exp Med 1998; 188:919–930.

48. Sperandio S, de Belle I, Bredesen DE. An alternate non apoptotic form of cell death. Proc Natl Acad Sci USA 2000; 97:14376–14381.

49. Chautan M, Chazal G, Cecconi F, Gruss P, Goldstein P. Interdigital cell death can occur through a necrotic and caspase-independent pathway. Curr Biol 1999; 9:967–970.

50. Marshansky V, et al. Proteasomes modulate balance among proapoptotic and antiapoptotic Bcl-2 family members and compromise functioning of the electron transport chain in leukemic cells. J Immunol 2001; 166:3130–3142.

51. Suzuki Y, Nakabayashi Y, Takahashi R. Ubiquitin-protein ligase activity of X-linked inhibitor of apoptosis protein promotes proteasomal degradation of caspase-3 and enhances its anti-apoptotic effect in Fas-induced cell death. Proc Natl Acad Sci USA 2001; 98:8662–8667.

52. Matsui T, Li L, del Monte F, Fukui Y, Franke T, Hajjar R, Rosenzweig A. Adenoviral gene transfer of activated PI 3-kinase and Akt inhibits apoptosis of hypoxic cardiomyocytes in vitro. Circulation 1999; 100:2373–2379.

53. Matsui T, Tao J, del Monte F, Lee K-H, Li L, Picard M, Force TL, Franke TF, Hajjar RJ, Rosenzweig A. Akt activation preserves cardiac function and prevents injury after transient cardiac ischemia in vivo. Circulation 2001; 104:330–335.

54. Hagl C, Tatton NA, Khaladj N, Zhang N, Nandor S, Insolia S, Weisz DJ, Spielvogel D, Griepp RB. Involvement of apoptosis in neurological injury after hypothermic circulatory arrest: a new target for therapeutic intervention?. Ann Thorac Surg 2001; 72:1457–1464.

55. Narula J, Baliga R. What's in a name? Would that which we call death by any other name be less tragic?. Ann Thorac Surg 2001; 72:1454–1456.

56. Nicotera P, Leist M, Ferrando-May E. Intracellular ATP, a switch in the decision between apoptosis and necrosis. Toxicol Lett 1998; 102:139–142.

4

Excitation-Contraction Coupling Mechanisms in Heart Failure

Federica del Monte and Roger J. Hajjar
Cardiovascular Research Center, Massachusetts General Hospital
Boston, Massachusetts, USA

SUMMARY

The behavior of the heart as it goes through each beat is governed by the contraction and relaxation cycle of individual cardiac myocytes. The process that begins contraction is known as excitation-contraction (E-C) coupling because it couples electrical signals on the membrane of the cardiac cell to activation of the myofilament and cross-bridge cycling. The cardiac action potential is produced by the coordinated interaction of many ion channels, which transduce physiological signals within and between cardiomyocytes. These cardiomyocytes are further regulated by a number of receptors that control the strength of the contraction on a beat-to-beat basis and their morphology in a chronic fashion. In heart failure, a number of steps in excitation-contraction coupling become abnormal. In this chapter, we will examine the role of these abnormalities in the development of heart failure.

EXCITATION-CONTRACTION COUPLING

In the mammalian heart, depolarization of the cell membrane leads to the opening of voltage gated L-type Ca^{2+} channels, located in the T-tubular regions of the myocytes, allowing the influx of trans-sarcolemmal influx of Ca^{2+} into the cell (Fig. 1) [1,2]. These channels are in close proximity to the Ca^{2+} release channels, known as ryanodine receptors (RyRs), which are located on the sarcoplasmic reticulum (SR), the major Ca^{2+} storing organelle in the cardiomyocyte. Ca^{2+} entering the cells through a single L-type Ca^{2+} channel induces the opening of one or a cluster of ryanodine receptors resulting in the local release of Ca^{2+} from the SR [1,2 1,3–5]. During membrane depolarization, a large number of L-type Ca^{2+} channels are opened, resulting in a large release of Ca^{2+} from the ryanodine receptors, raising cytosolic Ca^{2+} from 0.1–0.2 μM to 2–10 μM.

Recently, with the advent of confocal microscopy, a functional Ca^{2+} signaling and releasing unit has been characterized, namely the Ca^{2+} spark [6–20]. Ca^{2+} sparks were first identified as the ''elementary events'' of spontaneous increases in intracellular $[Ca^{2+}]$, which were detected by laser scanning confocal microscopy and the fluorescent Ca^{2+}

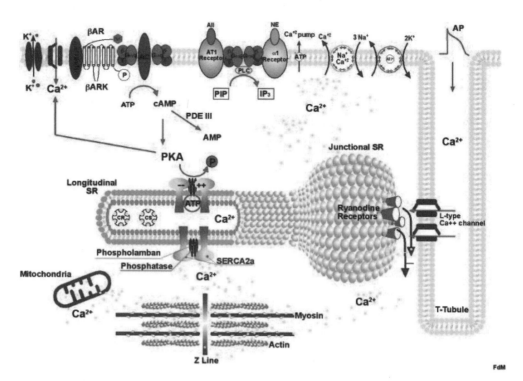

Figure 1 Depolarization of the membrane by the action potential leads to the opening of voltage gated L-type calcium (Ca^{2+}) channels allowing the entry of a small amount of Ca2$^+$ into the cell. Through a coupling mechanism between the L-type Ca^{2+} channel and the sarcoplasmic reticulum (SR) release channels (ryanodine receptors), a larger amount of Ca^{2+} is released activating the myofilaments leading to contraction. During relaxation, Ca^{2+} is reaccumulated back into the SR by the SR Ca^{2+} ATPase pump (SERCA2a) and extruded extracellularly by the sarcolemmal Na^+/Ca^{2+} exchanger. A number of sarcolemmal receptors affect calcium handling in cardiac myocytes. Agonists through G proteins increase adenyl cyclase activity resulting in cAMP production. This results in activation of PKA leading to phosphorylation of the L-type calcium channels, allowing an increase in calcium entry, phosphorylation of phospholamban, increasing SERCA2a activity, and phosphorylation of troponin I, decreasing the sensitivity of the myofilaments to Ca^{2+}. The phosphorylation effects of PKA induce a greater release of calcium from the SR and a faster relaxation. Digoxin inhibits the Na^+/K^+ ATPase pump increasing intracellular Na^+. This results in an increase in intracellular Ca^{2+} via the Na^+/Ca^{2+} exchanger, which leads to an enhanced Ca^{2+} loading of the SR and an increase in Ca^{2+} release. Phosphodiesterase inhibitors block the breakdown of cAMP, increasing its intracellular level activating PKA.

indicator fluo-3 as shown by Figure 2. Ca^{2+} sparks, which also can be produced by the Ca^{2+} entering through L-type Ca^{2+} channels during the E-C coupling process, therefore underlie the elementary Ca^{2+} signaling unit in excitation-contraction coupling at the individual junction. Functionally, the Ca^{2+} sparks represent Ca^{2+} releases from the SR through the opening of the SR Ca^{2+} release channels/ryanodine receptors. Ca^{2+} sparks are produced by $10 \sim 100$ RyRs based on the ratio of the Ca^{2+} sparks current and the single RyR channel current because the morphology of Ca^{2+} sparks vary even within a single cell. Ca^{2+} sparks are depicted/measured by their morphology and the frequency of occurrence. The information of the morphology includes the sizes of Ca^{2+} sparks (amplitude,

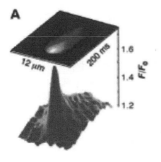

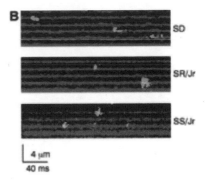

Figure 2 Unitary properties of SR Ca^{2+} release in rat heart cells. Signal-averaged Ca^{2+} sparks are shown as line-scan image (*top*) and a surface plot (*bottom*) from control cRDIc myocytes. The SR Ca^{2+} release takes place at the t-tubules in heart cells. Sulpho-rhodamine B identify the extracellular space in the t-tubules, whereas Ca^{2+} sparks were imaged simultaneously. (Adapted from Ref. 20a.)

width, and duration) and the kinetics is described by the spark's rising and decaying dynamics. The activity of individual ryanodine receptors and the number of the RyRs recruited during a spark play an important role in the spark morphology. Thus, the more active the Ca^{2+} release channels are, the more Ca^{2+} would be released and as a consequent, the increased size and the more frequent occurrence of Ca^{2+} sparks would be observed. Therefore, direct modifications that change the RyRs activity or the modulators that regulate RyR activity will have an impact on the size and frequency of Ca^{2+} sparks. SR Ca^{2+} content also regulates Ca^{2+} sparks because luminal [Ca^{2+}] plays a critical role in regulating RyR by increasing the activity of the RyRs and by sensitizing the threshold of RyR for activation to the stimulus. Ca^{2+} sparks can be triggered by the Ca^{2+} influx through the L-type Ca^{2+} sparks during voltage pulses. Thus, the kinetics, fidelity, and stoichiometry of coupling between L-type Ca^{2+} channels and RyR plays a critical role in determination of the signal transduction during the E-C coupling process. The distance of the cleft between the cell plasma membrane and the SR membrane, which is roughly 12 nm in normal cardiomyocytes, is critical for this kind of coupling and signal transduction. Extension of the distance between them, by pulling the plasma membrane under tight-seal conditions, decreases or abolishes the signaling reliability.

The release of Ca^{2+} into the myofibrillar space, in turn, results in cross-bridge formation and contraction [21–28]. The myofilaments are organized in a regular array of thick and thin filaments giving the typical striated appearance of the entire myocyte as shown by Figure 3. Each unit of this striated organization, known as the sarcomere, is composed of one unit of interacting thin and thick filaments. The thick filaments consist mainly of myosin heavy chains (MHC) and two pairs of light chains (Fig. 4). The "tail" of the molecule is coiled with two myosin heavy chains wound around each other. The "heads" of myosin include the globular region of one myosin molecule and two myosin light chains [24–28]. Each myosin head has an ATP (adenosine triphosphate)-binding area in close proximity to myosin ATPase, which breaks down ATP. Two myosin heavy chain isoforms exist in human mammalian myocardium, α-MHC and β-MHC. In human ventricular myocardium only 10% to 20% is α-MHC, while the β-MHC is more abundant. The thin filaments are composed of actin and troponin complex. Within the sarcomere, the actin polymers intertwine in a helical fashion. At intervals of 385 Å along the thin

Contractile proteins

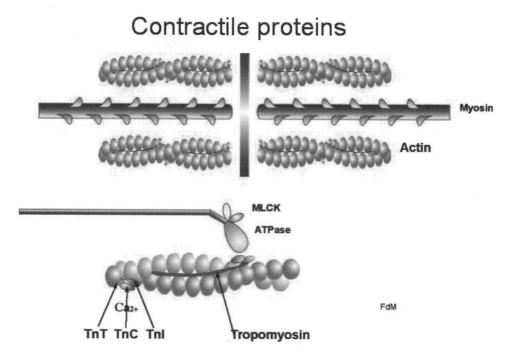

Figure 3   Contractile proteins in cardiac myocytes.

filaments are a group of three regulatory proteins called the troponin complex carried on a long helical molecule, tropomyosin. The troponin complexes are made up of one molecule each of troponin C, troponin I, and troponin T. The strength of the bond linking troponin I and actin varies depending on the intracellular Ca^{2+} level.

When the cytosolic Ca^{2+} is low the tropomyosin-troponin complex is positioned in such a way that the myosin heads cannot interact with actin. This is due to the bond linking troponin I to actin. When cytosolic calcium increases, it binds to troponin C strengthening the bond between troponin C and troponin I and weakening the bond linking troponin I to actin. This leads to a conformational change of the tropomyosin-troponin C complex that allows the myosin head to interact with actin. When Ca^{2+} binds to troponin C it exposes the active site on the thin filament, permitting the myosin head to bind weakly to the actin filaments. Subsequent ATP hydrolysis allows a strong binding of the myosin head to actin, which is followed by a power stroke that moves the actin molecule 5 nm to 10 nm, locking the myosin head into a rigor state. The myosin head releases ADP (adenosine diphosphate) and is ready to accept ATP, which starts the cycle again. ATP binding to the myosin head dissociates the thin and thick filaments.

Relaxation occurs when calcium detaches from troponin C and is reaccumulated back into the SR by the cardiac isoform of the Ca^{2+} ATPase pump (SERCA2a) and extruded extracellularly by the sarcolemmal Na^+/Ca^{2+} exchanger. The contribution of each of these mechanisms for lowering cytosolic Ca^{2+} varies among species. In humans ~75% of the Ca^{2+} is removed by SERCA2a and ~25% by the Na^+/Ca^{2+} exchanger. SERCA2a transports Ca^{2+} back to the luminal space of the SR against a Ca^{2+} gradient by an energy dependent mechanism (one molecule of ATP is hydrolyzed for the transport of two molecules of Ca^{2+}), where it binds to a calcium buffering protein, calsequestrin.

GENES

Lamin A/C

δ-sarcoglycan

Dystrophin

Desmin

Vinculin

Titin

Troponin-T

α-tropomyosin

ß-Myosin heavy chain

Actin

Mitochondrial DNA mutations

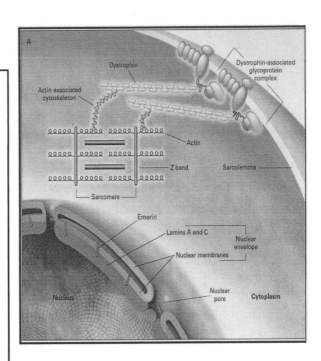

Figure 4 In failing hearts, the action potential duration is markedly prolonged and is associated with changes in ionic currents.

The Ca^{2+} pumping activity of SERCA2a is regulated by phospholamban. In its unphosphorylated state, phospholamban inhibits the Ca^{2+}-ATPase, whereas phosphorylation of phospholamban by cAMP-dependent protein kinase and by Ca^{2+}-calmodulin dependent protein kinase reverses this inhibition.

Electrical Activity in the Heart

A distinctive feature of the cardiac myocyte is its action potential (Fig. 5). At the cellular level, the formation of the heartbeat is directly regulated by the cardiac action potential, which depends on the coordinated actions of a large number of ion channels. Because different parts of the heart have different complements or densities of ion channels and pumps, the action potentials can differ between different myocardial regions. Figure 3 shows a human action potential from the anterior wall of the left ventricle with the approximate time course of the depolarizing and repolarizing currents carried by the different ion channels. Action potential conduction in the heart depends on the ion conductance activity of specific voltage-gated ion channels that mediate rapid, voltage-dependent changes in ion permeability causing a change in the membrane potential. The action potential is classically divided in five phases:

Phase 0: A rapid increase in Na^+ permeability mediated by voltage-sensitive Na^+ channels causes rapid depolarization during the initial phase of the action potential.
Phase 1: This is followed by a rapid repolarization governed by the transient outward current (I_{to}). The magnitude of I_{to} varies markedly within the different chambers and walls of the heart. I_{to} density is highest in atrial myocytes and epicardial

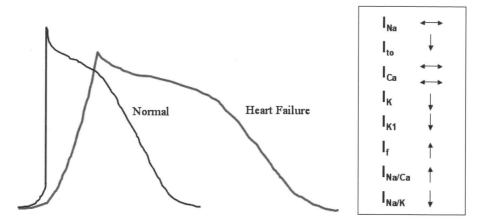

Figure 5 Action potential in cardiac myocytes. Different currents involved in the different phases of the action potential.

ventricular myocytes, giving rise to the short action potential, and very low in endocardial ventricular myocytes. Two separate potassium channel gene families contribute to the formation of I_{to}: Kv1.4, a member of the *shaker* family, and Kv4.2 and Kv4.3, members of the *shal* family, the latter playing a predominant role in the repolarization of the action potential in humans.

Phase 2: A slow repolarization phase ensues, which gives rise to the plateau of the action potential. Ca^{2+} enters the cells during this phase. The major determinants of the repolarization are the inactivation of the L-type Ca^{2+} current and the activation of the delayed rectifier K^+ currents (I_K).

Phase 3: Toward the end of the plateau, the rate of depolarization is markedly accelerated by the delayed rectifier current and the inward rectifier current (I_{K1}). Also contributing to the plateau currents are the Na^+/Ca^+ exchanger current and Na^+ currents through the Na^+/K^+ ATPase pump.

Phase 4: Spontaneous depolarization during diastole is a normal property of SA (sino-atrial) nodal, (atrio-ventricular), AV nodal, and Purkinje cells, but not atrial or ventricular myocytes. The hyperpolarization-activated inward current I_f and the delayed rectifier current (I_K), which gradually deactivates, favor net inward current, thus depolarizing the cell.

Regulation of Contractility in the Heart

A number of endogenous and exogenous factors regulate the strength of contraction in cardiomyocytes. Circulating and locally released catecholamines bind to myocardial β1 and β2 adrenoreceptors (Fig. 1). Both β1 and β2 adrenoreceptors activate adenylyl cyclase through stimulatory G proteins (Gsα), which results in the production of cAMP. Binding of cAMP to the regulatory subunit of protein kinase A triggers a conformational change that allows the catalytic subunits of the enzyme to dissociate and phosphorylate protein substrates at serine and threonine subunits. In cardiac cells, PKA (cAMP protein kinase A) phosphorylates

- the L-type Ca^{2+} channel resulting in increased Ca^{2+} entry
- phospholamban at its serine 16 site resulting in enhanced Ca^{2+} uptake into the SR
- troponin I resulting in enhanced detachment of Ca^{2+} from troponin C

The effects of PKA phosphorylation, therefore, increase the strength of the contraction and enhance relaxation thereby combining inotropic and lusitropic effects. The force-frequency relationship also contributes to the regulation of contractile strength in the heart. In a normal heart, increasing heart rate results in enhanced transsarcolemmal Ca^{2+} influx secondary to high frequency induced recruitment of Ca^{2+} currents, which results in more Ca^{2+} release from the SR and stronger contraction. In addition, length-dependent activation of the myofilaments serves as a largely Ca^{2+}-independent mechanism for the short-term regulation of the strength of contraction.

The cardiac ryanodine receptors RyR2 are also regulated by the β-adrenergic receptor (β-AR) signaling pathway. Activation of the sympathetic nervous system results in binding of norepinephrine to the β-AR and in elevation of cAMP levels and activation of PKA. Phosphorylation of RyR2 may not correlate directly with cellular cAMP levels, however. On the ryanodine receptor, there is a delicate balance between PKA phosphorylation and phosphatases (protein phosphatase 1 [PP1] and protein phosphatase 2 [PP2A]). In addition, there are other molecules, such as FKB 12.6, which bind the L-type calcium channel receptor to the RyR2 and stabilize this interaction. Upon β-AR activation, PP1 and PP2A levels in RyR2 complex and depletes FKBP12.6 from RyR2 complex, pathologically increasing Ca^{2+}-dependent activation of RyR2 and resulting in depletion of SR Ca^{2+} stores, and uncoupling of RyR2 from each other (reducing E-C coupling gain).

The angiotensin I and endothelin I receptors couple to heterotrimeric G Gq, which activates phospholipase C and inositol triphosphate (IP3), releasing Ca^{2+} from endoplasmic reticular stores. Both angiotensin and endothelin receptor activation cause modest increases in contractility, but their role (as detailed in the following text) is mainly centered on the induction of hypertrophy. β3 receptors have been recently identified in the heart and their function is mainly inhibitory on contractility.

CHANGES IN HEART FAILURE

In cardiomyocytes isolated from patients with heart failure, contraction and relaxation exhibit a similar set of abnormalities regardless of the etiology. These can be attributed to alterations in cellular processes within the myocytes including the sarcolemmal ionic channels, receptors, the intracellular pumps, the myofilaments, and the metabolic pathways that generate ATP.

Action Potential and Repolarizing Currents in Heart Failure

Changes in calcium-handling proteins and channel proteins governing cardiac repolarization have a significant impact on electrical activity in the failing heart (Fig. 4) [29,30]. Prolongation of the action potential duration is a prominent feature of heart failure. Various ionic currents have been shown to be altered in heart failure. The inward rectifier K^+ current (I_{K1}) and the transient outward K^+ current (I_{to}) are significantly reduced in heart failure. Associated with the reduction in I_{to}, there is a decrease in the expression of Kv4.2 and Kv4.3. Other changes in ionic currents are summarized in the side panel of Figure 6.

Calcium Handling in Failing Hearts

Abnormal calcium dynamics is a key causal component in the failing cardiomyocyte [3,22,23,31–39]. As shown in Figure 6, cardiomyocytes isolated from failing human hearts

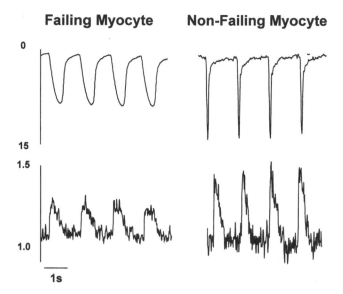

Figure 6 Recordings from cardiomyocytes isolated from a nonfailing heart and from failing heart infected stimulated at 1 Hz at 37°C. Failing cell had a characteristic decrease in contraction and prolonged relaxation along with a prolonged Ca^{2+} transient.

exhibit three important characteristics: (a) a decrease in systolic Ca^{2+}, (b) an increase in diastolic Ca^{2+}, and (c) a prolonged relaxation phase. There is elevated diastolic calcium, an inability to recruit a large amount of calcium at high loads and frequencies, and an inability to take up calcium during relaxation. In addition, a critical characteristic of a failing cardiac cell is the negative frequency response. Although in normal hearts, an increase in stimulation frequency at fixed preload induces a sharp rise in contractile response, in failing hearts, there is a decrease in contraction and calcium release with increasing frequency (Fig. 7).

Since calcium handling is regulated by the voltage-dependent Ca^{2+} channel, the SR Ca^{2+} release channels ryanodine, the SERCA2a/phospholamban complex, and the Na^+/Ca^{2+} exchanger, studies have focused on the relative changes in these proteins between myopathic and normal hearts (Table 1) [3,22,23,31-39].

The conductive properties of both the L-type Ca^{2+} channels and the ryanodine release channels from patients with dilated cardiomyopathy, as assayed by voltage clamp, are essentially normal, but their coupling may be defective, such that with failing myocardial cells, L-type Ca^{2+} channels have a reduced ability to activate the adjacent ryanodine receptors. It is still unclear whether all forms of heart failure have this type of coupling abnormality.

In both failing human hearts and in experimental models of heart failure, there is reduction in the expression and enzymatic activity of SERCA2a but an increase in Na^+/Ca^{2+} exchanger expression and activity. The enhanced expression of the exchanger has been hypothesized to be compensatory for the reduction of SERCA2a since the Na^+Ca^+ exchanger can operate to bring Ca^{2+} into the cell or extrude it from the cell. In fact, there is an increase in sensitivity to compounds that produce positive inotropic effects through raised intracellular Na^+, either by inhibiting the Na^+/K^{2+}-ATPase or by opening Na^+ channels, in failing human hearts.

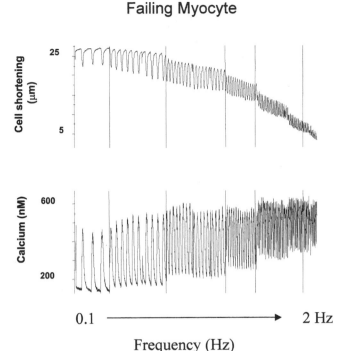

Figure 7 Recordings from same cardiomyocytes stimulated at increasing frequencies. Failing cardiomyocyte demonstrated a decrease in contraction amplitude and systolic Ca^{2+} and an increase in diastolic tone and Ca^{2+}

Changes of Ca^{2+} spark characteristics have been investigated in explanted failing human hearts as well as different animal models of cardiac hypertrophy and heart failure. Overall, a number of findings have been noted across different models of heart failure: (a) the efficiency of the signaling transduction between L-type Ca^{2+} channel and RyR was reduced [42]. This finding has been interpreted as a defective communication between L-type Ca^{2+} channels and RyRs, either because of the mismatch of the two Ca^{2+} channels, or the distance between LCC and RyR has been changed; (b) $[Ca^{2+}]_i$ transient is reduced secondary to a decrease in the SR Ca^{2+} load; (c) the frequency of Ca^{2+} sparks occurrence is reduced in failing myocytes while the triggering L-type Ca^{2+} current remains unchanged; and (d) the rising and decaying time is also elongated in failing myocytes [40]. All these changes in Ca^{2+} sparks suggest that several molecular mechanisms, including

Table 1 Changes in Ca^{2+} Cycling Proteins

•	↓	SERCA2a
•	←→	Phospholamban
•	↑	NCX Sodium-calcium exchange
•	←→	L-type Ca^{2+} Channel

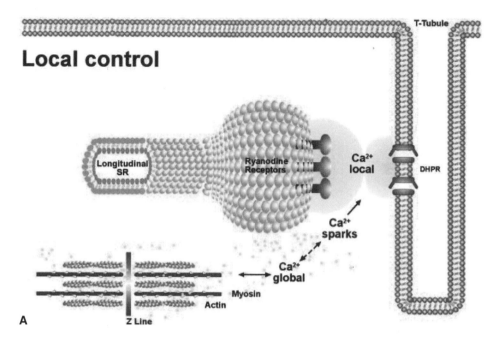

Figure 8 (**A**) Calcium spark is generated by the stochastic opening of the L-type calcium channels and the subsequent activation of RyR2. (**B**) In heart failure, the distance between the L-type calcium channels and RyR2 is increased, thereby decreasing the coupling and release mechanisms.

increased RyR activity (increased duration and width of Ca^{2+} sparks), reduction in SR Ca^{2+} content (reduced amplitude of Ca^{2+} sparks and the frequency of Ca^{2+} sparks responded to field stimulation), as well as the defective E-C coupling gain (reduced frequency of Ca^{2+} sparks responded to field stimulation) as shown in Figure 8.

In heart failure, the stimulation of the sympathetic nervous system results in phosphorylation of RyR2 by PKA. PKA phosphorylation modulates RyR2 function by changing the sensitivity of RyR2 to calcium resulting in ''leaky'' channels, which may cause diastolic Ca^{2+} release, and generating delayed afterdepolarizations. In addition, PKA hyperphosphorylation of RyR2s in failing hearts, functionally uncouples the channels from the L-type calcium channel, thereby reducing E-C coupling gain.

Contractile Proteins

A number of abnormalities occur at the level of the contractile proteins in failing myocardium. There is a decrease in the fast isoform of the myosin heavy chain (α-MHC) and an increase in the slower isoform β-MHC (Fig. 9). There is also a decrease in myosin light chain kinase. Furthermore, there is a 20% to 30% decrease in myofibrillar protein content. In nonfailing myocardium, there is one single predominant isoform for troponin T, referred to as Troponin T1. A second isoform (Troponin T2) increases substantially in ventricular myocardium of patients with heart failure. These isoform shifts and changes of the contractile proteins have direct consequences on the functional properties of muscle contraction. An increase in β-MHC results in a decrease in the cross-bridge cycling rate and an increase in energy conservation, because fewer ATP molecules are split. It also

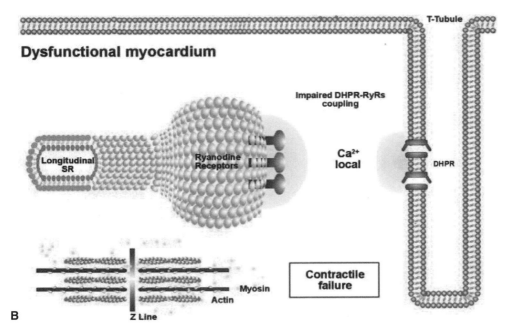

Figure 8 (continued)

leads to a slower contraction and relaxation phases, which are characteristic of failing myocardium. An increase in Troponin T2 leads to a decrease in the sensitivity of the myofilaments to Ca^{2+} and an abnormal response to agents targeting the myofilaments.

Energetics

In heart failure there is a mismatch between energy supply and demand. In both human and experimental models of heart failure, there are decreases in energy supplied by key enzymes involved in ATP-producing pathways, including creatine kinase, oxidative phosphorylation, and glycolysis, and high energy phosphate content and turnover rates are decreased. Cardiac muscle contains a large amount of phospho-creatine (PCr) and creatine kinase (CK). The creatine kinase system acts as an energy reserve system especially during

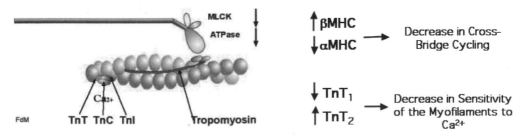

Figure 9 Changes in isoforms and ATPase activity in the myofibrillar process that contribute to the failing phenotype.

Table 2 Alterations of Membrane
Receptors in Failing Hearts

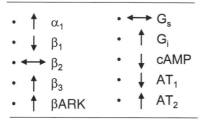

high work loads. A decrease in creatine kinase pharmacologically or genetically decreases the ability of cardiac muscle to increase contractile performance.

Abnormal β-receptor Signaling

β-adrenergic signaling defects in heart failure include down-regulation of myocardial β-adrenergic receptors, β-AR uncoupling, and an up-regulation of the β-AR kinase (β ARK1) as shown by Figure 8. As a consequence to these molecular changes, there is reduced functional responsiveness to β-adrenergic agonists and cAMP dependent inotropic agents. These alterations are described in detail in chapter 5.

CONCLUDING REMARKS

Through the window of excitation-contraction coupling, we can get a better understanding of heart failure on the cellular and molecular levels. Abnormal intracellular calcium handling seems to be the common pathway that induces a decrease in contractility and a worsening in arrhythmias. Our understanding of the key abnormalities in ionic changes within the cardiac cell in the failing heart may provide new therapeutic strategies for heart failure.

REFERENCES

1. Bers DM. Cardiac excitation-contraction coupling. Nature 2002; 415:198–205.
2. Bers DM, Weber CR. Na/Ca exchange function in intact ventricular myocytes. Ann N Y Acad Sci 2002; 976:500–512.
3. Gwathmey JK, Slawsky MT, Hajjar RJ, Briggs GM, Morgan JP. Role of intracellular calcium handling in force-interval relationships of human ventricular myocardium. J Clin Invest 1990; 85:1599–1613.
4. Bers DM. Calcium and cardiac rhythms: physiological and pathophysiological. Circ Res 2002; 90:14–17.
5. Piacentino V, Weber CR, Chen X, Weisser-Thomas J, Margulies KB, Bers DM, Houser SR. Cellular basis of abnormal calcium transients of failing human ventricular myocytes. Circ Res 2003; 92:651–658.
6. Pratusevich VR, Balke CW. Factors shaping the confocal image of the calcium spark in cardiac muscle cells. Biophys J 1996; 71:2942–2957.
7. Satoh H, Blatter LA, Bers DM. Effects of [Ca2 +]i, SR Ca2 + load, and rest on Ca2 + spark frequency in ventricular myocytes. Am J Physiol 1997; 272:H657–H668.
8. Yue DT. Quenching the spark in the heart. Science 1997; 276:755–756.

9. Bonev AD, Jaggar JH, Rubart M, Nelson MT. Activators of protein kinase C decrease Ca2+ spark frequency in smooth muscle cells from cerebral arteries. Am J Physiol 1997; 273: C2090–C2095.

10. Satoh H, Hayashi H, Blatter LA, Bers DM. BayK 8644 increases resting calcium spark frequency in ferret ventricular myocytes. Heart Vessels 1997(Suppl 12):58–61.

11. Smith GD, Keizer JE, Stern MD, Lederer WJ, Cheng H. A simple numerical model of calcium spark formation and detection in cardiac myocytes. Biophys J 1998; 75:15–32.

12. Parrington J, Coward K. The spark of life. Biologist (London) 2003; 50:5–10.

13. Zhuge R, Fogarty KE, Tuft RA, Walsh JV. Spontaneous transient outward currents arise from microdomains where BK channels are exposed to a mean Ca(2+) concentration on the order of 10 microM during a Ca(2+) spark. J Gen Physiol 2002; 120:15–27.

14. Shtifman A, Ward CW, Yamamoto T, Wang J, Olbinski B, Valdivia HH, Ikemoto N, Schneider MF. Interdomain interactions within ryanodine receptors regulate Ca2+ spark frequency in skeletal muscle. J Gen Physiol 2002; 119:15–32.

15. Gonzalez A, Kirsch WG, Shirokova N, Pizarro G, Stern MD, Rios E. The spark and its ember: separately gated local components of Ca(2+) release in skeletal muscle. J Gen Physiol 2000; 115:139–158.

16. Gyorke S. Ca2+ spark termination: inactivation and adaptation may be manifestations of the same mechanism. J Gen Physiol 1999; 114:163–166.

17. Fill M, Mejia-Alvarez R, Kettlun C, Escobar A. Ryanodine receptor permeation and gating: glowing cinders that underlie the Ca2+ spark. J Gen Physiol 1999; 114:159–161.

18. Imaizumi Y, Ohi Y, Yamamura H, Ohya S, Muraki K, Watanabe M. Ca2+ spark as a regulator of ion channel activity. Jpn J Pharmacol 1999; 80:1–8.

19. Izu LT, Wier WG, Balke CW. Theoretical analysis of the Ca2+ spark amplitude distribution. Biophys J 1998; 75:1144–1162.

20. Keizer J, Smith GD. Spark-to-wave transition: saltatory transmission of calcium waves in cardiac myocytes. Biophys Chem 1998; 72:87–100.

20a. Gómez AM, Valdivia HH, Cheng H, Miriam R, Lederer LF, Santana MB, Cannell SA, McCune RA, Altschuld RA, Lederer WJ. Defective excitation-contraction coupling in experimental cardiac hypertrophy and heart failure. Science 1997 May 2; 276:800–806.

21. Hajjar RJ, Schwinger RH, Schmidt U, Kim CS, Lebeche D, Doye AA, Gwathmey JK. Myofilament calcium regulation in human myocardium. Circulation 2000; 101:1679–1685.

22. Gwathmey JK, Kim CS, Hajjar RJ, Khan F, DiSalvo TG, Matsumori A, Bristow MR. Cellular and molecular remodeling in a heart failure model treated with the beta-blocker carteolol. Am J Physiol 1999; 276:H1678–H1690.

23. Gwathmey JK, Liao R, Helm PA, Thaiyananthan G, Hajjar RJ. Is contractility depressed in the failing human heart? [Review] [40 refs]. Cardiovas Drugs Ther 1995; 9:581–587.

24. Solaro RJ, Varghese J, Marian AJ, Chandra M. Molecular mechanisms of cardiac myofilament activation: modulation by pH and a troponin T mutant R92Q. Basic Res Cardiol 2002(97 Suppl 1):I102–I110.

25. Solaro RJ, Montgomery DM, Wang L, Burkart EM, Ke Y, Vahebi S, Buttrick P. Integration of pathways that signal cardiac growth with modulation of myofilament activity. J Nucl Cardiol 2002; 9:523–533.

26. Martin AF, Phillips RM, Kumar A, Crawford K, Abbas Z, Lessard JL, de Tombe P, Solaro RJ. Ca(2+) activation and tension cost in myofilaments from mouse hearts ectopically expressing enteric gamma-actin. Am J Physiol Heart Circ Physiol 2002; 283:H642–H649.

27. de Tombe PP, Solaro RJ. Integration of cardiac myofilament activity and regulation with pathways signaling hypertrophy and failure. Ann Biomed Eng 2000; 28:991–1001.

28. Wolska BM, Keller RS, Evans CC, Palmiter KA, Phillips RM, Muthuchamy M, Oehlenschlager J, Wieczorek DF, de Tombe PP, Solaro RJ. Correlation between myofilament response to Ca2+ and altered dynamics of contraction and relaxation in transgenic cardiac cells that express beta-tropomyosin. Circ Res 1999; 84:745–751.

29. Kaprielian R, Wickenden AD, Kassiri Z, Parker TG, Liu PP, Backx PH. Relationship between K+ channel down-regulation and [Ca2+]i in rat ventricular myocytes following myocardial infarction. J Physiol 1999; 517:229–245.

30. Kaprielian R, del Monte F, Hajjar RJ. Targeting Ca2+ cycling proteins and the action potential in heart failure by gene transfer. Basic Res Cardiol 2002(97 Suppl 1):I136–I145.

31. del Monte FEW, Lebeche D, Schmidt U, Rosenzweig A, Gwathmey JK, Lewandowski DE, Hajjar RJ. Improvement in survival and cardiac metabolism following gene transfer of SER-CA2a in a rat model of heart failure. Circulation 2001; 104:1424–9.

32. del Monte F, Harding SE, Dec GW, Gwathmey JK, Hajjar RJ. Targeting phospholamban by gene transfer in human heart failure. Circulation 2002; 105:904–907.

33. del Monte F, Harding SE, Schmidt U, Matsui T, Kang ZB, Dec GW, Gwathmey JK, Rosenzweig A, Hajjar RJ. Restoration of contractile function in isolated cardiomyocytes from failing human hearts by gene transfer of SERCA2a. Circulation 1999; 100:2308–2311.

34. DeSantiago J, Maier LS, Bers DM. Frequency-dependent acceleration of relaxation in the heart depends on CaMKII, but not phospholamban. J Mol Cell Cardiol 2002; 34:975–984.

35. Despa S, Islam MA, Pogwizd SM, Bers DM. Intracellular [Na+] and Na+ pump rate in rat and rabbit ventricular myocytes. J Physiol 2002; 539:133–143.

36. Despa S, Islam MA, Weber CR, Pogwizd SM, Bers DM. Intracellular Na(+) concentration is elevated in heart failure but Na/K pump function is unchanged. Circulation 2002; 105: 2543–2548.

37. Force T, Hajjar R, Del Monte F, Rosenzweig A, Choukroun G. Signaling pathways mediating the response to hypertrophic stress in the heart. Gene Expr 1999; 7:337–348.

38. Ginsburg KS, Weber CR, Despa S, Bers DM. Simultaneous measurement of [Na]i, [Ca]i, and I(NCX) in intact cardiac myocytes. Ann N Y Acad Sci 2002; 976:157–158.

39. Gwathmey JK, Hajjar RJ. Relation between steady-state force and intracellular [Ca2+] in intact human myocardium. Index of myofibrillar responsiveness to Ca2+. Circulation 1990; 82:1266–1278.

40. Yue DT. Quenching the spark in the heart [comment]. Science 1997; 276:755–756.

5

β-Adrenergic Signaling in Heart Failure

Stefan Engelhardt
Cardiovascular Research Center, Massachusetts General Hospital
Boston, Massachusetts, USA
DFG-Research Center for Experimental Biomedicine, University of Wuerzburg
Wuerzburg, Germany

INTRODUCTION

Activation of cardiac β-adrenergic receptors (AR) represents the body's most powerful principle to increase cardiac contractility and heart rate [1]. Since the description of the βAR as a distinct pharmacological entity [2] and the subdivision into β_1-adrenergic and β_2-adrenergic receptors by Lands and colleagues in 1967 [3], it has rapidly evolved into one of the most intensely studied receptor families. Pharmacological agents active at β-adrenergic receptors were soon introduced into clinical practice. Before the 1980s, heart failure was regarded and treated primarily from the standpoint of reduced contractility and cardiac output. Hence, positive inotropic agents, including β-receptor agonists, were used to treat heart failure patients with the result of inotropic benefit. Consequently, blockade of cardiac β-adrenergic receptors was regarded as a contraindication in heart failure treatment due to its negative inotropic effect. In recent years, a dramatic change in the perception of cardiac β-adrenergic signaling has occurred. Both experimental and clinical studies have shaped a novel picture of β-adrenergic signaling, including the propagation of cardiomyocyte hypertrophy and apoptosis, and the progression of heart failure. As a direct result of this altered perception, β-blockade in heart failure is now regarded as the single most effective therapeutic principle to treat chronic heart failure. This chapter will provide a brief overview about β-adrenergic receptors in the heart, and focus on recent developments in the understanding of β-adrenergic signaling and the use of β-blockers in heart failure.

β-ADRENERGIC RECEPTORS–MORE THAN REGULATORS OF CARDIAC CONTRACTILITY

Adrenergic receptors are a family of G-protein–coupled receptors with nine members, three α_1, three α_2, and three β: β_1, β_2, and β_3. When the first subdivision of adrenergic receptors was proposed in 1948 on the basis of pharmacological experiments [2], the α-subtype was defined as the one that causes smooth muscle contraction, whereas the β-subtype mediates smooth muscle relaxation. Twenty years later, β-receptors were subdivided, again on the basis of functional pharmacological experiments, into the β_1-subtype, which stimulates cardiac muscle, and the β_2-subtype, which relaxes smooth muscle [3].

The mammalian heart expresses all three β-adrenergic receptor subtypes (Fig. 1) [4–6]. In the healthy heart, the majority (i.e., 60%-80%) of receptors are of the β_1-subtype in most species, while the β_2-subtype accounts for a minor fraction of total βARs. A third β-adrenergic receptor subtype, the β_3-subtype, was initially thought to be limited to adipose tissue on the basis of ligand binding experiments [6], but was later detected also in the heart [5]–this subtype is generally perceived as less important due to its very low expression level and relatively minor functional effects. It is not precisely clear *where* the receptors are expressed in the heart, but there is evidence, that the β_1-subtype is preferentially located on cardiac myocytes, whereas the β_2-subtype is expressed to a significant extent on noncardiomyocyte cells, including vascular smooth muscle cells and synaptic nerve endings. Knockout mice of the β_1- and the β_2-subtypes [7] have helped to clarify a long-standing question as to whether a fourth β-receptor subtype exists [8]. The putative β_4-adrenergic receptor had been postulated on the basis of functional assays on isolated organs and ligand binding assays, in which high concentrations of the β-receptor antagonist CGP12177 produced cardiostimulatory effects [9]. This phenomenon could have been explained both by a distinct molecular entity, i.e., a fourth βAR-gene, or by an atypical state of either the β_1- or the β_2-adrenergic receptors. By the use of isolated atria from β_1- and β_2-knockout animals, it has been demonstrated by two independent groups that the pharmacology of the putative β_4-subtype is entirely dependent on the presence of the β_1-adrenergic receptor, i.e., must be an atypical state or binding site of the β_1-AR [10,11].

β_1- and β_2-adrenergic receptors are potent stimulators of cardiac contraction and relaxation in the human heart [1,12]. As direct effectors of the sympathetic nervous system,

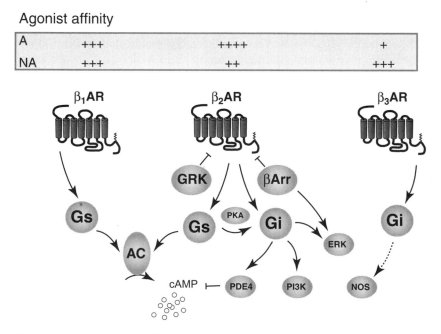

Figure 1 Agonist activation and coupling/signaling properties of β-adrenergic receptor subtypes. Abbreviations: A, adrenaline; NA, noradrenaline; GRK, G protein coupled receptor kinase; βArr, βArrestin; PDE, phosphodiesterase; PI3K, phosphatidylinositol-3-kinase; AC, adenylyl cyclase. (Adapted from Ref. [4])

they serve to rapidly adapt cardiac performance to an increased hemodynamic demand. Both receptor subtypes couple to the stimulatory G protein G_s, thereby activating adenylyl cyclase. The formation of the second messenger cAMP then leads to activation of PKA (cAMP protein kinase A) , which phosphorylates several key regulators of the cardiac excitation-contraction machinery. This includes phospholamban [14], the L-type Ca-channel [14,15] the ryanodine receptor [16], troponin T and I [17], myosin binding protein C [18] and the small protein phosphatase inhibitor-1 [19]. These events lead to rapid (within seconds) changes of the cardiomyocyte calcium transient and enhanced myofilament sensitivity for calcium, resulting in a potent inotropic effect.

In recent years, a debate has evolved surrounding whether the β_2-adrenergic receptor couples to the inhibitory G protein G_i and how this might be regulated [20,21]. Coupling of the β_2AR to G_i in addition to G_s has been demonstrated in several species, including mice and rats [22,23]. Interestingly, this dual coupling of the β_2AR to G_s and G_i proteins has been described as occurring sequentially (first G_s and then G_i). PKA-dependent phosphorylation of the β_2AR seems to represent the critical signal for this process [24,25]. In human myocardium, however, coupling of the β_2AR to G_i seems to be of minor importance compared with coupling to G_s [26]. In addition to coupling to G_i proteins, a rapidly increasing number of ''alternative'' signaling pathways have been described in recent years that are activated directly by the β_2AR. These include activation of the MAP (mitogen-activated kinases)-kinase–pathway, activation of phosphatidylinositol-3-kinase and phosphodiesterases (for recent reviews see [4,27,28]). Whether and how these signaling pathways contribute to the detrimental effects of chronic β-adrenergic signaling remains to be clarified.

Evidence is accumulating that a major part of the specificity of cellular signaling networks is achieved through a highly ordered spatial localization of the individual components (for a recent review see [29]). Studies on isolated cardiomyocytes and on isolated hearts have played a prominent role in proving the concept of subcellular compartmentation of signaling pathways. Early work from Keely and colleagues suggested that PKA-activation by prostaglandin E and isoproterenol exerted differential effects on target protein-phosphorylation [30]. Similar findings were then obtained in cardiac myocytes [31]. Also recently, cAMP-accumulation through the glucagon-like peptide-receptor was found to be completely uncoupled from inotropic effects in cardiac myocytes [32]. Experiments demonstrating different ''efficacies'' for cAMP generated through β-adrenergic receptor activation and directly through forskolin, further suggest spatial compartmentation of cellular signaling in cardiac myocytes [33]. Recently, this concept has been assessed through the use of electrophysiological and optical techniques. By using a local stimulation of cardiac β-adrenergic receptors and the L-type calcium channel as a readout system, Jurevicius and colleagues [34] proved spatial compartmentation of β-adrenergic signaling in frog cardiomyocytes. Zaccolo and co-workers extended these findings at the subcellular level in neonatal cardiac myocytes by using a fluorescence resonance energy transfer (FRET) approach, by which they defined the diffusion length of cAMP to be limited to approx. 1 μm [35].

There is evidence that differences in compartmentation between the β_1- and the β_2-adrenergic receptor subtype exist. These include the differential coupling to G_s and G_i proteins [22,36], potential differences in the PKA-phosphorylation pattern (which are still a matter of debate) [13,27,38–41] and differences in the inhibition of muscarinic receptor signaling through the β_1- and the β_2-subtypes [41–43]. The mechanisms underlying the spatial compartmentation of cardiomyocyte β-adrenergic signaling include differential localization at different compartments of the cardiomyocyte sarcolemma and the existence of large heterogeneous protein clusters, i.e., signalosomes, that might differ between the

β_1- and the β_2AR-subtypes [44]. Also the postreceptor signaling machinery is probably highly organized [45].

An aspect in cardiovascular research, which has long been neglected, is time as a critical parameter in signal transduction processes. The inherent properties of many experimental systems (e.g., isolated organs) make it necessary to limit studies to durations less than 24 hours. In fact, the majority of signal transduction work is performed within a time span of a few hours. Similarly, in clinical studies, an acute benefit (i.e., increased cardiac output) after administration of β-adrenergic agonists was long taken as a surrogate parameter for beneficial effects in heart failure. Accordingly, the negative hemodynamic effects of administration of a normal dose of a β-blocker to a patient with symptomatic heart failure were regarded as evidence for the beneficial effects of β-adrenergic receptor stimulation. It took experimental studies performed on a long-term time scale and long-term clinical studies, with end-points such as mortality, to discover that continuous β-adrenergic signaling is detrimental and that receptor blockade is beneficial when the sympathetic nervous system is activated. A model for such continuous overactivity of the β-adrenergic system are transgenic mice with cardiac overexpression of the human β_1-adrenergic receptor targeted to the ventricles of transgenic mice. β_1-adrenergic receptor transgenic mice display cardiomyocyte hypertrophy, followed by fibrosis, and finally heart failure [46,47]. In addition, the calcium transients in cardiomyocytes from these animals showed a delayed return to normal during diastole even at a very young age [48]. These changes were accompanied by an altered expression pattern of SR-proteins involved in calcium handling, in particular a marked reduction of the expression of junctin [49]. β_1-Receptor transgenic mice progressively develop cardiomyocyte hypertrophy (increase in cross-sectional areas by more than 300%), but the heart weight of these animals increases only to a moderate extent [46,49]. Thus, a dramatic loss of ventricular cardiomyocytes must take place. We found enhanced apoptosis in the left ventricular myocardium of these transgenic mice [48,50], and possible mechanisms of such apoptosis will be discussed in the following text.

These data indicate that the β_1-receptor system, which is ideally suited to provide short-term increases in cardiac function, causes marked structural and functional damage to the heart after extended periods of either receptor stimulation or overexpression. Thus, its chronic activation by the sympatho-adrenergic system in heart failure is most likely a maladaptive response.

Transgenic overexpression of the human β_2-adrenergic receptor targeted to the ventricles of transgenic mice has led to a multitude of new insights about β_2-adrenergic signaling in the heart. In the initial report by Milano and co-workers, a mouse model with 20 to 30 pmol of receptor/mg membrane protein was described. This led to marked enhancement of basal cardiac contractility, which could not be further augmented by β-agonist treatment [49]. Given that in the heart the β_2-subtype constitutes about 25% to 30% of the total β-adrenergic receptor number, which is normally 50 to 70 fmol/mg of membrane protein, this corresponds to a more than 1000-fold overexpression. This dramatic level of receptor density remarkably did not result in overt cardiac pathology [50] (it has to be taken into account, that increased mortality has been reported at old age [51]). Thus β_2-adrenergic receptor gene therapy was proposed to enhance myocardial function of failing hearts [52]. At least on a short-term basis, this concept was proven to effectively enhance myocardial contractility in a rabbit model of heart failure [53].

Overexpression of the human β_2-adrenergic receptor in surgical or genetic heart failure models has led to ambiguous results, however. First, the β_2TG4 mice described by Milano and colleagues have been subjected to aortic banding and myocardial infarction. While high-density overexpression of the β_2-adrenergic receptor worsened cardiac function after aortic banding [54], it rescued some of the consequences of myocardial infarction

[55]. This high level of β_2AR-overexpression clearly negatively affected the development of heart failure in several genetic heart failure models. Both in mice with cardiac overexpression of $G\alpha_q$ [58] and in mice carrying a mutation for cardiac troponin T [57], high-level overexpression of the β_2AR led to further impairment of cardiac structure and function. However, if lower levels of β_2AR-overexpression were used (30-fold), beneficial effects of β_2AR-overexpression could be demonstrated in the same model [56].

These observations were confirmed by a study of Liggett and co-workers who compared different levels of β_2AR overexpression on cardiac structure and function in transgenic mice [58]. This study shows that moderate (50-fold) overexpression was well tolerated, while very high densities of transgenic β_2AR receptors (350-fold) induced cardiac pathology. Thus, for the purpose of enhancing cardiac function by β_2ARs, there seems to exist an optimum of β_2AR overexpression with higher levels being detrimental.

TARGETS OF β-ADRENERGIC RECEPTOR STIMULATION

Although no direct comparison of cardiac overexpression of the β_1- or the β_2-adrenergic receptors has so far been done using identical mouse strains, the findings reported so far suggest remarkable differences between the two β-receptor subtypes.

The classic cAMP-signaling cascade is common to both receptor subtypes. Thus, if these differences are indeed true, they must be due to other receptor-specific signals. One obvious possible explanation is that these differences might be artifacts of overexpression, which might result in erroneous localization or protein coupling and tell us very little about the endogenous receptors. This caveat aside, a more interesting explanation might be provided by the different nonclassic signaling pathways previously discussed, which appear to be receptor-specific. In particular, coupling of the β_2-subtype to G_i may represent a potential protective signal that may be related to activation of alternative pathways including the activation of MAP-kinases [24,59,60]. Third, distinct temporal and spatial compartmentation of the classic cAMP pathway (see previous text) might explain why cAMP generated by the β_1-receptor might be different from cAMP generated by the β_2-receptor [61].

Whether these potential differences can actually be demonstrated under strictly identical conditions, and whether they are actually due to such differences in intracellular signaling, remains to be proven. However, the potential clinical implications are obvious. For example, it might suggest that β_1-selective antagonists might be superior to nonselective blockers in heart failure, because they would leave the β_2-receptor operational, or β_1-antagonists with agonistic activity at the β_2-subtype might be even better. On a more experimental level, increasing the expression of β_2-receptors either by means of gene transfer or by increasing the expression of the endogenous receptors might also turn out to be beneficial [53].

Continued stimulation of cardiomyocyte β-adrenergic receptors through infusion of β-adrenergic agonists [62], deletion of presynaptic norepinephrine-release controlling α_2-receptors [63], or overexpression of the β_1AR [47,48] in animal models (see above) leads to cardiac hypertrophy and remodeling that results, eventually, in clinically overt heart failure. Some of these effects could also be demonstrated in isolated primary cardiac myocyte cultures, in which chronic stimulation of the β_1AR, but not of the β_2AR lead to cardiomyocyte hypertrophy [64]. Despite the clarity of the results of these trials, it is still unclear what the precise signaling mechanisms are to explain these observations. Potential candidates that have been discussed for these effects include the induction of apoptosis [65], abnormal calcium-handling of the cardiomyocyte [49] and the sodium-proton-exchanger (NME) [66] (Fig. 2).

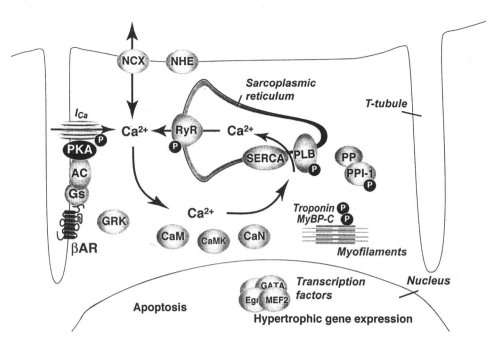

Figure 2   Calcium cycling in cardiac myocytes and regulation by PKA. Abbreviations: AC, adenylyl cyclase; RYR, ryanodine receptor; PLB, phospholamban; SERCA, sarcoplasmic reticulum calcium ATPase; CaM, calmodulin; CaMK, calmodulin-dependent kinase; CaN, calcineurin; GRK, G protein coupled receptor kinase; NCX, sodium-calcium exchanger; NHE, sodium-proton exchanger; PP, protein phosphatase. (Adapted from Ref. [4])

Induction of cardiomyocyte apoptosis by β-adrenergic stimulation was first described by Communal and colleagues [65], who found apoptotic cell death after stimulation of isolated rat cardiomyocytes with high doses of isoproterenol. In a follow-up study, the same authors described that the β₁- and the β₂-adrenergic receptor subtypes mediate opposing effects on cardiomyocyte apoptosis, with the β₁-subtype being proapoptotic and the β₂-subtype mediating antiapoptotic effects [67]. These results have been confirmed by several groups [68–70], including the studies of Xiao and co-workers [70], who isolated adult cardiomyocytes from β₁-/β₂-receptor double knockout mice and reintroduced the individual receptor subtypes by adenoviral gene transfer, resulting in "pure" β₁- and β₂-receptor expressing myocytes. While all these studies suggest that β₁-stimulation induces apoptosis and that concomitant β₂-stimulation has a protective effect, they differ as to the responsible intracellular signaling pathway. Whereas Communal and colleagues found β₂-mediated stimulation of p38 MAP-kinase to be responsible for the antiapoptotic effect [59], Xiao and co-workers, identified activation of Akt-kinase via Gᵢ as the crucial mediator [70]. Recently, the Colucci group demonstrated that the proapoptotic effect of β₁-receptor stimulation was largely dependent on the formation of reactive oxygen species [71], while results from the Xiao-group imply PKA-independent activation of CaMK [72]. These in vitro studies are paralleled by findings in transgenic mice where β₁-adrenergic receptor and Gαₛ-overexpression led to a dramatic increase in cardiomyocyte apoptosis [47,73].

In conclusion, a picture emerges that clearly links chronic β₁-receptor activation to cardiomyocyte apoptosis and suggests antiapoptotic properties for the β₂-subtype. However, the mechanistic link between receptor stimulation and apoptosis remains controversial. Nor is it clear whether β_1-receptor-mediated apoptosis really matters for the progression of heart failure. A study investigating the model of pacing-induced heart failure in dogs, a model characterized by very significant cardiomyocyte apoptosis, demonstrated that β-blocker treatment reduced apoptosis [74]. Thus, the issue of β_1-receptor-mediated apoptosis will remain an active area of research.

Functionally, the most important cardiac protein phosphorylated by PKA is phospholamban (PLB), a 52 amino acid phosphoprotein that controls SR-Ca^{2+}-uptake by inhibiting SERCA (sarcoplasmic reticulum calcium ATPase)-function [13]. PKA-mediated phosphorylation of PLB on Ser16 results in disinhibition of SERCA-function, thus causing enhanced calcium uptake into the SR (positive lusitropic effect of β_1-receptor stimulation). Interestingly, the positive lusitropic effect of β-adrenergic receptor stimulation was originally described to be completely absent in PLB-knockout mice [75]. Later, however, this view was modified because under lower external calcium concentrations the lusitropic and inotropic effect of β-adrenergic stimulation reappeared [76]. The relative contribution of phospholamban to diastolic calcium removal seems to be significantly lower in larger mammals compared with rodents [77]. In larger mammals the sarcolemmal sodium-calcium-exchanger mediates up to 30% of diastolic calcium extrusion, and the role of the exchanger becomes more important in failing hearts [78–80].

Even though phosphorylation of phospholamban is a major effector of PKA in cardiomyocytes, several lines of evidence suggest that it is not responsible for the detrimental effects of chronic β-adrenergic stimulation. Most importantly, knockout of phospholamban rescued several, but not all [81,82], heart failure models and also had remarkably beneficial effects in β_1-adrenergic receptor transgenic mice [85]. Thus, even with an inhibitory effect of PKA-phosphorylation on phospholamban function, complete inhibition of phospholamban by deletion of the gene can rescue β-adrenergically induced hypertrophy and heart failure. This suggests that inhibition of phospholamban by PKA cannot be the culprit for the detrimental effects of chronic β-adrenergic stimulation. In line with these observations, gene therapy approaches applying both inhibition of phospholamban [84,85] and augmentation of SERCA-expression [86,87] have been shown to remarkably ameliorate the failure phenotype in vitro and in animal models of heart failure. Phospholamban mutants have also been found in humans. Recently, a mutation of the phospholamban gene leading in its heterozygous state to impaired inhibition of the wild-type allele (and thus to impaired PKA-stimulation of SERCA), has been demonstrated to cause heart failure in a family with hereditary cardiomyopathy [88]. In contrast, Haghighi and colleagues recently described a human phospholamban mutation coding for a premature STOP-codon to cause heart failure both in the heterozygous and the homozygous state [89]. At present, it is unclear how these findings can be integrated with the data obtained in animals, except for the notion that any form of altered phospholamban function might be detrimental.

Recently, ryanodine receptor (RyR) hyperphosphorylation has been implicated in the pathogenesis of heart failure [16]. The authors found the RyR-receptor complex to be hyperphosphorylated by PKA, together with an increased open probability in failing human cardiomyocytes. However, others have more recently attributed the PKA-induced increase in sarcoplasmic Ca-release entirely to an indirect mechanism occurring through phospholamban phosphorylation [90], and RyR hyperphosphorylation in heart failure has also been disputed [91]. Thus, the regulation of RyR-function by PKA and its role in the pathogenesis of heart failure await further clarification [92].

Opening of the L-type Ca-channel by PKA-mediated phosphorylation serves both as a source of cytosolic calcium and (functionally dominating) as a trigger for SR-calcium-release through the RyR [79]. Although the whole-cell L-type Ca-current appears to be unaltered in heart failure, a markedly increased open probability has been described by single-channel recordings of individual channels at non-T-tubular localization [93]. Further PKA targets are myosin binding protein C (MyBPC) and troponin I located at the contractile apparatus. Phosphorylation of MyBPC may release an inhibitory effect of the N-terminal domain on myosin actin interaction [18], but its role in cardiac function remains unclear. Phosphorylation of troponin I enhances relaxation due to a reduction of myofilament sensitivity to calcium [94]. Functionally, this effect is overcome during systole by the massive increase of cytosolic calcium [77]. A functional imbalance between signaling elements that increase diastolic calcium (Ca^{2+}-channel, RyR, partly also NCX (sodium-calcium exchanger) and those that reduce it (SERCA, possibly also NCX) would elevate cytosolic free Ca^{2+}, as shown in failing cardiomyocytes [95]. It appears possible that this is a final pathway of many alterations that lead to heart failure. What might be the downstream mechanisms exerting the detrimental action of cytosolic calcium? During the last few years, a multitude of experimental results has refined our picture of how enhanced calcium levels might chronically harm cardiomyocytes (reviewed by Frey and colleagues [96]). Specifically, activation of calcineurin [97] and the calmodulin/CaM-kinase [98] pathway appear to be critically involved in Ca^{2+}-mediated cardiomyocyte hypertrophy.

Phosphatase activity has traditionally been regarded as an essentially unregulated mechanism, but recent evidence supports a more active role for phosphatases in cardiomyocytes [99]. First, phosphatase 2A has been found in β_2-receptor- ''signalosomes'' in neurons [44], and also together with the RyR-receptor at the T-tubular junction of the SR [16]. Second, heart failure is accompanied by an increase in global protein phosphatase (PP) activity [99]. Increased dephosphorylation is expected to aggravate the imbalance between phosphorylation and dephosphorylation resulting in a net decrease in steady-state phosphorylation of target proteins. An interesting link between PKA and PP1, the main protein phosphatase in the heart, is a small heat-stable PKA-substrate, the protein phosphatase inhibitor-1, (PPI-1). PPI-1 inhibits PP1 only in its PKA-phosphorylated form, and recent studies indicate that PPI-1 exerts an amplifier role in β-adrenergic signaling in cardiomyocytes [100,101]. PPI-1 mRNA, protein, and phosphorylation levels have been found to be reduced by 50%, 60% and 80%, respectively, in failing human hearts [101,102]. The reduction in PPI-1 can well explain the discrepancy between unchanged PP1-protein expression and increased global PP1 activity in failing hearts [99]. Furthermore, expression of a constitutively active inhibitor rescued function of isolated cardiomyocytes from failing hearts [100]. These observations suggest that PPI-1, via loss of its amplifier role, participates in β-adrenergic desensitization in heart failure. It will be interesting to delineate the downstream targets of this regulatory mechanism, i.e., to identify the proteins whose phosphorylation is most sensitive to control by PPI-1.

There is now increasing evidence, that the cardiac isoform of the sodium-proton-exchanger family is critically involved in the detrimental effects of β_1AR signaling. Although acute β-adrenergic receptor stimulation may *inhibit* NHE1 [103], its activation seems to play a major role in mediating the long-term hypertrophic response to β-adrenergic stimulation. In β_1-adrenergic receptor transgenic mice, NHE1 is upregulated, and pharmacological NHE1-inhibition prevented the development not only of hypertrophy and fibrosis, but also of heart failure in these mice [66]. Thus, cardiac NHE1 appears to be essential for the detrimental cardiac effects of chronic β_1-receptor stimulation. It may do so either by serving as a direct downstream target of sustained β_1-adrenergic receptor activation, or by playing a permissive role in the propagation of a detrimental signal that remains to be determined. The mechanism(s) by which NHE1-inhibition exerts its protective effect on β_1-adrenergic receptor induced cardiac hypertrophy is still unclear and an area of active investigation, but increasing evidence points toward a critical role of enhanced intracellular sodium concentration through NHE1 in cardiac hypertrophy [104]. Candidates for regulation of NHE1 involve Ca^{2+}-calmodulin dependent activation [105] and transcriptional up-regulation of the NHE1-gene [66].

CHANGES OF β-ADRENERGIC SIGNAL TRANSDUCTION IN HEART FAILURE

For almost two decades, the perception of β-adrenergic signaling in heart failure was dominated by the fact that it is desensitized in failing human hearts. Desensitization of β-adrenergic signal transduction in heart failure was first discovered by Bristow and co-workers [106]. Central findings to explain this phenomenon of reduced responsiveness to β-adrenergic stimulation were a reduction of the density of $β_1ARs$ in failing human myocardium [106], a decrease of NE–re-uptake [107] and finally an increase in G_i-protein expression [110] and in GRK2 (βARK)-activity [109], a receptor kinase that phosphorylates and thereby inactivates βARs. Table 1 gives an overview of the changes in protein expression of compounds of the β-adrenergic signaling system in heart failure. Originating from the traditional picture of βAR-signaling in the heart, this desensitization process was interpreted primarily as a loss of inotropy and therefore introduce detrimental for a compromised heart. As previously detailed, recent evidence supports a different view of the role of β-adrenergic receptor desensitization. The observed desensitization of βAR-receptors represents an adaptation process to the highly increased levels of catecholamines in heart failure. Thus, the β-adrenergic signal transduction cascade is operative, but with its sensitivity adjusted to high catecholamine levels. [Table 1] This would then have to be interpreted as a beneficial readjustment of the signaling cascade to minimize the detrimental effects of chronic stimulation of the myocardium.

The desensitization pattern of the two main cardiac βAR-subtypes, $β_1$ and $β_2$, is rather different. While the $β_1$-subtype shows prominent downregulation (by about 50%), the $β_2$-subtype is nearly unaffected in its density [110]. Remarkably, in cell culture experiments, the $β_2$-subtype desensitizes much faster than the $β_1$-subtype [111]. The reason for this discrepancy is unknown. The selective loss of the $β_1AR$-subtype in human heart failure leads to a $β_1$:$β_2$-ratio of approx. 1:1, thus enhancing the relative contribution of the $β_2AR$-subtype. However, it has to be taken into account that the relevant ligand in vivo, noradrenaline, which is released by sympathetic nerve endings, is significantly $β_1$-selective and that noradrenaline levels are enhanced in many heart failure patients. Thus, the overall signal will still be dominated by the $β_1$-subtype.

Table 1 Changes in Protein Expression of Components of the β-Adrenergic Signaling System in Heart Failure

β-Adrenergic Signaling Component	Change of Expression in Heart Failure
$β_1$-adrenergic receptor	↓
$β_2$-adrenergic receptor	↔
$β_3$-adrenergic receptor	↑
Stimulatory G protein, $G_sα$	↔↓
Inhibitory G protein, $G_iα$	↑
Adenylyl cyclase, AC	↔↓
G protein coupled receptor kinase, GRK	↑
SR calcium ATPase, SERCA	↓

A regulatory mechanism of cardiac β-adrenergic signaling, which has gained major interest in the recent years, is phosphorylation of the βAR through G protein coupled receptor kinases (GRKs), which switch off the capacity of an agonist-activated receptor to activate G proteins [112–114]. After the first description of elevated GRK activity and GRK2 (synonymous for βARK1 = βAR kinase1) expression in heart failure [109], numerous studies have confirmed elevated GRK2 activities in heart failure (reviewed by Lohse [115]). Elevated GRK activity is often regarded as a major factor contributing to the progression of heart failure through desensitization of the β-adrenergic signal transduction pathway. Evidence for this argument comes mainly from studies using a C-terminal peptide of GRK2 (termed βARKct) that not only has been demonstrated to effectively block desensitization of the βAR in vitro [116], but which also proved to be an effective therapeutic agent.

The prevailing view that GRK2-activity is generally detrimental in the heart largely relies on the perplexing success of a GRK2-peptide (βARKct) to prevent the heart failure phenotype in various heart failure models [51,57,117,118]. The βγ-scavenging properties of the βARKct-peptide results in reduced translocation of GRK2 to the membrane, thereby reducing receptor-phosphorylation [118]. This inhibition of βAR-desensitization is regarded as the protective mechanism that increases inotropy and prevents the internalization and coupling to "alternative" signaling mechanisms, such as the activation of src-dependent pathways [119].

Much evidence, however, points towards alternative mechanisms of action. First and foremost, the overwhelming clinical efficacy of β-blockers in the therapy of heart failure constitutes an obvious paradox to the "resensitization-hypothesis." In addition, the phenotype of $\beta_1 AR$-transgenic mice is closely mimicked by $G\alpha_s$ and PKA-transgenics, therefore, with proteins immanent to the "classic" signaling cascade further downstream of the $\beta_1 AR$. The receptor subtype proven capable of activating the "alternative" signaling mechanisms, i.e., the β_2-subtype, seems to be less detrimental when overexpressed [49,58].

Second, GRK2-transgenic mice obviously do not show signs of overt cardiac pathology or heart failure [120]. If enhanced GRK2-function would be a cornerstone of heart failure pathogenesis, these animals with strong overexpression of GRK2 should display a dramatic phenotype.

Third, a direct comparison of the beneficial effects of βARKct and β-blockers in a transgenic mouse model of heart failure demonstrated that β-blockers conferred a (very prominent) additional benefit toward the progression of heart failure in addition to βARKct alone (and vice versa), suggesting a unrelated mechanism of action for both therapeutic principles [118].

And finally, the protective actions of βARKct can be closely reproduced by other βγ-binding proteins such as phosducin which is a abequitous G protein resetator. Cardiac overexpression of a phosducin-mutant led to quantitatively indistinguishable beneficial effects on heart failure progression in a rabbit model of heart failure [121].

Thus, the beneficial effects of the βARKct-peptide might be significantly due to inhibition of βγ-mediated signaling pathways rather than pure resensitization of the βAR-system. According to this view, the beneficial effects of βARKct might be achieved not through but rather *despite* resensitization of the β_1-adrenergic receptor. Both β-blockade and βARkct might therefore be used as complimentary therapeutic principles for the treatment of heart failure.

β-BLOCKERS AS THERAPEUTIC PRINCIPLE IN HEART FAILURE

β-adrenergic receptor blockade is now regarded as the single most effective therapeutic principle in heart failure treatment [122]. Despite the discovery of antagonists for the β-adrenergic receptor almost half a century ago by Sir James Black and co-workers and their rapid introduction into clinical practice, β-blockers have been introduced into the treatment of heart failure only recently. As previously detailed, the reasons underlying this discrepancy are most probably due to the fact that short-term hemodynamic improvement was long regarded as a surrogate parameter of therapeutic effectiveness of a drug in heart failure. In addition, a major focus of β-adrenergic research focused on desensitization of cardiovascular β-adrenergic signaling in heart failure and on ways how to preclude this. Much credit is owed to a small group of Scandinavian cardiologists, who followed their own concept and started to treat small numbers of heart failure patients with β-blockers in the late 1970s [123]. It took a very long time for these pioneering studies to result in a large mortality trial [124]. From then on several large trials, among them some of the largest heart failure trials ever conducted, showed a marked benefit for this therapeutic principle in the treatment of heart failure [125,126].

As ACE (angiotensin-converting enzyme)-inhibitors had been successfully introduced into heart failure therapy in the meantime, the effect of β-blocker treatment in heart failure had to be tested not vs. placebo, but vs. the established treatment regime, including ACE-inhibitors. Despite this, β-blockade lead to impressive reductions of mortality (ranging from 35% to 60% [124–126]), with larger effects than ACE-inhibitors tested vs. placebo. In contrast to ACE-inhibitors, β-blockers not only reverse remodeling, but also increase systolic function after several months of treatment [127].

Obvious questions, such as how would β-blockade alone vs. placebo perform, or whether ACE-inhibitors would achieve a significant reduction in mortality on the background of β-blockade, have not been tested. Exciting evidence pertaining to these questions may be expected from CIBIS III, a trial containing a patient group that starts treatment for heart failure with the β-blocker bisoprolol alone, in the absence of ACE-inhibition. The competitive antagonism of β-blockers leads to–as expected from a dynamically regulated system–reversal of the agonist-induced desensitization processes, including upregulation of decreased β-receptor levels. Whether or not this phenomenon has meaningful effects remains to be defined.

Several large clinical trials with carvedilol, metoprolol, and bisoprolol have demonstrated a significant benefit in large placebo-controlled trials Chapter 13 [124–126]. On the contrary, two β-blockers (xamoterol and bucindolol) have failed to significantly reduce mortality or even increased mortality [128,129]. How might this be explained? The most likely explanation for the failure of xamoterol is the pronounced partial agonism exerted by this agents [130]. In the sensitive setting of β_1-adrenergic receptor transgenic mice, the potency of xamoterol to activate the β_1AR actually amounts to 48% of the full agonist isoproterenol [130]. Therefore, xamoterol acts as an agonist under nearly all circumstances in vivo, leading to chronic β_1AR-signaling and its negative consequences. The situation is different for bucindolol. Bucindolol led to a nonsignificant reduction of mortality in the BEST trial. Two main reasons might account for this finding. First, the study population of the BEST trial differed markedly from the other big heart failure trials. It included a high percentage of African-Americans and of women, and both of these groups are underrepresented in other trials [130]. In both groups, the beneficial effects of β-blockade were less pronounced compared with the effects in Caucasians [128]. Second, bucindolol might display some degree of partial agonism. This has been shown not only in several animal species, but recently for the human β_1-adrenergic receptor [131,132]. The reason why this property of bucindolol has not been detected in prior studies investigating bucindolol, may be attributed to the dependency of its partial agonist activity on the desensitization level of the receptor [132,133]. Thus, in myocardium from failing human hearts with desensitized β-receptors, bucindolol does display its partial agonist activity only after prior resensitization [132].

Given that partial agonism of β-blockers appears to be detrimental in heart failure, a property that might further contribute to their clinical efficacy is inverse agonism at the β_1-adrenergic receptor. β-adrenergic receptors show some degree of spontaneous activity, i.e., signaling in the absence of agonist. Under the assumption that every chronic β_1-adrenergic signal is detrimental for a diseased heart, β-blockers with inverse agonistic activity might be expected to be superior to β-blockers devoid of inverse agonism. Both metoprolol and bisoprolol–but not propranolol, xamoterol, and bucindolol–have recently been shown to exert inverse agonism at the β_1AR [130,134], showing a positive correlation of inverse agonism and clinical efficacy.

Carvedilol, however, does not possess this property, but has numerous other effects such as α_1AR-blocking and antioxidative effects. Thus, at present, the contribution of inverse agonism at the β_1AR to the clinical efficacy of a β-blocker is unclear. Carvedilol, as an unselective β-blocker with multiple other pharmacological effects, has recently been compared with the β_1-selective metoprolol in one of the largest clinical heart failure trials to date, COMET [135]. Carvedilol showed a 6% higher reduction in overall mortality (17% higher relative to metoprolol). It is difficult to draw a final conclusion from this study because carvedilol was compared with metoprolol-tartrate and not with the slow-release formulation metoprolol-succinate, which is the formulation proven to be effective in heart failure trials [126]. In addition, the dosage of carvedilol led to a significantly greater reduction of heart rate (short-term) and blood pressure (long-term) than did metoprolol. Thus, unequal dosage of the two agents relating to their β-blocking efficacy cannot be excluded. What can be concluded from this study is that at least 83% of the reduction in mortality through carvedilol is achieved through blocking chronic β_1AR-signaling.

MUTATIONS IN ADRENERGIC RECEPTOR GENES LEADING TO ALTERED SIGNALING PROPERTIES

In addition to the *general* principles of receptor regulation and dysregulation in health and disease there is increasing evidence that genetic polymorphisms of key proteins of the β-adrenergic signaling cascade can significantly influence the signaling properties of this system in *individual* patients [136,137]. Both the α_2-adrenergic receptor as the principal presynaptic regulator of noradrenaline-release and the β-adrenergic receptors as the principal effectors have been extensively studied, and numerous polymorphisms with potential significant clinical impact have been identified (Fig. 3). Among the multitude of receptor polymorphisms discovered to date, three appear to be of special relevance for the pathophysiology and treatment of heart failure. All three go in line with the hypothesis that enhanced β_1-adrenergic signaling is detrimental for the heart.

Among the presynaptic α_2-receptors, a deletion mutant of the α_{2C}-subtype has been shown to be significantly associated with both enhanced noradrenaline release and the risk of developing heart failure [138,139]. Similarly, a hypofunctional β_1-adrenergic receptor mutant (Gly389) has been associated with a better prognosis in heart failure patients. In CHO-cells transfected with the different receptor mutants, the Arg389 variant displayed a three-fold higher β-adrenergic-stimulatory adenylyl cyclase activity than the (less common) Gly389 variant. Whereas it is not undisputed whether the Arg389 polymorphism of the β_1-adrenergic receptor alone leads to a markedly increased risk per se [140], combination with the α_{2C}-deletion mutant has been demonstrated to significantly enhance the risk of heart failure [138]. Thus, the combination of disinhibited noradrenaline-release and a

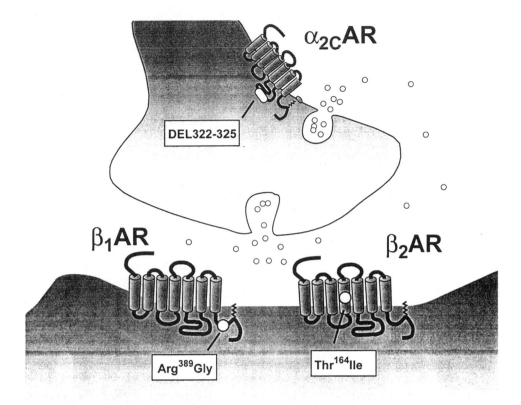

Figure 3 Important receptor polymorphisms potentially involved in heart failure. Three receptor polymorphisms of the β-adrenergic receptor system, that have been linked to heart failure prognosis.

hyperfunctional β₁-adrenergic receptor leading to a chronic enhancement of the β-adrenergic signaling cascade, increases the risk of developing heart failure, with about 2% of the general population carrying this combination.

Less than 3% of the average population are heterozygous carriers of the Ile164 variant of the β₂-adrenergic receptor. In contrast to the Arg389 polymorphism of the β₁-adrenergic receptor, this variant is hypofunctional with impaired agonist binding and adenylyl cyclase activation [141]. Comparison of the "wild-type" Gly164 β₂-adrenergic receptor and the Ile164 variant when overexpressed in the hearts of transgenic mice, confirmed this notion with the hypofunctional Ile164 transgenics being not significantly different from wild-type animals [142]. In principle, these findings can be reproduced after β-agonist-application in humans and the 164Ile mutant of the β₂-adrenergic receptor might be associated with decreased survival in heart failure [136].

Thus, the clinical data from the three best characterized variants of the βAR-signal transduction system support the experimental evidence that chronic β₁-adrenergic signaling is detrimental and β₂AR-signaling might be protective. It is reasonable to expect that our picture of genetic variations in receptors and other key proteins of the β-adrenergic signaling cascade will soon be refined with more variants to be discovered and more reliable clinical data to be obtained. This might, in the not too distant future, lead to individualized treatment regimens that take into account which patients will profit the most from β-blockade, and which patients will benefit most from alternative therapeutic regimens.

ACKNOWLEDGEMENTS

Studies in the authors' laboratories were supported by grants from the Deutsche Forschungsgemeinschaft (SFB 355, Leibniz award) and the Fonds der Chemischen Industrie.

REFERENCES

1. Brodde OE, Michel MC. Adrenergic and muscarinic receptors in the human heart. Pharmacol Rev 1999; 51:651–690.
2. Alquist RP. A study of the adrenotropic receptors. Am J Physiol 1948; 153:586–600.
3. Lands AM, Arnold A, McAuliff JP, Luduena FP, Brown TG. Differentiation of receptor systems activated by sympathamimetic amines. Nature 1967; 214:597–598.
4. Brodde OE. β-adrenoceptors in cardiac disease. Pharmacol Ther 1993; 60:405–430.
5. Gauthier C, Langin D, Balligand JL. β_3-adrenoceptors in the cardiovascular system. Trends Pharmacol Sci 2000; 21:426–431.
6. Arch JR, Ainsworth AT, Cawthorne MA, Piercy V, Sennitt MV, Thody VE, Wilson C, Wilson S. Atypical beta-adrenoceptor on brown adipocytes as target for anti-obesity drugs. Nature 1984; 309:163–5.
7. Rohrer DK, Chruscinski A, Schauble EH, Bernstein D, Kobilka BK. Cardiovascular and metabolic alterations in mice lacking both beta1- and beta2-adrenergic receptors. J Biol Chem 1999; 274:16701–16708.
8. Kaumann AJ, Molenaar P. Modulation of human cardiac function through 4 beta-adrenoceptor populations. Naunyn Schmiedebergs Arch Pharmacol 1997; 355:667–681.
9. Kaumann AJ. (-)-CGP 12177-induced increase of human atrial contraction through a putative third beta-adrenoceptor. Br J Pharmacol 1996; 117:93–98.
10. Konkar AA, Zhai Y, Granneman JG. β_1-adrenergic receptors mediate β_3-adrenergic-independent effects of CGP 12177 in brown adipose tissue. Mol Pharmacol 2000; 57:252–258.
11. Kaumann AJ, Engelhardt S, Hein L, Molenaar P, Lohse M. Abolition of (-)-CGP 12177-evoked cardiostimulation in double β_1/β_2-adrenoceptor knockout mice. Naunyn Schmiedebergs Arch Pharmacol 2001; 363:87–93.
12. Kaumann A, Bartel S, Molenaar P, Sanders L, Burrell K, Vetter D, Hempel P, Karczewski P, Krause EG. Activation of β_2-adrenergic receptors hastens relaxation and mediates phosphorylation of phospholamban, troponin I., and C-protein in ventricular myocardium from patients with terminal heart failure. Circulation 1999; 99:65–72.
13. Simmerman HK, Jones LR. Phospholamban: protein structure, mechanism of action, and role in cardiac function. Physiol Rev 1998; 78:921–947.
14. Zhao XL, Gutierrez LM, Chang CF, Hosey MM. The α_1-subunit of skeletal muscle L-type Ca channels is the key target for regulation by A-kinase and protein phosphatase-1C. Biochem Biophys Res Commun 1994; 198:166–173.
15. Gerhardstein BL, Puri TS, Chien AJ, Hosey MM. Identification of the sites phosphorylated by cyclic AMP-dependent protein kinase on the beta 2 subunit of L-type voltage-dependent calcium channels. Biochemistry 1999; 38:10361–10370.
16. Marx SO, Reiken S, Hisamatsu Y, Jayaraman T, Burkhoff D, Rosemblit N, Marks AR. PKA phosphorylation dissociates FKBP12.6 from the calcium release channel (ryanodine receptor): defective regulation in failing hearts. Cell 2000; 101:365–376.
17. Sulakhe PV, Vo XT. Regulation of phospholamban and troponin-I phosphorylation in the intact rat cardiomyocytes by adrenergic and cholinergic stimuli. Mol Cell Biochem 1995; 149-150:103–126.

18. Kunst G, Kress KR, Gruen M, Uttenweiler D, Gautel M, Fink RH. Myosin binding protein C., a phosphorylation-dependent force regulator in muscle that controls the attachment of myosin heads by its interaction with myosin S2. Circ Res 2000; 86:51–58.

19. Zhang ZY, Zhou B, Xie L. Modulation of protein kinase signaling by protein phosphatases and inhibitors. Pharmacol Ther 2002; 93:307–17.

20. Xiao RP, Cheng H, Zhou YY, Kuschel M, Lakatta EG. Recent advances in cardiac β_2-adrenergic signal transduction. Circ Res 1999; 85:1092–100.

21. Steinberg SF. The molecular basis for distinct β-adrenergic receptor subtype actions in cardiomyocytes. Circ Res 1999; 85:1101–1111.

22. Xiao RP, Avdonin P, Zhou YY, Cheng H, Akhter SA, Eschenhagen T, Lefkowitz RJ, Koch WJ, Lakatta EG. Coupling of beta2-adrenoceptor to Gi proteins and its physiological relevance in murine cardiac myocytes. Circ Res 1999; 84:43–52.

23. Xiao RP, Ji X, Lakatta EG. Functional coupling of the beta 2-adrenoceptor to a pertussis toxin-sensitive G protein in cardiac myocytes. Mol Pharmacol 1995; 47:322–329.

24. Daaka Y, Luttrell LM, Lefkowitz RJ. Switching of the coupling of the β_2-adrenergic receptor to different G proteins by protein kinase. A. Nature 1997; 390:88–91.

25. Devic E, Xiang Y, Gould D, Kobilka B. Beta-adrenergic receptor subtype-specific signaling in cardiac myocytes from β_1 and β_2 adrenoceptor knockout mice. Mol Pharmacol 2001; 60: 577–583.

26. Kaumann AJ, Sanders L, Lynham JA, Bartel S, Kuschel M, Karczewski P, Krause EG. b$_2$-adrenoceptor activation by zinterol causes protein phosphorylation, contractile effects and relaxant effects through a cAMP pathway in human atrium. Mol Cell Biochem 1996; 163–164: 113–123.

27. Hall RA, Lefkowitz RJ. Regulation of G protein-coupled receptor signaling by scaffold proteins. Circ Res. 2002; 91:672–680.

28. Lohse MJ, Engelhardt S, Eschenhagen T. β-adrenergic signaling in heart failure. Circ Res 2003:in press.

29. Steinberg SF, Brunton LL. Compartmentation of G protein-coupled signaling pathways in cardiac myocytes. Annu Rev Pharmacol Toxicol 2001; 41:751–773.

30. Keely SL. Activation of cAMP-dependent protein kinase without a corresponding increase in phosphorylase activity. Res Commun Chem Pathol Pharmacol 1977; 18:283–290.

31. Hayes JS, Brunton LL, Brown JH, Reese JB, Mayer SE. Hormonally specific expression of cardiac protein kinase activity. Proc Natl Acad Sci U S A 1979; 76:1570–1574.

32. Vila Petroff MG, Egan JM, Wang X, Sollott SJ. Glucagon-like peptide-1 increases cAMP but fails to augment contraction in adult rat cardiac myocytes. Circ Res 2001; 89:445–452.

33. Hohl CM, Li QA. Compartmentation of cAMP in adult canine ventricular myocytes. Relation to single-cell free Ca^{2+} transients. Circ Res 1991; 69:1369–1379.

34. Jurevicius J, Fischmeister R. cAMP compartmentation is responsible for a local activation of cardiac Ca^{2+} channels by β-adrenergic agonists. Proc Natl Acad Sci U S A 1996; 93: 295–299.

35. Zaccolo M, Pozzan T. Discrete microdomains with high concentration of cAMP in stimulated rat neonatal cardiac myocytes. Science 2002; 295:1711–1715.

36. Kuschel M, Zhou YY, Cheng H, Zhang SJ, Chen Y, Lakatta EG, Xiao RP. G$_i$ protein-mediated functional compartmentalization of cardiac β_2-adrenergic signaling. J Biol Chem 1999; 274:22048–22052.

37. Kuschel M, Zhou YY, Spurgeon HA, Bartel S, Karczewski P, Zhang SJ, Krause EG, Lakatta EG, Xiao RP. b$_2$-adrenergic cAMP signaling is uncoupled from phosphorylation of cytoplasmic proteins in canine heart. Circulation 1999; 99:2458–2465.

38. Bartel S, Krause EG, Wallukat G, Karczewski P. New insights into β_2-adrenoceptor signalling in the adult rat heart. Cardiovasc Res 2003; 57:694–703.

39. Molenaar P, Bartel S, Cochrane A, Vetter D, Jalali H, Pohlner P, Burrell K, Karczewski P, Krause EG, Kaumann A. Both β_2- and β_1-adrenergic receptors mediate hastened relaxation and phosphorylation of phospholamban and troponin I in ventricular myocardium of Fallot infants, consistent with selective coupling of β_2-adrenergic receptors to G$_s$-protein. Circulation 2000; 102:1814–1821.

40. Altschuld RA, Starling RC, Hamlin RL, Billman GE, Hensley J, Castillo L, Fertel RH, Hohl CM, Robitaille PM, Jones LR, et al. Response of failing canine and human heart cells to β_2-adrenergic stimulation. Circulation 1995; 92:1612–1618.

41. Aprigliano O, Rybin VO, Pak E, Robinson RB, Steinberg SF. β1-and β2-adrenergic receptors exhibit differing susceptibility to muscarinic accentuated antagonism. Am J Physiol 1997; 272:H2726–H2735.

42. Skeberdis VA, Jurevicius J, Fischmeister R. Pharmacological characterization of the receptors involved in the beta-adrenoceptor-mediated stimulation of the L-type Ca2 + current in frog ventricular myocytes. Br J Pharmacol 1997; 121:1277–1286.

43. Rau T, Nose M, Remmers U, Weil J, Weissmuller A, Davia K, Harding S, Peppel K, Koch WJ, Eschenhagen T. Overexpression of wild-type Ga$_{i2}$ suppresses b-adrenergic signaling in cardiac myocytes. Faseb J. 2003; 17:523–525.

44. Davare MA, Avdonin V, Hall DD, Peden EM, Burette A, Weinberg RJ, Horne MC, Hoshi T, Hell JW. A β_2-adrenergic receptor signaling complex assembled with the Ca^{2+} channel Cav1.2. Science 2001; 293:98–101.

45. Zaccolo M, Magalhaes P, Pozzan T. Compartmentalisation of cAMP and Ca^{2+} signals. Curr Opin Cell Biol 2002; 14:160–166.

46. Engelhardt S, Hein L, Wiesmann F, Lohse MJ. Progressive hypertrophy and heart failure in β_1-adrenergic receptor transgenic mice. ProcNatl Acad Sci U S A 1999; 96:7059–7064.

47. Bisognano JD, Weinberger HD, Bohlmeyer TJ, Pende A, Raynolds MV, Sastravaha A, Roden R, Asano K, Blaxall BC, Wu SC, Communal C, Singh K, Colucci W, Bristow MR, Port DJ. Myocardial-directed overexpression of the human β_1-adrenergic receptor in transgenic mice. J Mol Cell Cardiol 2000; 32:817–830.

48. Engelhardt S, Boknik P, Keller U, Neumann J, Lohse MJ, Hein L. Early impairment of calcium handling and altered expression of junction in hearts of mice overexpressing the β_1-adrenergic receptor. FASEBJ 2001; 15:2718–2720.

49. Milano CA, Allen LF, Rockman HA, Dolber PC, McMinn TR, Chien KR, Johnson TD, Bond RA, Lefkowitz RJ. Enhanced myocardial function in transgenic mice overexpressing the β_2-adrenergic receptor. Science 1994; 264:582–586.

50. Koch WJ, Lefkowitz RJ, Rockman HA. Functional consequences of altering myocardial adrenergic receptor signaling. AnnuRev Physiol 2000; 62:237–260.

51. Du XJ, Gao XM, Wang B, Jennings GL, Woodcock EA, Dart AM. Age-dependent cardiomyopathy and heart failure phenotype in mice overexpressing beta(2)-adrenergic receptors in the heart. CardiovascRes 2000; 48:448–454.

52. Lefkowitz RJ, Rockman HA, Koch WJ. Catecholamines, cardiac beta-adrenergic receptors, and heart failure. Circulation 2000; 101:1634–1637.

53. Akhter SA, Skaer CA, Kypson AP, McDonald PH, Peppel KC, Glower DD, Lefkowitz RJ, Koch WJ. Restoration of β-adrenergic signaling in failing cardiac ventricular myocytes via adenoviral-mediated gene transfer. ProcNatl Acad Sci U S A 1997; 94:12100–12105.

54. Du XJ, Autelitano DJ, Dilley RJ, Wang B, Dart AM, Woodcock EA. β_2-adrenergic receptor overexpression exacerbates development of heart failure after aortic stenosis. Circulation 2000; 101:71–77.

55. Du XJ, Gao XM, Jennings GL, Dart AM, Woodcock EA. Preserved ventricular contractility in infarcted mouse heart overexpressing β_2-adrenergic receptors. Am J Physiol Heart Circ Physiol 2000; 279:H2456–H2463.

56. Dorn GW, Tepe NM, Lorenz JN, Koch WJ, Liggett SB. Low- and high-level transgenic expression of β_2-adrenergic receptors differentially affect cardiac hypertrophy and function in Ga$_q$- overexpressing mice. Proc Natl Acad Sci U S A 1999; 96:6400–6405.

57. Freeman K, Lerman I, Kranias EG, Bohlmeyer T, Bristow MR, Lefkowitz RJ, Iaccarino G, Koch WJ, Leinwand LA. Alterations in cardiac adrenergic signaling and calcium cycling differentially affect the progression of cardiomyopathy. J Clin Invest 2001; 107:967–974.

58. Liggett SB, Tepe NM, Lorenz JN, Canning AM, Jantz TD, Mitarai S, Yatani A. Dorn GW 2nd. Early and delayed consequences of β_2-adrenergic receptor overexpression in mouse hearts: critical role for expression level. Circulation 2000; 101:1707–1714.

59. Communal C, Colucci WS, Singh K. p38 mitogen-activated protein kinase pathway protects adult rat ventricular myocytes against β-adrenergic receptor-stimulated apoptosis. J Biol Chem 2000; 275:19395–19400.

60. Luttrell LM, Ferguson SS, Daaka Y, Miller WE, Maudsley S, Della Rocca GJ, Lin F, Kawakatsu H, Owada K, Luttrell DK, Caron MG, Lefkowitz RJ. β-arrestin-dependent formation of β₂ adrenergic receptor-Src protein kinase complexes. Science 1999; 283:655–661.

61. Lohse MJ, Engelhardt S. Protein kinase A transgenes: the many faces of cAMP. Circ Res 2001; 89:938–940.

62. Rona G. Catecholamine cardiotoxicity. J Mol Cell Cardiol 1985; 17:291–306.

63. Hein L, Altman JD, Kobilka BK. Two functionally distinct α_2-adrenergic receptors regulate sympathetic neurotransmission. Nature 1999; 402:181–184.

64. Schafer M, Frischkopf K, Taimor G, Piper HM, Schluter KD. Hypertrophic effect of selective β₁-adrenoceptor stimulation on ventricular cardiomyocytes from adult rat. Am J Physiol Cell Physiol 2000; 279:C495–C503.

65. Communal C, Singh K, Pimentel DR, Colucci WS. Norepinephrine stimulates apoptosis in adult rat ventricular myocytes by activation of the β-adrenergic pathway. Circulation 1998; 98:1329–1334.

66. Engelhardt S, Hein L, Keller U, Klambt K, Lohse MJ. Inhibition of Na^+-H^+-exchange prevents hypertrophy, fibrosis, and heart failure in β₁-adrenergic receptor transgenic mice. Circ Res 2002; 90:814–819.

67. Communal C, Singh K, Sawyer DB, Colucci WS. Opposing effects of β₁- and β₂-adrenergic receptors on cardiac myocyte apoptosis: role of a pertussis toxin-sensitive G protein. Circulation 1999; 100:2210–2212.

68. Chesley A, Lundberg MS, Asai T, Xiao RP, Ohtani S, Lakatta EG, Crow MT. The β₂-adrenergic receptor delivers an antiapoptotic signal to cardiac myocytes through G_i-dependent coupling to phosphatidylinositol 3'-kinase. Circ Res 2000; 87:1172–1179.

69. Zaugg M, Xu W, Lucchinetti E, Shafiq SA, Jamali NZ, Siddiqui MA. β-adrenergic receptor subtypes differentially affect apoptosis in adult rat ventricular myocytes. Circulation 2000; 102:344–350.

70. Zhu WZ, Zheng M, Koch WJ, Lefkowitz RJ, Kobilka BK, Xiao RP. Dual modulation of cell survival and cell death by β₂-adrenergic signaling in adult mouse cardiac myocytes. Proc Natl Acad Sci U S A 2001; 98:1607–1612.

71. Remondino A, Kwon SH, Communal C, Pimentel DR, Sawyer DB, Singh K, Colucci WS. β-adrenergic receptor-stimulated apoptosis in cardiac myocytes is mediated by reactive oxygen species/c-Jun NH2-terminal kinase-dependent activation of the mitochondrial pathway. Circ Res 2003; 92:136–138.

72. Zhu WZ, Wang SQ, Chakir K, Yang D, Zhang T, Brown JH, Devic E, Kobilka BK, Cheng H, Xiao RP. Linkage of β₁-adrenergic stimulation to apoptotic heart cell death through protein kinase A-independent activation of Ca^{2+}/calmodulin kinase II. J Clin Invest 2003; 111: 617–625.

73. Geng YJ, Ishikawa Y, Vatner DE, Wagner TE, Bishop SP, Vatner SF, Homcy CJ. Apoptosis of cardiac myocytes in Gsα transgenic mice. Circ Res 1999; 84:34–42.

74. Sabbah HN, Sharov VG, Gupta RC, Todor A, Singh V, Goldstein S. Chronic therapy with metoprolol attenuates cardiomyocyte apoptosis in dogs with heart failure. J Am Coll Cardiol 2000; 36:1698–1705.

75. Luo W, Grupp IL, Harrer J, Ponniah S, Grupp G, Duffy JJ, Doetschman T, Kranias EG. Targeted ablation of the phospholamban gene is associated with markedly enhanced myocardial contractility and loss of β-agonist stimulation. Circ Res 1994; 75:401–409.

76. Serikov VB, Petrashevskaya NN, Canning AM, Schwartz A. Reduction of Ca_i^{2+} restores uncoupled β-adrenergic signaling in isolated perfused transgenic mouse hearts. Circ Res 2001; 88:9–11.

77. Bers DM. Cardiac excitation-contraction coupling. Nature 2002; 415:198–205.

78. Hasenfuss G, Schillinger W, Lehnart SE, Preuss M, Pieske B, Maier LS, Prestle J, Minami K, Just H. Relationship between Na^+-Ca^{2+}-exchanger protein levels and diastolic function of failing human myocardium. Circulation 1999; 99:641–648.

79. Movsesian MA, Karimi M, Green K, Jones LR. $Ca^{(2+)}$-transporting ATPase, phospholamban, and calsequestrin levels in nonfailing and failing human myocardium. Circulation 1994; 90: 653–657.

80. Schwinger RH, Bohm M, Schmidt U, Karczewski P, Bavendiek U, Flesch M, Krause EG, Erdmann E. Unchanged protein levels of SERCA II and phospholamban but reduced Ca^{2+} uptake and Ca^{2+}-ATPase activity of cardiac sarcoplasmic reticulum from dilated cardiomyopathy patients compared with patients with nonfailing hearts. Circulation 1995; 92:3220–3228.

81. Song Q, Schmidt AG, Hahn HS, Carr AN, Frank B, Pater L, Gerst M, Young K, Hoit BD, McConnell BK, Haghighi K, Seidman CE, Seidman JG, Dorn GW, Kranias EG. Rescue of cardiomyocyte dysfunction by phospholamban ablation does not prevent ventricular failure in genetic hypertrophy. J Clin Invest 2003; 111:859–867.

82. Delling U, Sussman MA, Molkentin JD. Re-evaluating sarcoplasmic reticulum function in heart failure. Nat Med 2000; 6:942–943.

83. Engelhardt S, Hein L, Kranias E, Lohse MJ. Phospholamban is critically involved in β-adrenergic receptor induced hypertrophy and heart failure. Naunyn-Schmiedeberg's Arch. Pharmacol 2003; 367:R93.

84. Hoshijima M, Ikeda Y, Iwanaga Y, Minamisawa S, Date MO, Gu Y, Iwatate M, Li M, Wang L, Wilson JM, Wang Y, Ross J, Chien KR. Chronic suppression of heart-failure progression by a pseudophosphorylated mutant of phospholamban via in vivo cardiac rAAV gene delivery. Nat Med 2002; 8:864–871.

85. del Monte F, Harding SE, Dec GW, Gwathmey JK, Hajjar RJ. Targeting phospholamban by gene transfer in human heart failure. Circulation 2002; 105:904–907.

86. del Monte F, Harding SE, Schmidt U, Matsui T, Kang ZB, Dec GW, Gwathmey JK, Rosenzweig A, Hajjar RJ. Restoration of contractile function in isolated cardiomyocytes from failing human hearts by gene transfer of SERCA2a. Circulation 1999; 100:2308–2311.

87. del Monte F, Williams E, Lebeche D, Schmidt U, Rosenzweig A, Gwathmey JK, Lewandowski ED, Hajjar RJ. Improvement in survival and cardiac metabolism after gene transfer of sarcoplasmic reticulum Ca^{2+}-ATPase in a rat model of heart failure. Circulation 2001; 104: 1424–1429.

88. Schmitt JP, Kamisago M, Asahi M, Li GH, Ahmad F, Mende U, Kranias EG, MacLennan DH, Seidman JG, Seidman CE. Dilated cardiomyopathy and heart failure caused by a mutation in phospholamban. Science 2003; 299:1410–1413.

89. Haghighi K, Kolokathis F, Pater L, Lynch RA, Asahi M, Gramolini AO, Fan GC, Tsiapras D, Hahn HS, Adamopoulos S, Liggett SB, Dorn GW, MacLennan DH, Kremastinos DT, Kranias EG. Human phospholamban null results in lethal dilated cardiomyopathy revealing a critical difference between mouse and human. J Clin Invest 2003; 111:869–876.

90. Li Y, Kranias EG, Mignery GA, Bers DM. Protein kinase A phosphorylation of the ryanodine receptor does not affect calcium sparks in mouse ventricular myocytes. Circ Res 2002; 90: 309–316.

91. Jiang MT, Lokuta AJ, Farrell EF, Wolff MR, Haworth RA, Valdivia HH. Abnormal Ca^{2+} release, but normal ryanodine receptors, in canine and human heart failure. Circ Res 2002; 91:1015–1022.

92. Eisner DA, Trafford AW. Heart failure and the ryanodine receptor: does Occam's razor rule?. Circ Res 2002; 91:979–981.

93. Schroder F, Handrock R, Beuckelmann DJ, Hirt S, Hullin R, Priebe L, Schwinger RH, Weil J, Herzig S. Increased availability and open probability of single L-type calcium channels from failing compared with nonfailing human ventricle. Circulation 1998; 98:969–976.

94. Kentish JC, McCloskey DT, Layland J, Palmer S, Leiden JM, Martin AF, Solaro RJ. Phosphorylation of troponin I by protein kinase A accelerates relaxation and crossbridge cycle kinetics in mouse ventricular muscle. Circ Res 2001; 88:1059–1065.

95. Beuckelmann DJ, Nabauer M, Erdmann E. Intracellular calcium handling in isolated ventricular myocytes from patients with terminal heart failure. Circulation 1992; 85:1046–1055.

96. Frey N, McKinsey TA, Olson EN. Decoding calcium signals involved in cardiac growth and function. Nat Med 2000; 6:1221–1227.

97. Molkentin JD, Lu JR, Antos CL, Markham B, Richardson J, Robbins J, Grant SR, Olson EN. A calcineurin-dependent transcriptional pathway for cardiac hypertrophy. Cell 1998; 93: 215–228.

98. Zhang T, Maier LS, Dalton ND, Miyamoto S, Ross J, Bers DM, Brown JH. The {delta}C isoform of CaMKII is activated in cardiac hypertrophy and induces dilated cardiomyopathy and heart failure. Circ Res 2003.

99. Neumann J. Altered phosphatase activity in heart failure, influence on Ca^{2+} movement. BasicRes Cardiol 2002; 97(Suppl 1):I91–I95.

100. Carr AN, Schmidt AG, Suzuki Y, del Monte F, Sato Y, Lanner C, Breeden K, Jing SL, Allen PB, Greengard P, Yatani A, Hoit BD, Grupp IL, Hajjar RJ, DePaoli-Roach AA, Kranias EG. Type 1 phosphatase, a negative regulator of cardiac function. Mol Cell Biol 2002; 22: 4124–4135.

101. El-Armouche A, Rau T, Zolk O, Ditz D, Pamminger T, Zimmermann WH, Jackel E, Harding SE, Boknik P, Neumann J, Eschenhagen T. Evidence for protein phosphatase inhibitor-1 playing an amplifier role in β-adrenergic signaling in cardiac myocytes. FASEBJ 2003; 17: 437–439.

102. El-Armouche A, Pamminger T, Ditz D, Zolk O, Eschenhagen T. Decreased protein and phosphorylation level of the protein phosphatase inhibitor-1 in failing human hearts. Cardiovasc Res 2004; 61:87–93.

103. Lagadic-Gossmann D, Vaughan-Jones RD. Coupling of dual acid extrusion in the guinea-pig isolated ventricular myocyte to α_1- and β-adrenoceptors. J Physiol 1993; 464:49–73.

104. Baartscheer A, Schumacher CA, van Borren MM, Belterman CN, Coronel R, Fiolet JW. Increased Na^+/H^+-exchange activity is the cause of increased Na_i^+ and underlies disturbed calcium handling in the rabbit pressure and volume overload heart failure model. Cardiovasc Res 2003; 57:1015–1024.

105. Wakabayashi S, Ikeda T, Iwamoto T, Pouyssegur J, Shigekawa M. Calmodulin-binding autoinhibitory domain controls ''pH-sensing'' in the Na^+/H^+ exchanger NHE1 through sequence-specific interaction. Biochemistry 1997; 36:12854–12861.

106. Bristow MR, Ginsburg R, Minobe W, Cubicciotti RS, Sageman WS, Lurie K, Billingham ME, Harrison DC, Stinson EB. Decreased catecholamine sensitivity and β-adrenergic-receptor density in failing human hearts. N Engl J Med 1982; 307:205–211.

107. Bohm M, La Rosee K, Schwinger RH, Erdmann E. Evidence for reduction of norepinephrine uptake sites in the failing human heart. J Am Coll Cardiol 1995; 25:146–153.

108. Neumann J, Schmitz W, Schols H, Von Meyerinck L, Doring V, Kalmar P. Increased in myocardiol G_i-proteins in heart failure. Lancet 1988; 2:936–937.

109. Ungerer M, Bohm M, Elce JS, Erdmann E, Lohse MJ. Altered expression of β-adrenergic receptor kinase and β_1-adrenergic receptors in the failing human heart. Circulation 1993; 87: 454–463.

110. Bristow MR, Ginsburg R, Umans V, Fowler M, Minobe W, Rasmussen R, Zera P, Menlove R, Shah P, Jamieson S, et al. β_1- and β_2-adrenergic-receptor subpopulations in nonfailing and failing human ventricular myocardium: coupling of both receptor subtypes to muscle contraction and selective β_1-receptor down-regulation in heart failure. Circ Res 1986; 59: 297–309.

111. Lohse MJ. Molecular mechanisms of membrane receptor desensitization. BiochimBiophys Acta 1993; 1179:171–188.

112. Lohse MJ, Krasel C, Winstel R, Mayor F. G-protein-coupled receptor kinases. Kidney Int 1996; 49:1047–1052.

113. Penn RB, Pronin AN, Benovic JL. Regulation of G protein-coupled receptor kinases. Trends-Cardiovasc Med 2000; 10:81–89.

114. Pitcher JA, Freedman NJ, Lefkowitz RJ. G protein-coupled receptor kinases. AnnuRev Biochem 1998; 67:653–692.

115. Lohse MJ. G-protein coupled receptor kinases and the heart. TrendsCardiovasc. Med 1995; 5:63–68.

116. Inglese J, Luttrell LM, Iniguez-Lluhi JA, Touhara K, Koch WJ, Lefkowitz RJ. Functionally active targeting domain of the β-adrenergic receptor kinase: an inhibitor of Gbg-mediated stimulation of type II adenylyl cyclase. ProcNatl Acad Sci U S A 1994; 91:3637–3641.

117. Rockman HA, Chien KR, Choi DJ, Iaccarino G, Hunter JJ, Ross J, Lefkowitz RJ, Koch WJ. Expression of a β-adrenergic receptor kinase 1 inhibitor prevents the development of myocardial failure in gene-targeted mice. ProcNatl Acad Sci U S A 1998; 95:7000–7005.

118. Harding VB, Jones LR, Lefkowitz RJ, Koch WJ, Rockman HA. Cardiac βARK1 inhibition prolongs survival and augments β-blocker therapy in a mouse model of severe heart failure. ProcNatl Acad Sci U S A 2001; 98:5809–5814.

119. Rockman HA, Koch WJ, Lefkowitz RJ. Seven-transmembrane-spanning receptors and heart function. Nature 2002; 415:206–212.

120. Koch WJ, Rockman HA, Samama P, Hamilton RA, Bond RA, Milano CA, Lefkowitz RJ. Cardiac function in mice overexpressing the b-adrenergic receptor kinase or a βARK inhibitor. Science 1995; 268:1350–1353.

121. Li Z, Laugwitz KL, Pinkernell K, Pragst I, Baumgartner C, Hoffmann E, Rosport K, Münch G, Moretti A, Humrich J, Lohse MJ, Ungerer M. Effects of two bg-binding proteins - N-terminally truncated phosducin and β-adrenergic receptor kinase C terminus (βARKct)- in heart failure. GeneTher 2003 :in press.

122. Bristow MR. β-adrenergic receptor blockade in chronic heart failure. Circulation 2000; 101: 558–569.

123. Waagstein F, Hjalmarson A, Varnauskas E. Effect of chronic β-adrenergic receptor blockade in congestive cardiomyopathy. Br Heart J 1975; 37.

124. Packer M, Bristow MR, Cohn JN, Colucci WS, Fowler MB, Gilbert EM, Shusterman NH. The effect of carvedilol on morbidity and mortality in patients with chronic heart failure. N Engl J Med 1996; 334:1349–1355.

125. CIBIS II Investigators and Committees: The Cardiac Insufficiency Bisoprolol Study II (CIBIS-II): a randomised trial. Lancet 1999; 353:9–13.

126. MERIT-HF Study Group Effect of metoprolol CR/XL in chronic heart failure: Metoprolol CR/XL randomised intervention trial in congestive heart failure (MERIT-HF). Lancet 1999; 353:2001–2007.

127. Gilbert EM, Abraham WT, Olsen S, Hattler B, White M, Mealy P, Larrabee P, Bristow MR. Comparative hemodynamic, left ventricular functional, and antiadrenergic effects of chronic treatment with metoprolol versus carvedilol in the failing heart. Circulation 1996; 94: 2817–2825.

128. Beta-Blocker Evaluation of Survival Trial Investigators A Trial of the beta-blocker bucindolol in patients with advanced chronic heart failure. N Engl J Med 2001; 344:1659–1667.

129. Xamoterol in Severe Heart Failure Study Group: Xamoterol in severe heart failure.. Lancet 1990; 336:1–6.

130. Engelhardt S, Grimmer Y, Fan GH, Lohse MJ. Constitutive activity of the human β_1-adrenergic receptor in β_1-receptor transgenic mice. MolPharmacol 2001; 60:712–717.

131. Andreka P, Aiyar N, Olson LC, Wei JQ, Turner MS, Webster KA, Ohlstein EH, Bishopric NH. Bucindolol displays intrinsic sympathomimetic activity in human myocardium. Circulation 2002; 105:2429–2434.

132. Maack C, Böhm M, Vlaskin L, Dabew E, Lorenz K, Schäfers HJ, Lohse MJ, Engelhardt S. Partial agonist activity of bucindolol is dependent on the activation state of thes human β_1-adrenergic receptor. Circulation 2003; 108:348–353.

133. Chidiac P, Nouet S, Bouvier M. Agonist-induced modulation of inverse agonist efficacy at the β_2-adrenergic receptor. MolPharmacol 1996; 50:662–669.

134. Maack C, Cremers B, Flesch M, Hoper A, Sudkamp M, Bohm M. Different intrinsic activities of bucindolol, carvedilol and metoprolol in human failing myocardium. BrJ Pharmacol 2000; 130:1131–1139.

135. Poole-Wilson PA, Swedberg K, Cleland JG, Di Lenarda A, Hanrath P, Komajda M, Lubsen J, Lutiger B, Metra M, Remme WJ, Torp-Pedersen C, Scherhag A, Skene A. Comparison of carvedilol and metoprolol on clinical outcomes in patients with chronic heart failure in the Carvedilol Or Metoprolol European Trial (COMET): randomised controlled trial. Lancet 2003; 362:7–13.

136. Small KM, McGraw DW, Liggett SB. Pharmacology and physiology of human adrenergic receptor polymorphisms. AnnuRev Pharmacol Toxicol 2003; 43:381–411.

137. Hein L. Physiological significance of beta-adrenergic receptor polymorphisms: in-vivo or in-vitro veritas? Pharmacogenetics 2001; 11:187–189.

138. Small KM, Wagoner LE, Levin AM, Kardia SL, Liggett SB. Synergistic polymorphisms of β_1- and α_{2C}-adrenergic receptors and the risk of congestive heart failure. N Engl J Med 2002; 347:1135–1142.

139. Brede M, Wiesmann F, Jahns R, Hadamek K, Arnolt C, Neubauer S, Lohse MJ, Hein L. Feedback inhibition of catecholamine release by two different α_2-adrenoceptor subtypes prevents progression of heart failure. Circulation 2002; 106:2491–2416.

140. O'Shaughness KM, Fu B, Dickerson C, Thurston D, Brown MJ. The gain-of-function G389R variant of the β_1-adrenoceptor does not influence blood pressure or heart rate response to β-blockade in hypertensive subjects. ClinSci (Lond) 2000; 99:233–238.

141. Liggett SB. Pharmacogenetics of β_1- and β_2-adrenergic receptors. Pharmacology 2000; 61: 167–173.

142. Turki J, Lorenz JN, Green SA, Donnelly ET, Jacinto M, Liggett SB. Myocardial signaling defects and impaired cardiac function of a human β_2-adrenergic receptor polymorphism expressed in transgenic mice. ProcNatl Acad Sci U S A 1996; 93:10483–10488.

6

Ventricular Remodeling and Secondary Valvular Dysfunction in Heart Failure Progression

Judy Hung, Khurram Shahzad, Ronen Beeri, and Robert A. Levine
Cardiac Unit, Massachusetts General Hospital
Boston, Massachusetts, USA

Heart failure (HF) remains an important public health problem affecting an estimated 5 million people in the United States. The prevalence of heart failure is increasing, with about 750,000 new HF cases diagnosed each year [1,2]. It is estimated that heart failure accounts for about 6.5% of the nation's total health care budget and results in more than $20 billion in health care administration cost [2,3].

As heart disease progresses to heart failure, the heart size increases, cardiac function deteriorates and symptoms of HF become evident. This clinical syndrome is, in fact, the result of changes to the heart's cellular matrix and molecular components as well as to the mediators that drive hemostatic control. Ventricular remodeling encompasses many such changes and is defined by the International Forum on Remodeling as genomic expression that results in molecular, cellular, and interstitial changes and is manifested clinically as changes in size, shape, and function of the heart resulting from cardiac load or injury[4].

Ventricular remodeling can be either pathological or physiological [4]. Pathological remodeling may occur after myocardial infarction, with pressure overload (hypertension or aortic stenosis), in inflammatory myocardial disease (myocarditis), with idiopathic dilated cardiomyopathy, or with volume overload (valvular regurgitation). Pathological remodeling appears to result from failed attempts to compensate for loss of contractile function. Initial ventricular dilatation and hypertrophy are compensatory changes that may ultimately progress to heart failure. Physiological remodeling, however, is a compensatory change in the proportions and function of the heart, such as can occur in athletes.

PATHOGENESIS OF VENTRICULAR REMODELING

Etiologies of remodeling may vary but they share many common pathways in terms of mechanical, biological, and molecular events. Although cardiac myocytes are thought to be the major target of these events, other components, such as the interstitium, fibroblasts, collagen, and coronary vasculature, also play an important role in adverse cardiac remodeling. Neurohumoral activation, hemodynamic load, and other factors also influence the process of remodeling.

Adverse ventricular remodeling most frequently occurs after myocardial infarction. In postinfarct animal models and in humans, LV (left ventricle) remodeling usually begins as early as the first few hours postinfarction and progresses over time [5–8]. Processes that occur postinfarction leading to ventricular remodeling include: lengthening of cardiomyocytes with resultant myocyte slippage [6–10], ventricular wall thinning [6–10], infarct expansion [6,11–13], followed by inflammatory response and reabsorption of necrotic tissue [6] leading to scar formation. Continued expansion of infarct zone [13] leads to LV deformation and dilatation [6,9,13]. Compensatory myocyte hypertrophy in noninfarcted regions ensues [6,9,10,12], and there is excessive accumulation of collagen in the cardiac interstitium [14].

Although the precise mechanisms of all the pathways and cells involved in LV remodeling remain unclear, the following general scenario has been proposed at a molecular level. With stretching of the myocytes, local norepinephrine activity, angiotensin II and endothelin release are augmented. These changes, in turn, stimulate expression of altered proteins and myocyte hypertrophy. This sequence of events leads to further deterioration in cardiac performance and increased neurohormonal activation. In addition, collagen synthesis is stimulated by the increased activation of aldosterone and cytokines, which leads to fibrosis and remodeling of the extracellular matrix [4].

FUNCTIONAL CHANGES

The initial remodeling phase after a myocardial infarction (MI) is characterized by repair of the necrotic area with scar tissue formation. These changes may, to some extent, be considered beneficial since there is an improvement in or maintenance of LV function and cardiac output [15,16]. However, the cellular rearrangement of the ventricular wall is associated with hypertrophy of the remaining noninfarcted myocardium, LV dilatation, and a significant increase in LV volume. These changes might augment LV function early on but this beneficial effect is transient, and at some point the hypertrophied myocardium fails and progressive ventricular dilatation ensues.

The time, course, and extent of remodeling are influenced by a variety of factors including the severity of the underlying disease, secondary events (e.g.; recurrent ischemia), neuroendocrine activation, genotype, and treatment [6,17,18]. In postinfarct animal models and humans following myocardial infarction, the extent of remodeling is roughly related to infarct size [18,19]. In a human study, left ventricular end-diastolic and end-systolic volumes increased progressively from hospital discharge to 1 year after an initial, moderately large, anterior wall transmural infarction, but remained stable in patients with an initial small, inferior wall infarction [18] (Fig. 1). In patients with progressive postinfarction dilatation, the end-systolic volume index increases progressively and LV ejection fraction (LVEF) declines, due in part to loss of function in initially normally contracting myocardium [9,13]. All these changes are important predictors of all-cause mortality [20](Fig. 1).

Diastolic dysfunction and changes in the passive elastic properties of the ventricular walls have been well documented in a rat postinfarction heart failure model. The pressure-volume relationship is displaced rightward with a profound increase in operating end-diastolic volume [1]. The degree of LV remodeling after MI has also been found to be age-dependent in a rat model [21] of heart failure.

Antecedent hypertension has been found to be associated with more extensive ventricular remodeling and the development of HF after a myocardial infarction. This was

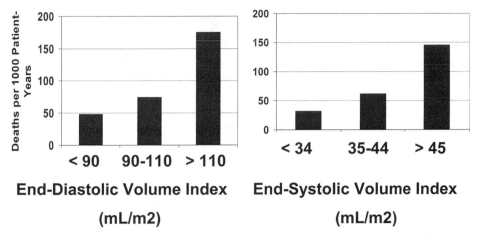

Figure 1 The relationship between left ventricular size as assessed by the left ventricular end-diastolic dimension (LVEDD) and left ventricular end-systolic dimension (LVESD) following acute myocardial infarction and survival. Ml, milliliters; M2, meters2. (From Ref. 19a.)

demonstrated in a series of 1093 post-MI patients, where hypertensive patients were found to have significantly higher plasma levels of neurohormones and significantly greater increase in LV volumes (i.e., remodeling) at 5 months post-MI. Improvement in LVEF was observed in normotensive patients at 5 months post-MI, whereas hypertensive patients were found to be at an increased risk of developing HF requiring hospitalization at a mean follow-up of 2 years [22].

NEUROHORMONAL ACTIVATION

Neurohormonal activation is an important cause of ventricular remodeling [17,23–26,26a]. Although initially adaptive, neurohormonal activation may be deleterious over the long-term, in part by contributing to pathologic remodeling [27]. With HF progression, gradual increases in the release of renin, norepinephrine, and antidiuretic hormone occur that are proportional to the severity of the cardiac dysfunction [25,27](Fig. 2). Plasma

Heart Failure Progression

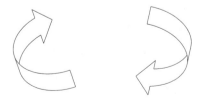

Renin, Norepinephrine, ADH

Figure 2 Heart failure leads to release of neurohumoral factors such as renin, norepinephrine, and ADH, resulting in further heart failure progression.

norepinephrine levels are elevated in both asymptomatic left ventricular dysfunction and overt HF [24,25] and higher levels of circulating plasma norepinephrine correlate with a poorer long-term prognosis [23,25,28]. Plasma BNP (brain natriuretic peptide) concentrations are also increased in HF patients and correlate with symptom severity and prognosis [29]. In contrast to the deleterious effect of angiotensin II and norepinephrine, BNP release from cardiac myocytes in the failing heart may protect against pathologic remodeling [30].

Many human studies have revealed that the angiotensin converting enzyme (ACE) inhibitors improve survival in HF by slowing and in some cases even reversing certain parameters of cardiac remodeling [31–33]. Both systemic and locally generated angiotensin II are believe to participate in this process, which in part acts via alterations in gene expression [34–37]. It appears to be an important mediator of the cellular responses to stretch, with local production by cardiac myocytes [38]. In human myocardial tissue, ACE is markedly increased at the edge of the infarct scar [39], while in an animal model, there is increased expression of angiotensin 1 (AT1) receptor mRNA in noninfarcted viable areas [40]. AT1 receptors have been identified on cardiac myocytes and human fibroblasts cultured from cardiomyopathic and ischemic hearts [41,42]. Acting through these AT1 receptors, angiotensin Il increases protein synthesis and induces hypertrophy in cardiac myocytes [36,38] and collagen synthesis by fibroblasts [38,43,44], an effect that can be reduced by ACE inhibition [45].

Harada and colleagues demonstrated that more marked LV enlargement and remodeling occurs in wild-type mice than in AT1A receptor knockout mice following a large myocardial infarction. In this study, all of the wild-type mice developed HF compared with none of the knockout mice [40]. Further support for the role of the cardiomyocyte AT1 receptor in cardiac remodeling comes from the observation that transgenic mice with overexpression of the AT1 receptor limited to the cardiac myocyte, develop cardiac hypertrophy and remodeling without a change in the systemic blood pressure [45]. Animal models have shown that remodeling is minimized or, in established disease, reversed by angiotensin II receptor antagonists, which block the AT1 receptor [46,47]. The clinical importance of angiotensin mediated remodeling has been demonstrated with the observation that the AT1 receptor antagonist valsartan was equally effective to the ACE inhibitor captopril in preventing mortality and hospitalization for heart failure in patients with a myocardial infarction complicated by LV dysfunction. [47a]

Aldosterone secretion is enhanced by angiotensin II, which may also participate in adverse remodeling. Aldosterone extracted by the mineralocorticoid receptors in hearts after a myocardial infarction, and the secondary hyperaldosteronism state commonly seen in HF, may contribute to the postinfarction remodeling via stimulation of collagen synthesis by myocardial fibroblasts [48], hence, resulting in myocardial hypertrophy and fibrosis [49–51]. Aldosterone has also been shown to activate matrix metalloproteinase 12 (MMP-12) [elastase], which could contribute to further degradation of the cytoskeletal support structure. Spironolactone, which competes for the mineralocorticoid receptor, can reduce fibrosis and, therefore, influence remodeling [52, 52a].

Myocytes stretch in HF also stimulates an increase in local production or release of norepinephrine, BNP, and endothelin. These neurohormonal changes stimulate protein expression and myocyte hypertrophy. Increases in angiotensin II, aldosterone, and cytokines stimulate collagen synthesis, which leads to fibrosis, resulting in remodeling of the extracellular matrix. The end result is further deterioration in cardiac performance and increased neurohormonal activation.

Stretch sensors located on the cell membrane respond to deformation of the cell membrane and include: (a) integrins; a family of membrane proteins linking the cytoskeleton to the extracellular matrix; (b) stretch-activated ion channels (SACs) (c) Na+/H+

exchangers; and (d) heterotrimeric G proteins [52b,52c,52d,52e,52f].Although the exact mechanisms remain incompletely understood, these stretch sensors, when activated, induce a number of signaling pathways involved in the remodeling process [52f]. There are three major signaling pathways that are stretch mediated: (a) P13-K dependant signaling; (b) JAK/STAT signaling; and (c) calcium mediated stretch-activated channels [52f,52g].

CELLULAR AND SUBCELLULAR CHANGES IN REMODELING

The cellular and subcellular basis for remodeling is of critical importance, and not completely understood. A number of subcellular and cellular changes, including extracellular matrix degradation, myocyte hypertrophy, loss of myocytes due to apoptosis [53–55] or necrosis [56], fibroblast proliferation [57] and fibrosis [58,59], are thought to play key roles in remodeling. (Fig. 3)

EXTRACELLULAR MATRIX DEGRADATION

The components of the myocardium involved in the remodeling process include the cardiac myocytes and the extracellular matrix (ECM), which provides the scaffolding to maintain normal myocyte architecture. The extracellular matrix is composed of basement membrane proteoglycans and fibrillar collagen, particularly subtypes I and III. Maintenance of myocyte shape, alignment, and architecture is critically dependent on the supporting extracellular matrix. Recent evidence has demonstrated that the ECM plays an active role in the remodeling process by not only providing structural support proteins but also as an important interface for cellular signaling. In particular, integrins, a family of transmembrane proteins, appear to be critically important in the transduction of extracellular signals as well as being anchors for cellular adhesion in the ECM [60]. In response to myocardial injury and decreased contractile dysfunction, a number of cellular, biomechani-

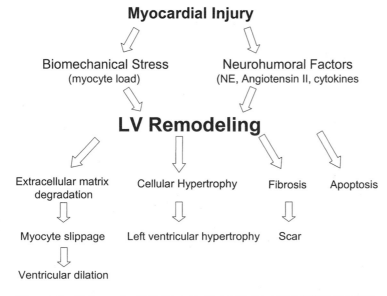

Figure 3 Schematic of factors involved in the remodeling process.

cal, and humoral factors, particularly cytokines, such as tumor necrosis factor (TNF-α) and interleukin-1, are activated, leading to modulation of matrix metalloproteinase activation. Matrix metalloproteinases are an important family of enzymes that help shape remodeling in several disease states [61,62]; at least 20 different matrix metalloproteinases have been identified, including collagenases, gelatinases, and stromelysins and membrane-type metalloproteinases.

The release and activation of matrix metalloproteinases are mediated by biomechanical factors and neurohumoral/cytokine activation. Matrix metalloproteinases cause extracellular matrix degradation, which results in the weakening of the myocyte and myofibril scaffolding network. Inevitably, this degradation of the support scaffolding leads to myocyte stretch, with lengthening and thinning of the myocyte and myocyte "slippage" or loss of the normal myocyte architecture [63–67]. These changes lead to ventricular thinning and infarct expansion, which may lead to wall stress and, in turn, promote further structural remodeling.

MYOCYTE HYPERTROPHY AND APOPTOSIS

Hypertrophy of the surviving myocytes is an important adaptive response to loss of contractile function. The processes, which lead to myocyte hypertrophy, are complex, involving several cellular signaling pathways (Chapter 2). Both neurohormonal and mechanical factors play important roles in stimulating myocyte hypertrophy. A decrease in cardiac function leads to increased levels of norepinephrine and activation of the renin-angiotensin system, leading to release of angiotensin II. Both norepinephrine and angiotensin II stimulate myocyte hypertrophy. Mechanical stress, such as increased stretch or tension resulting from changes in load, also plays an important role in the hypertrophic response. Angiotensin II and mechanical stress induce a number of cellular signaling pathways important in the development of cellular hypertrophy. Both angiotension II and mechanical stress stimulate the release of endothelin-1, which is a vasoactive peptide released by endothelial cells. In turn, endothelin-1 activates a family of enzymes called mitogen-activated kinases (MAP kinases), which mediate the cellular pathways leading to hypertrophy. In addition to the signaling pathways mediated by endothelin-1 and MAP kinases, the gp130 and calcineurin-mediated signaling pathways also appear to play important regulatory roles in myocyte hypertrophy [65, 67–69](Fig. 4).

Hypertrophy of the noninfarcted myocardium is an important early adaptive mechanism to loss of contractile function and initially results in compensated function. However,

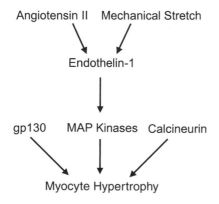

Figure 4   Schematic showing the mediators of myocyte hypertrophy.

at some critical stage that is not yet fully understood, these prohypertrophic signaling mechanisms may be downregulated or even exhausted, shifting the signaling balance from compensation to failure. This loss of contractile function eventually leads to the development of clinical heart failure. In addition to myocyte hypertrophy, myocyte apoptosis, in which cells embark on a suicide pathway to death, is increasingly recognized as playing an important role in the remodeling process [66,70–72]. Apoptosis is induced when adjacent myocardial necrosis occurs, and appears to be initiated, in part, by cytokines such as TNFα and oxidative stress [4, 73,74] (Chapter 3). Caspases, a family of serine proteases, are the intracellular mediators of apoptosis and execute cellular death by cleavage of cellular proteins. Caspases are activated in the cardiac myocyte by two main signaling pathways: (i) activation of death receptors on the cell surface, and (ii) apoptotic mediators released by mitochondria [66,75–79]. Interestingly, the rate of apoptosis is noted to be increased in noninfarcted myocardium, although it remains at a relatively low overall rate [66]. In addition, the rate of apoptosis appears to correlate with degree of ventricular thinning and dilatation, and development of heart failure [80], suggesting that apoptosis plays an important role in the remodeling process and its prevention may be an important therapeutic intervention.

FIBROSIS

The remodeling process induces changes in collagen production of the extracellular matrix. Fibroblasts are activated by myocardial necrosis, mediated by cytokines released by myocytes and macrophages. In turn, matrix metalloproteinases released by activated fibroblasts promote the increase of collagen subtype I and III production, resulting in fibrosis and scar formation within the necrotic region. There is also evidence that increased collagen production and subsequent fibrosis occurs in noninfarcted regions as well [81–83]. The gradual fibrosis of noninfarcted regions contributes to the development of heart failure.

REMODELING CHANGES ON THE MACROSCOPIC LEVEL

These changes in the extracellular matrix and myocyte architecture lead to changes at the macroscopic level, which involve ventricular dilatation, ventricular hypertrophy, and changes in ventricular shape, such as the development of a less elliptical and more spherical ventricle, and LV scar and LV aneurysm formation. Ultimately, these changes in the LV geometry result in adverse ventricular mechanics and inefficiencies in ventricular contraction, further increasing myocardial oxygen demand and wall stress and resulting in contractile dysfunction and heart failure. With infarction, myocardial necrosis occurs, with eventual replacement of the necrotic region with scar [84], a process that is generally completed by 6 to 8 weeks. Shortly following myocardial infarction, ventricular dilatation of the noninfarcted myocardium occurs. Initially this is an important adaptive response aimed at maintaining cardiac output via the Frank-Starling mechanism. Ventricular dilatation increases the end-diastolic dimension and allows the ventricle to maintain the same stroke volume despite loss of contractile function. However, dilatation of the ventricle results in increased wall stress according to Laplace's law, which states that wall stress increases proportionately with the radius of a sphere (Fig. 5A). Increased wall stress leads to an increase in myocardial oxygen demand, which reduces the efficiency of contraction. In response to ventricular dilatation and increased wall stress, myocytes hypertrophy leading to an increase in wall thickness; thus, reducing wall stress back toward normal (Fig. 5B). As ventricular dilatation progresses, however, this adaptive mechanism is eventually overwhelmed resulting in decreased contractile function and heart failure.

Increased wall tension with dilatation

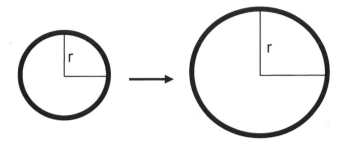

Laplace's Law: Wall Stress = Radius/Wall Thickness

Figure 5A   Illustration of Laplace's law. Wall stress increases proportionately with the radius of a sphere.

Continued expansion of infarcted tissue begins acutely after myocardial infarction. A more gradual remodeling process, however, also involves dilatation of the noninfarcted regions [4,85], which while initially compensatory, ultimately becomes maladaptive, changing the normally ellipsoid shape of the LV to a larger, more spherical, and poorly contracting ventricle (Fig. 6) [8, 86,87].A more spherical LV results in detrimental ventricular mechanics and is associated with an adverse prognosis [4,88–93]. In addition to global changes in LV shape, segmental deformation, such as LV aneurysm formation, also produces deleterious effects on LV function. The development of a LV aneurysm is a serious complication of myocardial infarction and is associated with increased mortality. The incidence of LV aneurysm post-myocardial-infarction is approximately 10% to 30% [94–96], although this appears to be decreasing in the era of thrombolytics and primary angioplasty [97]. An LV aneurysm is defined as a focal area of thinned and scarred myocardium. Pathologically, this area has no contractile elements and is composed entirely of scar tissue (Fig. 7). The presence of an LV aneurysm creates an area of noncontractile

Decreased wall tension with hypertrophy of the walls

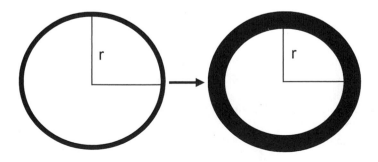

Laplace's Law: Wall Stress = Radius/2xWall Thickness

Figure 5B   In response to ventricular dilation and increased wall stress, cells hypertrophy, which increases wall thickness to limit increases in wall stress.

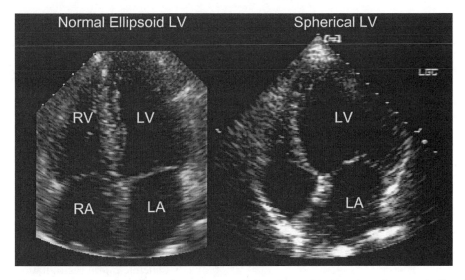

Figure 6 Left ventricular sphericity by echocardiographic imaging. A normal ellipsoid left ventricle is shown in the left panel. The right panel depicts a patient with multiple myocardial infarcts whose ventricle has lost the normal elliptical shape and become more spherical. LV, left ventricle, LA, left atrium; RV, right ventricle; RA, right atrium.

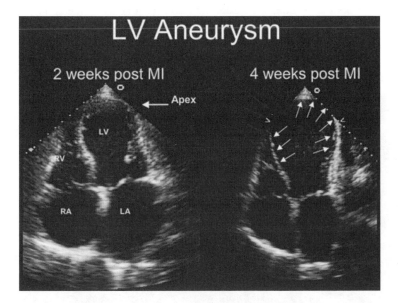

Figure 7 Echocardiographic image of a left ventricular aneurysm. These echocardiographic images show the development of an apical aneurysm in a patient following an anterior myocardial infarction. The left panel shows mild dilation of the left ventricular apex 2 weeks following infarction. Four weeks following infarction, there has been interval focal thinning and dilation of the apex (*right panel, arrows*). LV, left ventricle; LA, left atrium; RV, right ventricle; RA, right atrium.

tissue, leading to stagnant blood flow and inefficient LV contraction. The formation of an LV aneurysm is not only influenced by the molecular and cellular changes initiated by myocardial injury but also by hemodynamic variables, such as heart rate and loading of the ventricle [98]. In addition to loss of contractile function and decrease in ventricular mechanics with the formation of an LV aneurysm, studies have demonstrated decreased function of the border zones of an LV aneurysm. This may occur because of an increase in wall stress at the border zone of the aneurysm, resulting in increased myocardial oxygen consumption, further reducing the efficiency of left ventricular function [99,100]. In addition to reduction in mechanical function, LV aneurysms are predisposed to the formation of thrombus and can serve as foci for ventricular arrhythmias.

SECONDARY VALVULAR DYSFUNCTION

The LV remodeling process leads to secondary valvular dysfunction, primarily mitral regurgitation (MR). Mitral regurgitation in this setting, in which the mitral leaflets are morphologically normal, is often referred to as functional or ischemic mitral regurgitation and is characterized by valve leaflets that coapt apically within the left ventricle, restricting leaflet closure in a pattern known as incomplete mitral leaflet closure (Fig. 8) [101]. Functional mitral regurgitation develops in up to 20% of patients following myocardial infarction [102,103] and is present in up to 50% of patients with dilated cardiomyopathy [104–106]. Functional mitral regurgitation is associated with an adverse prognosis; the development of mitral regurgitation following myocardial infarction nearly doubling mortality [107,108]. This relationship seems to be associated in a quantitative manner, as a greater degree of mitral regurgitation correlates with higher mortality [108]. It is important to emphasize that the mitral valve function should be understood in terms of its relationship to its ventricular support structures and not as freestanding leaflets attached at the annulus. The mitral valve apparatus includes both anterior and posterior mitral leaflets, the mitral annulus, papillary muscles, and associated chordae tendineae. The mitral leaflets are at-

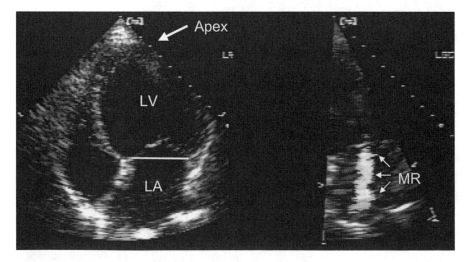

Figure 8 Incomplete mitral leaflet closure. Instead of normal coaptation at the annular plane, mitral leaflets coapt apically (*left panel*) resulting in mitral regurgitation (*arrows, right panel*).

tached to the mitral annulus and tethered to the ventricle by the papillary muscles via the chordae tendineae. The posteromedial and anterolateral papillary muscles, located along the inferior and posterolateral surfaces of the left ventricle, both give off chordae to each mitral leaflet. The papillary muscles and chordae tendineae serve an important function, anchoring the leaflets at the annular level during coaptation. The mechanism underlying functional mitral regurgitation relates to changes in the mitral valve geometry resulting from the underlying LV remodeling process. Although a spectrum of morphological abnormalities of the LV and papillary muscles exists, considerable evidence points to the central and predominant role of tethering as the final common pathway in inducing functional MR [109–113].

With infarction, the papillary muscles and surrounding left ventricle remodel, becoming thinned and dilated, resulting in posterolateral displacement of the papillary muscles. Posterolateral displacement of the papillary muscles leads to stretching of the chordae tendineae and increased tethering forces on the mitral valve leaflets. In turn, an increase in mitral leaflet tethering leads to restricted mitral leaflet closure where instead of normal leaflet coaptation at the level of the annulus, the leaflets coapt apically restricting leaflet closure, leading to regurgitation (Fig. 9). Because of the posterior-lateral location of the papillary muscles, infarctions in these walls have a greater incidence of mitral regurgitation compared with anterior infarctions [114]. In patients who develop diffuse LV dysfunction, either from a myopathic process or multiple infarctions, there is global LV dilatation leading to papillary muscle displacement as well.

Dilatation of the mitral annulus also plays a role in the development of functional mitral regurgitation [115]. Annular dilation results in stretching of the mitral leaflets, restricting closure of the mitral leaflets.

Mitral regurgitation can itself initiate and worsen LV remodeling. Mitral regurgitation alters left ventricular loading [116], increases wall stress, which can then induce eccentric LV hypertrophy and dilatation [117]. This can result in further distortion of the

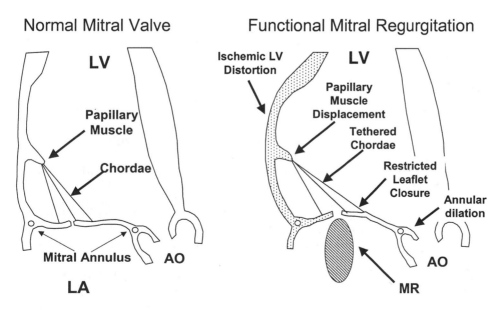

Figure 9 Schematic of the mechanism of functional mitral regurgitation. Levine RA, Hung J. JACC 2003; 42:1929–1932.

mitral valve apparatus and worsening of the mitral regurgitation leading to a vicious cycle in which mitral regurgitation begets more mitral regurgitation [118,119]. In addition, mitral regurgitation induces neurohumoral and cytokine promoters of adverse remodeling [120–122].

REMODELING AND VALVULAR DYSFUNCTION OF THE RIGHT VENTRICLE

Most of what is known about the remodeling process has been described or demonstrated in the left ventricle. Less is known about the right ventricular remodeling process, although there is evidence that right ventricular dilatation, hypertrophy, and decreased contractility occur following LV myocardial infarction [123,124]. Tricuspid regurgitation resulting from right ventricular remodeling is present in approximately 30% of patients with cardiomyopathy and is associated with an adverse prognosis [106,125].

THERAPEUTIC TARGETS

Ventricular remodeling is an important aspect of disease progression in heart failure; hence, it is emerging as an important therapeutic target. LV remodeling involves a myriad of molecular and cellular processes that are initiated in response to myocardial injury. These processes provide a useful framework for targeting therapy to prevent or limit the deleterious effects of LV remodeling on myocardial function. ACE inhibitors, which antagonize the effects of angiotensin II, have well-known beneficial effects on LV remodeling and survival. Experimental evidence has demonstrated favorable remodeling effects with the use of inhibitors of matrix metalloproteinases, caspases, and cytokines, suggesting a potential role for therapy aimed at the signaling pathways responsible for the LV remodeling process [126–128].

In summary, left ventricular remodeling occurs as an adaptive responsive to loss of myocardial function and involves molecular and cellular responses that are initially adaptive, but ultimately result in deleterious effects on ventricular function.

REFERENCES

1. McFate SW. Epidemiology of congestive heart failure. Am J Cardiol 1985; 55(Suppl A): 3–8.
2. American Heart Association. Heart Disease and Stroke Statistics--2001 Update. Dallas, TX: American Heart Association, 2001.
3. Bristow MR. New approaches to therapy for congestive heart failure. American Heart Association Twenty-First Science Writers Forum, Clearwater, FL, January 1994.
4. Cohn JN, Ferrari R, Sharpe N. Cardiac remodeling-concepts and clinical implications: a consensus paper from an international forum on cardiac remodeling. Behalf of an International Forum on Cardiac Remodeling. J Am Coll Cardiol 2000; 5(3):569–582.
5. Hochman JS, Bulkley BH. Expansion of acute myocardial infarction: an experimental study. Circulation 1982; 65(7):1446–1450.
6. Weisman HF, Bush DE, Mannisi JA, Bulkley BH. Global cardiac remodeling after acute myocardial infarction: a study in the rat model. J Am Coll Cardiol 1985; 5:1355–1362.
7. Korup E, Dalsgaard D, Nyvad O, Jensen TM, Toft E, Berning J. Comparisons of degrees of left ventricular dilation within 3 hours and up to 6 days after onset of first acute myocardial infarction. Am J Cardiol 1997; 80:449–453.

8. Giannuzzi P, Temporelli PL, Bosimini F, Lucci D, Maggioni AP, Tavazzi L, Badano L, Stoian I, Piazza R, Heyman I, Levantesi G, Cervesado E, Geraci E, Nicolosi GL. Heterogeneity of left ventricular remodeling after acute myocardial infarction. Am Heart J 2001; 141:131.

9. McKay RG, Pfeffer MA, Pasternak RC, Markis JE, Come PC, Nako S, Alderman JD, Ferguson JJ, Nicolosi GL. Left ventricular remodeling after myocardial infarction: a corollary to infarct expansion. Circulation. 1986; 74:693–702.

10. Anversa P, Olivetti G, Capasso JM. Cellular basis of ventricular remodeling after myocardial infarction. Am J Cardiol 1991; 68:7D–16D.

11. Hutchins GM, Bulkley BH. Infarct expansion extension: two different complications of acute myocardial infarction. Am J Cardiol 1978; 41:1127–1133.

12. Olivetti G, Capasso JM, Sonnenblick EH, Anversa P. Side-to-side slippage of myocytes in ventricular wall remodeling acutely after myocardial infarction in rats. Circ Res 1990; 67: 23–34.

13. Gaudron P, Eilles C, Kugler I, Ertl G. Progressive left ventricular dysfunction and remodeling after myocardial infarction. Circulation 1993; 87:755–763.

14. Weber KT, Brilla CG. Pathological hypertrophy and the cardiac interstitium: fibrosis and the renin-angiotensin-aldosterone system. Circulation 1991; 83:1849–1865.

15. Ning XH, Zhang J, Liu J, Ye Y, Chen SH, From AH, Bache RJ, Portman MA. Signaling and expression for mitochondrial membrane proteins during left ventricular remodeling and contractile failure after myocardial infarction. J Am Coll Cardiol 2000; 36:282–287.

16. Cohen MV, Yang XM, Neumann T, Heusch G, Downey JM. Favorable remodeling enhances recovery of regional myocardial function in the weeks after infarction in ischemically preconditioned hearts. Circulation 2000; 102:579–583.

17. Jugdutt BI. Effect of captopril and enalapril on left ventricular geometry, function and collagen during healing after anterior and inferior myocardial infarction in a dog model. J Am Coll Cardiol 1995; 25:1718–1725.

18. Rumberger JA, Behrenbeck T, Breen JR, Reed JE, Gersh BJ. Nonparallel changes in global left ventricular chamber volume and muscle mass during the first year after transmural myocardial infarction in humans. J Am Coll Cardiol 1993; 21:673–682.

19. Anversa P, Olivetti G, Capasso JM. Cellular basis of ventricular remodeling after myocardial infarction. Am J Cardiol 1991; 68:7D–16D.

19a. Hammemeister KE, De Rowen TA and HT Dodge. Variables predictive of survival in patients with coronary disease. Selection by univariate and multivariate analysis from the clinical, electrocardiographic, exercise, arteriographic, and quantitative angiographic evaluations. Circulation 1979; 59:421–30.

20. White HD, Norris RM, Brown MA, Brandt PW, Whillock RM, Wild CJ. Left ventricular end-systolic volume as the major determinant of survival after recovery from endomyocardial infarction. Circulation 1987; 76:44–51.

21. Raya TE, Gaballa M, Anderson P, Goldman S. Left ventricular function and remodeling after myocardial infarction in aging rats. Am J Physiol 1997; 273(6 Pt 2):H2652–H2658.

22. Richards AM, Nicholls MG, Troughton RW, Lainchbury JG, Elliott J, Frampton C, Espexer EA, Crozier IG, Yandle TG, Turner J. Antecedent hypertension and heart failure after myocardial infarction. J Am Coll Cardiol 2002; 39:1182–1188.

23. Cohn JN, Levine TB, Olivari MT, Garberg V, Lura D, Francis GS, Simon AB, Rector T. Plasma norepinephrine as a guide to prognosis in patients with chronic congestive heart failure. N Engl J Med 1984; 311:819–823.

24. Chidsey C, Braunwald E, Morrow AG, Mason DT. Myocardial norepinephrine concentrations in man. N Engl J Med 1963; 269:653–658.

25. Francis GS, Benedict C, Johnstone DE, Kirlin PC, Nicklas J, Liang CS, Kubo SH, Rudin-Toretsky E, Yusuf S. Comparison of neuroendocrine activation in patients with left ventricular dysfunction with and without congestive heart failure. Circulation 1990; 82:1724–1729.

26. Torre-Amione G, Kapadia S, Benedict C, Oral H, Young JB, Mann DL. Proinflammatory cytokine levels in patients with depressed left ventricular ejection fraction: a report from the Studies of Left Ventricular Dysfunction (SOLVD). J Am Coll Cardiol 1996; 27:1201–1206.

26a. Vaughn DE, Rouleau JL, Ridker PM, Arnold JM, Menapace FJ, Pfeffer MA. Effects of ramipril on plasma fibrinolytic balance in patients with acute anterior myocardial infarction. Heart Study Investigators. Circulation 1997 Jul 15; 96(2):442–447.

27. Packer M. The neurohormonal hypothesis: a theory to explain the mechanism of disease progression in heart failure. J Am Coll Cardiol 1992; 20:248–254.

28. Vantrimpont P, Rouleau JL, Ciampi A, Harel F, de Champlain J, Bichet D, Maye LA, Pfeffer M. Two-year course and significance of neurohumoral activation in the Survival and Ventricular Enlargement (SAVE) study. Eur Heart J 1998; 19:1552–1563.

29. Maeda K, Tsutamoto T, Wada A, Mabuchi N, Hayashi M, Tsutsui T, Ohnishi M, Sawaki M, Fujii M, Matsumoto T, Kinoshita M. High levels of plasma brain natriuretic peptide and interleukin-6 after optimized treatment for heart failure are independent risk factors for morbidity and mortality in patients with congestive heart failure. J Am Coll Cardiol 2000; 36:1587–1593.

30. Tamura N, Ogawa Y, Chusho H, Nakamura K, Nakao K, Suda M, Kasahara M, Hashimoto R, Katsuura G, Mukoyama M, Itoh H, Saito Y, Tanaka I, Otani H, Katsuki M. Cardiac fibrosis in mice lacking brain natriuretic peptide. Proc Natl Acad Sci U S A 2000; 97: 4239–4224.

31. Konstam MA, Rousseau MF, Kronenberg MW, Udelson JE, Melin J, Stewart D, Dolan N, Edens TR, Ahn S, Kinan D, et al. Effects of the angiotensin converting enzyme inhibitor enalapril on the long-term progression of left ventricular dysfunction in patients with heart failure. SOLVD Investigators. Circulation 1992; 86:431–438.

32. Konstam MA, Kronenberg MW, Rousseau MF, Udelson JE, Melin J, Stewart D, Dolan N, Edens TR, Ahn S, Kinan D, et al. Effects of the angiotensin converting enzyme inhibitor enalapril on the long-term progression of left ventricular dilatation in patients with asymptomatic systolic dysfunction. SOLVD (Studies of Left Ventricular Dysfunction) Investigators. Circulation 1993; 88:(5 PT 1):2277–2283.

33. Greenberg B, Quinones MA, Koilpillai C, Limacher M, Shindler D, Benedict C, Shelton B. Effects of long-term enalapril therapy on cardiac structure and function in patients with left ventricular dysfunction. Results of the SOLVD echocardiography substudy. Circulation 1995; 91:2573–2581.

34. Ning XH, Zhang J, Liu J, Ye Y, Chen SH, From AH, Bache RJ, Portman MA. Signaling and expression for mitochondrial membrane proteins during left ventricular remodeling and contractile failure after myocardial infarction. J Am Coll Cardiol 2000; 36:282–287.

35. Reiss K, Capasso JM, Huang HE, Meggs LG, Li P, Anversa P. ANG II receptors, c-myc, and c-jun in myocytes after myocardial infarction and ventricular failure. Am J Physiol 1993: 264(3 PT 2)H760–769.

36. Sadoshima J, Izumo S. Molecular characterization of angiotensin II—induced hypertrophy of cardiac myocytes and hyperplasia of cardiac fibroblasts. Critical role of the AT1 receptor subtype. Circ Res 1993; 73:413–423.

37. Everett AD, Tufro-McReddie A, Fisher A, Gomez RA. Angiotensin receptor regulates cardiac hypertrophy and transforming growth factor-beta 1 expression. Hypertension 1994; 23: 587–592.

38. Sadoshima J, Xu Y, Slayter HS, Izumo S. Autocrine release of angiotensin II mediates stretch-induced hypertrophy of cardiac myocytes in vitro. Cell 1993; 75:977–984.

39. Hokimoto S, Yasue H, Fujimoto K, Yamamoto H, Nakao K, Kaikita K, Sakata R, Miyamoto E. Expression of angiotensin-converting enzyme in remaining viable myocytes of human ventricles after myocardial infarction. Circulation 1996; 94:1513–1518.

40. Harada K, Sugaya T, Murakami K, Yazaki Y, Komuro I. Angiotensin II type 1A receptor knockout mice display less ventricular remodeling and improved survival after myocardial infarction. Circulation 1999; 100:2093–2999.

41. Hafizi S, Wharton J, Morgan K, Allen SP, Chester AH, Catravas JD, Polak JM, Yacoub MH. Expression of functional angiotensin-converting enzyme and AT1 receptors in cultured human cardiac fibroblasts. Circulation 1998; 98:2553.

42. Matsusaka T, Katori H, Inagami T, Fogo A, Ichikawa I. Communication between myocytes and fibroblasts in cardiac remodeling in angiotensin chimeric mice. J Clin Invest 1999; 103: 1451–1458.

43. McEwan PE, Gray GA, Sherry L, Webb DJ, Kenyon CJ. Differential effects of angiotensin II on cardiac cell proliferation and intramyocardial perivascular fibrosis in vivo. Circulation 1998; 98:2765–2773.

44. Kawano H, Do YS, Kawano Y, Starnes V, Barr M, Law RE, Hsueh WA. Angiotensin II has multiple profibrotic effects in human cardiac fibroblasts. Circulation 2000; 101:1130–1137.

45. Paradis P, Dali-Youcef N, Paradis FW, Thibault G, Nemer M. Overexpression of angiotensin II type I receptor in cardiomyocytes induces cardiac hypertrophy and remodeling. Proc Natl Acad Sci U S A 2000; 97:931–936.

46. van Kats JP, Duncker DJ, Haitsma DB, Schuijt MP, Niebuur R, Stubenitsky R, Boomsma F, Schalekamp MA, Verdouw PD, Danser AH. Angiotensin-converting enzyme inhibition and angiotensin II type 1 receptor blockade prevent cardiac remodeling in pigs after myocardial infarction. Role of tissue angiotensin II. Circulation 2000; 102:1556–1563.

47. Tamura T, Said S, Harris J, Lu W, Gerdes AM. Reverse remodeling of cardiac myocyte hypertrophy in hypertension and failure by targeting of the renin-angiotensin system. Circulation 2000; 102:253–259.

47a. Pfeffer MA, McMurray JJV, Velazquez ES, Rouleau JL, Kober L, Maggioni AP, Solomon SD, Swedberg K, Van de Werf F, White H, Leimberger JD, Henis M, Edwards S, Zelenkofske S, Sellers MA, Califf RM; Valsartan in Acute Myocardial Infarction Trial Investigators. Valsartan, captopril, or both in myocardial infarction complicated by heart failure, left ventricular dysfunction, or both. N Eng J Med 2003; 349:1893–1906.

48. Brilla CG, Zhou G, Matsubara L, Weber KT. Collagen metabolism in cultured adult rat cardiac fibroblasts: response to angiotensin II and aldosterone. J Mol Cell Immunol 1994; 26:809–820.

49. Hayashi M, Tsutamoto T, Wada A, Maeda K, Mabuchi N, Tsutsui T, Matsui T, Fujii M, Matsumoto T, Yamamoto T, Horie H, Ohnishi M, Kinoshita M. Relationship between transcardiac extraction of aldosterone and left ventricular remodeling in patients with first acute myocardial infarction: extracting aldosterone through the heart promotes ventricular remodeling after acute myocardial infarction. J Am Coll Cardiol 2001; 38:1375–1382.

50. Lijnen P, Petrov V. Induction of cardiac fibrosis by aldosterone. J Mol Cell Cardiol 2000; 32:865–879.

51. Fullerton MJ, Funder JW. Aldosterone and cardiac fibrosis: in vitro studies. Cardiovasc Res 2000; 1994:1863–1867.

52. Zannad F, Alla F, Dousset B, Perez A, Pitt B. Limitation of excessive extracellular matrix turnover may contribute to survival benefit of spironolactone therapy in patients with congestive heart failure. Insights from the Randomized Aldactone Evaluation Study (RALES). Circulation 2000; 102:2700–2706.

52a. Pitt B, Remme W, Zannad F, Neaton I, Martinez F, Roniker R, Bittman R, Hurley S, Kleinman J, Gatlin M. for the EPERENONE Study Investigators. Eplerenone in patients with left ventricle dysfunction after myocardial Infarction NEJM 2003; 348:309–21.

52b. Ingber D. Integrins as mechanochemical transducers. Opin Cell Biol 1991; 3:841–848.

52c. Hu H, Sachs F. Stretch-activated ion channels in the heart. J Mol Cell Cardiol 1997; 29: 1511–1523.

52d. Akhter SA, Luttrell LM, Rockman HA, Iaccarino G, Lefkowitz RJ, Koch WJ. Targeting the receptor-Gq interface to inhibit in vivo pressure overload myocardial hypertrophy. Science 1998; 280:574–577.

52e. Gudi SRP, Lee AA, Clark CB, Frangos JA. Equibiaxial strain and strain rate stimulate early activation of G proteins in cardiac fibroblasts. Am J Physiol 1998; 274:C1424–C1428.

52f. Force T, Michael A, Kilter H, Haq S. Stretch-activated pathways and left ventricular remodeling. J Cardiac Fail 2002; 8(No 6 Suppl):S351–S358.

52g. Dostal DE, Hunt RA, Kule CE, Bhat GJ, Karoor V, McWhinney CD, Baker KM. Molecular mechanisms of angiotensin II in modulating cardiac function: intracardiac effects and signal transduction pathways. J Mol Cell Cardiol 1997; 29:2893–2902.

53. Sharov VG, Sabbah HN, Shimoyama H, Goussev AV, Lesch M, Goldstein S. Evidence of cardiocyte apoptosis in myocardium of dogs with chronic heart failure. Am J Pathol 1996; 143:141–149.

54. Teiger E, Than VD, Richard L, Wisnewsky C, Tea BS, Gaboury H, Tremblay J, Schwartz K, Hamet P. Apoptosis in pressure overload-induced heart hypertrophy in the rat. J Clin Invest 1996; 97:2891–2897.

55. Olivetti G, Abbi R, Quaini F, Kajstura J, Cheng W, Nitahara JA, Quaini E, Di Loreto C, Beltrami CA, Krajewski S, Reed JC, Anversa P. Apoptosis in the failing human heart. N Engl J Med 1997; 336:1131–1141.

56. Tan LB, Jalil JE, Pick R, Janieki JS, Weber KT. Cardiac myocyte necrosis induced by angiotensin II.. Circ Res 1991; 69:1185–1195.

57. Villarreal FJ, Kim NN, Ungab GD, Printz MP, Dillmann WH. Identification of functional angiotensin II receptors on rat cardiac fibroblasts. Circulation 1993; 88:2849–2861.

58. Anderson KR, Sutton MG, Lie JT. Histopathological types of cardiac fibrosis in myocardial disease. J Pathol 1979; 128:79–85.

59. Weber KT, Pick R, Silver MA, Moe GW, Janicki JS, Zucker IH, Armstrong PW. Fibrillar collagen and remodeling of dilated canine left ventricle. Circulation 1990; 82:1387–1401.

60. Ross RS, Borg TK. Integrins and the myocardium. Circ Res 2001; 88(11):1112–1119.

61. Spinale FG, Coker ML, Thomas CV, Walker JD, Mukherjee R, Hebbar L. Time-dependent changes in matrix metalloproteinase activity and expression during the progression of congestive heart failure: relation to ventricular and myocyte function. Circ Res 1998 Mar 9; 82(4): 482–495.

62. Mann DL, Spinale FG. Activation of matrix metalloproteinases in the failing human heart: breaking the tie that binds. Circulation 1998 Oct 27; 98(17):1699–1702.

63. Weisman HF, Bush DE, Mannisi JA, Weisfeldt ML, Healy B. Cellular mechanisms of myocardial infarct expansion. Circulation 1988 Jul; 78(1):186–201.

64. Rubin SA, Fishbein MC, Swan HJ. Compensatory hypertrophy in the heart after myocardial infarction in the rat. J Am Coll Cardiol 1983 Jun; 1(6):1435–1441.

65. Sutton MG, Sharpe N. Left ventricular remodeling after myocardial infarction: pathophysiology and therapy. Circulation 2000 Jun 27; 101(25):2981–2988.

66. Mani K, Kitsis RN. Myocyte apoptosis: programming ventricular remodeling. J Am Coll Cardiol 2003 Mar 5; 41(5):761–764.

67. Dorn GW, Mann DL. Signaling pathways involved in left ventricular remodeling: summation. J Card Fail 2002 Dec; 8(6 Suppl):S387–S388.

68. Bueno OF, Molkentin JD. Involvement of extracellular signal-regulated kinases 1/2 in cardiac hypertrophy and cell death. Circ Res 2002 Nov 1; 91(9):776–781.

69. Wilkins BJ, Molkentin JD. Calcineurin and cardiac hypertrophy: where have we been? Where are we going?. J Physiol 2002 May 15; 541(Pt 1):1–8.

70. Palojoki E, Saraste A, Eriksson A, Pulkki K, Kallajoki M, Voipio-Pulkki LM, Tikkanen I. Cardiomyocyte apoptosis and ventricular remodeling after myocardial infarction in rats. Am J Physiol Heart Circ Physiol 2001 Jun; 280(6):H2726–2731.

71. Sharov VG, Sabbah HN, Shimoyama H, Goussev AV, Lesch M, Goldstein S. Evidence of cardiocyte apoptosis in myocardium of dogs with chronic heart failure. Am J Pathol 1996 Jan; 148(1):141–149.

72. Teiger E, Than VD, Richard L, Wisnewsky C, Tea BS, Gaboury L, Tremblay J, Schwartz K, Hamet P. Apoptosis in pressure overload-induced heart hypertrophy in the rat. J Clin Invest 1996 Jun 15; 97(12):2891–2897.

73. Polunovsky VA, Wendt CH, Ingbar DH, Peterson MS, Bitterman PB. Induction of endothelial cell apoptosis by TNF alpha: modulation by inhibitors of protein synthesis. Exp Cell Res 1994 Oct; 214(2):584–594.

74. Ferrari R, Agnoletti L, Comini L, Gaia G, Bachetti T, Cargnoni A, Ceconi C, Curello S, Visioli O. Oxidative stress during myocardial ischaemia and heart failure. Eur Heart J. 1998 Feb; 19 Suppl B:B2–B11.

75. Ashkenazi A, Dixit VM. Death receptors: signaling and modulation. Science 1998 Aug 28; 281(5381):1305–1308.

76. Mani K, Kitsis RN. Myocyte apoptosis: programming ventricular remodeling. J Am Coll Cardiol 2003 Mar 5; 41(5):761–764.

77. Green DR, Reed JC. Mitochondria and apoptosis. Science 1998 Aug 28; 281(5381): 1309–1312.

78. Bialik S, Geenen DL, Sasson IE, Cheng R, Horner JW, Evans SM, Lord EM, Koch CJ, Kitsis RN. Related articles, links myocyte apoptosis during acute myocardial infarction in the mouse localizes to hypoxic regions but occurs independently of p53. J Clin Invest 1997 Sep 15; 100(6):1363–1372.

79. Jeremias I, Kupatt C, Martin-Villalba A, Habazettl H, Schenkel J, Boekstegers P, Debatin KM. Involvement of CD95/Apo1/Fas in cell death after myocardial ischemia. Circulation 2000 Aug 22; 102(8):915–920.

80. Abbate A, Biondi-Zoccai GG, Bussani R, Dobrina A, Camilot D, Feroce F, Rossiello R, Baldi F, Silvestri F, Biasucci LM, Baldi A. Increased myocardial apoptosis in patients with unfavorable left ventricular remodeling and early symptomatic post-infarction heart failure. J Am Coll Cardiol 2003 Mar 5; 41(5):753–760.

81. Cleutjens JP, Verluyten MJ, Smiths JF, Daemen MJ. Collagen remodeling after myocardial infarction in the rat heart. Am J Pathol 1995 Aug; 147(2):325–238.

82. Cleutjens JP, Kandala JC, Guarda E, Guntaka RV, Weber KT. Regulation of collagen degradation in the rat myocardium after infarction. J Mol Cell Cardiol 1995 Jun; 27(6):1281–1292.

83. Volders PG, Willems IE, Cleutjens JP, Arends JW, Havenith MG, Daemen MJ. Interstitial collagen is increased in the noninfarcted human myocardium after myocardial infarction. J Mol Cell Cardiol 1993 Nov; 25(11):1317–1323.

84. Reimer KA, Jennings RB. The changing anatomic reference base of evolving myocardial infarction. Underestimation of myocardial collateral blood flow and overestimation of experimental anatomic infarct size due to tissue edema, hemorrhage and acute inflammation. Circulation 1979 Oct; 60(4):866–876.

85. Pfeffer MA, Braunwald E. Ventricular remodeling after myocardial infarction: experimental observations and clinical implications. Circulation 1990; 81:1161–1172.

86. Picard MH, Wilkins GT, Ray PA, Weyman AE. Progressive changes in ventricular structure and function during the year after acute myocardial infarction. Am Heart J 1992; 124:24–31.

87. Pfeffer MA. Left ventricular remodeling after acute myocardial infarction. Annu Rev Med 1995; 46:455–466.

88. Kono T, Sabbah HN, Rosman H, Alam M, Jafri S, Stein PD, Goldstein S. Left ventricular shape is the primary determinant of functional mitral regurgitation in heart failure. J Am Coll Cardiol 1992; 20:1594–1598.

89. White HD, Norris RM, Brown MA, Brandt PW, Whitlock RM, Wild CJ. Left ventricular end-systolic volume as the major determinant of survival after recovery from myocardial infarction. Circulation 1987; 76:44–51.

90. Menicanti L, Dor V, Buckberg GD, Athanasuleas CL, Di Donato M. Inferior wall restoration: anatomic and surgical considerations. Semin Thorac Cardiovasc Surg 2001 Oct; 13(4): 504–513.

91. Buckberg GD. The structure and function of the healthy helical and failing spherical heart. Overview: the ventricular band and its surgical implications. Semin Thorac Cardiovasc Surg 2001 Oct; 13(4):298–300.

92. Torrent-Guasp F, Buckberg GD, Clemente C, Cox JL, Coghlan HC, Gharib M. The structure and function of the helical heart and its buttress wrapping. I. The normal macroscopic structure of the heart. Semin Thorac Cardiovasc Surg 2001 Oct; 13(4):301–319.

93. Torrent-Guasp F, Ballester M, Buckberg GD, Carreras F, Flotats A, Carrio I, Ferreira A, Samuels LE, Narula J. Spatial orientation of the ventricular muscle band: physiologic contribution and surgical implications. J Thorac Cardiovasc Surg 2001 Aug; 122(2):389–392.

94. Visser CA, Kan G, Meltzer RS, Koolen JJ, Dunning AJ. Incidence, timing and prognostic value of left ventricular aneurysm formation after myocardial infarction: a prospective, serial echocardiographic study of 158 patients. Am J Cardiol 1986 Apr 1; 57(10):729–732.

95. Arvan S, Badillo P. Contractile properties of the left ventricle with aneurysm. Am J Cardiol 1985 Feb 1; 55(4):338–341.

96. Kirklin JW, Barratt-Boyes BG. Left Ventricular Aneurysm. In: Cardiac Surgery. New York: Churchill Livingstone Inc., 1993: Chapter 8:383–401.

97. Tikiz H, Balbay Y, Atak R, Terzi T, Genc Y, Kutuk E. The effect of thrombolytic therapy on left ventricular aneurysm formation in acute myocardial infarction: relationship to successful reperfusion and vessel patency. Clin Cardiol 2001 Oct; 24(10):656–662.

98. Bartel T, Vanheiden H, Schaar J, Mertzkirch W, Erbel R. Biomechanical modeling of hemodynamic factors determining bulging of ventricular aneurysms. Ann Thorac Surg 2002 Nov; 74(5):1587–1588.

99. Moustakidis P, Maniar HS, Cupps BP, Absi T, Zheng J, Guccione JM, Sundt TM, Pasque MK. Altered left ventricular geometry changes the border zone temporal distribution of stress in an experimental model of left ventricular aneurysm: a finite element model study. Circulation 2002 Sep 24; 106(12 Suppl 1):I168–I175.

100. Jackson BM, Gorman JH, Moainie SL, Guy TS, Narula N, Narula J, John-Sutton MG, Edmunds LH, Gorman RC. Extension of borderzone myocardium in postinfarction dilated cardiomyopathy. J Am Coll Cardiol 2002 Sep 18; 40(6):1160–1167.

101. Godley RW, Wann LS, Rogers EW, Feigenbaum H, Weyman AE. Incomplete mitral leaflet closure in patients with papillary muscle dysfunction. Circulation 1981 Mar; 63(3):565–571.

102. Barzilai B, Gessler C, Perez JE, Schaab C, Jaffe AS. Significance of Doppler-detected mitral regurgitation in acute myocardial infarction. Am J Cardiol 1988 Feb 1; 61(4):220–223.

103. Lehmann KG, Francis CK, Dodge HT. Mitral regurgitation in early myocardial infarction. Incidence, clinical detection, and prognostic implications. TIMI Study Group. Ann Intern Med 1992 Jul 1; 117(1):10–17.

104. Stevenson LW, Bellil D, Grover-McKay M, Brunken RC, Schwaiger M, Tillisch JH, Schelbert HR. Effects of afterload reduction (diuretics and vasodilators) on left ventricular volume and mitral regurgitation in severe congestive heart failure secondary to ischemic or idiopathic dilated cardiomyopathy. Am J Cardiol 1987 Sep 15; 60(8):654–658.

105. Junker A, Thayssen P, Nielsen B, Andersen PE. The hemodynamic and prognostic significance of echo-Doppler-proven mitral regurgitation in patients with dilated cardiomyopathy. Cardiology 1993; 83(1–2):14–20.

106. Koelling TM, Aaronson KD, Cody RJ, Bach DS, Armstrong WF. Prognostic significance of mitral regurgitation and tricuspid regurgitation in patients with left ventricular systolic dysfunction. Am Heart J 2002 Sep; 144(3):524–529.

107. Lamas GA, Mitchell GF, Flaker M, Smith SC, Gersh BJ, Basta L, Moye L, Braunwald E, Pfeffer MA. For the Survival And Ventricular Enlargement investigators: clinical significance of mitral regurgitation after acute myocardial infarction. Circulation 1997; 96:827–833.

108. Grigioni F, Enriquez-Sarano M, Zehr KJ, Bailey KR, Tajik AJ. Ischemic mitral regurgitation: long-term outcome and prognostic implications with quantitative doppler assessment. Circulation 2001; 103:1759–1764.

109. Rankin JS, Hickey MSJ, Smith LR, Muhlbaier L, Reves JG, Pryor DB, Wechsler AS. Ischemic mitral regurgitation. Circulation 1989; 79(6 PT 2):I116–I121.

110. Otsuji Y, Handschumacher MD, Schwammenthal E, Jiang L, Song JK, Guerrero JL, Vlahakes GJ, Levine RA. Insights from three-dimensional echocardiography into the mechanism of functional mitral regurgitation: direct in vivo demonstration of altered leaflet tethering geometry. Circulation 1997 Sep 16; 96(6):1999–2008.

111. Otsuji Y, Handschumacher MD, Liel-Cohen N, Tanabe H, Jiang L, Schwammenthal E, Guerrero JL, Nicholls LA, Vlahakes GJ, Levine RA. Mechanism of ischemic mitral regurgitation with segmental left ventricular dysfunction: three-dimensional echocardiographic studies in models of acute and chronic progressive regurgitation. J Am Coll Cardiol 2001 Feb; 37(2): 641–648.

112. Yiu SF, Enriquez-Sarano M, Tribouilloy C, Seward JB, Tajik AJ. Determinants of the degree of functional mitral regurgitation in patients with systolic left ventricular dysfunction: A quantitative clinical study. Circulation 2000 Sep 19; 102(12):1400–1406.

113. He S, Fontaine AA, Schwammenthal E, Yoganathan AP, Levine RA. Integrated mechanism for functional mitral regurgitation: leaflet restriction versus coapting force: in vitro studies. Circulation 1997 Sep 16; 96(6):1826–1834.

114. Kumanohoso T, Otsuji Y, Yoshifuku S, Matsukida K, Koriyama C, Kisanuki A, Minagoe S, Levine RA, Tei C. Mechanism of higher incidence of ischemic mitral regurgitation in

patients with inferior myocardial infarction: quantitative analysis of left ventricular and mitral valve geometry in 103 patients with prior myocardial infarction. J Thorac Cardiovasc Surg 2003 Jan; 125(1):135–143.

115. Boltwood CM, Tei C, Wong M, Shah PM. Quantitative echocardiography of the mitral complex in dilated cardiomyopathy: the mechanism of functional mitral regurgitation. Circulation 1983 Sep; 68(3):498–508.

116. Carabello BA. Mitral valve regurgitation. Curr Probl Cardiol 1998 Apr; 23(4):202–241.

117. Spinale FG, Ishihra K, Zile MR, DeFryte G, Crawford FA, Carabello BA. Structural basis for changes in left ventricular function and geometry because of chronic mitral regurgitation and after correction of volume overload. J Thorac Cardiovasc Surg 1993; 106:1147–1157.

118. Corin WJ, Monrad ES, Murakami T, Nonogi H, Hess OM, Krayenbuehl HP. The relationship of afterload to ejection performance in chronic mitral regurgitation. Circulation 1987 Jul; 76(1):59–67.

119. Zile MR, Gaasch WH, Levine HJ. Left ventricular stress-dimension-shortening relations before and after correction of chronic aortic and mitral regurgitation. Am J Cardiol 1985 Jul 1; 56(1):99–105.

120. Talwar S, Squire IB, Davies JE, Ng LL. The effect of valvular regurgitation on plasma cardiotrophin-1 in patients with normal left ventricular systolic function. Eur J Heart Fail 2000 Dec; 2(4):387–391.

121. Dell'Italia LJ, Meng QC, Balcells E, Straeter-Knowlen IM, Hankes GH, Dillon R, Cartee RE, Orr R, Bishop SP, Oparil S, et al. Increased ACE and chymase-like activity in cardiac tissue of dogs with chronic mitral regurgitation. Am J Physiol 1995 Dec; 269(6 Pt 2): H2065–H2073.

122. Kapadia SR, Yakoob K, Nader S, Thomas JD, Mann DL, Griffin BP. Elevated circulating levels of serum tumor necrosis factor-alpha in patients with hemodynamically significant pressure and volume overload. J Am Coll Cardiol 2000 Jul; 36(1):208–212.

123. Hirose K, Shu NH, Reed JE, Rumberger JA. Right ventricular dilatation and remodeling the first year after an initial transmural wall left ventricular myocardial infarction. Am J Cardiol 1993 Nov 15; 72(15):1126–1130.

124. Nahrendorf M, Hu K, Fraccarollo D, Hiller KH, Haase A, Bauer WR, Ertl G. Time course of right ventricular remodeling in rats with experimental myocardial infarction. Am J Physiol Heart Circ Physiol 2003 Jan; 284(1):H241–H248.

125. Hung J, Koelling T, Semigran MJ, Dec GW, Levine RA, Di Salvo TG. Usefulness of echocardiographic determined tricuspid regurgitation in predicting event-free survival in severe heart failure secondary to idiopathic-dilated cardiomyopathy or to ischemic cardiomyopathy. Am J Cardiol 1998 Nov 15; 82(10):1301–1303.

126. Rohde LE, Ducharme A, Arroyo LH, Aikawa M, Sukhova GH, Lopez-Anaya A, McClure KF, Mitchell PG, Libby P, Lee RT. Matrix metalloproteinase inhibition attenuates early left ventricular enlargement after experimental myocardial infarction in mice. Circulation 1999 Jun 15; 99(23):3063–3070.

127. Nishigaki K, Minatoguchi S, Seishima M, Asano K, Noda T, Yasuda N, Sano H, Kumada H, Takemura M, Noma A, Tanaka T, Watanabe S, Fujiwara H. Plasma Fas ligand, an inducer of apoptosis, and plasma soluble Fas, an inhibitor of apoptosis, in patients with chronic congestive heart failure. J Am Coll Cardiol 1997 May; 29(6):1214–1220.

128. Susin SA, Zamzami N, Castedo M, Hirsch T, Marchetti P, Macho A, Daugas E, Geuskens M, Kroemer G. Bcl-2 inhibits the mitochondrial release of an apoptogenic protease. J Exp Med 1996 Oct 1; 184(4):1331–1341.

7

Neurohormonal and Cytokine Activation in Heart Failure

Dennis M. McNamara
Heart Failure & Transplantation Program, University of Pittsburgh Medical Center, Pittsburgh, Pennsylvania, USA

When the whole body experiences changes, whether alternations of cold and heat, or changes of color, protracted disease is announced. Hippocrates. (470–410, B.C.) [1]

SYNOPSIS

Heart failure, regardless of severity, is characterized by activation of the renin-angiotensin-aldosterone system (RAAS) and sympathetic nervous system (SNS). The complex interaction of the RAAS and SNS suggests they act as two arms of a single common pathway. More recently, a wide variety of proinflammatory cytokines, including tumor necrosis factor (TNF) and interleukin-6, have been shown to be related to heart failure severity and outcome. TNF appears to be particularly important in the transition from compensated to decompensated heart failure. Natriuretic peptides represent an additional hormonal response designed to control plasma volume and are released by elevated ventricular filling pressures of fluid overload. Higher brain natriuretic peptide (BNP) levels predict a poorer prognosis and may provide an easy method to monitor the effectiveness of heart failure therapies in the near future. Genetic heterogenicity as reflected by single nucleotide polymorphisms (SNPs) appear to affect the response of heart failure patients to pharmacologic therapies. Common deletion/insertion polymorphisms of the ACE D-allele, beta-2 adrenergic receptor, and nitric oxide synthase have been demonstrated to influence outcome and may lead to individualization of pharmacologic therapies in the future.

INTRODUCTION

Whether ischemic, viral, or inflammatory in etiology, the pathological processes leading to the clinical syndrome of heart failure begin with myocardial injury. The hemodynamic consequences of the initial injury, a decline in contractility, and the reduction of cardiac output elicit a complex humoral response involving the central nervous system, the kidney, and the vascular endothelium. Progression to the syndrome of heart failure is determined by both the degree of myocardial injury and the nature and magnitude of the resultant humoral activation. Pharmacologic interventions targeted to improve cardiac contractility have not improved clinical outcomes [2,3]. In contrast, all therapies that improve heart failure survival inhibit aspects of the systemic response [4,5,6].

The systemic response has two major components: the sympathetic nervous system and the renin angiotensin aldosterone pathway [7], which are collectively referred to as neurohormonal activation [8]. Additional circulating mediators, such as natruretic peptides and nitric oxide [9], also play a role in the circulatory adaptations to the heart failure state. Finally, myocardial injury and the heart failure syndrome stimulate the production of cytokines, circulating peptide mediators of inflammation such as tumor necrosis factor (TNF) and interleukin-6 (IL-6) [10]. For both neurohormonal and cytokine activation, these reflex pathways are designed for acute injury and have maladaptive consequences in the chronic heart failure state. Understanding their impact on progressive myocardial dysfunction and subsequent vascular adaptation is critical to deciphering the systemic nature of the heart failure syndrome. Investigation of the complex interactions of these pathways is essential for the optimal application of clinical therapeutics [11,12,13]. The variability among patients in heart failure progression likely reflects genetic differences in the neurohormonal response, and the delineation of the genomic basis for this heterogeneity may allow highly specific tailoring of therapy for individual patients.

RENIN ANGIOTENSIN ALDOSTERONE SYSTEM

The renin-angiotensin-aldosterone system (RAAS) is a compensatory pathway primarily designed for preservation of renal blood flow [14,15]. A decrease in renal perfusion pressure results in the secretion of renin by juxtaglomerular cells lining the afferent renal arterioles. This release is also under the control of the autonomic nervous system through beta-adrenergic receptors in the kidney. Renin, an aspartyl protease, cleaves a propeptide produced by the liver, angiotensinogen, to form the decapeptide angiotensin-I. The angiotensin converting enzyme (ACE), a dipeptidyl carboxypeptidase bound to the plasma membrane of endothelial cells, cleaves the two C terminal amino acids to form the vasoactive octapeptide angiotensin-2, the primary effector of the system (Fig. 1). Receptors for angiotensin-II are divided into

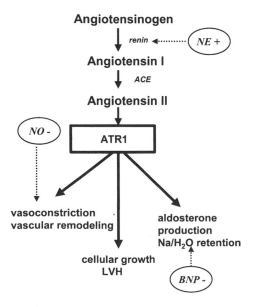

Figure 1   Renin angiotensin pathway: physiologic effects of angiotensin II and interactions with other neurohormones. ACE, angiotensin converting enzyme; NE, norepinephrine; NO, nitric oxide; ATR1, angiotensin receptor type 1; BNP, brain natruretic peptide.

subtypes, AT-1 and AT-2, based on antagonist binding affinity [16]. AT-1 is the predominant subtype in the vascular endothelium and the primary target for pharmacologic blockade [17]. Binding of angiotensin-II to AT-1 receptors results in increased release of intracellular calcium from the sarcoplasma reticulum through activation of protein kinase C (PKC). Binding of angiotensin-II in the vasculature results in vasoconstriction, an increase in systemic vascular resistance and restoration of blood pressure.

During acute declines in renal perfusion, such as from blood loss or dehydration, this compensatory pathway has salutary effects on renal perfusion; however, in chronic heart failure the rise in systemic vascular resistance increases myocardial work, decreases cardiac output, and results in compensatory left ventricular hypertrophy [7,18]. In addition, angiotensin-II has direct effects on the myocardium that increase remodeling of the extracellular matrix [19], induces myocyte hypertrophy, and initiates apoptosis and interstitial fibrosis (Fig. 2) [20,21,22,23]. This worsens myocardial relaxation and contributes to diastolic dysfunction [24]. The impact of angiotensin-II on the myocardium and the peripheral vasculature decreases cardiac output and renal blood flow and, thus, leads to further increases in renin-angiotensin activation and a progressive decline in cardiac function.

The potential benefit of renin-angiotensin inhibition was first demonstrated in postinfarction animal models, in which ACE inhibitors decreased left ventricular remodeling after myocardial infarction. These preclinical models provided the rationale for landmark clinical investigations, which demonstrated that the ACE inhibitor captopril limited left ventricular remodeling [26,27] and improved clinical outcomes in patients after significant myocardial infarction. The improvement of heart failure survival with ACE inhibitors has been consistently demonstrated in clinical trials [4,27] supporting the central role renin-angiotensin activation plays in progression of heart failure. However, the impact of ACE inhibitors in heart failure reflects more than simple reductions in circulating angiotensin-II, as the therapeutic effects persist while the decline in angiotensin-II is transient [28,29] and incomplete, even at high doses [30].

In addition to the effects on the vasculature and the myocardium, angiotensin-II increases plasma volume by initiating production of the minerocorticoid aldosterone by the adrenal cortex [31]. Aldosterone acts on the distal tubules of the renal nephron and activates a sodium potassium exchange pump. This results in the retention of sodium and water at the expense of increased kaluresis. As with the other compensatory action of RAAS, with acute volume loss the elevations in aldosterone result in a restoration of

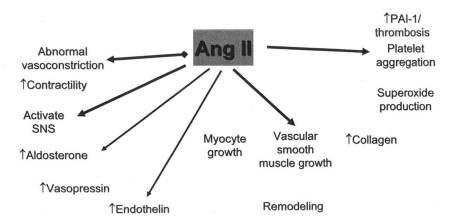

Figure 2 Potentially deleterious pathophysiologic effects of angiotensin II in chronic heart failure.

plasma volume, however, in chronic heart failure this increase exacerbates fluid overload and peripheral edema. In addition aldosterone, like angiotensin-II [32], has a direct effect on vascular and ventricular remodeling, and chronic excess leads to increase fibrosis in the atria, ventricles, kidneys and the perivasculature. Both angiotensin 2 and aldosterone contribute to adverse ventricular remodeling and progressive heart failure [33]. The addition of aldosterone receptor antagonists to a background of ACE inhibitor therapy improves survival in patients with severe chronic heart failure [34] and in subjects with left ventricular dysfunction postmyocardial infarction [35] (Chapter 15). In contrast, attempts to improve survival with the addition of angiotensin receptor blockers to ACE inhibitors have not been successful [36].

Through control of vascular tone and plasma volume, the two primary effectors of the RAAS play a central role in regulating blood pressure. Recently, a homologue of the angiotensin converting enzyme, ACE2, has been cloned and mapped to a position on the X chromosome [37,38]. It has significant cardiac expression [39], primarily in the endocardium and cleaves the C terminal amino acid from the vasoconstrictive octapeptide angiotensin-II to form a 7 amino acid peptide with vasodilatory properties. Overexpression in transgenic models produces a hypotensive phenotype, and decreased expression has been demonstrated in hypertensive rat models. While it is clear that ACE2 plays a counter regulatory role to ACE in terms of blood pressure control, the role of this second ACE enzyme in the inhibition and modulation of neurohormonal activation in heart failure remains uncertain.

SYMPATHETIC ACTIVATION

Increased sympathetic nerve activity plays a central role in the physiological maladaptations of chronic heart failure [40]. The decline in cardiac output and stroke volume is sensed by vascular baroreceptors and results in an increase in sympathetic nerve activity and release of norepinephrine. Sympathetic activation, the "fight or flight response" of the autonomic nervous system, improves cardiac output through increased heart rate, myocardial contractility and stroke volume. In the peripheral vasculature, sympathetic activation increases systemic resistance and blood pressure. Stimulation of beta-adrenergic receptors in the kidney increase renin release and angiotenin-II production, further increasing vascular resistance and afterload.

The augmentation of cardiac function by sympathetic activation is primarily mediated through beta-adrenergic receptors [41]. The predominant receptor subtypes in the myocardium are beta-1 and beta-2. Agonist binding of both subtypes results in increased cyclic adenosine monophosphate (cAMP) and the activation of several cAMP-dependent protein kinases and phosphorylation of intracellular proteins [42]. Beta-1 receptors are the predominant subtype in the nonfailing heart, comprising roughly 80% of the beta-adrenergic receptors [43]. However, chronic sympathetic stimulation results in significantly more downregulation of beta-1 receptors than beta-2 and, therefore, in the failing heart the relative percentage of beta-2 receptors increases to approximately 40%. While beta 2 receptors are less downregulated, they are inactivated by repetitive agonist stimulation and, as a result, become less responsive to adrenergic agonists in heart failure.

In addition to the effects on cardiac beta receptors, chronic adrenergic stimulation has significant deleterious effects on cardiac function. The increase in cardiac contractility and heart rate increases myocardial metabolic demands, worsens ischemia, and has proarrhythmic effects. In addition, catecholamine stimulation of myocardial cells has direct cytotoxic effects and results in cell damage and cell death [44,45]. Therefore, though norepinephrine acutely increases myocardial contractility, chronic stimulation of beta-adrenergic receptors worsens cardiac function and results in progression of the clinical syndrome of left ventricular dysfunction, worsening pulmonary edema, and death.

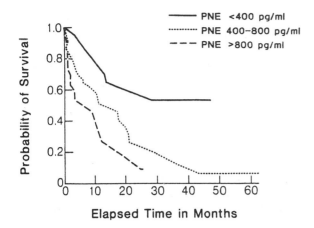

Figure 3   Survival in chronic heart failure by plasma norepinephrine level (PNE). (From Ref. 46.)

In clinical heart failure, increasing severity of functional limitations and NYHA (New York Heart Association) class is associated with increasing levels of plasma norepinephrine. Higher levels of circulating norepinephrine are associated with poorer survival in subjects with heart failure despite identical degrees of depression of left ventricular function (Fig. 3) [46]. The importance of sympathetic activation in the progression of left ventricular dysfunction is best evidenced by clinical studies of beta adrenergic blockade, which consistently demonstrate an improvement of left ventricular ejection fraction of 6 to 10 EF units after several months of therapy [47]. This degree of improvement in LVEF far exceeds that achieved with any other pharmacologic therapeutics.

INTERACTION OF RENIN ANGIOTENSIN AND SYMPATHETIC ACTIVATION

The complex interaction of renin angiotensin and sympathetic activation in the pathophysiology of congestive heart failure suggests they act as two aspects of a single common pathway. The release of renin is regulated by the sympathetic nervous system through beta-receptors in the kidney, and therapy with beta-blockers results in reductions in plasma renin and circulating angiotensin-II. The effectiveness of beta-blockers as antihypertensives relates as much to their reductions in plasma renin as to their blockade of cardiac adrenoreceptors. This has led to some speculation that the beneficial effects of beta-blockers in heart failure may reflect their actions as ''renin inhibitors'' [48].

In a similar fashion, treatment with angiotensin converting enzyme inhibitors reduces sympathetic activation characteristic of the heart failure state. Treatment with ACE inhibitors reduces circulating plasma norepinephrine, and leads to increases in the myocardium cardiac beta-receptor density [49]. Studies of pharmacologic perturbation of both renin angiotensin pathway and sympathetic activation demonstrate that it is impossible to inhibit either system without having significant impact on the other, and suggest they represent interdependent aspects of a single compensatory pathway of neurohormonal activation.

CYTOKINE ACTIVATION

Cardiac inflammation plays a significant role in the initiation of myocardial injury, subsequent ventricular remodeling, and the progression of left ventricular dysfunction [50].

Cytokines, circulating peptides initially isolated from cells of the immune system, are important mediators of systemic inflammation. Tumor necrosis factor (TNF) is a 17 kDa polypeptide that activates endothelial cells, recruits inflammatory cells, and enhances the production of other proinflammatory cytokines. Initially called ''cachectin'' [51], it promotes weight loss and muscle wasting in end-stage malignancy. The similar wasting phenotype in end-stage cardiac cachexia led to investigation of TNF in severe chronic heart failure, where it was found to be markedly elevated [52].

The cytokine hypothesis proposes that heart failure progression is an inflammatory process and that elaboration of proinflammatory cytokines worsens left ventricular dysfunction and facilitates the development of the clinical syndrome [10]. As with the neurohormonal mediators norepinephrine and angiotensin, clinical trial data demonstrate that increasing levels of circulating TNF correlated with increasing levels of functional limitations in heart failure [53]. Early in the disease process, much of circulating TNF is derived from immune cell line such as activated macrophages. However, late in disease progression the heart itself becomes a secretory organ and much of the TNF is produced by the cardiac myocytes themselves (Fig. 4) [54]. TNF appears to be particularly important in the transition from compensated to decompensated heart failure.

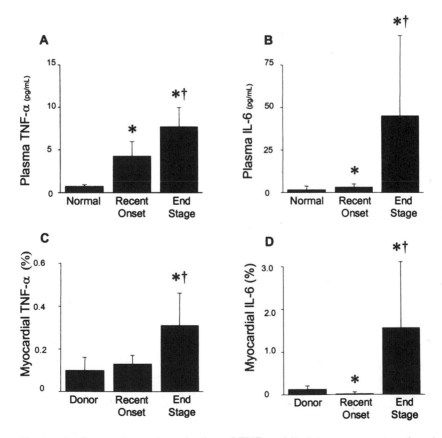

Figure 4 Comparison of production of TNF and IL-6 in new onset and end-stage heart failure. (**A**) Plasma and myocardial TNF-α (*A, C*) and IL-6 (*B, D*) levels in recent onset cardiomyopathy and end-stage patients. (Plasma levels: protein [pg/ml]; myocardial levels: mRNA expressed as percent of GAPDH mRNA level.) [a] Significantly different (p<0.05) from normal or donor group. [b] Significantly different (p<0.05) from recent onset group.

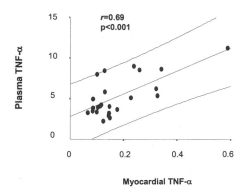

Figure 4 (continued) **(B)** Correlation of plasma TNF-α (pg/ml) with myocardial mRNA levels (percent of GAPDH mRNA level); r = 0.69, p<0.001. (From Ref. 54; pp. 819--824.)

The effects of TNF on myocardial function have been evaluated extensively in animal models. Transgenic mice with cardiac specific overexpression of TNF develop an early inflammatory myocarditis that later progresses to myocyte hypertrophy, left ventricular dilatation, and progressive left ventricular dysfunction [55]. In the transgenic model, TNF activates expression of matrix metalloproteinases [56], which contribute to LV remodeling and dilatation. Exogenously administered TNF in animal models at concentrations comparable to those observed in clinical heart failure, produces significant declines in myocardial contractility, worsening left ventricular function, and increasing pulmonary edema [57]. In a model of exogenously infused TNF, rats developed time-dependent progressive left ventricular enlargement accompanied by significant degradation of the extracellular matrix [58].

The negative inotropic effects of TNF on cardiac myocytes are mediated through increased expression of inducible nitric oxide synthase (NOS2) and the production of nitric oxide [59,60]. Chronic adrenergic stimulation induces myocardial TNF expression [61], which in turn attenuates beta-adrenergic responsiveness. Blockade of TNF with soluble TNF receptor limits cardiac inflammation [62] in animal models, and led to the hypothesis that inhibition of TNF activation would improve LV function and clinical outcomes [63]. However, while initial small clinical studies suggested soluble receptor improved function in chronic heart failure [64,65], two larger randomized multicenter studies failed to prove benefit [10].

In murine models of myocarditis, TNF appears to limit viral injury as TNF knockout mice have less cardiac inflammation but also less viral clearing and more myocyte cell death [66]. Myocardial expression of TNF is elevated in human myocarditis, and in clinical investigations of recent onset cardiomyopathy, higher levels of circulating TNF at presentation predicted a higher probability of subsequent recovery of LV function [67]. These studies suggest a cardioprotective role for TNF in early heart failure pathogenesis that appears quite distinct from the deleterious impact evident in end-stage disease [68].

Interleukin-6, (IL-6) is also significantly elevated in heart failure, particularly in end-stage disease [69]. Initially thought to be proinflammatory like TNF, recent evidence suggests more of an immune modulatory role [70]. IL-6 knockout mice stimulated with lipopolysaccharide produce more TNF than wild-type litter mates, suggesting IL-6 limits TNF production. Murine transgenic models with chronic IL-6 overexpression are at greater risk for viral injury [71]. In contrast, animals treated with short-term exogenous IL-6 appear protected from viral injury. In addition to potential immune modulatory interactions with TNF,

IL-6 has direct effects on the myocardium and decreases contractility, induces myocyte hypertrophy, activates matrix metalloproteinases, and contributes to LV remodeling [72].

In clinical investigations, IL-6 levels correlate with measures of myocardial function including LVEF, NYHA class and cardiac hemodynamics [67,69]. Myocardial expression of IL-6 is evident in severe end-stage heart failure but not in mild to moderate disease, suggesting that cardiac IL-6 production occurs later in the disease process than TNF [54]. Higher circulating levels of IL-6 are associated with a poorer prognosis [73,74]. IL-6 plays a central role in the acute phase response, inducing production of C-reactive protein (CRP) and fibrinogen. CRP levels are also markedly elevated in heart failure and predict poor outcomes.

As with neurohormonal activation, cytokine-mediated cardiac inflammation begins as an appropriate acute response to myocardial injury but has significant maladaptive consequences in chronic heart failure. Proinflammatory cytokines, in particular TNF, may have cardioprotective effects in myocarditis and recent onset cardiomyopathy. However, in end-stage disease, increased production of inflammatory cytokines by the myocardium facilitates progression from compensated to decompensated heart failure. Unlike neurohormonal activation, direct inhibition of the cytokine response has not demonstrated clinical benefit in randomized trials.

REGULATION OF PLASMA VOLUME

Natruretic peptides represent an additional hormonal response designed to control plasma volume and are activated in heart failure by excess fluid retention [75]. Increased atrial and ventricular filling pressures, dilatation, and wall stress result in the secretion of peptides that act on the kidney, increase natruresis and decrease plasma volume [76]. Brain natruretic peptide (BNP) is a 32-amino acid peptide synthesized by the ventricle. BNP is markedly elevated in congestive heart failure and correlates with cardiac filling pressures. Higher levels of BNP in subjects with heart failure predict a poor prognosis [77,78,79a] (Fig. 5). In addition to natruresis, BNP induces vasodilatation, decreases renin-angiotensin and sympathetic activation [79]. Therefore, as neurohormonal activation drives the heart failure pathway forward, the increase in secretion of BNP driven by fluid overload diminishes their impact and serves as an important counter regulatory mechanism.

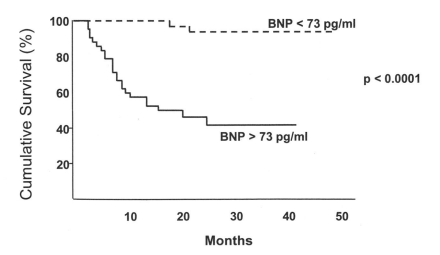

Figure 5   Survival rates for patients with left ventricular dysfunction stratified by initial mean plasma BNP concentration. BNP, brain natriuretic peptide. (From Ref. 79a.)

VASCULAR REACTIVITY

Heart failure leads to endothelial dysfunction [80,81] and changes in the peripheral vasculature. Elevations in angiotensin-II increase peripheral vascular resistance initially preserving perfusion pressure. Over time vascular remodeling becomes evident with smooth muscle cell hypertrophy, cellular proliferation, and interstitial fibrosis that results ultimately in the loss of capillary vascular volume. Similar vascular changes occur in the pulmonary vasculature, driven by chronic elevations in pulmonary capillary wedge pressure, and leads to pulmonary hypertension. In addition to angiotensin-II, several important mediators are released by the endothelium that help regulate vascular tone: the endothelins and the nitric oxide pathway.

The primary mediator of endothelium-dependent vasodilatation, initially functionally described as endothelium derived relaxation factor (EDRF), is now known to be nitric oxide and its derivatives. Nitric oxide (NO), a freely diffusible gas with a short half-life, is produced from arginine from a family of enzymes, the nitric oxide synthases [9]. Endothelial nitric oxide synthase (NOS3) is the primary source of vascular NO production and is a constitutively active enzyme. However, in heart failure inducible nitric oxide (NOS2) is upregulated and may be an important source of circulating NO [82].

The primary effect of NO on vascular function is vasodilatation. In heart failure, this results in decreased peripheral resistance and reduced after load, and the effects of NO on the vasculature improves cardiac performance and limits disease progression. In addition, at least some of the beneficial effects of ACE inhibitors in heart failure are mediated through nitric oxide dependent mechanisms [83]. ACE inhibitors limit postinfarction LV remodeling in wild-type animals but not in NOS3 knockout mice, suggesting the protective effects of therapy require the presence of NOS3 [84,85]. The impact of ACE inhibitors on endothelial function can be limited by pretreatment with N-monomethyl-L-arginine (LMNNA), an inhibitor of NO production [86]. While ACE inhibitors improve endothelial function by increasing NO production, circulating TNF impairs the action of NOS3 [87], and may tip the balance towards vasoconstriction and endothelial dysfunction.

Expression of NOS3 in the myocardium is increased in heart failure and affects myocardial function as well as vascular reactivity [88,89]. Nitric oxide is an important mediator of the impact of both cytokine and neurohormonal activation on myocyte function. Tumor necrosis factor (TNF) induces expression of NOS2 in cardiac myocytes, and the negative inotropic effect of this cytokine is mediated through increased NO. Nitric oxide also improves myocyte relaxation [90] and calcium homeostasis. In addition, nitric oxide reduces beta-receptor responsiveness to catecholamine stimulation and, therefore, may diminish the effects of sympathetic activation on myocyte function [91,92]. Though the effects of NO on endothelial function is clearly a protective mechanism in heart failure, the impact of NO on the cardiac myocyte itself is more complex with both deleterious and potentially cardioprotective effects.

Endothelin-1 is a 21 amino acid peptide released by the endothelium [93]. Endothelin-1 is upregulated in circulating plasma but not in cardiac tissues in heart failure, suggesting local production of endothelin-1 is responsible for heart failure elevations. Endothelium causes potent vasoconstriction mediated by type A endothelin receptors [94]. Endothelin is promitogenic and promotes cell division and hypertrophy among smooth muscle cells and increased matrix production, leading to the permanent vascular changes of chronic heart failure. Activation of a separate class of endothelin receptors, type B, acts in a counter regulatory manner and stimulates nitric oxide production and vascular relaxation [95].

CLINICAL HETEROGENEITY IN HEART FAILURE: IMPACT OF GENETIC DIVERSITY

Clinical outcomes in congestive heart failure are significantly heterogeneous, and two patients with similar degrees of initial myocardial injury after infarction may progress to the syndrome of heart failure at markedly different rates. Much of the clinical heterogeneity may reflect genetic differences in the degree of neurohormonal activation. Patients predisposed to greater degrees of renin-angiotensin and sympathetic activation would be predicted to progress more rapidly toward worsening heart failure, and have significantly poorer outcomes. The potential use of genomic information to predict outcomes and target therapy is the subject of increasing investigation.

The common deletion/insertion polymorphism of the angiotensin-converting enzyme has been extensively studied [96]. The ACE D-allele, named for a 287 base pair deletion in intron-16, has been consistently linked to higher levels of ACE activity and circulating angiotensin-2 [97,98]. Several studies have demonstrated that for patients with congestive heart failure, subjects homozygous for the D-allele have the poorest survival (Fig. 6). This impact appears independent of etiology and has been demonstrated in patients with idiopathic dilated cardiomyopathy [99] and postmyocardial infarction [77]. The genetic tendency toward poorer survival with the ACE D allele and higher ACE activity can be reduced by treatment with high dose ACE inhibitors. In addition, the adverse impact of the ACE D allele can be effectively eliminated by beta-blockers [100]. This powerful pharmacogenetic interaction of the ACE D-allele and beta-blocker therapy supports the role of beta-blockers as renin inhibitors and is an additional example of the complex interdependence of renin angiotensin and sympathetic activation.

Genetic heterogeneity of beta-adrenergic receptors also appears to affect heart failure outcomes [101]. Three common polymorphisms exist for the beta-2 receptor, two in the

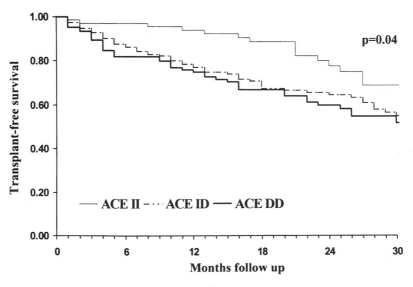

Figure 6   Effect of genetic heterogeneity on clinical outcomes in heart failure, and interactions with therapy. (**A**). Comparison of transplant-free survival by ACE genotype in 328 subjects with chronic heart failure. ACE D allele associated with poor outcomes, p = 0.044.

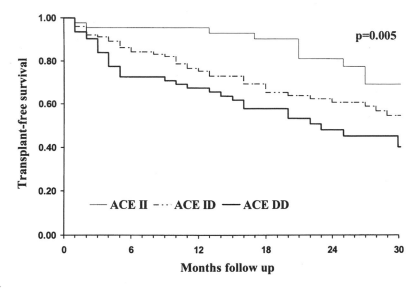

Figure 6 (continued) **(B)** Similar comparison in the 208 patients not treated with beta-blockers at the time of study entry. Impact of ACE D allele is much more significant in this subset, p = 0.005. (From Ref. 100.)

extracellular portion at codons 16 and 27, and one in the transmembrane core at position 164 (Fig. 7). An isoleucine residue at codon 164 (Ile164) results in a receptor less responsive to agonist stimulation than with the wild-type receptor with threonine at this position. This less active Ile164 variant is associated with significantly poor outcomes in subjects with heart failure [102] (Fig. 8). In the beta-1 receptor the serine/glycine polymorphism

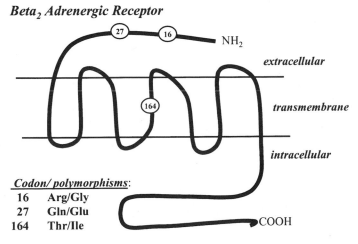

Figure 7 Structure and common polymorphisms of the β_2 adrenergic receptor. Arg, arginine; Gly, glycine; Gln, glutamine; Glu, glutamate; Thr, threonine; Ile, Isoleucine; NH_2, amino terminus; COOH, carboxyl terminus. Ile164 variant in the transmembrane region (3% to 5% of the general population) causes a loss of function and is associated with poor survival in chronic heart failure. (From Ref. 101.)

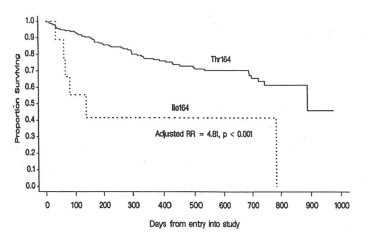

Figure 8 Effect of beta-2 receptor polymorphism on outcome in chronic heart failure. Thr, threonine; Ile, isoleucine; RR, risk ratio. (From Ref. 102.)

at codon 49 in the extracellular portion of the receptor appears to affect the degree of receptor downregulation in response to agonists. Clinically, this polymorphism appears to influence heart failure outcomes and responsiveness to beta-blocker therapy [103]. As with the ACE D-allele, beta-receptor heterogeneity that functionally modifies the impact of neurohormonal activation appears to influence heart failure progression. Recently, polymorphisms of endothelial nitric oxide synthase have also been shown to predict survival in heart failure populations (Fig. 9). Future investigations will clarify the potential use of

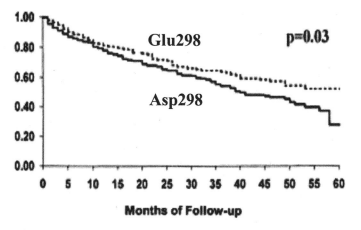

Figure 9 Effect of endothelial nitric oxide synthase (NOS) polymorphism on survival in chronic heart failure. Influence of Asp 298 codon substitution for Glu 298 for the entire population (n = 469;). Patients with ischemic cardiomyopathy (n = 146;). Asp, asparate; Glu, glutamine; NOS, nitric oxide synthase. (From Ref. 104.)

genetic background both for predicting heart failure outcomes and for targeting specific medical therapies.

SUMMARY

Heart failure begins with myocardial injury but progresses as a systemic illness. The compensatory pathways designed to respond to acute injury lead to maladaptive consequences in the chronic heart failure state, including progressive myocardial dysfunction and regression of the vascular bed. This pathological progression is driven by circulating mediators, in particular angiotensin-II and norepinephrine. Natruretic peptides play a significant role in the regulation of plasma volume and the downregulation neurohormonal activation. In the vasculature, nitric oxide, endothelin-1, and angiotensin-II are important mediators of vascular tone. Beginning with the initial myocardial injury, cardiac inflammation is mediated by cytokines that can worsen both cardiac and endothelial dysfunction as the heart failure state progresses. Although these pathways have been described separately, they are critically interdependent in the systemic response to heart failure (Table 1). All medical interventions in heart failure that improve survival directly inhibit neurohor-

Table 1 Neurohormones: Initiation, Impact and Interaction

	Initiation	Impact in Heart Failure	Interactions
RAAS			
Angiotensin II	Low cardiac output (renal perfusion) Beta-receptor stimulation	Increased vascular resistance (afterload) Cardiac myocyte hypertrophy Plasma expansion (aldosterone)	Sympathetic activation increases renin release BNP reduces RAAS activation
Sympathetic activation			
Norepinephrine	Baroreceptors (decreased stroke volume)	Increased myocardial work, cardiotoxicity, ischemia, arrhythmias	Increases renin release. Nitric oxide modulates beta receptor activation
Cytokine activation			
TFN alpha	Myocardial injury	Decrease contractility chronic: worsen LV remodeling acute: facilitate viral clearing	Induce expression of NOS 2 in cardiac myocytes
Natriuretic Peptides			
BNP	Ventricular pressure and wall stretch, increased volume	Sodium excretion, vasodilation	Inhibits RAAS activation
Nitric Oxide pathway			
Nitric oxide	Constitutively active if endothelium intact (NOS 3) Cytokine induction of NOS 2	Vasodilation Decrease contractility Improve myocardial relaxation	TNF induces NOS 2 NO decreases adrenergic reponsiveness

monal activation. Further investigation of the interactions of these pathways should lead to improved therapeutics. Given the importance of genetic diversity in the neurohormonal response, targeting of medical therapeutics to genetic background should an important addition to the treatment of heart failure in the near future.

ACKNOWLEDGEMENT

The author gratefully acknowledges the assistance of Mrs. Marge Altvater in the preparation of this manuscript.

REFERENCES

1. Thomas Coar. The Aphorisims of Hippocrates. 0: Longman and Co., 1822.
2. Cohn JN, Goldstein SO, Greenberg BH, et al. A dose-dependent increase in mortality with vesnarinone among patients with severe heart failure. Vesnarinone Trial Investigators. N Engl J Med 1998; 339(25):1810–1816.
3. Thackray S, Easthaugh J, Freemantle N, Cleland JG. The effectiveness and relative effectiveness of intravenous inotropic drugs acting through the adrenergic pathway in patients with heart failure-a meta-regression analysis. Eur J Heart Fail 2002; 4(4):515–529.
4. Pfeffer MA, Braunwald E, Moye LA, Basta L, Brown EJ, Cuddy TE, Davis BR, Geltman EM, Goldman S, Flaker GC, et al. Effect of captopril on mortality and morbidity in patients with left ventricular dysfunction after myocardial infarction. Results of the survival and ventricular enlargement trial. The SAVE Investigators. New Engl J Med 1992; 327:669–677.
5. The SOLVD Investigators. Effect of enalapril on survival in patients with reduced left ventricular ejection fractions and congestive heart failure. New Engl J Med 1991; 325:293–302.
6. Hjalmarson A, Goldstein S, Fagerberg B, Wedel H, Waagstein F, Kjekshus J, Wikstrand J, El Allaf D, Vitovec J, Aldershvile J, Halinen M, Dietz R, Neuhaus KL, Janosi A, Thorgeirsson G, Dunselman PH, Gullestad L, Kuch J, Herlitz J, Rickenbacher P, Ball S, Gottlieb S, Deedwania P. the MERIT-HF Study Group. Effects of controlled-release metoprolol on total mortality, hospitalizations, and well-being in patients with heart failure: the Metoprolol CR/XL Randomized Intervention Trial in congestive heart failure (MERIT-HF). JAMA 2000; 283:1295–1302.
7. Dzau VJ. Tissue renin-angiotensin system in myocardial hypertrophy and failure. Arch Int Med 1993; 153:937–942.
8. Packer M. The neurohormonal hypothesis: a theory to explain the mechanism of disease progression in heart failure. J Am Coll Cardiol 1992; 20:248–254.
9. Kelly RA, Balligand J-L, Smith TW. Nitric oxide and cardiac function. Circulation 1996; 79(3):363–380.
10. Mann DL. Inflammatory mediators and the failing heart. Circ Res 2002; 91:988–998.
11. Mehra MR, Uber PA, Francis GS. Heart failure therapy at a crossroad: are there limits to the neurohormonal model?. J Am Coll Cardiol 2003; 41:1606–1610.
12. Massie BM. Neurohormonal blockade in chronic heart failure. J Am Coll Cardiol 2002; 39(1): 79–82.
13. Gottlieb SS. The neurohormonal paradigm: have we gone too far?. J Am Coll Cardiol 2003; 41(9):1458–1459.
14. Lavoie JL, Sigmund CD. Mini-review: overview of the renin-angiotensin system—an endocrine and paracrine system. Endocrinology 2003; 144:2179–2183.
15. Volpe M, Savoia C, DePaolis P, et al. The renin-angiotensin system as a risk factor and therapeutic target for cardiovascular and renal disease. J Am Soc Nephrol 2002; 13: S173–S178.
16. Opie LH, Sack MN. Enhanced angiotensin II activity in heart failure. Reevaluation of the counterregulatory hypothesis of receptor subtypes. Circ Res 2001; 88:654–658.
17. Manohar P, Pina IL. Therapeutic role of angiotensin II receptor blockers in the treatment of heart failure. Mayo Clin Proc 2003; 78:334–338.

18. Shah M, Ali V, Lamba S, et al. Pathophysiology and clinical spectrum of acute congestive heart failure. Rev Cardiovasc Med 2001; 2(suppl 2):S2–S6.

19. Weber KT. Extracellular matrix remodeling in heart failure. A role for denovo angiotensin II generation. Circulation 1997; 96:4065–4082.

20. Valgimigli M, Curello S, Ceconi C, et al. Neurohormones, cytokines and programmed cell death in heart failure: a new paradigm for the remodeling heart. Cardiovasc Drugs Ther 2001; 15:529–537.

21. Ichihara S, Senbonmatsu T, Price E, et al. Angiotensin II type 2 receptor is essential for left ventricular hypertrophy and cardiac fibrosis in chronic angiotensin II-induces hypertension. Circulation 2001; 104:346–351.

22. Sadoshima J, Izumo S. Molecular characterization of angiotensin II-induced hypertrophy of cardiac myocytes and hyperplasia of cardiac fibroblasts. Critical role of the AT1 receptor subtype. Circ Res 1993; 73:413–423.

23. Sackner-Bernstein JD. Activation and release of degradative proteinases within the myocardium are the trigger for ventricular remodeling in chronic heart failure. Med Hypotheses 2002; 58(1):18–23.

24. Pouleur H, Rousseau MF, vanEyll C, et al. Effects of long-term enalapril therapy on left ventricular diastolic properties in patients with depressed ejection fraction. Circulation 1993; 88:481–491.

25. Pfeffer MA, Lamas GA, Vaughan DE, et al. Effect of captopril on progressive ventricular dilatation after anterior myocardial infarction. N Engl J Med 1988; 319:80–86.

26. Pfeffer MA, Pfeffer JM, Lamas GA. Development and prevention of congestive heart failure following myocardial infarction. Circulation 1993; 87(5S) Suppl 1):IV120–IV125.

27. The CONSENSUS Trial Study Group. Effects of enalapril on mortality in severe congestive heart failure. N Engl J Med 1987; 316(23):1429–1435.

28. Roig E, Perez-Villa F, Morales M, et al. Clinical implications of increased plasma angiotensin II despite ACE inhibitor therapy in patients with congestive heart failure. Eur Heart J 2000; 21:53–57.

29. Farquharson CAJ, Struthers AD. Gradual reactivation over time of vascular tissue angiotensin I to angiotensin II conversion during chronic lisinopril therapy in chronic heart failure. J Am Coll Cardiol 2002; 39(5):767–775.

30. Tang WH, Vagelos RH, Yee Y-G, et al. Neurohormonal and clinical responses to high- versus low-dose enalapril therapy in chronic heart failure. J Am Coll Cardiol 2002; 39(1):69–78.

31. Weber KT. Aldosterone in congestive heart failure. N Engl J Med 2001; 345(23):1689–1697.

32. Brasier AR, Recinos A III, Eledrisi M. Vascular inflammation and the renin-angiotensin system. Arterioscler Thromb Vasc Biol 2002; 22:1257–1266.

33. Mehra MR, Uber PA, Potluri S. Renin angiotensin aldosterone and adrenergic modulation in chronic heart failure: contemporary concepts. Am J Med Sci 2002; 324(5):267–275.

34. Pitt B, Zannad F, Remme WJ, et al. The effect of spironolactone on morbidity and mortality in patients with severe heart failure. N Engl J Med 1999; 341(10):709–717.

35. Pitt B, Remme W, Zannad F, et al. Eplerenone a selective aldosterone blocker, in patients with left ventricular dysfunction after myocardial infarction. N Engl J Med 2003; 348(14): 1309–1321.

36. Cohn JN, Tognoni G. the Valsartan Heart Failure Investigators. A randomized trial of the angiotensin-receptor blocker valsartan in chronic heart failure. N Engl J Med 2001 Dec 6; 345(23):1667–1675.

37. Tipnis SR, Hooper NM, Hyde R, Karran E, Christie G, Turner AJ. A human homolog of angiotensin-converting enzyme. Cloning and functional expression as a captopril-insensitive carboxypeptidase. J Biol Chem 2000; 275:33238–33243.

38. Donoghue M, Hsieh F, Baronas E, Godbout K, Gosselin M, Stagliano N, Donovan M, Woolf B, Robison K, Jeyaseelan R, Breitbart RE, Acton S. A novel angiotensin-converting enzyme-related carboxypeptidase (ACE2) converts angiotensin I to angiotensin 1-9. Circ Res 2000; 87:E1–E9.

39. Crackower MA, Sarao R, Oudit GY, Yagil C, Kozieradzki I, Scanga SE, Oliveira-dos-Santos AJ, da Costa J, Zhang L, Pei Y, Scholey J, Ferrario CM, Manoukian AS, Chappell MC, Backx PH, Yagil Y, Penninger JM. Angiotensin-converting enzyme 2 is an essential regulator of heart function. Nature 2002; 417:822–828.

40. Felder RB, Francis J, Zhang Z-H et al. Heart failure and the brain: new perspectives. Am J Physiol Regul Integr Comp Physiol 2004; 284:R259–R276.

41. Steinberg SF. The molecular basis for distinct β-adrenergic receptor subtype actions in cardiomyocytes. Circ Res 1999; 85(11):1101–1111.

42. Feldman AM, McTiernan C. New insight into the role of enhanced adrenergic receptor-effector coupling in the heart. Circulation 1999; 100(6):579–582.

43. Bristow MR. β-adrenergic receptor blockade in chronic heart failure. Circulation 2000; 101(5):558–569.

44. Zaugg M, Xu W, Lucchinetti E, et al. β-adrenergic receptor subtypes differentially affect apoptosis in adult rat ventricular myocytes. Circulation 2000; 102:344–350.

45. Lefkowitz RJ, Rockman HA, Koch WJ. Catecholamines, cardiac β-adrenergic receptors, and heart failure. Circulation 2000; 101:1634–1637.

46. Cohn JN, Levine TB, Olivari M. Plasma norepinephrine as a guide to prognosis in patients with chronic heart failure. N Engl J Med 1984; 311(13):819–23.

47. Bristow MR, Gilbert EM, Abraham WT, et al. MOCHA Investigators. Carvedilol produces dose-related improvements in left ventricular function and survival in subjects with chronic heart failure. Circulation 1996 Dec 1; 94(11):2807–2816.

48. Roden DM, Brown NJ. Pre-prescription genotyping: not yet ready for prime time, but getting there. Circulation 2001 Mar 27; 103(12):1608–1610.

49. Gilbert EM, Sandoval A, Larrabee P, Renlund DG, O'Connell JB, Bristow MR. Lisinopril lowers cardiac adrenergic drive and increases beta-receptor density in the failing human heart. Circulation 1993 Aug; 88(2):472–480.

50. Ferrari R. The role of TNF in cardiovascular disease. Pharmacological Res 1999; 40(2): 97–105.

51. Sharma R, Anker SD. Cytokines, apoptosis and cachexia: the potential for TNF antagonism. Int J Cardol 2002; 85:161–171.

52. Levine B, Kalman J, Mayer L, Fillit HM, Packer M. Elevated circulating levels of tumor necrosis factor in severe chronic heart failure. N Engl J Med 1990 Jul 26; 323(4):236–241.

53. Koller-Strametz J, Pacher R, Frey B, et al. Circulating tumor necrosis factor-α levels in chronic heart failure: relation to its soluble receptor interleukin-6, and neurohumoral variables. J Heart Lung Transplant 1998; 17:356–362.

53a. Tsutamoto T, Wada A, Maeda K, Hisanagg T, Maeda Y, Fukai D, Onishi M, Sugimoto Y, Kinoshita M. Attenuation of endogenous cardiac natriuretic peptide system in chronic heart failure: prognostic role of brain natiuretic peptide concentration in patients with chronic symptomatic left ventricular dysfunction. Circulation 1997; 96:509–516.

54. Kubota T, Miyagishima M, Alvarez R, et al. Expression of proinflammatory cytokines in the failing human heart: comparison of recent-onset and end-stage congestive heart failure. J Heart Lung Transplantation 2000; 19(9):819–824.

55. Kubota T, McTiernan CF, Frye CS, et al. Dilated cardiomyopathy in transgenic mice with cardiac-specific overexpression of tumor necrosis factor-alpha. Circ Res 1997 Oct; 81(4): 627–635.

56. Sivasubramanian N, Coker ML, Kurrelmeyer KM, et al. Left ventricular remodeling in transgenic mice with cardiac restricted overexpression of tumor necrosis factor. Circulation 2001; 104:826–831.

57. Bozkurt B, Kribbs SB, Clubb FJ, et al. Pathophysiologically relevant concentrations of tumor necrosis factor-alpha promote progressive left ventricular dysfunction and remodeling in rats. Circulation 1998 Apr 14; 97(14):1382–1391.

58. Bradham WS, Bozkurt B, Gunasinghe H, et al. Tumor necrosis factor-alpha and myocardial remodeling in progression of heart failure: a current perspective. Cardiovasc Res 2002; 53: 822–830.

59. Funakoshi H, Kubota T, Machida Y, et al. Involvement of inducible nitric oxide synthase in cardiac dysfunction with tumor necrosis factor-α. Am J Physiol Heart Circ Physiol 2002(282): H2159–H2166.

60. Ferdinandy P, Danial H, Ambrus I, et al. Peroxynitrite is a major contributor to cytokine-induced myocardial contractile failure. Circ Res 2000; 87(3):241–247.

61. Murray DR, Prabhu SD, Chandrasekar B. Chronic β-adrenergic stimulation induces myocardial proinflammatory cytokine expression. Circulation 2000; 101:2338–2341.

62. Kubota T, Bounoutas GS, Miyagishima M, et al. Soluble tumor necrosis factor receptor abrogates myocardial inflammation but not hypertrophy in cytokine-induced cardiomyopathy. Circulation 2000; 101:2518–2525.

63. Francis GS. TNF-α and heart failure. The difference between proof of principle and hypothesis testing. Circulation 1999; 99:3213–3214.

64. Bozkurt B, Torre-Amione G, Warren MS, et al. Results of targeted anti-tumor necrosis factor therapy with etanercept (ENBREL) in patients with advanced heart failure. Circulation 2001 Feb 27; 103(8):1044–1047.

65. Deswal A, Bozkurt B, Seta Y et al. Safety and efficacy of a soluble P75 tumor necrosis factor receptor (Enbrel, etanercept) in patients with advanced heart failure. Circulation; 1999 Jun 29; 99(25):3224–3226.

66. Wada H, Saito K, Kanda T, et al. Tumor necrosis factor-α (TNF-α) plays a protective role in acute viral myocarditis in mice. A study using mice lacking TNF-α. Circulation 2001; 103:743–749.

67. McNamara DM, Starling R, Dec GW, et al. Plasma cytokines in acute cardiomyopathy: evolution over time, correlations with functional studies, and potential role in recovery. Circulation 2000; [abstr] 102(18):2020.

68. Mann D. Tumor necrosis factor and viral myocarditis. The fine line between innate and inappropriate immune responses in the heart. Circulation 2001; 103:626–629.

69. MacGowan GA, Mann DL, Kormos RL, et al. Circulating interleukin-6 in severe heart failure. Am J Cardiol 1997; 79:1128–1131.

70. Mann DL. Interleukin-6 and viral myocarditis: the yin-yang of cardiac innate immune responses. J Mol Cell Cardiol 2001; 33:1551–1553.

71. Tanaka T, Kanda T, McManus BM, et al. Overexpression of interleukin-6 aggravates viral myocarditis: impaired increase in tumor necrosis factor-α. J Mol Cell Cardiol 2001; 33(9): 1627–1635.

72. Wollert KC, Drexler H. The role of interleukin-6 in the failing heart. Heart Fail Reviews; 2001:95–103.

73. Vasan RS, Sullivan LM, Roubenoff R, et al. Inflammatory markers and risk of heart failure in elderly subjects without prior myocardial infarction. The Framingham Heart Study. Circulation 2003; 107:1486–1491.

74. Roig E, Orus J, Pare C, et al. Serum interleukin-6 congestive heart failure secondary to idiopathic dilated cardiomyopathy. Am J Cardiol 1998; 82(5):688–690.

75. Kalra PR, Bolger AP, Coats AJ, et al. The regulation and measurement of plasma volume in heart failure. J Am Coll Cardiol 2002; 39:1901–1908.

76. Braunwald E, Bristow MR. Congestive heart failure: fifty years of progress. Circulation 2000; 102:IV14–IV23.

76a. Lemos JA, Morrow D, Bentley JH, et al. The prognostic value of B-type natriuretic peptide in patients with acute coronary syndromes. N Engl J Med 2001; 345:1014–1021.

77. Palmer BR, Pilbrow AP, Yandle TG, et al. Angiotensin-converting enzyme gene polymorphism interacts with left ventricular ejection fraction and brain natriuretic peptide levels to predict mortality after myocardial infarction. J Am Coll Cardiol 2003; 41:729–736.

78. Latini R, Masson S, deAngelis N, et al. Role of brain natriuretic peptide in the diagnosis and management of heart failure: current concepts. J Card Fail 2002; 8(5):288–299.

79. Shi SJ, Ngyuyen HT, Sharma GD, et al. Genetic disruption of atrial natriuretic peptide receptor-A alters renin and angiotensin II levels. Am J Renal Physiol 2001; 281:F665–F673.

80. Fang ZY, Marwick TH. Vascular dysfunction and heart failure: epiphenomenon or etiologic agent? Am Heart J 2002; 143:383–390.

81. Mathier MA, Rose GA, Fifer MA, et al. Coronary endothelial dysfunction in patients with acute-onset idiopathic dilated Cardiomyopathy. J Am Coll Cardiol 1998; 32:216–224.
82. Drexler H. Nitric oxide synthases in the failing human heart. A doubled-edged sword?. Circulation 1999; 99:2972–2975.
83. Nikolaidis LA, Doverspike A, Huerbin R, et al. Angiotensin-converting enzyme inhibitors improve coronary flow reserve in dilated Cardiomyopathy by a bradykinin-mediated, nitric oxide-dependent mechanism. Circulation 2002; 105:2785–2790.
84. Yang X-P, Liu YH, Shesely EG, et al. Endothelial nitric oxide gene knockout mice. Cardiac phenotypes and the effect of angiotensin-converting enzyme inhibitor on myocardial ischemia/reperfusion injury. Hypertension 1999; 34:24–30.
85. Liu YH, Xu J, Yang XP, Shesely E, Carretero OA. Effect of ACE inhibitors and angiotensin II type 1 receptor antagonists on endothelial NO synthase knockout mice with heart failure. Hypertension 2002; 39(2 Pt 2):375–381.
86. Wittstein IS, Kass DA, Pak PH, et al. Cardiac nitric oxide production due to angiotensin-converting enzyme inhibition decreases beta-adrenergic myocardial contractility in patients with dilated cardiomyopathy. J Am Coll Cardiol 2001; 38:429–435.
87. Agnoletti L, Curello S, Bachetti T, et al. Serum from patients with severe heart failure downregulates eNOS and is proapoptotic: role of tumor necrosis factor-α. Circulation 1999; 100(19):1983–1991.
88. Kojda G, Kottenberg K. Regulation of basal myocardial function by N. O.. Cardiovasc Res 1999; 41:514–523.
89. Paulus WJ, Frantz S, Kelly RA. Nitric oxide and cardiac contractility in human heart failure. Time for reappraisal. Circulation 2001; 104:2260–2262.
90. Heymes C, Vanderheyden M, Bronzwaer JGF, et al. Endomyocardial nitric oxide synthase and left ventricular preload reserve in dilated cardiomyopathy. Circulation 1999; 99:3009–3016.
91. Hare JM, Givertz MM, Creager MA, et al. Increased sensitivity to nitric oxide synthase inhibition in patients with heart failure. Potentiation of β-adrenergic inotropic responsiveness. Circulation 1998; 97:161–166.
92. Ashley EU, Sears CE, Bryant SM, et al. Cardiac nitric oxide synthase 1 regulates basal and adrenergic contractility in murine ventricular myocytes. Circulation 2002; 105:3011–3016.
93. Teerlink JR. The role of endothelin in the pathogenesis of heart failure. Curr Cardiol Rep 2002; 4(3):206–212.
94. Greenberg B. Endothelin and endothelin receptor antagonists in heart failure. Congest Heart Fail 2002; 8(5):257–261.
95. Alonso D, Radomski MW. The nitric oxide-endothelin 1 connection. Heart Fail Rev 2003; 8(1):107–115.
96. Rigat B, Hubert C, Corvol P, Soubrier F. PCR detection of the insertion/deletion polymorphism of the human angiotensin converting enzyme gene (DCP) (dipeptidyl carboxypeptidase 1). Nucleic Acids Res 1992; 20(1433).
97. Tiret L, Rigat B, Visvikis S, Breda SC, Corvol P, Cambien F, et al. Evidence, from combined segregation and linkage analysis, that a variant of the angiotensin I-converting enzyme (ACE) gene controls plasma ACE levels. Am J Hum Genet 1992; 51:197–205.
98. Danser AH, Derkx FH, Hense HW, Jeunemaitre X, Riegger GA, Schunkert H. Angiotensinogen (M235T) and angiotensin-converting enzyme (I/D) polymorphisms in association with plasma renin and prorenin levels. J Hypertens 1998; 16:1879–1883.
99. Andersson B, Sylven C. The DD genotype of the angiotensin-converting enzyme gene is associated with increased mortality in idiopathic heart failure. J Am Coll Cardiol 1996; 28(1):162–167.
100. McNamara DM, Holubkov R, Janosko K, et al. Pharmacogenetic interactions between β-blocker therapy and the angiotensin-converting enzyme deletion polymorphism in patients with congestive heart failure. Circulation 2001; 103(12):1644–1648.
101. McNamara DM, MacGowan GA, London B. Clinical importance of β-adrenoceptor polymorphisms in cardiovascular disease. Am J Pharmacogenomics 2002; 2(2):73–78.
102. Liggett SB, Wagoner LE, Craft LL, et al. The Ile164 beta2-adrenergic receptor polymorphism adversely affects the outcome of congestive heart failure. J Clin Invest 1998 Oct 15; 102(8):1534–1539.

103. Borjesson M, Magnusson Y, Hjalmarson A, Andersson B. A novel polymorphism in the gene coding for the β_1 adrenergic receptor associated with survival in patients with heart failure. Eur Heart J 2000; 21:1810–1812.

104. McNamara DM, Holobkov R, Postava L, et al. Effect of the Asp298 variant of endothelial synthase on survival for patients with congestive heart failure. Circulation 2003; 107: 1598–1602.

8

Cardiomyopathies in the Adult (Dilated, Hypertrophic, and Restrictive)

Richard Rodeheffer
Mayo Clinic School of Medicine
Rochester, Minnesota, USA

INTRODUCTION

The World Health Organization Classification system restricts the term cardiomyopathy to idiopathic conditions and, in contrast, refers to myocardial disease of known cause (e.g., "ischemic" or "hypertensive" or "valvular" cardiomyopathy) as specific heart muscle disease [1]. Although this conceptual approach is nosologically coherent from a pathologist's viewpoint, it does not group patients according to common clinical features, such as the type of the cardiac dysfunction and the presenting signs and symptoms. A traditional classification, based on gross morphology and the principal form of functional cardiac impairment, is to divide the cardiomyopathies into the dilated, hypertrophic, and restrictive types. (Fig. 1) The cardinal features of the dilated forms are multichamber dilation with marked impairment of systolic function, as well as reduced diastolic function. The features of the hypertrophic forms are atrial dilatation, marked left ventricular muscle hypertrophy with vigorous systolic function, severely impaired ventricular diastolic relaxation and compliance, and a small left ventricular volume. The restrictive forms display atrial enlargement, normal ventricular chamber size, preserved systolic function, and markedly impaired diastolic filling.

DILATED CARDIOMYOPATHY

Morphology and Pathology

In dilated cardiomyopathy there is uniform involvement of all the myocardium. In its fully evolved form, therefore, dilated cardiomyopathy manifests impressive cardiomegaly (Fig. 1). Although there is impairment of muscle function during both diastole and systole, the dominant feature is that of decreased systolic ejection. A small minority of patients present with globally reduced contractile function with only mild chamber dilatation. On gross examination biventricular dilatation is predominant, the atrioventricular valve rings are dilated, and there is modest myocardial hypertrophy. Histological evaluation reveals myocyte hypertrophy, variable degrees of diffuse fibrosis (particularly in the subendocardium), occasional lymphocytes and, rarely, focal myocyte necrosis.

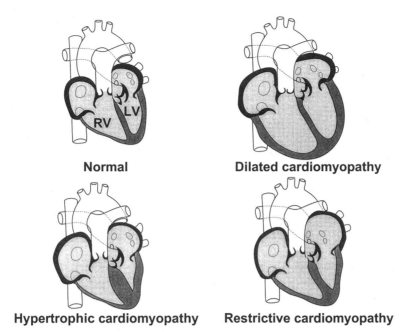

Figure 1 Morphologic characteristics of the three principle forms of cardiomyopathy.

Epidemiology and Natural History

The incidence of dilated cardiomyopathy is based on autopsy series and population-based studies. Data from Sweden and Minnesota suggest five to eight cases per 100,000 persons per year [2,3]. Pediatric surveillance registries indicate an annual incidence of 0.6 to 0.7 cases per 100,000 children per year, with most patients presenting in the first year of life, and the disease being less common in whites than nonwhites [4,5]. Although the incidence has been reported to be increasing, some of this apparent increase could be related to ascertainment bias consequent to widespread application of noninvasive diagnostic tools, such as echocardiography [3]. The age- and sex-adjusted prevalence rate is estimated at 36.5 per 100,000 population [3]. Among adults, there is evidence that blacks have a two- to three-fold greater prevalence than whites [6].

Prognosis has been assessed in a population-based cohort and in referral cohorts. Dilated cardiomyopathy patients identified in the community appear to have better survival than those referred to tertiary hospitals, likely as a result of the referral bias that results from tertiary hospital clinic patients being at a more advanced stage of their disease (Fig. 2) [7]. Even among referral cohorts, however, there is evidence of improved survival beginning in the 1980s [8]. Factors associated with poor survival in dilated cardiomyopathy are similar to those associated with early death in heart failure in general: severe hemodynamic derangement, advanced neurohumoral activation, NYHA (New York Heart Association) Class III—IV symptom severity; and marked ventricular dilatation and severe depression of left ventricular ejection fraction.

Etiology

Four chamber dilatation with depressed contractile function is a final common pathway that may result from a range of myocardial stresses or injuries [9]. The source of injury

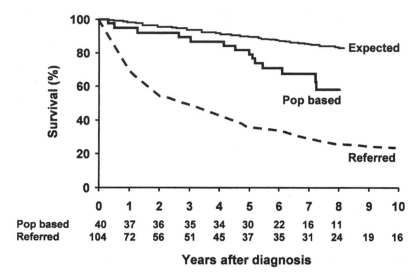

Figure 2 Survival in idiopathic dilated cardiomyopathy: comparison of referral patients and community patients (From Ref. 7.)

may be known, as in the secondary dilated cardiomyopathies (e.g., inflammatory injury, metabolic deficiency states, excessive stimulation by hyperactive endogenous endocrine systems, or exogenous toxins); or the nature of the injury may be unknown, as in truly idiopathic dilated cardiomyopathy (Table 1). In this discussion of dilated cardiomyopathy etiology, three topics warrant additional comment: viral myocarditis, familial dilated cardiomyopathy, and alcoholic cardiomyopathy.

Table 1 Principle Causes of Nonischemic, Nonvalvular Dilated Cardiomyopathy

1. METABOLIC
   Nutritional deficiency (carnitine, selenium, thiamine)
   Endocrine (hyperthyroidism, hypothyroidism, acromegaly,
   pheochromocytoma, diabetes)
   Hemochromatosis
2. INFLAMMATORY
   Viral, spirochetal, parasitic infection
   Collagen vascular disease
   Giant cell myocarditis
   Eosinophilic myocarditis
   Sarcoidosis
3. TOXIC EXPOSURE
   Alcohol
   Cobalt
   Adriamycin, cyclophosphamide
   Chloroquine
4. FAMILIAL DILATED CARDIOMYOPATHY
5. POSTPARTUM DILATED CARDIOMYOPATHY
6. IDIOPATHIC

It is widely believed that viral infection can cause a lymphocytic myocarditis with widespread myocyte injury, and that this process can lead ultimately to dilated cardiomyopathy [10–12]. There are epidemiological data and experimental animal models of viral myocarditis that lend support to this hypothesis. Nevertheless, compelling microbiological evidence proving this relationship has been difficult to obtain in humans. There is circumstantial evidence in the form of high serum viral antibody titers and persistence of viral genome in human dilated cardiomyopathy myocytes, but definitive evidence of progression to dilated cardiomyopathy has been elusive [10,13–15]. The proposed mechanism of viral injury involves persistence of virus, a sustained host immunologic response to the virus, and the development of a low-grade chronic active myocarditis that results in progressive myocyte destruction. Persons with disordered immune regulation or impaired myocyte responses to persistent virus could be at risk of evolving into chronic dilated cardiomyopathy (Fig. 3). The outcome of acute viral myocarditis may depend on the intensity of inflammation at presentation; paradoxically, cases manifesting more intense and widespread inflammation appear to have a more favorable prognosis [16]. Viral myocarditis should be distinguished from other infectious myocarditides, from lymphocytic myocarditis that may be associated with systemic collagen vascular disease, and from other forms of inflammatory injury, such as giant cell and eosinophilic myocarditis.

The second area of particular interest is that of familial dilated cardiomyopathy, a condition that until a decade ago was believed to be rare. Systematic studies in the 1990s, involving echocardiographic and electrocardiographic screening of the first degree relatives of idiopathic dilated cardiomyopathy patients, revealed that at least 20% to 25% of presumably sporadic idiopathic dilated cardiomyopathy cases were actually familial [17–20]. Importantly, 83% of these familial dilated cardiomyopathy cases would not have been identified as such on the basis of the family history alone, i.e., other affected family members were only identified as having dilated cardiomyopathy by echocardiographic screening [17]. To date, more than ten gene mutations leading to dilated cardiomyopathy have been identified, and it is highly probable that more will be reported in the coming

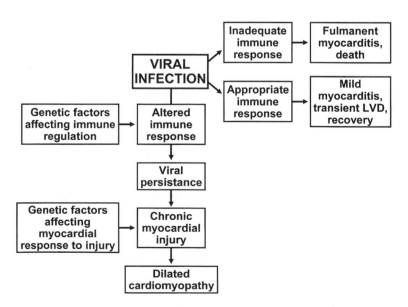

Figure 3   Proposed mechanism for viral injury leading to dilated cardiomyopathy.

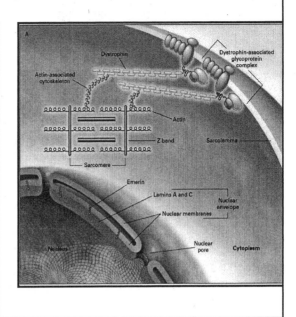

GENES
Lamin A/C
δ-sarcoglycan
Dystrophin
Desmin
Vinculin
Titin
Troponin-T
α-tropomyosin
ß-myosin heavy chain
Actin
Mitochondrial DNA mutations

Figure 4   Cytoskeletal and sarcomeric protein mutations associated with dilated cardiomyopathy. (Adapted from Ref. 41.)

years. Unlike hypertrophic disease (see following text), in which mutations generally involve sarcomeric contractile and regulatory proteins (β-myosin, actin, troponin, tropomyosin), the mutations associated with dilated cardiomyopathies usually involve cytoskeletal and nuclear envelop proteins (e.g., lamin A/C, emerin, dystrophin). Skeletal myopathy may also accompany common heritable forms of dilated cardiomyopathy, such as the muscular dystrophies (Duchenne, Beckers) and mitochondrial myopathies.

The third area deserving of additional comment is alcoholic cardiomyopathy. Alcohol depresses myocardial contractility, and the risk of developing dilated cardiomyopathy is related to the volume and duration of alcohol consumption [21–24]. Women appear to be susceptible at a lower level of alcohol exposure than men [23]. Abstinence from alcohol has been observed to allow recovery of ventricular function if achieved early in the course of alcoholic cardiomyopathy. Avoidance of significant alcohol consumption is recommended in all dilated cardiomyopathy patients, whether or not alcohol toxicity is believed to be the primary underlying etiology.

Clinical Presentation

Dilated cardiomyopathy can present at any age, though it is more common to present in infancy or during the fourth to sixth decades. There may be an asymptomatic phase, lasting months to years, during which the disease is occasionally discovered by chance if cardiomegaly is detected on a chest radiograph, bundle branch block, or abnormal ST-T changes are noted on an EKG (electrocardiogram), or ectopic beats are found on a routine physical examination. Although the common presenting symptoms of dyspnea, fatigue, and fluid retention may seem to evolve over only a few days or weeks, it is typically difficult to determine when the onset of ventricular dysfunction actually occurred. Some patients appear to develop symptoms after a viral infection syndrome but proof of a viral inflammatory injury to the heart is usually difficult to establish. In patients who present in atrial fibrillation, it may be difficult to determine if the atrial fibrillation is secondary to a previously established but undiagnosed cardiomyopathy, or whether the ventricular systolic dysfunction and dilatation are due to prolonged tachycardia [25,26].

Typical symptoms of advanced disease include exertional or supine dyspnea, effort fatigue, and edema. Physical findings depend on the stage of disease, with cardiac enlargement, S4 and S3 gallop, functional mitral and tricuspid regurgitation murmurs, jugular venous distention, pulmonary rales, liver enlargement, and edema suggesting serious decompensation. Prominent right ventricular failure signs are evidence of end-stage deterioration. In addition to physical findings indicative of circulatory decompensation, one should be alert to noncardiac findings that may provide clues to etiology, such as signs of thyroid dysfunction, hemochromatosis, sarcoidosis, pheochromocytoma or alcoholism.

Evaluation

The goals of clinical assessment are to establish etiology and estimate prognosis. In screening for secondary causes of dilated cardiomyopathy measuring TSH (thyroid-stimulating hormone), creatinine, phosphorous, calcium, potassium, ferritin, complete blood count, and HIV serology may provide valuable clues. The electrocardiogram may disclose left bundle branch block, sometimes an early precursor of dilated cardiomyopathy, or clinically silent tachyarrhythmias. Nonsustained ventricular tachycardia is detectable in most patients if ambulatory monitoring is performed, and tends to be more severe as the disease progresses. The chest radiograph, in addition to providing information on cardiac size and pulmonary congestion, may also show signs of pulmonary infection or other thoracic disease such as sarcoidosis.

Measurement of ventricular function is essential. While this may be performed by echocardiographic, radionuclide, or angiographic means, the echocardiogram has merit in that it provides a wealth of corollary information, such as LV (left ventricle) mass, regional wall and valve function, chamber sizes, and the presence of pericardial effusion. When monitoring for changes in ventricular function, it is helpful to perform serial measurements using the same methodology.

Since coronary disease can present as a dilated cardiomyopathy without a history of documented myocardial infarction, it is important to exclude occult ischemic disease. In dilated cardiomyopathy, stress echocardiography or thallium scintigraphy may show regional abnormalities even in the absence of significant coronary occlusions. Therefore, a low threshold for performing coronary angiography in persons over 35 years of age is appropriate.

The use of endocardial biopsy should be selective. Knowledge of histology may point toward a specific etiology in approximately 15% of dilated cardiomyopathy cases seen in referral centers, but in only a few of these is an effective etiology-specific therapy available [9]. Examples of potentially treatable conditions include sarcoidosis, eosinophilic hypersensitivity myocarditis, and giant cell myocarditis. At this time we lack evidence that immunosuppressive treatment improves survival or ventricular function in lymphocytic myocarditis [27]. In general, the biopsy is more likely to yield useful clinical information in patients with acute or subacute onset of symptoms and prominent ventricular arrhythmias [28].

Right heart catheterization provides prognostic information when it is performed after a comprehensive medical treatment program is established. If PCW (pulmonary capillary wedge) and RA (right atrium) pressures remain high despite optimal medical therapy, the prognosis is particularly worrisome.

Treatment

The approach to management of dilated cardiomyopathy is similar to that of systolic heart failure in general—neurohormonal blockade with angiotensin converting enzyme inhibitors or angiotensin II receptor blockers, beta-adrenergic blockers and aldosterone blockade, digoxin, diuretics, biventricular pacing, ventricular assist devices, and cardiac transplantation. Patients having sustained ventricular arrhythmias should receive internal defibrillators; current ongoing clinical trials may provide further information on the value of prophylactic defibrillator implantation in those with nonsustained ventricular tachycardia.

Patients with treatable underlying etiologic conditions, such as myocardial ischemia, hypertension, sustained atrial tachyarrhythmias, etc., should have optimal therapy for those conditions. Concomitant anemia or obstructive sleep apnea needs to be aggressively managed. Avoidance of cardiotoxins, such as alcohol, is advised and moderate aerobic conditioning exercise is recommended. Warfarin anticoagulation is important for preventing emboli in those with atrial fibrillation; for patients in sinus rhythm with severely depressed systolic function the value of anticoagulation is being evaluated in controlled clinical trials at this time.

Patients with apparent idiopathic dilated cardiomyopathy need genetic counseling to alert them to the 20% to 25% probability that they may have a heritable condition. Although longitudinal data are not yet available, it is prudent to offer periodic screening with EKG and echocardiography to adult first-degree relatives of the dilated cardiomyopathy patient, perhaps repeated every 5 years.

HYPERTROPHIC CARDIOMYOPATHY

Morphology and Pathology

Hypertrophic cardiomyopathy is an hereditary condition characterized by regional left ventricular hypertrophy, normal or hyperdynamic systolic function, markedly impaired diastolic relaxation and compliance, left atrial enlargement, and a small left ventricular chamber volume [29–31]. Although a minority of patients have a detectable intraventricular pressure gradient across the outflow tract, the degree of increase in left ventricular mass is out of proportion to the increase in wall stress associated with the pressure gradient. The distribution of left ventricular hypertrophy is variable, and often includes especially prominent thickening of the intraventricular septum and anterolateral wall or, less commonly, the apex. Concentric left ventricular hypertrophy is not a common presentation. The histology is notable for widespread myocyte hypertrophy and disarray, scattered fibrosis, and reduced intramuscular coronary artery lumen size [32,33].

Epidemiology and Natural History

In population-based studies the age- and sex-adjusted annual incidence of hypertrophic cardiomyopathy has been estimated at 2.5 per 100,000 persons, approximately half the frequency of dilated cardiomyopathy [3]. Among children, hypertrophic cardiomyopathy also presents less commonly than dilated cardiomyopathy [4, 5].

The natural history of hypertrophic cardiomyopathy is not uniform, and may depend significantly on the specific underlying genetic defect responsible for the condition in an individual patient. In population-based community studies, many patients are found to be asymptomatic and have mortality similar to age-matched controls [34]. (Fig. 4) If they develop at all, symptoms are usually mild for many years. In contrast, patients reported from tertiary hypertrophic cardiomyopathy referral centers tend to have advanced symptoms, severe hypertrophy, and annual mortality rates in the range of 3% [35–37]. The higher mortality reported from these specialty clinics represents, no doubt, the effect of significant referral bias. A minority of patients, perhaps 5%, progress to a "burned out" HCM (hypertrophic cardiomyopathy) characterized by LV dilatation, and reduced LV ejection fraction [38]. The most common mode of death is sudden, particularly in younger patients in whom the disease is not suspected [39–42]. A history of syncope or the presence of high-risk mutations have predictive value for sudden cardiac death [42,43]. Severe dyspnea, marked (> 30 mm) left ventricular hypertrophy, chest pain, or a very high intraventricular gradient are predictors of poor prognosis [43,44]. Finally, evidence for severely impaired coronary vasodilation is a marker for increased mortality [45]. (Table 2)

Etiology

The etiology of hypertrophic cardiomyopathy has been an area of dramatic research progress over the last decade [30,31,36,37]. There is evidence that abnormal intracellular calcium flux, associated with abnormalities in sarcomere proteins or calcium channel function, results in increased intracellular calcium concentration. Subendocardial ischemia, a consequence of high intramural wall stress and reduced coronary luminal diameter, may also play a secondary role.

The greatest advances in HCM research in the last decade have been in elucidation of its genetic basis. Most cases, perhaps all, are caused by an inherited or sporadic mutation. Mendelian autosomal dominant patterns of inheritance are characteristic, but there is considerable genetic heterogeneity (i.e., HCM can be caused by mutations at scores of different

Table 2   Factors Associated with Increased Risk of Sudden Cardiadc Death in Hypertrophic Cardiomyopathy

GENETIC
Family history of sudden death
Specific mutations of sarcomeric proteins (i.e., Arg403Gln mutation of β-myosin heavy chain or Arg92Gln mutation of troponin T)
CLINICAL
Prior cardiac arrest
Recurrent syncope
Ventricular tachycardia on monitoring
MORPHOLOGIC
Extreme left ventricular hypertrophy (≥30 mm)
HEMODYNAMIC
Left ventricular outflow pressure gradient > 30 mm Hg
Decline in blood pressure during exercise testing
Limited myocardial coronary blood flow reserve

Source: Adapted from Cannon (2003)

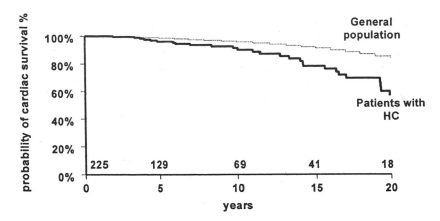

Figure 5 Kaplan-Meier survival curve for 225 patients with hypertrophic cardiomyopathy (HC) and age-matched controls in a community based population study. Numbers on the horizontal axis refer to number of patients at each follow-up interval. (From Ref. 35.)

loci). At this time, more than 150 different mutations have been associated with HCM phenotypes involving mutations in genes coding for sarcomere proteins, including beta cardiac myosin heavy chain, troponin T, and α-tropomyosin [35–37]. (Fig. 5) In addition to genotypic heterogeneity, there is phenotypic heterogeneity in HCM. Some mutations in the β-myosin heavy chain and troponin T appear to be characterized by a higher risk of sudden death, such as the Arg403Gln β–myosin heavy chain mutation or Arg92Gln troponin T mutation [6,41–43,49]. However, the frequency with which these "malignant" mutations are found in large referral clinics may be low, on the order of 1% of patients [48]. While some families do appear to manifest an unusually high frequency of sudden death, it is clear that all patients with the same mutation may not be at equally high risk. Confounding factors may influence the phenotypic manifestations of the genetic mutation, such as variable penetrance within families, modifier genes, and the role of other nongenetic factors [48,49].

Genetic mutations give rise to gross abnormalities of cardiac structure and function. The hypertrophic walls, hypercontractility state, and the small LV chamber size combine to produce systolic intracavitary pressure gradients and small stroke volume. Diastolic dysfunction, caused by a reduced rate of diastolic relaxation and increased chamber stiffness, is a more universal characteristic of HCM than are systolic intracavitary pressure gradients, which are demonstrable in only 30% to 40% of cases. Prolonged relaxation, likely related to high intracellular calcium concentration and subendocardial ischemia, combines with decreased distensibility due to hypertrophy and fibrosis to produce high diastolic filling pressures and atrial enlargement. Mitral regurgitation, usually proportional to the intracavitary pressure gradient, is often a feature [29]. Finally, in addition to these hemodynamic abnormalities there is significant impairment of coronary microvascular dilatation [45].

Clinical Presentation

The age of presentation is variable and may depend in part on the specific underlying mutation, with many myosin-binding protein C mutations not becoming phenotypically evident until the fifth decade [47]. Many patients are asymptomatic when discovered by genetic screening of relatives of an index case. Symptomatic patients present most commonly with effort dyspnea, but may also have angina, palpitations, syncope, and fatigue. Unfortunately, an initial manifestation may be sudden cardiac death, as observed in young athletes [37–39].

Physical examination usually features a sustained left ventricular impulse. It may include a ventricular gallop, and patients with intracavitary pressure gradients usually have a prominent systolic murmur associated with a bifid carotid upstroke. The murmur is typically midsystolic and harsh along the left sternal border, suggestive of aortic outflow tract obstruction, and more holosystolic at the apex due to mitral regurgitation. Maneuvers that increase peripheral resistance (e.g., squatting) reduce murmur intensity and, conversely, maneuvers that reduce afterload (standing from the squatting position) augment murmur intensity.

Evaluation

The evaluation aims to establish the diagnosis and, if possible, determine prognosis. The electrocardiogram usually demonstrates left ventricular hypertrophy. Echocardiography is the fundamental diagnostic tool, providing information on the distribution and extent of ventricular hypertrophy (septal, apical, or concentric), the presence and magnitude of an intraventricular pressure gradient, the severity of mitral regurgitation, systolic anterior motion of the mitral valve, the size of the LV chamber, and the degree of diastolic dysfunction. Echocardiographic evaluation in suspected or known cases should always assess for the presence and severity of an outflow tract gradient at rest and during provocative maneuvers (e.g., Valsalva, premature ventricular beats).

Most patients can be effectively diagnosed with echocardiography, and routine cardiac catheterization is not indicated. However, coronary angiography is necessary to exclude concomitant coronary disease in older patients with chest pain. A number of hemodynamic abnormalities are observed, including an intraventricular pressure gradient that varies with afterload and displays postextrasystolic potentiation (increased intracavitary gradient during the postextrasystolic beat), increased LVEDP (left ventricular end-diastolic pressure) and atrial *a*-wave, diminished aortic pressure during beats with increased intraventricular pressure gradient (Brockenbrough effect), and a bifid aortic peak systolic pressure form.

Management

Treatment has been offered primarily to patients who have symptoms associated with left ventricular outflow tract obstruction (i.e., approximately 30% to 40% of patients) and is directed toward reduction of symptoms and prevention of sudden death. Agents that increase myocardial contractility and intraventricular pressure gradient should be avoided. Diuretics should be used with caution since excessively decreased ventricular preload may result in increased intracavitary gradients and orthostatic hypotension.

Beta blockers are the first-line agents, their benefits being related to preventing tachycardia, reducing left ventricular cavitary gradient, improving diastolic filling, and reducing myocardial oxygen consumption [30]. Approximately half of patients report improvement in angina or dyspnea with beta blockade [51–53]. A reasonable therapeutic goal is to keep the heart rate at 60 bpm at rest, and this may require relatively high doses.

In patients whose symptoms persist despite beta-blockers, the calcium channel blocker verapamil may be employed to further reduce contractility, heart rate, and intracavitary gradient. Care should be taken to monitor cardiac conduction and blood pressure after starting verapamil. Occasional patients who remain symptomatic on beta-blockers or verapamil may benefit from the addition of disopyramide, which possesses potent negative inotropic effects.

Atrial fibrillation typically results in an abrupt increase in heart rate and dyspnea, as well as hypotension. Prompt treatment by electrical cardioversion may be needed, and amiodarone added to help maintain sinus rhythm. Patients with a past history of paroxysmal or chronic atrial fibrillation are at particularly high risk of thromboembolic complications and should be maintained on systemic anticoagulation.

Implantation of DDD pacemaker devices in patients with high intracavitary gradients results in a reduction in gradient and symptoms, and improved exercise capacity in a small minority (approximately 15%) of cases [54,55]. However, the benefits are highly variable and DDD pacing is now most often applied in those also needing pacing for conventional indications, such as symptomatic bradyarrhythmias or in those who are not candidates for surgical myectomy.

In patients felt to be at high risk for sudden death ICD (implantable cardioverter defibruillator) implantation is warranted [56]. Risk factors for sudden death, most commonly due to ventricular arrhythmias, include younger age, previously sustained ventricular tachycardia, or a family history of sudden death with HCM [42,43]. Early data suggest that some mutations may especially predispose to sudden death, but confirmatory information on larger numbers of families will be necessary to clarify these observations and better allow the use of genetic information to play a role in the decision to implant an ICD (36,37,41–43). Antiarrhythmic drugs, such as amiodarone, have not been prospectively studied in HCM and have significant long-term side effects. Patients should be advised to avoid vigorous physical activity, since HCM is a well-recognized substrate for sudden death in apparently healthy athletes [39–42].

Surgical septal myectomy has traditionally been offered to patients whose symptoms cannot be controlled medically, with the goal of reducing intracavitary outflow tract gradient [57,58]. Effective surgery eliminates or reduces the mitral regurgitation and relieves symptoms. These benefits occur in 80% to 90% of patients and are long-lasting [58]. However, surgery does not appear to reduce the risk of sudden death in most studies.

Percutaneous alcohol ablation of the septum has recently been employed as a catheter-based alternative to surgical myectomy [30,59,60]. Injection of alcohol into the first septal perforator produces focal myocardial infarction in the basal septum and, thereby, reduces the outflow tract obstruction. The most common complication of the procedure is complete heart block resulting from conduction system damage, occurring in about 10% of patients. While 3-year follow-up data are quite encouraging, the long-term benefits and risks of alcohol septal ablation are as yet unknown.

As HCM has a genetic basis, echocardiographic screening of first-degree relatives every 3 to 5 years is recommended. Evidence for hypertrophy is most likely to appear during puberty or early adulthood. Patients with LV cavitary obstruction are at increased risk for bacterial endocarditis and antibiotic endocarditis prophylaxis is prudent.

RESTRICTIVE CARDIOMYOPATHY

Morphology and Pathology

Restrictive cardiomyopathy (RCM) is characterized by severe diastolic dysfunction, relatively preserved systolic function and left ventricular cavity size, and biatrial enlargement [61]. Its physiology is very similar to that constrictive pericarditis [62]. Several different processes may produce severely impaired ventricular filling and restrictive cardiomyopa-

Table 3 Principle Causes of Restrictive Cardiomyopathy

1. INFILTRATIVE AND STORAGE DISEASES
   Amyloidosis
   Gaucher or Hurler diseases
   Gaucher, Hurler, or Fabry diseases; and glycogen storage
     disorders
2. NONINFILTRATIVE
   Sarcoidosis
   Scleroderma
   Radiation
   Endomyocardial fibrosis
   Hypereosinophilic syndrome
   Carcinoid syndrome
   Metastatic malignancy

thy, including infiltrative conditions (most commonly amyloidosis), diffuse myocardial fibrosis, and endocardial fibrosis (Table 3).

The histology of RCM depends upon the cause of the myocardial restriction. Infiltrative disorders, such as amyloidosis, sarcoidosis, or Gaucher, Hurler, or Fabry diseases, each have a distinct infiltrative histology. Extensive myocardial fibrosis may be idiopathic, secondary to radiation, eosinophilic myocarditis, or progressive systemic sclerosis (Fig. 6). Dense endocardial fibrosis may be a consequence of hypereosinophilic syndrome or radiation.

Epidemiology, Natural History, and Etiology

Different etiologic events can lead to the final common pathway of RCM. Therefore, the epidemiology and natural history of RCM depend on the particular etiology [61,63,64]. Several of the more common will be considered.

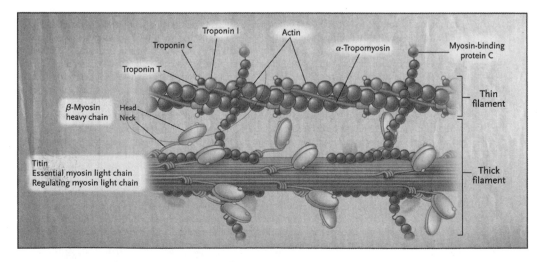

Figure 6 Sacromeric proteins subject to mutations resulting in hypertrophic cardiomyopathy and their frequency in reported series. (Adapted from Ref. 46.)

Cardiac amyloidosis may be considered a paradigm for infiltrative cardiomyopathy leading to restrictive physiology. Amyloidosis occurs as a consequence of the widespread multiorgan deposition of amyloid protein, most commonly caused by a plasma cell dyscrasia that results in excessive production of an immunoglobulin light chain fragment (AL amyloid). Cardiac involvement is common in ''primary'' AL amyloidosis and contributes seriously to the overall morbidity and mortality of the disease. Early manifestations include thickening of the left ventricular walls and biatrial enlargement. Initially, ejection fraction is maintained, but with progressive amyloid infiltration it begins to decrease and the prognosis for survival is then usually less than a year.

Cardiac amyloidosis often presents as right heart failure, with ascites, increased central venous pressure, edema, pleural effusions, and exercise intolerance. Concomitant renal involvement may produce nephrotic magnitude proteinuria, which aggravates the symptoms of fluid retention. The diagnosis is based on the typical echocardiographic features previously described, as well as increased myocardial echogenicity (''speckling'') and Doppler evidence of impaired diastolic function. While endocardial biopsy can confirm the diagnosis, an amyloid positive tissue biopsy from elsewhere (e.g., fat aspirate, mucosal, or rectal biopsy), combined with identification of an amyloid protein in serum or urine, are usually sufficient to explain the echocardiographic findings. Treatment, in selected cases, may involve autologous bone marrow stem cell transplantation, or cardiac transplantation [65].

Eosinophilic heart disease includes disorders in which hypereosinophilia and/or eosinophilic myocarditis are associated with endocardial or myocardial fibrosis. Hypereosinophilic syndrome is usually associated with cardiac involvement and has been known as Löffler endocarditis [66–68]. The disorder is characterized by thromboembolic events, widespread arteritis, and eosinophilic myocarditis. Both ventricles are subject to mural thrombosis and dense fibrotic thickening. Damage to valvular support may produce significant mitral regurgitation, and biatrial enlargement predisposes to atrial fibrillation. In equatorial Africa, a similar disease, known as endomyocardial fibrosis (EMF), is not associated with peripheral eosinophilia [68–71]. EMF may involve either or both ventricles and sometimes responds favorably to surgical resection of fibrotic endocardium [71].

Hemochromatosis, while generally classified with infiltrative cardiomyopathies, usually does not present with restrictive physiology. Rather, its clinical picture is more typical of the dilated cardiomyopathies [72,73]. Patients with hepatic dysfunction, diabetes mellitus, and dilated ventricles should be evaluated with serum iron, iron binding capacity, and ferritin levels.

Idiopathic restrictive cardiomyopathy is diagnosed if no other potential etiology can be identified. It is characterized by marked biatrial enlargement and predominantly affects the elderly. Survival rates at 5 and 10 years have been reported to be 64% and 37%, respectively [63] (Fig. 7). Patients who present with systemic or pulmonary venous congestion and atrial fibrillation have a particularly poor prognosis.

Clinical Presentation

The clinical features of restrictive cardiomyopathy may be difficult to distinguish from those of constrictive pericarditis, and include abdominal distention, dependent edema, exercise intolerance, low systemic blood pressure, anorexia, and hepatic congestion. Because cardiac restriction may affect right-sided filling as much as left-sided filling, pulmonary congestion symptoms, such as paroxysmal nocturnal dyspnea, are not prominent symptoms.

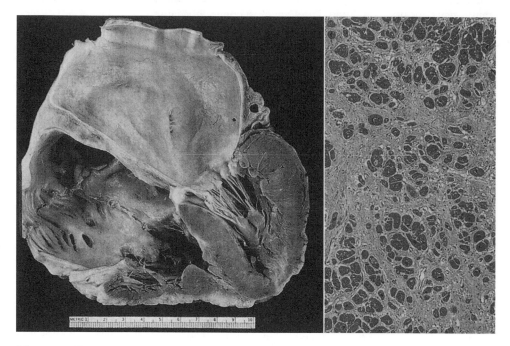

Figure 7 Pathology of idiopathic restrictive cardiomyopathy. (left panel): Gross specimen demonstrates prominent biatrial enlargement and normal ventricular size. (right panel): Light microscopy showing marked interstitial fibrosis; Hematoxylin and eosin staining, magnification X 120. (From Ref. 59a)

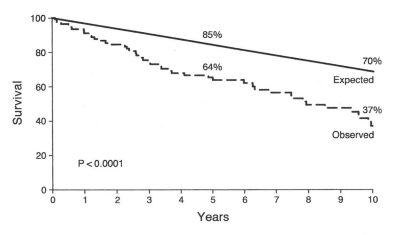

Figure 8 Kaplan Meier survival curve for a cohort of patients (n = 94) with idiopathic restrictive cardiomyopathy compared to expected survival in age- and sex-matched patients. (From Ref. 63.)

The physical examination is dominated by signs of "right-sided" heart failure—jugular venous distention, which increases on inspiration, hepatic enlargement, icterus, ascites, and anasarca. The left ventricle may be palpable, the P_2 augmented, and S_3 or S_4 gallops are common.

Evaluation

The workup centers on determining the etiology and distinguishing restrictive cardiomyopathy from constrictive pericarditis, the latter requiring surgical pericardiectomy. To distinguish constrictive from restrictive disease, thorough noninvasive imaging and invasive hemodynamic evaluating may be needed. Echocardiography is valuable to assess systolic and diastolic function and to look for evidence of amyloidosis. MR (magnetic resonance) imaging or CT (computed tomography) scanning may provide important information on pericardial thickness and calcification. An optimal catheterization study should include simultaneous high-fidelity ventricular pressure measurements and respirometry recordings. In restrictive disease, respiratory maneuvers produces concordant changes in RV (right ventricle) and LV systolic pressures, whereas constriction usually results in discordant respiratory variation in ventricular systolic pressures (i.e., greater ventricular interdependence) [62]. The measurement of ventricular interdependence appears to be more sensitive and specific for identification of constrictive pericarditis than does measurement of more traditional hemodynamic parameters [62]. Finally, endocardial biopsy may provide useful diagnostic information, such as extensive myocardial fibrosis, amyloid infiltration, or evidence of sarcoidosis or storage disease; in constrictive pericarditis the myocardium is normal.

Management

The approach to management is a challenging one. Attempts to treat the underlying etiology (amyloidosis—prednisone and melphalan immunosuppression or autologous stem cell transplantation; hypereosinophilic syndrome—corticosteroids) should be undertaken. General measures include employing as much diuretic as needed to control fluid retention without producing clinically significant orthostatic hypotension. If tachycardia is contributing to impaired diastolic filling, beta blockade may be beneficial. The onset of atrial fibrillation can produce an abrupt increase in symptoms, and urgent efforts to restore sinus rhythm may need to be undertaken. Inotropic agents are of little benefit.

SUMMARY

The cardiomyopathies present a diverse group of diseases, but can be usefully categorized into three clinical classes: dilated, hypertrophic, and restrictive. Within each class a variety of specific etiologies give rise to similar morphology and pathophysiology. Clinical efforts need to be directed toward proper classification, identification of the etiology, and selection of appropriate therapy. Advances in genomic medicine may soon permit more accurate identification of patients with mild symptomatic disease, identify those at high risk of adverse outcomes, and help guide individualized treatment strategies.

REFERENCES

1. Richardson P, McKenna W, Bristow M, Maisch B, Mautner B, O'Connell J, Olsen E, Thiene G, Goodwin J, Gyarfas I, Martin I, Nordet P. Report of the 1995 World Health Organization/

International Society and Federation of Cardiology Task Force on the Definition and Classification of Cardiomyopathies. Circulation 1996; 93:841.

2. Torp A. Incidence of congestive cardiomyopathy. Postgrad Med J 1978; 54:435–437.

3. Codd MB, Sugrue DD, Gersh BJ, Melton LJ. Epidemiology of idiopathic dilated and hypertrophic cardiomyopathy: a population-based study in Olmsted County, Minnesota, 1975–1984. Circulation 1989; 80:564–572.

4. Nugent AW, Piers BS, Daubeney EF, Chondros P, Carlin JB, Cheung M, Wilkinson LC, Davis AM, Kahler SG, Chow CW, Wilkinson JL, Weinitraub RG. The epidemiology of childhood cardiomyopathy in Australia. N Engl J Med 2003; 348:1639–1646.

5. Lipschultz SE, Sleeper LA, Towbin JA, Lowe AM, Orav EJ, Cox GF, Lurie PR, McCoy KL, McDonald MA, Messere JE, Colan SD. The incidence of pediatric cardiomyopathy in two regions of the United States. N Engl J Med 2003; 348:1647–1655.

6. Coughlin SS, Szklo M, Baughman K, Pearson TA. The epidemiology of idiopathic dilated cardiomyopathy in a biracial community. Am J Epidemiol 1990; 131:48–56.

7. Sugrue DD, Rodeheffer RJ, Codd MB, Ballard DI, Fuster V, Gersh BJ. The clinical course of idiopathic dilated course of idiopathic dilated cardiomyopathy. Am Inter Med 1992: 117: 117–123.

8. Redfield MM, Gersh BJ, Bailey KR, Ballard DJ, Rodeheffer RJ. Natural history of idiopathic dilated cardiomyopathy: effect of referral bias and secular trend. J Am Coll Cardiol 1993; 22: 1921–1926.

9. Kasper EK, Agema WRP, Hutchins GM, Deckers JW, Hare JM, Baughman KL. The causes of dilated cardiomyopathy: A clinicopathologic review of 673 consecutive patients. J Am Coll Cardiol 1994; 23:586–590.

10. Feldman AM, McNamara D. Myocarditis. N Engl J Med 2000; 373:1388–1398.

11. Liu P, Martino T, Opavsky MA, Penninger J. Viral myocarditis: balance between viral infection and immune response. Can J Cardiol 1996; 12:935–943.

12. Kawai C. From myocarditis to cardiomyopathy: mechanisms of inflammation and cell death. Circulation 1999; 99:1091–1100.

13. Why HJR, Meany BT, Richardson PJ, Olsen EGJ, Bowles NE, Cunningham L, Freeke CA, Archard LC. Clinical and prognostic significance of detection of enteroviral RNA in the myocardium of patients with myocarditis or dilated cardiomyopathy. Circulation 1994; 89: 2582–2589.

14. Li Y, Bourlet T, Andreoletti L, Mosnier JF, Peng T, Yang Y, Archard LC, Pozzetto B, Zhang H. Enteroviral capsid protein VP1 is present in myocardial tissues from some patients with myocarditis or dilated cardiomyopathy. Circulation 2000; 101:231–234.

15. Archard LC, Bowles NE, Cunningham L, Freeke CA, Olsen ECJ, Rose ML, Meany B, Why HJF, Richardson PJ. Molecular probes for detection of persisting enterovirus infection of human heart and their prognostic value. Eur Hrt J 1991; 12:56–59.

16. McCarthy RE, Boehmer JP, Hruban RH, Hutchins GM, Kasper EK, Hare JM, Baughman KL. Long-term outcome of fulminant myocarditis as compared with acute (nonfulminant) myocarditis. N Engl J Med 2000; 342:690–695.

17. Michels VV, Moll PP, Miller FA, Tajik AJ, Chu JS, Driscoll DJ, Burnett JC, Rodeheffer RJ, Chesebro JH, Tazelaar HD. The frequency of familial dilated cardiomyopathy in a series of patients with idiopathic dilated cardiomyopathy. N Engl J Med 1992; 326:77–82.

18. Keeling PJ, Gang Y, Smith G, Seo H, Bent SE, Murday V, Caforio ALP, McKenna WJ. Familial dilated cardiomyopathy in the United Kingdom. Br Heart J 1995; 73:417–421.

19. Grunig E, Tasman JA, Kucherer H, Franz W, Kubler W, Katus HA. Frequency and phenotypes of familial dilated cardiomyopathy. J Am Coll Cardiol 1998; 31:186–194.

20. Baig MK, Goldman JH, Caforio ALP, Coonar AS, Keeling PJ, McKenna WJ. Familial dilated cardiomyopathy: cardiac abnormalities are common in asymptomatic relatives and may represent early disease. J Am Coll Cardiol 1998; 31:195–201.

21. Regan TJ. Alcohol and the cardiovascular system. JAMA 1990; 264:377–381.

22. Urbano-Marquez A, Estruch R, Navarro-Lopez F, Grau JM, Mont L, Rubin E. The effects of alcoholism on skeletal and cardiac muscle. N Engl J Med 1989; 320:409–415.

23. Urbano-Marquez A, Estruch R, Fernandez-Sola J, Nicolas JM, Pare JC, Rubin E. The greater risk of alcoholic cardiomyopathy and myopathy in women compared with men. JAMA 1995; 274:149–154.

24. Kupari M, Koskinen P. Relation of left ventricular function to habitual alcohol consumption. Am J Cardiol 1993; 72:1418–1424.

25. Grogan M, Smith HC, Gersh BJ, Wood DL. Left ventricular dysfunction due to atrial fibrillation in patients initially believed to have idiopathic dilated cardiomyopathy. Am J Cardiol 1992; 69:1570–1573.

26. Kajstura J, Zhang X, Liu Y, Szoke E, Cheng W, Olivetti G, Hintze TH, Anversa P. The cellular basis of pacing-induced dilated cardiomyopathy. Myocyte cell loss and myocyte cellular reactive hypertrophy. Circulation 1995; 92(8):2306–2317.

27. Mason JW, O'Connell JB, Herskowitz A, Rose NR, McManus BM, Billingham ME, Moon TE. A clinical trial of immunosuppression therapy for myocarditis. The Myocarditis Treatment Trail Investigators. N Engl J Med 1995; 333:269–275.

28. Cooper LT, Berry GJ, Shabetai R. Idiopathic giant-cell myocarditis—natural history and treatment. N Engl J Med 1997; 336(26):1860–1866.

29. Wigle ED, Rakowski H, Kimball BP, Williams WG. Hypertrophic cardiomyopathy. Clinical spectrum and treatment. Circulation 1995; 92:1680–1692.

30. Braunwald E, Seidman CE, Sigwart U. Contemporary evaluation and management of hypertrophic cardiomyopathy. Circulation 2002; 106(11):1312–1316.

31. Maron BJ. Hypertrophic cardiomyopathy. A systematic review. JAMA 2002; 287(10): 1308–1320.

32. Maron BJ, Wolfson JK, Epstein SE, Roberts WC. Intramural (''small vessel'') coronary artery disease in hypertrophic cardiomyopathy. J Am Coll Cardiol 1986; 8:545–557.

33. Maron BJ, Anan TJ, Roberts WC. Quantitative analysis of the distribution of cardiac muscle cell disorganization in the left ventricular wall of patients with hypertrophic cardiomyopathy. Circulation 1981; 63:882–894.

34. Cannan CR, Reeder GS, Bailey KR, Melton LJ, Gersh BJ. Natural history of hypertrophic cardiomyopathy. A population-based study, 1976 through 1990. Circulation 1995; 92: 2488–2495.

35. Kofflard MJM, TenCate PJ, van der Lee C, van Domburg RT, Hypertrophic cardiomyopathy in a large community-based population: clinical outcome and identification of risk factors for sudden cardiac death and clinical deterioration. J Am Coll Cardiol 2003; 41:989.

36. Roberts R, Sigwart U. New concepts in hypertrophic cardiomyopathies, part I. Circulation 2001; 104(17):2113–2116.

37. Roberts R, Sigwart U. New concepts in hypertrophic cardiomyopathies, part II. Circulation 2001; 104(18):2249–2252.

38. Spirito P, Maron BJ, Bonow RO, Epstein SE. Occurrence and significance of progressive left ventricular wall thinning and relative cavity dilatation in hypertrophic cardiomyopathy. Am J Cardiol 1987; 60:123–129.

39. Maron BJ, Shirani J, Poliac LC, Mathenge R, Roberts WC, Mueller FO. Sudden death in young competitive athletes. Clinical, demographic, and pathological profiles. JAMA 1996; 276:199–204.

40. Spirito P, Seidman CE, McKenna WJ, Maron BJ. The management of hypertrophic cardiomyopathy. N Engl J Med 1997; 336:775–785.

41. Maron BJ. Sudden death in young athletes. N Engl J Med 2003; 349:1064–1075.

42. Watkins H. Sudden death in hypertrophic cardiomyopathy. N Engl J Med 2000; 342:422–424.

43. Cannon RO. Assessing risk in hypertrophic cardiomyopathy. N Engl J Med 2003; 349:11.

44. Maron MS, Olivotto I, Betocchi S, Casey SA, Lesser JR, Losi MA, Cecchi F, Maron BJ. Effect of left ventricular outflow tract obstruction in clinical outcome in hypertrophic cardiomyopathy. N Engl J Med 2003; 348:295–303.

45. Cecchi F, Olivotto I, Gistri R, Lorenzoni R, Chiriatti G, Camici PG. Coronary microvascular dysfunction and prognosis in hypertrophic cardiomyopathy. N Engl J Med 2003; 349: 1027–1035.

46. Nabel E. Cardiovascular disease. N Engl J Med 2003; 349:60–72.
47. Anan R, Greve G, Thierfelder L, Watkins H, McKenna WJ, Solomon S, Vecchio C, Shono H, Nakao S, Tanaka H, et al. Prognostic implications of novel beta cardiac myosin heavy chain gene mutations that cause familial hypertrophic cardiomyopathy. J Clin Invest 1994; 93:280–285.
48. Ackerman MJ, VanDriest SL, Ommen SR, Will ML, Nishimura RA, Tajik AJ, Gersh BJ. Prevalence and age-dependence of malignant mutations in the beta-myosin heavy chain and troponin T genes in hypertrophic cardiomyopathy: a comprehensive outpatient perspective. J Am Coll Cardiol 2002; 39:2042–2048.
49. Van Driest SL, Ackerman MJ, Ommen SR, Shakur R, Will ML, Nishimura RA, Tajik AJ, Gersh BJ. Prevalence and severity of "benign" mutations in the β-myosin heavy chain, cardiac troponin T, and α-tropomyosin genes in hypertrophic cardiomyopathy. Circulation 2002; 106: 3085–3090.
50. Niimura H, Patton KK, McKenna WJ, Soults J, Maron BJ, Seidman JG, Seidman CE. Sarcomere protein gene mutations in hypertrophic cardiomyopathy of the elderly. Circulation 2002; 105:446–451.
51. Maron BJ, Bonow RO, Cannon RO, Leon MB, Epstein SE. Hypertrophic cardiomyopathy. Interrelations of clinical manifestations, pathophysiology and therapy. N Engl J Med 1987; 316:780–789.
52. Maron BJ, Bonow RO, Cannon RO, Leon MB, Epstein SE. Hypertrophic cardiomyopathy. Interrelations of clinical manifestations, pathophysiology and therapy. N Engl J Med 1987; 316:844–852.
53. Louie EK, Edwards LC. Hypertrophic cardiomyopathy. Prog Cardiovascular Dis 1994; 36: 275.
54. Maron BJ, Nishimura RA, McKenna WJ, Rakowski H, Josephson ME, Kieval RS. Assessment of permanent dual-chamber pacing as a treatment for drug-refractory symptomatic patients with obstructive hypertrophic cardiomyopathy. A randomized, double-blind, crossover study (M-PATHY). Circulation 1999; 99(22):2927–2933.
55. Ommen SR, Nishimura RA, Squires RW, Schaff HV, Danielson GK, Tajik AJ. Comparison of dual-chamber pacing versus septal myectomy for the treatment of patients with hypertrophic obstructive cardiomyopathy: a comparison of objective hemodynamic and exercise end points. J Am Coll Cardiol 1999; 34(1):191–196.
56. Maron BJ, Shen WK, Link MS, Epstein AE, Almquist AK, Daubert JP, Bardy GH, Favale S, Rea RF, Boriani G, Estes NA, Spirito P. Efficacy of implantable cardioverter-defibrillators for the prevention of sudden death in patients with hypertrophic cardiomyopathy. New Engl J Med 2000; 342:365–673.
57. Schulte HD, Borisov K, Gams E, Gramsch-Zabel H, Losse B, Schwartzkopff B. Management of symptomatic hypertrophic obstructive cardiomyopathy-long-term results after surgical therapy. Thorac Cardiovasc Surg 1999; 47:213–218.
58. Merrill WH, Friesinger GC, Graham TP, Byrd BF, Drinkwater DC, Christian KG, Bender HW. Long-lasting improvement after septal myectomy for hypertrophic obstructive cardiomyopathy. Ann Thorac Surg 2000; 69:1732–1735; discussion 1735–1736.
59. Braunwald E. Induced septal infarction: a new therapeutic strategy for hypertrophic obstructive cardiomyopathy. Circulation 1997; 95(8):1981–1982.
60. Braunwald E. Hypertrophic cardiomyopathy–the benefits of a multidisciplinary approach. N Engl J Med 2002; 347(17):1306–1307.
61. Kushwaha SS, Fallon JT, Fuster V. Restrictive cardiomyopathy. N Engl J Med 1997; 336: 267–276.
62. Hurrell DG, Nishimura RA, Higano ST, Appleton CP, Danielson GK, Holmes DR, Tajik AJ. Value of dynamic respiratory changes in left and right ventricular pressures for the diagnosis of constrictive pericarditis. Circulation 1996; 93:2007–2013.
63. Ammash NM, Seward JR, Bailey KR, Edwards WD, Tajik A. Clinical profile and outcome of idiopathic restrictive cardiomyopathy. Circulation 2000; 2490–2496.
64. Ammash NM, Seward JB, Bailey KR, Edwards WD, Tajik AJ. Clinical profile and outcome of idiopathic restrictive cardiomyopathy. Circulation 2000; 101:2490–2496.

65. Hirota Y, Shimizu G, Kita Y, Nakayama Y, Suwa M, Kawamura K, Nagata S, Sawayama T, Izumi T, Nakano T, et al. Spectrum of restrictive cardiomyopathy: Report of the national survey in Japan. Am Heart J 1990; 120:188.

66. McGregor CGA, Rodeheffer RJ, Daly RC, Kyle RA, Gertz MA, Edwards BS, Olson LJ, Frantz RP, Dearani JA. Heart transplantation for AL amyloidosis. J Heart Lung Transplantation 2000; 19:51.

67. Parrillo JE. Heart disease and the eosinophil. N Engl J Med 1990; 323:1560–1561.

68. deMello DE, Liapis H, Jureidini S, Nouri S, Kephart GM, Gleich GJ. Cardiac localization of eosinophil-granule major basic protein in acute necrotizing myocarditis. N Engl J Med 1990; 323:1542–1545.

69. Weller PF, Bubley GJ. The idiopathic hypereosinophilic syndrome. Blood 1994; 83: 2759–2779.

70. Gupta PN, Valiathan MS, Balakrishnan KG, Kartha CC, Ghosh MK. Clinical course of endomyocardial fibrosis. Br Heart J 1989; 62:450–454.

71. Shaper AG. What's new in endomyocardial fibrosis?. Lancet 1993; 342:255–256.

72. Barretto AC, Lemos da Luz P, de Oliveira SA, Stolf NAG, Mady C, Bellotti G, Jatene AD, Pilegii F. Determinants of survival in endomyocardial fibrosis. Circulation 1989; 80(suppl I): I-177–I-182.

73. Olson LJ, Edwards WD, McCall JT, Ilstrup DM, Gersh BJ. Cardiac iron deposition in idiopathic hemochromatosis: histologic and analytic assessment of 14 hearts from autopsy. JACC 1987; 10:1239–1243.

74. Olson LJ, Baldus WP, Tajik AJ. Echocardiographic features of idiopathic hemochromatosis. Am J Cardiol 1987; 60:885–889.

9

Heart Failure with Normal Systolic Function

Johan Sundström and Ramachandran S. Vasan
National Heart, Lung and Blood Institute's Framingham Heart Study, Framingham, Massachusetts, USA

INTRODUCTION

Approximately 30% to 50% of patients with heart failure are reported to have a normal or nearly normal left ventricular systolic function [1–7]. This condition has been labeled diastolic heart failure (DHF), and shares several characteristics with systolic heart failure, including reduced exercise performance, neuroendocrine activation, reduced quality of life [8], and a considerably increased mortality risk [1,9]. In this chapter, we will review the pathophysiology, diagnosis, differential diagnosis, and prognosis of DHF. Treatment of DHF is discussed in Chapter 17.

PATHOPHYSIOLOGY OF DIASTOLIC HEART FAILURE

DHF is defined as overt congestive heart failure due to the inability of the left ventricle to fill adequately at normal filling pressures [10]. Left ventricular diastolic dysfunction is a progressive condition characterized by an increased resistance to ventricular filling and, thus, an increasing dependence on higher ventricular preload in order to maintain adequate stroke volume. In diastolic dysfunction, the left ventricular diastolic pressure-volume relation is shifted upward (Fig. 1) so that for any given left ventricular end-diastolic volume, left ventricular end-diastolic pressure is increased with a corresponding increase in left atrial and pulmonary venous pressure. This, in combination with the reduced forward cardiac output, triggers neurohormonal activation, and eventually symptoms and signs of pulmonary and systemic congestion [8].

From a pathophysiological perspective, left ventricular filling is determined by an early diastolic rapid-filling phase dependent on active *relaxation* of the ventricle, (an energy-dependent process in which the sarcoplasmic reticulum calcium ATPase pump ($SRCa^{++}ATPase$) plays a key role [11] and a late diastolic passive-filling phase determined by the viscoelastic *compliance* of the ventricle (defined as change in volume for a given change in pressure during diastolic filling). Reduced ventricular relaxation and/or decreased compliance are the hallmarks of diastolic dysfunction, which eventually leads to DHF [10].

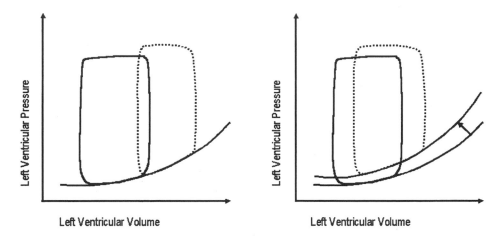

Figure 1 Two sets of pressure-volume loops, the dashed ones have increased filling pressures compared to the solid ones. Left panel illustrates how an increased left ventricular volume may shift the pressure-volume loop to the right, to a steeper portion of the same curve. Right panel curve illustrates how an increased myocardial stiffness or pericardial restraint may shift the diastolic pressure-volume curve upward and to the left. (Adapted from Ref. 66. Copyright 1997 American College of Cardiology Foundation.)

Impaired relaxation can be caused by factors such as delayed inactivation of contraction, diminished ventricular load dependence, and increased nonuniformity of relaxation [12–14]. Ventricular compliance has a multitude of determinants, including diastolic suction, passive filling, pericardial restraint, ventricular interaction, viscoelastic properties, and possibly coronary vascular engorgement. In addition, abnormalities involving increased myocardial stiffness or increased pericardial restraint would tend to shift the diastolic pressure-volume relation upward and to the left, whereas an increased left ventricular volume would move the ventricle to the right to a steeper segment of the pressure-volume curve (Fig. 1), both ultimately leading to elevated left ventricular filling pressure.

Relaxation abnormalities are early manifestations in hypertensive and coronary disease, and can be induced by acute processes such as ischemia. Abnormal ventricular compliance is often a later stage in the progression of diastolic dysfunction (Fig. 2) and is frequently the result of chronic processes, such as hypertrophy or infiltrative disorders. Thus, several contributory factors for reduced ventricular relaxation and/or compliance are extrinsic to the heart [10,12–15]. Overt congestive DHF is often a result of a combination of an acute precipitating factor and an underlying state of subclinical left ventricular diastolic dysfunction.

Recently, it has been questioned whether diastolic dysfunction is a cause or a consequence of elevated ventricular filling pressures. Investigators have evaluated the left ventricular pressure-volume curves in patients with congestive heart failure and normal left ventricular ejection fraction, and reported a range of patterns. An upward and leftward shift of the pressure-volume curve was not present in several patients [16]. Additional investigations are warranted to confirm these findings.

Increased vascular stiffness with age (abnormal ventriculo-vascular coupling, i.e., a stiffer heart ejecting into a stiffer vascular tree) [17–19] has also emerged as a major pathophysiological abnormality underlying DHF [8,20,21]. Increased vascular stiffness is associated with augmentation of the pulsatile load on the heart. At any given level of mean arterial pressure, an increase in pulsatile load, and, therefore, total hemodynamic load, may result

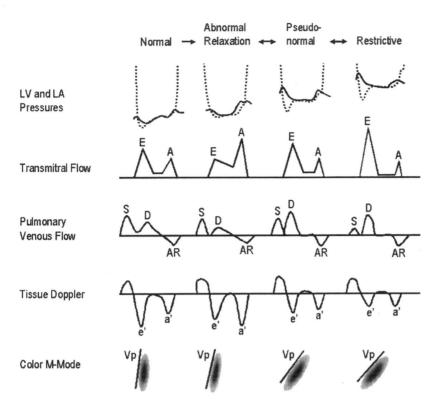

Figure 2   Progression of diastolic heart failure from a normal ventricle via abnormal relaxation and a pseudonormal pattern to a restrictive pattern, illustrated by ventricular and atrial pressures and corresponding transmitral and pulmonary venous flow velocities, tissue Doppler velocities, and color M-mode patterns. LV, left ventricular; LA, left atrial; E, early peak filling velocity; A, peak filling velocity during atrial systole; S, peak systolic pulmonary venous flow velocity; D, peak diastolic pulmonary venous flow velocity; AR, retrograde flow during atrial systole; e', peak early myocardial velocity; a', peak myocardial velocity during atrial systole; Vp, ventricular flow propagation velocity. See Table 3 for diagnostic cut-off values.

from an increase in characteristic impedance of the aorta, which directly impacts early systolic pressure and peak LV (left ventricle) force and wall stress, or from premature return of the reflected pressure wave during systole, which increases late systolic LV load and has a deleterious effect on diastolic function [22–24].

At a cellular level, numerous myocardial and extramyocardial factors may promote diastolic functional abnormalities [25]. These are reviewed in detail elsewhere [25]. Briefly, myocardial factors include altered cardiomyocyte function and alterations in the extracellular matrix. Cardiomyocyte factors include changes in calcium homeostasis (changes in sarcolemmal channels for short- and long-term calcium transport; changes in $SRCa^{++}ATPase$; changes in phosphorylation state of phospholamban, calsequestrin, and calmodulin that can influence $SRCa^{++}ATPase$), alterations in myofilaments and cytoskeleton, and abnormalities in myocardial energetics. Changes in the content of fibrillar collagen in the matrix may predispose to diastolic dysfunction. Extramyocardial factors include alterations in afterload (vascular stiffness, previously discussed), and in pericardial restraint.

The cellular changes that mediate diastolic dysfunction, in turn are influenced by numerous signaling pathways involving endocrine, paracrine, and autocrine factors [26–28].

Briefly, these include neurohumoral activation (renin-angiotensin-aldosterone,and natri-uretic peptide pathways), sympathetic nervous system, cytokines of the gp130 family, growth factors, proteolytic enzymes (matrix metalloproteinases), and cardiac endothelial ni-tric oxide pathways [26–31].

DIAGNOSING DIASTOLIC HEART FAILURE

A person can be said to have DHF when there is [32]:

a. Objective evidence of congestive heart failure
b. Objective evidence of normal left ventricular systolic function
c. Objective evidence of left ventricular diastolic dysfunction
d. Resolution of symptoms with treatment directed at the etiology of the diastolic dysfunction

Objective Evidence of Congestive Heart Failure

Congestive heart failure is a syndrome identified by a combination of clinical signs and symptoms that lacks a universally accepted definition. A number of diagnostic definitions using clinical criteria exist [33–38]. These definitions have variable sensitivities and speci-ficities for heart failure depending on the severity of heart failure diagnosed and the desired degree of certainty in the diagnosis [39,40]. Although primarily intended for epidemiological purposes, a definition such as the Framingham Heart Study Heart Failure Criteria [33] can be helpful for clinicians (Table 1).

The clinical diagnosis of heart failure is especially imprecise in the setting of primary care [41,42]. Recently, investigators have raised the possibility that a majority of general practice patients diagnosed with DHF have, in fact, been misdiagnosed, and have either obe-sity or pulmonary disease as the etiology of breathlessness [43,44]. In hospital-based set-tings, objective evidence of heart failure typically consists of a combination of the clinical signs and symptoms of heart failure and laboratory blood and x-ray tests, with or without documentation of elevated left ventricular filling pressures or a low cardiac index [45,46]. Measurement of B-type natriuretic peptide in the emergency care setting has been shown to

Table 1 Framingham Heart Study Criteria for Congestive Heart Failure

Major Criteria[a]	Minor Criteria
Paroxysmal nocturnal dyspnea	Bilateral ankle edema
Jugular venous distension	Nocturnal cough
Pulmonary rales	Dyspnea on ordinary exertion
Radiographic cardiomegaly	Hepatomegaly
Acute pulmonary edema	Pleural effusion
Third heart sound	Decrease in vital capacity by 1/3
Central Venous Pressure >16 cm H_2O	Heart rate $\geq$120 beats/minute
Hepatojugular reflex	
Autopsy: pulmonary edema, visceral congestion or cardiomegaly	
Weight loss $\geq$4.5 Kg in 5 days in response to treatment for congestive heart failure	

[a]Two major, or one major plus two minor criteria required for diagnosis of congestive heart failure. (From Ref. 33.)

be a useful adjunct for the diagnosis of congestive heart failure in patients with acute dyspnea [47,48].

In the differential diagnostic decision between congestive heart failure and other noncardiac reasons for dyspnea, the clinician should pay attention to the following features (Table 2). *Symptoms* of heart failure include exertional dyspnea, paroxysmal nocturnal dyspnea and orthopnea, which are all indicative of pulmonary venous hypertension. *Signs* of heart failure comprise a displaced apical impulse (indicating cardiac enlargement), S3 or S4 gallops (suggestive of elevated left ventricular end-diastolic pressure), increased pulmonic component of the second heart sound (indicative of pulmonary arterial hypertension), elevated jugular venous pressure, hepatomegaly with positive hepatojugular reflux, and peripheral edema (correlates of right ventricular failure). X-ray features of heart failure include enlargement of the cardiac silhouette, alveolar or interstitial pulmonary edema, pulmonary vascular redistribution, Kerley B lines, and pleural effusion. Interobserver reproducibility of some of the key clinical signs that distinguish cardiac from noncardiac causes of dyspnea is only fair, especially among nonspecialists, rendering the diagnosis of heart failure challenging sometimes. If diagnostic uncertainty persists, pulmonary and thyroid function tests, exercise tolerance test, as well as catheterization and angiography may aid in the differential diagnosis [45,46]. Right heart catheterization may be indicated if the clinical presentation is equivocal and there is the following: echocardiographic evidence of pulmonary hypertension; radiographic evidence of interstitial lung disease; unexplained peripheral edema.

Objective Evidence of Normal Left Ventricular Systolic Function

The second step in diagnosing DHF requires verifying the presence of a normal or near normal left ventricular systolic function. The clinical differentiation of normal from reduced

Table 2 Features Distinguishing Cardiac from Pulmonary Causes of Dyspnea

---

Features more common in cardiac dyspnea[a]
  History of paroxysmal nocturnal dyspnea
  History of myocardial infarction, high blood pressure, or valve disease
  Displaced apical impulse
  S3 or S4 gallop
  Cardiac murmur
  Elevated jugular venous pressure
  Cardiac enlargement, interstitial edema, pulmonary vascular redistribution on x-ray
  Echocardiography: left ventricular dilation, hypertrophy, wall motion abnormalities, pulmonary hypertension
  Cardiopulmonary exercise: low anerobic threshold; lack of desaturation with exercise
  Right heart cardiac catheterization: elevated right-sided filling pressures, increased right ventricular systolic/pulmonary systolic pressure, elevated pulmonary capillary wedge pressure
Features more common in pulmonary causes of dyspnea[a]
  History of chronic bronchitis; cough/dyspnea relieved with expectoration of sputum
  Absence of signs noted above that favor cardiac dyspnea
  Pulmonary function tests indicate an airway obstruction pattern
  Cardiopulmonary exercise: significant desaturation, development of bronchospasm with falling forced expiratory volume in 1 sec
  Right heart cardiac catheterization: normal pulmonary capillary wedge pressure, pulmonary arterial pressure may be elevated if pulmonary hypertension is present

---

[a]Both conditions may coexist resulting in a mixed pattern.

left ventricular systolic function is notoriously difficult. No single clinical symptom or sign has an acceptable positive or negative predictive value to be clinically useful for distinguishing systolic from DHF [49]. An electrocardiographic anterior Q-wave, or a left bundle branch block pattern or a history of coronary revascularization would favor an increased probability of systolic dysfunction in a patient with heart failure, whereas a markedly elevated blood pressure would support the presence of DHF [50]. B-type natriuretic peptide levels are elevated in patients with predominant diastolic dysfunction [51], but is not useful in differentiating between diastolic and systolic dysfunction [52].

It is therefore important to perform an imaging study to estimate left ventricular systolic function in all heart failure patients [45,46]. For this purpose, imaging techniques such as echocardiography or radionuclide angiography, and in the case of patients undergoing cardiac catheterization, contrast ventriculography, have been used. The use of ejection phase indices is mostly used, although they are limited by their variation with cardiac loading conditions [53,54]. The demonstration of a left ventricular ejection fraction of 0.50 or greater on an imaging study strongly favors a diagnosis of DHF [32].

Objective Evidence of Left Ventricular Diastolic Dysfunction

Left ventricular diastolic dysfunction is defined as the inability of the left ventricle to fill adequately at a pressure less than 12 mm Hg [55]. Because most symptoms of congestive heart failure are due to an elevation of diastolic filling pressure, almost all patients with manifest heart failure by definition have diastolic dysfunction. Thus, the most common cause of left ventricular diastolic dysfunction is left ventricular systolic dysfunction. Isolated diastolic dysfunction is present when there is objective evidence of diastolic dysfunction with a normal systolic function. The clinical presentation of these patients ranges from congestive heart failure with preserved systolic function at one end, to exercise intolerance due to a failure to increase end-diastolic volume with exercise (resulting in elevated pulmonary venous pressure) in a subject who is asymptomatic at rest, at the other end [56]. An intermediate subset of subjects includes those who are critically dependent on an enhanced atrial contribution to ventricular filling; atrial arrhythmias can precipitate heart failure in such individuals [56].

Definitive determination of diastolic function involves assessing left ventricular diastolic pressure-volume relations using cardiac catheterization [13]. An upward or rightward shift of the diastolic pressure-volume relation indicates diastolic dysfunction. This invasive analysis, albeit the gold standard for researchers, is not feasible to obtain routinely in clinical practice. Accordingly, attention has been focused on noninvasive methods of assessment of diastolic function, including imaging modalities such as echocardiography [14,57,58], radionuclide angiography [59,60], computed tomography [61], and magnetic resonance imaging [62].

It has recently been demonstrated that virtually all heart failure patients with normal echocardiographic systolic function have evidence of abnormal left ventricular diastolic function on comprehensive invasive assessment [63]. Doppler echocardiography is the imaging modality of choice in assessing DHF, as it provides information on valve disease (important to exclude prior to the diagnosis of DHF); tricuspid regurgitation (for assessing the degree of pulmonary arterial hypertension); rare causes of DHF (such as constrictive pericardial disease and hypertrophic or infiltrative cardiomyopathy); as well as features supporting the presence of left ventricular diastolic dysfunction. The latter include increased left ventricular mass, presence of concentric left ventricular hypertrophy, left atrial enlargement, and altered Doppler transmitral and pulmonary venous flow patterns [64–68].

Doppler echocardiography can be used to determine isovolumic relaxation time (IVRT), the time from aortic valve closure to the onset of mitral inflow. Normal transmitral

Doppler flow consists of an early diastolic wave during the phase of rapid filling (E wave) and a late diastolic wave during atrial systole (A wave) separated by a period of diastasis. The transmitral flow patterns can provide information on impaired relaxation (a decreased peak E wave, a prolonged deceleration time of the early filling peak [time from peak of the E wave to its nadir], and a compensatory increased A wave) and abnormal compliance (a high E wave, a rapid deceleration, and a low A wave velocity, see Figure 2), aided by information obtained from pulmonary venous flow velocities. The normal pulmonary venous flow consists of forward flow during systole (S wave) and diastole (D wave), and retrograde flow during atrial systole (AR). The S/D pulmonary venous flow velocity ratio is increased in isolated relaxation abnormality conditions, and decreased together with increased retrograde flow during atrial contraction (AR) in compliance abnormalities [66].

These flow patterns are driven by instantaneous transmitral pressure gradients, and vary with age, loading conditions, heart rate, and ventricular systolic function [67], and exhibit a circadian variation [69]. Thus, although diastolic flow patterns can indicate the possible presence of diastolic functional abnormalities [64,67], the diastolic filling patterns must be distinguished from diastolic function itself. In addition, transmitral flow pattern pathology may progress over time. The first stage is thought to be isolated impaired relaxation, and as left atrial pressure increases, the early filling velocity component becomes increasingly dominant, and the pathology progresses via a *pseudonormal* stage (when the transmitral pattern appears normal due to restoration of the height of the E wave by elevated atrial pressure) to a restrictive pattern (Fig. 2) [66]. A pseudonormal transmitral waveform can be readily distinguished from a normal pattern if pulmonary venous flows are available.

Other echocardiographic modalities for assessment of diastolic function, such as tissue Doppler imaging, color-M-mode, and strain rate imaging, will likely contribute to increasing diagnostic certainty of DHF in the future [68,70]. Tissue Doppler imaging can quantitate the velocity of mitral annular motion in systole and diastole [71]. During systole, the descent of the mitral annulus is a measure of the longitudinal function of the left ventricle. The diastolic velocity of the mitral annulus is influenced by the relaxation of the surrounding myocardial segment. With the sample volume placed sequentially at the medial and lateral mitral annulus, the early diastolic velocities (e') and late diastolic velocities (a') can be obtained and averaged. Color M-mode Doppler echocardiography evaluates all velocities along a scan line aligned with the mitral inflow [68,70,72]. The velocity of flow propagation into the left ventricle (Vp) can be determined by the slope of the color wave front. A left ventricle with normal relaxation demonstrates rapid flow propagation, whereas a slowly relaxing ventricle is associated with blunted flow propagation. Proposed critical values for some of these echocardiographic measures are summarized in Table 3.

A newer technique for assessing regional myocardial function in systole and diastole is strain rate imaging (SRI) [72,73]. Strain rate imaging uses tissue Doppler to measure velocities along a scan line oriented parallel to a myocardial segment. Strain rate is the differential between myocardial velocities at two points normalized by the distance between them; a positive strain rate corresponds to myocardial lengthening or thinning, whereas a negative strain rate corresponds to myocardial shortening or thickening [72,73]. Regional abnormalities of diastolic function are evidenced by reduced early diastolic strain rate and slower propagation of ventricular relaxation from the base to the apex during diastole.

Radionuclide ventriculography can also provide information on diastolic volumes, early and late diastolic filling rates, and diastolic time intervals. Thus, reliable measurements can be obtained regarding the peak diastolic filling rate, the time to peak filling, proportion of filling that occurs during early diastole, and the atrial contribution to diastolic filling [59].

Table 3 Echocardiographic Diastolic Function Criteria

Parameter		Normal	Delayed Relaxation	Pseudo-normal	Restrictive
Transmitral	E/A	>1	<1	1–2	>2
Flow	DT, ms	<220	>220	150–200	<150
	IVRT, ms	<100	>100	60–100	<60
Pulmonary	S/D	≥1	≥1	<1	<1
Venous	AR, ms	<35	<35	>35	>35
Flow	AR-A dur, ms	<20	<20	20–30	>30
Tissue	e', cm/s	>8	<8	<8	<8
Doppler	E/e'	<10	<10	≥10	≥10
Color M-Mode	Vp, cm/s	>45	<45	<45	<45

E, early peak filling velocity; A, peak filling velocity during atrial systole; A dur, duration of the A wave; DT, deceleration time; IVRT, isovolumic relaxation time; S, peak systolic pulmonary venous flow velocity; D, peak diastolic pulmonary venous flow velocity; AR, retrograde flow during atrial systole; e', peak early myocardial velocity; a', peak myocardial velocity during atrial systole; Vp, early diastolic ventricular flow propagation velocity. See Figure 2 for graphic illustration of patterns. (Adapted from Ref. 70. Copyright 1998 American College of Cardiology Foundation.)

Cardiac magnetic resonance imaging is an accurate and reproducible method for measuring cardiac volumes, wall thickness, and left ventricular mass [62]. Phase contrast magnetic resonance imaging may be used to assess diastolic flow patterns and ventricular filling [74]. Currently, however, magnetic resonance imaging is only indicated in heart failure when other imaging techniques have not provided adequate diagnostic information [46].

It remains to be proven if detailed assessment of diastolic function provides information that will influence management of a heart failure patient with known systolic function.

Clinical Improvement by Treating Precipitating Factors

When treating a patient with an acute episode of DHF, the aims should include relief of symptoms, reversing the congestive state, rectification of the acute precipitating factors, and initiating treatment of identifiable underlying causes.

The distinction between precipitating factors and the underlying etiology of DHF is important to make. The precipitating factors are events or conditions that by themselves do not cause diastolic left ventricular dysfunction, but can cause acute decompensation in an otherwise compensated patient with subclinical diastolic dysfunction. Typical treatments of precipitating factors include treatment of acute hypertension, antibiotic treatment of bacterial pneumonias, and restitution of sinus rhythm in atrial fibrillation.

Merely stating that a given patient has DHF gives less information and guidance for treatment than stating that, for example, a patient has DHF with concentric left ventricular hypertrophy, precipitated by an episode of atrial fibrillation, with uncontrolled chronic hypertension as the underlying cause. Such a comprehensive diagnostic description includes specific components at which therapy should be directed. Thus, the patient would need diuresis, control of ventricular rate or reversion to sinus rhythm, control of HTN (hypertension), and might be helped by regression of left ventricular hypertrophy (chapter 17 for detailed approach).

Diagnosing Diastolic Heart Failure at the Bedside

Because definitive demonstration of abnormal left ventricular pressure-volume relations requires cardiac catheterization, development of diagnostic criteria for DHF using noninvasive technology that can be used in routine clinical practice is imperative. A rational approach would be to suggest that the source of heart failure symptoms is likely to be left ventricular diastolic dysfunction in patients with a normal left ventricular ejection fraction without valve disease and noncardiac causes of the symptoms. Since therapy of diastolic heart failure remains empirical, it would be difficult to evaluate the fourth criterion mentioned.

In 1998, a European study group proposed criteria for the diagnosis of DHF [75], although the clinical utility of these criteria was limited because of the need for evidence of abnormal left ventricular relaxation, filling, diastolic distensibility, or diastolic stiffness. In 1999, our group offered an alternative approach to diagnosis of DHF that accepts diagnostic uncertainty and makes diagnosis of the condition more clinically feasible [32]. We have since modified our original classification scheme, dropping an initial requirement for estimation of left ventricular ejection fraction within 72 hours of heart failure onset, as left ventricular ejection fraction has been shown to be relatively constant over the course of a week in patients with acute DHF [76]. This classification approach was suggested for patients who do not have heart failure attributable to valvular heart disease, cor pulmonale or volume overload. According to these criteria (Table 4), a patient who meets the following three conditions can be said to have *definite DHF*: (a) there is objective evidence of heart failure; (b) there is objective evidence of normal left ventricular systolic function; and (c) there is objective evidence of left ventricular diastolic dysfunction. In the absence of a cardiac catheterization, we proposed that patients can be categorized as having *probable DHF* if the etiology of heart failure is deemed likely to be diastolic dysfunction (Table 4) in heart failure patients with a normal left ventricular ejection fraction (provided mitral valve disease, cor pulmonale, volume overload and noncardiac causes of symptoms are excluded). If only the first two criteria are fulfilled, the patient may be said to have *presumed DHF*.

PREVALENCE

In 31 hospital-based reports, the proportion of heart failure patients with *presumed DHF* (satisfying our first two criteria) varied from 13% to 74%, with a majority of studies reporting values of approximately 40% [1]. Studies including elderly subjects had a high proportion (about 45%), whereas studies focusing on middle-aged patients with chronic heart failure reported a lower proportion (about 15%). Studies with a mixed sample of patients with acute and chronic heart failure reported intermediate estimates (usually 25% to 40%). Hypertension and coronary artery disease were frequently associated with DHF in these studies [1].

Only six of these 31 studies assessed *probable DHF* using noninvasive methods. The prevalence of DHF in these studies ranged from 23% to 42%, with four of the six studies reporting estimates of about 25% [1]. Two other studies [77,78] reported case series of patients with *definite DHF* by cardiac catheterization without angiographic evidence of coronary artery disease. Systemic hypertension was the underlying substrate for diastolic dysfunction in most patients.

Table 4 Modified Criteria for Diastolic Heart Failure

	Criterion	Objective Evidence
Definite Diastolic Heart Failure	Objective evidence of congestive heart failure	Includes clinical symptoms, signs, supporting tests (such as chest x-ray), a typical clinical response to treatment with diuretics, with or without documentation of elevated left ventricular filling pressure (at rest, on exercise, or in response to a volume load) or a low cardiac index
	Objective evidence of normal left ventricular systolic function	A left ventricular ejection fraction ≥ 0.50
	Objective evidence of left ventricular diastolic dysfunction	Abnormal left ventricular relaxation/filling/distensibility indices on cardiac catheterization
Probable Diastolic Heart Failure	Objective evidence of congestive heart failure	As above
	Objective evidence of normal left ventricular systolic function	As above
	Objective evidence of left ventricular diastolic dysfunction is lacking	Factors increasing likelihood of diastolic heart failure are evidence of: Markedly elevated blood pressure[a] during the episode of heart failure Echocardiographic concentric LVH without wall motion abnormalities A tachyarrhythmia with a shortened diastolic filling period Precipitation of event by a small amount of intravenous fluid infusion Clinical improvement in response to therapy directed at the etiology of diastolic dysfunction (such as lowering blood pressure, reducing heart rate, or restoring the atrial booster mechanism)
Presumed Diastolic Heart Failure	Objective evidence of congestive heart failure	As above
	Objective evidence of normal left ventricular systolic function	As above

Rule out valve disease before applying this scheme.
[a]defined as systolic pressure >160 mm Hg or diastolic pressure >100–105 mm Hg (50).

In epidemiologic investigations of DHF in the community, the proportion of heart failure patients with *presumed DHF* varied from 44% to 71% [2–4,9,79], which is considerably higher than that reported by hospital-based studies. This difference may be attributed to the high proportion of elderly ambulatory subjects with heart failure and absence of referral bias in the community-based investigations.

The prevalence of echocardiographically determined isolated diastolic dysfunction ranged between 3% and 20% (depending on criteria used) in community-based studies, suggesting that diastolic dysfunction is at least as prevalent as systolic dysfunction in the community [79–81].

THE ETIOLOGY

DHF is more frequent in the elderly and occurs more often in women than men. Hypertension and coronary disease are the most common underlying causes of DHF [1,2,7,9,82], and diabetes and obesity are additional important risk factors [2,83]. Prevention and treatment of hypertension and coronary disease decreases the incidence of heart failure [84–86], and recent guidelines suggest that blood pressure goals could be lower in patients with hypertension and DHF than for patients with hypertension alone [45].

Following is a list of important clinical conditions in which isolated diastolic dysfunction is frequently associated with heart failure (summarized in Table 5). The individual factors impairing diastolic ventricular function are often not per se sufficient to precipitate heart failure, but several such factors acting in concert may cause decompensation and an episode of overt heart failure. Thus, the incidence of atrial fibrillation with tachycardia in a previously compensated patient with diabetes and left ventricular hypertrophy may precipitate heart failure, as may an episode of exertional angina in an individual with uncontrolled hypertension, and a blood transfusion in an anemic elderly patient.

Hypertension

Hypertension is a leading cause of heart failure, with a population attributable risk for heart failure estimated to be 59% in women and 39% in men [87]. Heart failure risk decreases by approximately 50% with antihypertensive treatment [88]. Heart failure in hypertensive subjects often develops in the absence of a myocardial infarction, suggesting an important role of ventricular diastolic dysfunction in these subjects [87]. The clinical

Table 5 Conditions Associated with High Prevalence of Diastolic Heart Failure

Hypertension
Left ventricular hypertrophy
Myocardial fibrosis
Coronary artery disease
Diabetes
Obesity
Female sex
Advanced age
Aortic stenosis
Hypertrophic cardiomyopathy
Restrictive cardiomyopathy
Sustained tachycardia
Constrictive pericarditis
Hypothyroidism
Hypervolemia

presentation of DHF in hypertensives is varied. Some patients present with severe uncontrolled hypertension and acute pulmonary edema [76,89], which can be reversed by lowering blood pressure [76,89]. At the other end of the spectrum are hypertensives with left ventricular hypertrophy who are asymptomatic under resting conditions, but who may experience exertional dyspnea due to a relative inability to augment their ventricular enddiastolic volume upon exercise [90].

The mechanisms underlying DHF seen in hypertensives have been extensively investigated. In adult patients with diastolic [91,92], isolated systolic [93], borderline isolated systolic [94], and combined systolic and diastolic hypertension [95], as well as in children with hypertension [96], an abnormal diastolic filling pattern characterized by impaired early diastolic ventricular filling with an enhancement in late diastolic filling (due to atrial systole) has been reported, indicating subnormal left ventricular relaxation with normal ventricular compliance [97]. A prolonged isovolumic relaxation time has also been demonstrated in hypertensive persons [98]. Patients with DHF have stiff large arteries and an increased blood pressure lability [8,20,99]. In addition, hypertension is associated with left atrial enlargement, depression of atrial contractile function, and increased risk for atrial fibrillation [100,101], which can precipitate overt heart failure in patients with underlying ventricular diastolic dysfunction [56].

Possible contributing factors for the diastolic dysfunction observed in hypertensive patients include myocardial fibrosis and left ventricular hypertrophy (see following text), although they do not always accompany hypertension [102,103]. Blood pressure reduction with an ACE-inhibitor combined with spironolactone [104], or an ACE-inhibitor alone [105], has been demonstrated to result in decreases in both left ventricular mass and plasma levels of fibrosis markers. This may suggest that increased myocardial collagen content is partly responsible for the increased left ventricular mass and diastolic dysfunction in left ventricular hypertrophy. On the other hand, with similar effects on blood pressure, ACE-inhibitor treatment decreased myocardial collagen content and improved diastolic function but had no effect on left ventricular mass, whereas hydrochlorothiazide treatment reduced myocyte diameter but did not reduce fibrosis [106]. This may indicate that left ventricular mass is mainly determined by loading conditions, whereas myocardial fibrosis and diastolic dysfunction may be the detrimental effects of certain neurohormonal agents [106]. The hypothesis that left ventricular hypertrophy and myocardial fibrosis are regulated independently of each other and, to some extent, of blood pressure is supported by some experimental evidence [107–109].

Mediators that promote hypertrophy have been extensively detailed elsewhere [110]. They include vasoactive peptides, growth factors, hormones and neurotransmitters (endothelin, angiotensin II, fibroblast growth factor, insulin-like growth factor, cardiotrophin-1) [110]. Estrogens and the natriuretic peptides are antihypertrophic. The prohypertrophic factors trigger intracellular signaling cascades that activate fetal gene programs and a hypertrophic response [110]. Signalling pathways activated in hypertension include members of the mitogen-activated protein kinase (MAPK) superfamily (the p38 MAPK, the extracellular regulated kinases [ERK] and c-Jun kinases), the gp130 family (the JAK/STAT pathway), and the calcineurin pathway [110].

Left Ventricular Hypertrophy

Early diastolic filling abnormalities in hypertensives correlates with increased left ventricular mass [91,93,111,112]. Left ventricular hypertrophy is one of the most common causes of isolated diastolic dysfunction, and an important independent risk factor for heart failure [65,113,114]. A common precursor of DHF is a condition referred to as hypertensive *hypertrophic cardiomyopathy of the elderly.* [115]. This term refers to elderly patients who are frequently female, have systolic hypertension, and present with marked ventricular hypertrophy, a supernormal left ventricular ejection fraction, and a propensity for developing pulmonary edema.

Myocardial Fibrosis

Myocardial fibrosis with increased interstitial collagen deposition is another mechanism behind diastolic dysfunction in hypertensive subjects. There is a strong relation between left ventricular stiffness and myocardial collagen content [106,116] and plasma levels of fibrosis markers [117] in hypertensive persons. Improvement of diastolic function during antihypertensive treatment is related to regression in myocardial collagen content [106,116].

Coronary Artery Disease

Acute ischemia can cause DHF [118], illustrated by the fact that patients with unstable angina frequently have elevated pulmonary capillary wedge pressure during episodes of ischemia, with normal ventricular systolic function [119]. Similar observations have been made during pacing-induced tachycardia, during exertional angina [118], and during coronary angioplasty [120]. The dyspnea associated with short episodes of angina is believed to indicate a transient elevation in left ventricular filling pressure due to ischemia-induced abnormalities of myocardial distensibility [118], which is also exemplified by the episodes of acute pulmonary congestion observed in elderly subjects with chronic coronary disease during episodes of acute ischemia, so called *flash pulmonary edema* [121,122].

The type of acute ischemia may determine the left ventricular function, as isolated diastolic dysfunction is commonly found during episodes of *demand* ischemia, such as exercise, in contrast to the combined systolic and diastolic ventricular dysfunction more often found in *supply* ischemia, such as coronary occlusion [118].

Diabetes

Diabetic patients are at greater risk of developing DHF, due partly to the diabetic state itself [123], and partly to the increased myocardial mass [124] and concomitant coronary disease that frequently accompany diabetes [56].

A characteristic feature of type-2 diabetes is whole-body insulin resistance, which is related to increased left ventricular relative wall thickness and concentric remodeling [125,126]. In contrast, myocardial insulin sensitivity appears to be increased with increased left ventricular relative wall thickness [126]. An increased myocardial insulin-mediated glucose uptake may be involved in the pathogenesis of the growth of the left ventricular walls in diabetic persons, supported by the experimental observation that induced hyperinsulinaemia leads to marked ventricular hypertrophy [127].

Diabetic persons are subject to an increased cross-linking of collagen by advanced glycation end-products. This takes place both in the arterial walls and in the myocardium, and leads to a decreased arterial compliance and increased myocardial stiffness [128], both of which contribute to diastolic dysfunction [21]. Arterial and myocardial stiffness can be improved by treatment with advanced glycation end-product cross-link breakers [129].

Obesity

Obesity is an independent predictor of both systolic and DHF [83]. Severe obesity is associated with heart failure with preserved left ventricular systolic function [130]. Contributory factors may be impairment of ventricular relaxation and increased chamber stiffness (elevated left ventricular mass) [131], as well as the increased left ventricular relative wall thickness, which frequently accompanies central obesity-related insulin resistance [125] (see previous text).

Aging

A decline in left ventricular diastolic function has been associated with aging [18]. Elderly subjects demonstrate higher left ventricular end-diastolic pressures in the presence of smaller end-diastolic volumes [132]. This age-related diastolic dysfunction renders elderly subjects vulnerable to overt heart failure (with normal left ventricular systolic function) when an additional stress (such as ischemia, elevated blood pressure, volume overload, sustained tachycardia or atrial fibrillation) is superimposed.

Aortic Stenosis

Aortic valvular stenosis patients frequently present with heart failure symptoms with a normal left ventricular ejection fraction, suggesting an important role of diastolic dysfunction in the pathogenesis of the symptoms [133]. Obstruction of forward flow, especially upon obstruction, contributes to exertional dyspnea and fatigue. Surgical correction of the aortic stenosis relieves heart failure symptoms and regresses the left ventricular hypertrophy, supporting a causal relation between valvular obstruction, left ventricular hypertrophy, diastolic dysfunction, and the heart failure symptoms.

Hypertrophic Cardiomyopathy

Patients with hypertrophic cardiomyopathy are characterized by a variable degree of left ventricular hypertrophy, which is frequently asymmetric and exhibits myocardial fiber disarray and dynamic ventricular outflow tract obstruction (see Chapter 8). The echocardiographic features display a spectrum of abnormalities including asymmetrical septal hypertrophy, variable degree of dynamic left ventricular outflow obstruction, systolic anterior motion of the mitral valve, and a hypokinetic thick septum with vigorous posterior wall motion. Myocardial scarring has recently been demonstrated on gadolinium-enhanced magnetic resonance imaging [134].

The condition is inherited as an autosomal dominant trait. Mutations in genes coding for the beta-myosin heavy chain (40%), cardiac troponin T (15%), I, alpha tropomyosin (5%), myosin binding protein C (20%), myosin light chain 1 and 2, cardiac alpha actin, and titin have been reported [135,136].

The hallmark of this condition is left ventricular diastolic dysfunction [56], due to increased chamber stiffness and a slower and asynchronous relaxation. The onset of atrial fibrillation can precipitate acute pulmonary edema in these subjects [137]. The causal role of isolated diastolic dysfunction in the genesis of the dyspnea and episodes of pulmonary congestion often found in these patients, is confirmed by the relief of symptoms by beta-blockers and calcium channel antagonists (which improve diastolic function) and surgical myotomy-myectomy [138].

Restrictive Cardiomyopathy

Characteristic of this condition is a left ventricle with normal volume and systolic function but decreased compliance. The left ventricle fills rapidly in early diastole with little or no further filling in late diastole [139]. These patients initially exhibit isolated diastolic dysfunction, but may develop a variable degree of systolic dysfunction over time. This condition often results from endocardial abnormalities, such as Loffler's endocarditis or endomyocardial fibrosis, or myocardial infiltration, due to amyloidosis, sarcoidosis, hemochromatosis or cardiac transplant rejection. The hemodynamic and echocardiographic features that help distinguish restrictive cardiomyopathies from constrictive pericarditis are noted in the next section. Right ventricular transvenous endomyocardial biopsies may be required to identify the etiology of restriction.

Constrictive Pericarditis

Constrictive pericarditis is a recognized cause of restricted ventricular filling with markedly elevated filling pressures and normal systolic function [119,140]. The pathophysiological abnormalities underlying constrictive pericarditis stem from the encasement of the heart in an inflexible fibrotic case, and are three-fold [141]: (a) there is a dissociation of the intrathoracic and intracardiac pressures with respiration because of a noncompliant pericardium. The gradient between the pulmonary veins and the left-sided chambers decreases with inspiration; there is a reduction in velocity of pulmonary venous flow with inspiration and a decrease in left-sided filling; (b) there is increased ventricular interdependence that results in a leftward shift in the septum during inspiration (when left-sided filling is reduced) and a rightward shift of the septum with expiration. Hence, during expiration transtricuspid flow decreases, there may be diastolic flow-reversal in hepatic veins; (c) impairment in mid-late diastolic filling results in rapid filling in early diastole with a reduction in diastolic flow thereafter. In contrast, in cardiac tamponade the diastolic filling is impaired throughout diastole [141].

Cardiac catheterization demonstrates a dip and plateau ventricular diastolic pressure tracing (square root sign). The right atrial pressure tracing shows a prominent x and y descent (M shape), which may be reflected in the jugular veins. A hallmark of constrictive pericarditis is near equalization of the diastolic pressures in all chambers of the heart. This feature is often not seen in restrictive cardiomyopathies in which the degree of involvement of the two ventricles may be different. Consequently, three criteria have been proposed to distinguish constrictive physiology from restriction [142]. Findings that favor a diagnosis of constrictive pericarditis include: (a) a difference between right ventricular end-diastolic pressure and left ventricular end-diastolic pressure of 5 mm Hg or less; (b) a right ventricular systolic pressure of 50 mm Hg or less; and (c) a ratio of right ventricular end-diastolic pressure to right ventricular systolic pressure greater than or equal to 1:3 [142].

Echocardiographic findings that may help distinguish the two conditions include presence of a thickened pericardium and increased respiratory variation in transmitral flow (25% or greater decrease with inspiration) in constrictive pericarditis, and the demonstration of reduced myocardial longitudinal velocities on Doppler tissue imaging in patients with restriction [141]. A pericardial thickness of more than 3 mm on computed tomography or magnetic resonance imaging suggests a diagnosis of pericardial constriction.

Hypothyroidism

Hypothyroidism decreases the activity of the sarcoplasmic reticulum calcium ATPase pump, which slows the removal of calcium from the cytosol and frequently leads to an impaired relaxation with normal systolic function [11]. There are some conflicting data

on the prevalence of diastolic filling abnormalities in patients with subclinical hypothyroidism and the response of these abnormalities to thyroid hormone replacement [143,144].

PROGNOSIS OF DIASTOLIC HEART FAILURE

DHF increases mortality risk considerably, and DHF and systolic heart failure have been
associated with hazard ratios for mortality of 4.06 and 4.31, respectively, compared to
age- and sex-matched controls [9]. DHF has been shown [1,145], albeit not uniformly
[146], to be associated with a better long-term survival than systolic heart failure (Fig.
3). In the Framingham Heart Study, DHF was associated with an annual mortality rate of
8.7% compared with 18.9% for systolic heart failure [9], with reported annual mortality
rates for DHF ranging between 1.3% and 19% in other studies [1,145]. In the elderly, the
mortality attributable to DHF is higher than that due to systolic heart failure, because left
ventricular function is more often normal than impaired in elderly persons with heart
failure [1,147]. Among patients with DHF, age seems to be the most important prognostic
factor [10].

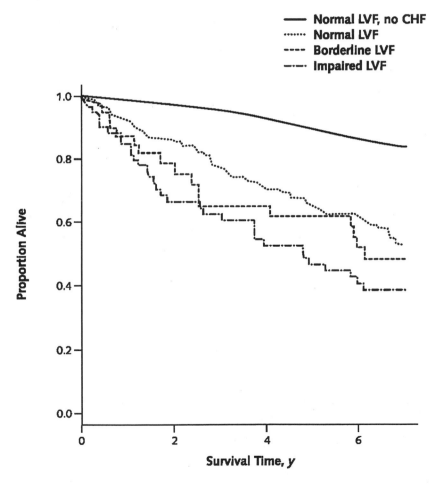

Figure 3 Unadjusted Kaplan-Meier survival curves for persons without congestive heart
failure (upper curve) and for those with congestive heart failure (lower three curves) based
on left ventricular systolic function (LVF). (From Ref. 147.)

SUMMARY

In one out of two to three patients with congestive heart failure, isolated diastolic dysfunction is believed to be the cause of the symptoms. DHF is defined as overt congestive heart failure due to the inability of the left ventricle to fill adequately at normal filling pressures, with an upward shift of the left ventricular diastolic pressure-volume relation, and resulting increase in left ventricular end-diastolic pressure.

A person can be said to have *definite DHF* when there is objective evidence of heart failure, objective evidence of normal left ventricular systolic function, and objective evidence of left ventricular diastolic dysfunction; *probable DHF* if a cardiac catheterization is lacking but the etiology of heart failure is deemed likely to be diastolic dysfunction (provided mitral valve disease, cor pulmonale, volume overload, and noncardiac causes of symptoms are excluded); and *presumed DHF* if only the first two criteria are fulfilled.

DHF is more common in women and in the elderly, and hypertension and coronary disease are the most common underlying causes of DHF, followed by diabetes and obesity. DHF increases mortality risk considerably but may have a better long-term prognosis than systolic heart failure.

The primary pathophysiological abnormality in individuals with congestive heart failure and a normal left ventricular ejection fraction has hitherto been assumed to be diastolic dysfunction. Recently, researchers have questioned this notion. Additional investigations are warranted to identify the primary abnormalities in these individuals and to develop clinical diagnostic tests for the condition that are easy to perform and interpret, and that have acceptable performance characteristics.

REFERENCES

1. Vasan RS, Benjamin EJ, Levy D. Prevalence, clinical features and prognosis of diastolic heart failure: an epidemiologic perspective. J Am Coll Cardiol 1995; 26:1565–1574.
2. Devereux RB, Roman MJ, Liu JE, Welty TK, Lee ET, Rodeheffer R, et al. Congestive heart failure despite normal left ventricular systolic function in a population-based sample: the Strong Heart Study. Am J Cardiol 2000; 86:1090–1096.
3. Kitzman DW, Gardin JM, Gottdiener JS, Arnold A, Boineau R, Aurigemma G, et al. Importance of heart failure with preserved systolic function in patients > or = 65 years of age. CHS Research Group. Cardiovascular Health Study. Am J Cardiol 2001; 87:413–419.
4. Kupari M, Lindroos M, Iivanainen AM, Heikkila J, Tilvis R. Congestive heart failure in old age: prevalence, mechanisms and 4-year prognosis in the Helsinki Ageing Study. J Intern Med 1997; 241:387–394.
5. Mosterd A, Hoes AW, de Bruyne MC, Deckers JW, Linker DT, Hofman A, et al. Prevalence of heart failure and left ventricular dysfunction in the general population; The Rotterdam Study. Eur Heart J 1999; 20:447–455.
6. Nielsen OW, Hilden J, Larsen CT, Hansen JF. Cross sectional study estimating prevalence of heart failure and left ventricular systolic dysfunction in community patients at risk. Heart 2001; 86:172–178.
7. Senni M, Tribouilloy CM, Rodeheffer RJ, Jacobsen SJ, Evans JM, Bailey KR, et al. Congestive heart failure in the community: a study of all incident cases in Olmsted County, Minnesota, in 1991. Circulation 1998; 98:2282–2289.
8. Kitzman DW, Little WC, Brubaker PH, Anderson RT, Hundley WG, Marburger CT, et al. Pathophysiological characterization of isolated diastolic heart failure in comparison to systolic heart failure. JAMA 2002; 288:2144–2150.
9. Vasan RS, Larson MG, Benjamin EJ, Evans JC, Reiss CK, Levy D. Congestive heart failure in subjects with normal versus reduced left ventricular ejection fraction: prevalence and mortality in a population-based cohort. J Am Coll Cardiol 1999; 33:1948–1955.

10. Zile MR, Brutsaert DL. New concepts in diastolic dysfunction and diastolic heart failure: Part I: diagnosis, prognosis, and measurements of diastolic function. Circulation 2002; 105: 1387–1393.

11. Angeja BG, Grossman W. Evaluation and management of diastolic heart failure. Circulation 2003; 107:659–663.

12. Brutsaert DL, Rademakers FE, Sys SU, Gillebert TC, Housmans PR. Analysis of relaxation in the evaluation of ventricular function of the heart. Prog Cardiovasc Dis 1985; 28:143–163.

13. Mirsky I. Assessment of diastolic function: suggested methods and future considerations. Circulation 1984; 69:836–841.

14. Nishimura RA, Housmans PR, Hatle LK, Tajik AJ. Assessment of diastolic function of the heart: background and current applications of Doppler echocardiography. Part I. Physiologic and pathophysiologic features. Mayo Clin Proc 1989; 64:71–81.

15. Brutsaert DL, Sys SU, Gillebert TC. Diastolic failure: pathophysiology and therapeutic implications. J Am Coll Cardiol 1993; 22:318–325.

16. Burkhoff D, Maurer MS, Packer M. Heart failure with a normal ejection fraction: is it really a disorder of diastolic function?. Circulation 2003; 107:656–658.

17. Chen CH, Nakayama M, Nevo E, Fetics BJ, Maughan WL, Kass DA. Coupled systolic-ventricular and vascular stiffening with age: implications for pressure regulation and cardiac reserve in the elderly. J Am Coll Cardiol 1998; 32:1221–1227.

18. Lakatta EG, Levy D. Arterial and cardiac aging: major shareholders in cardiovascular disease enterprises: Part II: the aging heart in health: links to heart disease. Circulation 2003; 107: 346–354.

19. Lakatta EG, Levy D. Arterial and cardiac aging: major shareholders in cardiovascular disease enterprises: Part I: aging arteries: a ''set up'' for vascular disease. Circulation 2003; 107: 139–146.

20. Hundley WG, Kitzman DW, Morgan TM, Hamilton CA, Darty SN, Stewart KP, et al. Cardiac cycle-dependent changes in aortic area and distensibility are reduced in older patients with isolated diastolic heart failure and correlate with exercise intolerance. J Am Coll Cardiol 2001; 38:796–802.

21. Kawaguchi M, Hay I, Fetics B, Kass DA. Combined ventricular systolic and arterial stiffening in patients with heart failure and preserved ejection fraction: implications for systolic and diastolic reserve limitations. Circulation 2003; 107:714–720.

22. Kass DA, Kelly RP. Ventriculo-arterial coupling: concepts, assumptions, and applications. Ann Biomed Eng 1992; 20:41–62.

23. Kass DA. Age-related changes in ventricular-arterial coupling: pathophysiologic implications. Heart Fail Rev 2002; 7:51–62.

24. Kass DA, Saeki A, Tunin RS, Recchia FA. Adverse influence of systemic vascular stiffening on cardiac dysfunction and adaptation to acute coronary occlusion. Circulation 1996; 93: 1533.

25. Apstein CS, Morgan JP. Cellular mechanisms underlying left ventricular diastolic dysfunction. In: Gaasch WH , LeWinter MM, Eds. Left Ventricular Diastolic Dysfunction and Heart Failure. Philadelphia. PA: Lea & Febiger, 1994:3–24.

26. Brutsaert DL. Cardiac endothelial-myocardial signaling: its role in cardiac growth, contractile performance, and rhythmicity. Physiol Rev 2003; 83:59–115.

27. Kurrelmeyer K, Kalra D, Bozkurt B, Wang F, Dibbs Z, Seta Y, et al. Cardiac remodeling as a consequence and cause of progressive heart failure. Clin Cardiol 1998; 21:114–119.

28. Swynghedauw B. Molecular mechanisms of myocardial remodeling. Physiol Rev 1999; 79: 215–262.

29. Dorn GW. Adrenergic pathways and left ventricular remodeling. J Card Fail 2002; 8: S370–S373.

30. Dorn II, Mann DL. Signaling pathways involved in left ventricular remodeling: summation. J Card Fail 2002; 8:S387–S388.

31. Francis GS. Cellular and subcellular basis for remodeling: summation. J Card Fail 2002; 8: S450–S451.

32. Vasan RS, Levy D. Defining diastolic heart failure: a call for standardized diagnostic criteria. Circulation 2000; 101:2118–2121.

33. McKee PA, Castelli WP, McNamara PM, Kannel WB. The natural history of congestive heart failure: the Framingham study. N Engl J Med 1971; 285:1441–1446.

34. Wilhelmsen L, Eriksson H, Svardsudd K, Caidahl K. Improving the detection and diagnosis of congestive heart failure. Eur Heart J 1989; 10 Suppl:C:13–C18.

35. Walma EP, Hoes AW, Prins A, Boukes FS, van der DE. Withdrawing long-term diuretic therapy in the elderly: a study in general practice in The Netherlands. Fam Med 1993; 25: 661–664.

36. Carlson KJ, Lee DC, Goroll AH, Leahy M, Johnson RA. An analysis of physicians' reasons for prescribing long-term digitalis therapy in outpatients. J Chronic Dis 1985; 38:733–739.

37. Schocken DD, Arrieta MI, Leaverton PE, Ross EA. Prevalence and mortality rate of congestive heart failure in the United States. J Am Coll Cardiol 1992; 20:301–306.

38. Gheorghiade M, Beller GA. Effects of discontinuing maintenance digoxin therapy in patients with ischemic heart disease and congestive heart failure in sinus rhythm. Am J Cardiol 1983; 51:1243–1250.

39. Marantz PR, Alderman MH, Tobin JN. Diagnostic heterogeneity in clinical trials for congestive heart failure. Ann Intern Med 1988; 109:55–61.

40. Mosterd A, Deckers JW, Hoes AW, Nederpel A, Smeets A, Linker DT, et al. Classification of heart failure in population based research: an assessment of six heart failure scores. Eur J Epidemiol 1997; 13:491–502.

41. Remes J, Miettinen H, Reunanen A, Pyorala K. Validity of clinical diagnosis of heart failure in primary health care. Eur Heart J 1991; 12:315–321.

42. Wheeldon NM, MacDonald TM, Flucker CJ, McKendrick AD, McDevitt DG, Struthers AD. Echocardiography in chronic heart failure in the community. Q J Med 1993; 86:17–23.

43. Banerjee P, Banerjee T, Khand A, Clark AL, Cleland JGF. Diastolic heart failure: neglected or misdiagnosed?. J Am Coll Cardiol 2002; 39:138–141.

44. Caruana L, Petrie MC, Davie AP, McMurray JJ. Do patients with suspected heart failure and preserved left ventricular systolic function suffer from ''diastolic heart failure'' or from misdiagnosis? A prospective descriptive study. B Med J 2000; 321:215–218.

45. Hunt SA, Baker DW, Chin MH, Cinquegrani MP, Feldmand AM, Francis GS, et al. ACC/ AHA Guidelines for the Evaluation and Management of Chronic Heart Failure in the Adult: Executive Summary A Report of the American College of Cardiology/American Heart Association Task Force on Practice Guidelines (Committee to Revise the 1995 Guidelines for the Evaluation and Management of Heart Failure): Developed in Collaboration With the International Society for Heart and Lung Transplantation; Endorsed by the Heart Failure Society of America. Circulation 2001; 104:2996–3007.

46. Remme WJ, Swedberg K. Guidelines for the diagnosis and treatment of chronic heart failure. Eur Heart J 2001; 22:1527–1560.

47. Maisel AS. B-type natriuretic peptide (BNP) levels: diagnostic and therapeutic potential. Rev Cardiovasc Med 2001; 2 Suppl 2:S13–S18.

48. Maisel AS, Krishnaswamy P, Nowak RM, McCord J, Hollander JE, Duc P, et al. Rapid measurement of B-type natriuretic peptide in the emergency diagnosis of heart failure. N Engl J Med 2002; 347:161–167.

49. Thomas JT, Kelly RF, Thomas SJ, Stamos TD, Albasha K, Parrillo JE, et al. Utility of history, physical examination, electrocardiogram, and chest radiograph for differentiating normal from decreased systolic function in patients with heart failure. Am J Med 2002; 112:437–445.

50. Badgett RG, Lucey CR, Mulrow CD. Can the clinical examination diagnose left-sided heart failure in adults?. JAMA 1997; 277:1712–1719.

51. Lubien E, DeMaria A, Krishnaswamy P, Clopton P, Koon J, Kazanegra R, et al. Utility of B-natriuretic peptide in detecting diastolic dysfunction: comparison with Doppler velocity recordings. Circulation 2002; 105:595–601.

52. Krishnaswamy P, Lubien E, Clopton P, Koon J, Kazanegra R, Wanner E, et al. Utility of B-natriuretic peptide levels in identifying patients with left ventricular systolic or diastolic dysfunction. Am J Med 2001; 111:274–279.

53. Smith N, McAnulty JH, Rahimtoola SH. Severe aortic stenosis with impaired left ventricular function and clinical heart failure: results of valve replacement. Circulation 1978; 58:255–264.

54. Zile MR, Gaasch WH, Carroll JD, Levine HJ. Chronic mitral regurgitation: predictive value of preoperative echocardiographic indexes of left ventricular function and wall stress. J Am Coll Cardiol 1984; 3:235–242.

55. Little WC, Downes TR. Clinical evaluation of left ventricular diastolic performance. Prog Cardiovasc Dis 1990; 32:273–290.

56. Shah PM, Pai RG. Diastolic heart failure. Curr Probl Cardiol 1992; 17:781–868.

57. Nishimura RA, Abel MD, Hatle LK, Tajik AJ. Assessment of diastolic function of the heart: background and current applications of Doppler echocardiography. Part II. Clinical studies. Mayo Clin Proc 1989; 64:181–204.

58. Appleton CP, Galloway JM, Gonzalez MS, Gaballa M, Basnight MA. Estimation of left ventricular filling pressures using two-dimensional and Doppler echocardiography in adult patients with cardiac disease. Additional value of analyzing left atrial size, left atrial ejection fraction and the difference in duration of pulmonary venous and mitral flow velocity at atrial contraction. J Am Coll Cardiol 1993; 22:1972–1982.

59. Clements IP, Sinak LJ, Gibbons RJ, Brown ML, O'Connor MK. Determination of diastolic function by radionuclide ventriculography. Mayo Clin Proc 1990; 5:1007–1019.

60. Harizi RC, Bianco JA, Alpert JS. Diastolic function of the heart in clinical cardiology. Arch Intern Med 1988; 148:99–109.

61. Rumberger JA, Weiss RM, Feiring AJ, Stanford W, Hajduczok ZD, Rezai K, et al. Patterns of regional diastolic function in the normal human left ventricle: an ultrafast computed tomographic study. J Am Coll Cardiol 1989; 14:119–126.

62. Buchalter MB, Weiss JL, Rogers WJ, Zerhouni EA, Weisfeldt ML, Beyar R, et al. Noninvasive quantification of left ventricular rotational deformation in normal humans using magnetic resonance imaging myocardial tagging. Circulation 1990; 81:1236–1244.

63. Zile MR, Gaasch WH, Carroll JD, Feldman MD, Aurigemma GP, Schaer GL, et al. Heart failure with a normal ejection fraction: is measurement of diastolic function necessary to make the diagnosis of diastolic heart failure?. Circulation 2001; 104:779–782.

64. Cohen GI, Pietrolungo JF, Thomas JD, Klein AL. A practical guide to assessment of ventricular diastolic function using Doppler echocardiography. J Am Coll Cardiol 1996; 27: 1753–1760.

65. Gardin JM, McClelland R, Kitzman D, Lima JA, Bommer W, Klopfenstein HS, et al. M-mode echocardiographic predictors of six- to seven-year incidence of coronary heart disease, stroke, congestive heart failure, and mortality in an elderly cohort (the Cardiovascular Health Study). Am J Cardiol 2001; 87:1051–1057.

66. Nishimura RA, Tajik AJ. Evaluation of diastolic filling of left ventricle in health and disease: Doppler echocardiography is the clinician's Rosetta Stone. J Am Coll Cardiol 1997; 30:8–18.

67. Oh JK, Appleton CP, Hatle LK, Nishimura RA, Seward JB, Tajik AJ. The noninvasive assessment of left ventricular diastolic function with two-dimensional and Doppler echocardiography. J Am Soc Echocardiogr 1997; 10:246–270.

68. Ommen SR, Nishimura RA. A clinical approach to the assessment of left ventricular diastolic function by Doppler echocardiography: update 2003. Heart 2003; 89 Suppl 3:iii18–iii23.

69. Voutilainen S, Kupari M, Hippelainen M, Karppinen K, Ventila M. Circadian variation of left ventricular diastolic function in healthy people. Heart 1996; 75:35–39.

70. Garcia MJ, Thomas JD, Klein AL. New Doppler echocardiographic applications for the study of diastolic function. J Am Coll Cardiol 1998; 32:865–875.

71. Isaaz K. Tissue Doppler imaging for the assessment of left ventricular systolic and diastolic functions. Curr Opin Cardiol 2002; 17:431–442.

72. Yip G, Abraham T, Belohlavek M, Khandheria B. Clinical applications of strain rate imaging. J Am Soc Echocardiogr 2003; 16:1334–1342.

73. Trambaiolo P, Tonti G, Salustri A, Fedele F, Sutherland G. New insights into regional systolic and diastolic left ventricular function with tissue doppler echocardiography: from qualitative analysis to a quantitative approach. J Am Soc Echocardiogr 2001; 14:85–96.

74. Fyrenius A, Wigstrom L, Bolger AF, Ebbers T, Ohman KP, Karlsson M, et al. Pitfalls in Doppler evaluation of diastolic function: insights from 3-dimensional magnetic resonance imaging. J Am Soc Echocardiogr 1999; 12:817–826.

75. European Study Group on Diastolic Heart Failure. How to diagnose diastolic heart failure. Eur Heart J 1998; 19:990–1003.

76. Gandhi SK, Powers JC, Nomeir AM, Fowle K, Kitzman DW, Rankin KM, et al. The pathogenesis of acute pulmonary edema associated with hypertension. N Engl J Med 2001; 344:17–22.

77. Brogan WCIII, Hillis LD, Flores ED, Lange RA. The natural history of isolated left ventricular diastolic dysfunction. Am J Med 1992; 92:627–630.

78. Kitzman DW, Higginbotham MB, Cobb FR, Sheikh KH, Sullivan MJ. Exercise intolerance in patients with heart failure and preserved left ventricular systolic function: failure of the Frank-Starling mechanism. J Am Coll Cardiol 1991; 17:1065–1072.

79. Redfield MM, Jacobsen SJ, Burnett JC, Mahoney DW, Bailey KR, Rodeheffer RJ. Burden of systolic and diastolic ventricular dysfunction in the community: appreciating the scope of the heart failure epidemic. JAMA 2003; 289:194–202.

80. Fischer M, Baessler A, Hense HW, Hengstenberg C, Muscholl M, Holmer S, et al. Prevalence of left ventricular diastolic dysfunction in the community. Results from a Doppler echocardiographic-based survey of a population sample. Eur Heart J 2003; 24:320–328.

81. Rodeheffer RJ. Epidemiology and screening of asymptomatic left ventricular dysfunction. J Card Fail 2002; 8:S253–S257.

82. Vasan RS, Levy D. The role of hypertension in the pathogenesis of heart failure. A clinical mechanistic overview. Arch Intern Med 1996; 156:1789–1796.

83. Kenchaiah S, Evans JC, Levy D, Wilson PW, Benjamin EJ, Larson MG, et al. Obesity and the risk of heart failure. N Engl J Med 2002; 347:305–313.

84. Prevention of stroke by antihypertensive drug treatment in older persons with isolated systolic hypertension. Final results of the systolic hypertension in the elderly program (SHEP). SHEP Cooperative Research Group. JAMA 1991; 265:3255–3264.

85. Dahlof B, Lindholm LH, Hansson L, Schersten B, Ekbom T, Wester PO. Morbidity and mortality in the Swedish trial in old patients with hypertension (STOP-Hypertension). Lancet 1991; 338:1281–1285.

86. Kjekshus L, Pederesen T. Lowering cholesterol with simvastatin may prevent development of heart failure in patients with coronary heart disease [abstr]. J Am Coll Cardiol 1995; 25:282A.

87. Levy D, Larson MG, Vasan RS, Kannel WB, Ho KK. The progression from hypertension to congestive heart failure. JAMA 1996; 275:1557–1562.

88. Moser M, Hebert PR. Prevention of disease progression, left ventricular hypertrophy and congestive heart failure in hypertension treatment trials. J Am Coll Cardiol 1996; 27:1214–1218.

89. Given BD, Lee TH, Stone PH, Dzau VJ. Nifedipine in severely hypertensive patients with congestive heart failure and preserved ventricular systolic function. Arch Intern Med 1985; 145:281–285.

90. Cuocolo A, Sax FL, Brush JE, Maron BJ, Bacharach SL, Bonow RO. Left ventricular hypertrophy and impaired diastolic filling in essential hypertension. Diastolic mechanisms for systolic dysfunction during exercise. Circulation 1990; 81:978–986.

91. Inouye I, Massie B, Loge D, Topic N, Silverstein D, Simpson P, et al. Abnormal left ventricular filling: an early finding in mild to moderate systemic hypertension. Am J Cardiol 1984; 53:120–126.

92. Smith VE, Schulman P, Karimeddini MK, White WB, Meeran MK, Katz AM. Rapid ventricular filling in left ventricular hypertrophy: II. Pathologic hypertrophy. J Am Coll Cardiol 1985; 5:869–874.

93. Pearson AC, Gudipati C, Nagelhout D, Sear J, Cohen JD, Labovitz AJ. Echocardiographic evaluation of cardiac structure and function in elderly subjects with isolated systolic hypertension. J Am Coll Cardiol 1991; 17:422–430.

94. Sagie A, Benjamin EJ, Galderisi M, Larson MG, Evans JC, Fuller DL, et al. Echocardiographic assessment of left ventricular structure and diastolic filling in elderly subjects with borderline

isolated systolic hypertension (the Framingham Heart Study). Am J Cardiol 1993; 72: 662–665.

95. Fouad FM, Slominski JM, Tarazi RC. Left ventricular diastolic function in hypertension: relation to left ventricular mass and systolic function. J Am Coll Cardiol 1984; 3:1500–1506.

96. Snider AR, Gidding SS, Rocchini AP, Rosenthal A, Dick M, Crowley DC, et al. Doppler evaluation of left ventricular diastolic filling in children with systemic hypertension. Am J Cardiol 1985; 56:921–926.

97. Devereux RB. Left ventricular diastolic dysfunction: early diastolic relaxation and late diastolic compliance. J Am Coll Cardiol 1989; 13:337–339.

98. Andren B, Lind L, Hedenstierna G, Lithell H. Left ventricular diastolic function in a population sample of elderly men. Echocardiography 1998; 15:433–450.

99. Kawaguchi M, Hay I, Fetics B, Kass DA. Combined ventricular systolic and arterial stiffening in patients with heart failure and preserved ejection fraction: implications for systolic and diastolic reserve limitations. Circulation 2003; 107:714–720.

100. Barbier P, Alioto G, Guazzi MD. Left atrial function and ventricular filling in hypertensive patients with paroxysmal atrial fibrillation. J Am Coll Cardiol 1994; 24:165–170.

101. Benjamin EJ, Levy D, Vaziri SM, D'Agostino RB, Belanger AJ, Wolf PA. Independent risk factors for atrial fibrillation in a population-based cohort. The Framingham Heart Study. JAMA 1994; 271:840–844.

102. Volders PG, Willems IE, Cleutjens JP, Arends JW, Havenith MG, Daemen MJ. Interstitial collagen is increased in the non-infarcted human myocardium after myocardial infarction. J Mol Cell Cardiol 1993; 25:1317–1323.

103. Brilla CG, Pick R, Tan LB, Janicki JS, Weber KT. Remodeling of the rat right and left ventricles in experimental hypertension. Circ Res 1990; 67:1355–1364.

104. Sato A, Takane H, Saruta T. High serum level of procollagen type III amino-terminal peptide contributes to the efficacy of spironolactone and angiotensin-converting enzyme inhibitor therapy on left ventricular hypertrophy in essential hypertensive patients. Hypertens Res 2001; 24:99–104.

105. Sasaguri M, Noda K, Tashiro E, Notomo J, Tsuji E, Koga M, et al. The regression of left ventricular hypertrophy by imidapril and the reduction of serum procollagen type III aminoterminal peptide in hypertensive patients. Hypertens Res 2000; 23:317–322.

106. Brilla CG, Funck RC, Rupp H. Lisinopril-mediated regression of myocardial fibrosis in patients with hypertensive heart disease. Circulation 2000; 102:1388–1393.

107. Jalil JE, Doering CW, Janicki JS, Pick R, Shroff SG, Weber KT. Fibrillar collagen and myocardial stiffness in the intact hypertrophied rat left ventricle. Circ Res 1989; 64: 1041–1050.

108. Weber KT, Brilla CG. Pathological hypertrophy and cardiac interstitium. Fibrosis and renin-angiotensin-aldosterone system. Circulation 1991; 83:1849.

109. Yamamoto K, Masuyama T, Sakata Y, Nishikawa N, Mano T, Yoshida J, et al. Myocardial stiffness is determined by ventricular fibrosis, but not by compensatory or excessive hypertrophy in hypertensive heart. Cardiovasc Res 2002; 55:76–82.

110. Lips DJ, de Windt LJ, van Kraaij DJ, Doevendans PA. Molecular determinants of myocardial hypertrophy and failure: alternative pathways for beneficial and maladaptive hypertrophy. Eur Heart J 2003; 24:883–896.

111. Bonaduce D, Breglio R, Conforti G, De Luca N, Montemurro MV, Arrichiello P, et al. Myocardial hypertrophy and left ventricular diastolic function in hypertensive patients: an echo Doppler evaluation. Eur Heart J 1989; 10:611–621.

112. Ren JF, Pancholy SB, Iskandrian AS, Lighty GW, Mallavarapu C, Segal BL. Doppler echocardiographic evaluation of the spectrum of left ventricular diastolic dysfunction in essential hypertension. Am Heart J 1994; 127:906–913.

113. Aronow WS, Ahn C, Kronzon I, Koenigsberg M. Congestive heart failure, coronary events and atherothrombotic brain infarction in elderly blacks and whites with systemic hypertension and with and without echocardiographic and electrocardiographic evidence of left ventricular hypertrophy. Am J Cardiol 1991; 67:295–299.

114. Gottdiener JS, Arnold AM, Aurigemma GP, Polak JF, Tracy RP, Kitzman DW, et al. Predictors of congestive heart failure in the elderly: the Cardiovascular Health Study. J Am Coll Cardiol 2000; 35:1628–1637.
115. Topol EJ, Traill TA, Fortuin NJ. Hypertensive hypertrophic cardiomyopathy of the elderly. N Engl J Med 1985; 312:277–283.
116. Diez J, Querejeta R, Lopez B, Gonzalez A, Larman M, Martinez Ubago JL. Losartan-dependent regression of myocardial fibrosis is associated with reduction of left ventricular chamber stiffness in hypertensive patients. Circulation 2002; 105:2512–2517.
117. Lindsay MM, Maxwell P, Dunn FG. TIMP-1: a marker of left ventricular diastolic dysfunction and fibrosis in hypertension. Hypertension 2002; 40:136–141.
118. Grossman W. Diastolic dysfunction in congestive heart failure. N Engl J Med 1991; 325:1557–1564.
119. Grossman W. Diastolic function and heart failure: an overview. Eur Heart J 1990; 11 Suppl C:2–7.
120. Bronzwaer JG, de Bruyne B, Ascoop CA, Paulus WJ. Comparative effects of pacing-induced and balloon coronary occlusion ischemia on left ventricular diastolic function in man. Circulation 1991; 84:211–222.
121. Dodek A, Kassebaum DG, Bristow JD. Pulmonary edema without cardiomegaly: ischemic cardiomyopathy and the small stiff heart. Am Heart J 1973; 85:281–284.
122. Kunis R, Greenberg H, Yeoh CB, Garfein OB, Pepe AJ, Pinkernell BH, et al. Coronary revascularization for recurrent pulmonary edema in elderly patients with ischemic heart disease and preserved ventricular function. N Engl J Med 1985; 313:1207–1210.
123. Bouchard A, Sanz N, Botvinick EH, Phillips N, Heilbron D, Byrd BFIII, et al. Noninvasive assessment of cardiomyopathy in normotensive diabetic patients between 20 and 50 years old. Am J Med 1989; 87:160–166.
124. Galderisi M, Anderson KM, Wilson PW, Levy D. Echocardiographic evidence for the existence of a distinct diabetic cardiomyopathy (the Framingham Heart Study). Am J Cardiol 1991; 68:85–89.
125. Sundstrom J, Lind L, Nystrom N, Zethelius B, Andren B, Hales CN, et al. Left ventricular concentric remodeling rather than left ventricular hypertrophy is related to the insulin resistance syndrome in elderly men. Circulation 2000; 101:2595–2600.
126. Sundstrom J, Lind L, Valind S, Holmang A, Bjorntorp P, Andren B, et al. Myocardial insulin-mediated glucose uptake and left ventricular geometry. Blood Press 2001; 10:27–32.
127. Holmang A, Yoshida N, Jennische E, Waldenstrom A, Bjorntorp P. The effects of hyperinsulinaemia on myocardial mass, blood pressure regulation and central haemodynamics in rats. Eur J Clin Invest 1996; 26:973–978.
128. Badenhorst D, Maseko M, Tsotetsi OJ, Naidoo A, Brooksbank R, Norton GR, et al. Cross-linking influences the impact of quantitative changes in myocardial collagen on cardiac stiffness and remodelling in hypertension in rats. Cardiovasc Res 2003; 57:632–641.
129. Kass DA, Shapiro EP, Kawaguchi M, Capriotti AR, Scuteri A, deGroof RC, et al. Improved arterial compliance by a novel advanced glycation end-product crosslink breaker. Circulation 2001; 104:1464–1470.
130. Alexander JK. The cardiomyopathy of obesity. Prog Cardiovasc Dis 1985; 27:325–334.
131. Mureddu GF, de Simone G, Greco R, Rosato GF, Contaldo F. Left ventricular filling pattern in uncomplicated obesity. Am J Cardiol 1996; 77:509–514.
132. Downes TR, Nomeir AM, Smith KM, Stewart KP, Little WC. Mechanism of altered pattern of left ventricular filling with aging in subjects without cardiac disease. Am J Cardiol 1989; 64:523–527.
133. Dineen E, Brent BN. Aortic valve stenosis: comparison of patients with to those without chronic congestive heart failure. Am J Cardiol 1986; 57:419–422.
134. Choudhury L, Mahrholdt H, Wagner A, Choi KM, Elliott MD, Klocke FJ, et al. Myocardial scarring in asymptomatic or mildly symptomatic patients with hypertrophic cardiomyopathy. J Am Coll Cardiol 2002; 40:2156–2164.
135. Arad M, Seidman JG, Seidman CE. Phenotypic diversity in hypertrophic cardiomyopathy. Hum Mol Genet 2002; 11:2499–2506.

136. Van Driest SL, Ellsworth EG, Ommen SR, Tajik AJ, Gersh BJ, Ackerman MJ. Prevalence and spectrum of thin filament mutations in an outpatient referral population with hypertrophic cardiomyopathy. Circulation 2003; 108:445–451.

137. Robinson K, Frenneaux MP, Stockins B, Karatasakis G, Poloniecki JD, McKenna WJ. Atrial fibrillation in hypertrophic cardiomyopathy: a longitudinal study. J Am Coll Cardiol 1990; 15:1279–1285.

138. Seiler C, Hess OM, Schoenbeck M, Turina J, Jenni R, Turina M, et al. Long-term follow-up of medical versus surgical therapy for hypertrophic cardiomyopathy: a retrospective study. J Am Coll Cardiol 1991; 17:634–642.

139. Katritsis D, Wilmshurst PT, Wendon JA, Davies MJ, Webb-Peploe MM. Primary restrictive cardiomyopathy: clinical and pathologic characteristics. J Am Coll Cardiol 1991; 18: 1230–1235.

140. Brockington GM, Zebede J, Pandian NG. Constrictive pericarditis. Cardiol Clin 1990; 8: 645–661.

141. Myers RB, Spodick DH. Constrictive pericarditis: clinical and pathophysiologic characteristics. Am Heart J 1999; 138:219–232.

142. Vaitkus PT, Kussmaul WG. Constrictive pericarditis versus restrictive cardiomyopathy: a reappraisal and update of diagnostic criteria. Am Heart J 1991; 122:1431–1441.

143. Arem R, Rokey R, Kiefe C, Escalante DA, Rodriguez A. Cardiac systolic and diastolic function at rest and exercise in subclinical hypothyroidism: effect of thyroid hormone therapy. Thyroid 1996; 6:397–402.

144. Biondi B, Fazio S, Palmieri EA, Carella C, Panza N, Cittadini A, et al. Left ventricular diastolic dysfunction in patients with subclinical hypothyroidism. J Clin Endocrinol Metab 1999; 84:2064–2067.

145. Gustafsson F, Torp-Pedersen C, Brendorp B, Seibaek M, Burchardt H, Kober L. Long-term survival in patients hospitalized with congestive heart failure: relation to preserved and reduced left ventricular systolic function. Eur Heart J 2003; 24:863–870.

146. Senni M, Redfield MM. Heart failure with preserved systolic function; a different natural history?. J Am Coll Cardiol 2001; 38:1277–1282.

147. Gottdiener JS, McClelland RL, Marshall R, Shemanski L, Furberg CD, Kitzman DW, et al. Outcome of congestive heart failure in elderly persons: influence of left ventricular systolic function. The Cardiovascular Health Study. Ann Intern Med 2002; 137:631–639.

10
The Clinical Syndrome of Heart Failure

Thomas DiSalvo
Massachusetts General Hospital and Harvard Medical School
Boston, Massachusetts, USA

INTRODUCTION

Heart failure (HF) remains the only common cardiovascular syndrome increasing in prevalence and incidence [1]. Despite significant advances in pharmacological and device therapies, morbidity and mortality for those afflicted with HF remains high [2]. Following a brief discussion of epidemiology and pathophysiology, this chapter focuses on the clinical syndrome of HF with particular emphasis on clinical presentation and diagnosis.

EPIDEMIOLOGY

Definition

Given pathophysiological and clinical heterogeneity, it is not surprising that there is not yet any firm consensus definition of the clinical syndrome of HF (Table 1) [3]. Over the past several decades, basic and clinical research elucidating the complex and continuous interplay of adaptive and maladaptive myocyte, myocardial extracellular matrix, hemodynamic, biochemical, energetic, genetic, neurohormonal, renal, pulmonary, skeletal muscle, vascular endothelial alterations and adaptations in HF has rendered consensus definition even more challenging [4]. However, virtually all clinical instances of HF may be broadly conceptualized as a primary failure of the heart to render sufficient pressure-volume work over the range of physiological resting and exercise pressure-volume conditions, and thereby maintain organ perfusion at ventricular filling pressures below the threshold for the precipitation of systemic or pulmonary venous congestion.

Classification

Heart failure may be classified as either predominantly systolic or diastolic [3]. Almost all instances of systolic HF also exhibit diastolic abnormalities; most instances of diastolic HF also exhibit systolic abnormalities, usually inadequate systolic functional reserve [5,6]. The cardiomyopathies have traditionally been classified as either dilated, restrictive, or hypertrophic [7]. Neither classification schema necessarily provides sufficient insight into disease etiology, severity, or prognosis.

Table 1 Definitions of Heart Failure

"A condition in which the heart fails to discharge its contents adequately"—*Thomas Lewis, 1933*

"A state in which the heart fails to maintain an adequate circulation for the needs of the body despite a satisfactory filling pressure"—*Paul Wood, 1950*

"A pathophysiological state in which an abnormality of cardiac function is responsible for the failure of the heart to pump blood at a rate commensurate with the requirements of the metabolizing tissues"—*Eugene Braunwald, 1980*

"Heart failure is the state of any heart disease in which, despite adequate ventricular filling, the heart's output is decreased or in which the heart is unable to pump blood at a rate adequate for satisfying the requirements of the tissues with functional parameters remaining within normal limits"—*H. Denolin, H. Kuhn, H.P. Krayenbuehl, F. Loogen, A. Reale, 1983*

"A clinical syndrome caused by an abnormality of the heart and recognized by a characteristic pattern of hemodynamic, renal, neural and hormonal responses"—*Philip A. Poole-Wilson, 1985*

"...syndrome ... which arises when the heart if chronically unable to maintain an appropriate blood pressure without support"—*Peter Harris, 1987*

"A syndrome in which cardiac dysfunction is associated with reduced exercise tolerance, a high incidence of ventricular arrhythmias and shortened life expectancy"—*Jay Cohn, 1988*

"Symptoms of heart failure, objective evidence of cardiac dysfunction and response to treatment directed towards heart failure"—*Task Force of ESC, 1995*

"Heart failure is a complex clinical syndrome that can result from any cardiac disorder that impairs the ability of the ventricle to eject blood"—*Consensus Recommendations for the Management of Chronic Heart Failure, 1999* (From Ref. 10.)

"Heart failure is a complex clinical syndrome that can result from any structural of functional cardiac disorder that impairs the ability of the ventricle to fill with or eject blood"—*ACC/AHA Consensus Guidelines, 2001* (From Ref. 2.)

Source: Adapted from Ref. 59, page 270.

It is important to distinguish HF from states of extreme or supra-physiological circulatory pressure or volume overload (e.g., acute severe hypertension, severe anemia, arteriovenous fistula) or from the occasional metabolic (e.g., hypoxemia, acidosis), endocrinologic (e.g., hypo- or hyperthyroidism), and diverse medical conditions (e.g., sepsis) associated with transient and reversible myocardial dysfunction [2,3]. In such instances, transient signs and/or symptoms of HF may appear in the absence of true myocardial dysfunction or disease.

Incidence and Prevalence

Heart failure is the only common cardiovascular disease with rising incidence and prevalence [8,9]. In the United States, HF afflicts approximately 4.8 million people [10] with approximately 400,000 to 700,000 new symptomatic cases, and 250,000 deaths annually. Between 1.5% and 2% of the U.S. population has symptomatic HF, with a prevalence of 6% to 10% in those more than age 65 years [11]. In the Framingham Heart Study, the lifetime HF risk for men and women free of HF at age 40 was 21% for men and 20.3% for women [12]. In the Framingham cohort, the incidence of HF declined for women but not men between 1950 and 1999 [13]. There is a marked age-dependence in HF prevalence and incidence with elderly patients being disproportionately afflicted [14]. Given the recent and continued successes in managing coronary artery disease, the incidence and prevalence of HF will likely only increase in the future [8].

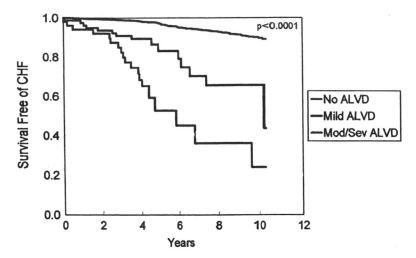

Figure 1 Kaplan-Meier curves for survival free of symptomatic heart failure. Referent group consists of subjects with normal left ventricular systolic function (LVEF > 50%). Mild ALVD indicates mild asymptomatic left ventricular systolic dysfunction (LVEF 40% to 50%). Mod/ Sev ALVD indicates moderate to severe asymptomatic left ventricular systolic dysfunction (LVEF < 40%). (From Ref. 15.)

The largest pool of patients with HF are, in fact, minimally symptomatic [15]. Up to 3% to 6% of the general population may have asymptomatic left ventricular systolic dysfunction and be at high risk of developing symptomatic HF within 5 years (Fig. 1) [10,15,16]. Up to 20% of the asymptomatic general population may have evidence of diastolic dysfunction by screening echocardiography [16]. The recent recognition and importance of these phenomena for public health and cardiovascular disease prevention inform the rationale for the recent "redefinition" of HF by the ACC/AHA (American College of Cardiology/American Heart Association) consensus guidelines [2]. The recent ACC/AHA reclassification seeks to emphasize the large number of "at-risk" future HF patients in the United States, and empowers physicians to deploy HF preventative strategies analogous to the life-long prevention and management strategies deployed in the management of patients with risk factors for coronary artery disease and its sequelae. In the current ACC/AHA classification schema, patients in HF stage "A" (high risk for HF but without structural heart disease) and HF stage "B" (structural heart disease without symptoms of HF) are, in fact, without symptoms or signs of heart HF [2]. Reducing the morbidity and mortality of HF in the future may well rest upon the success with which physicians extend the recommended life-long preventative strategies to at-risk patients long before the symptoms, signs, and overt echocardiographic features of HF supervene.

Economics

Heart failure poses an enormous societal financial burden with an estimated cost of between $20 and $40 billion dollars annually in the United States [10]. Care of HF consumes approximately 11% of total expenditure for cardiovascular disease [17,18]. The elderly bear a disproportionate economic burden given the rising prevalence of heart HF with age [14].

Table 2 Risk Factors for Heart Failure

Coronary artery disease
Hypertension
Heavy alcohol use
Familial or genetic cardiomyopathy
Significant mitral of aortic valvular heart
    disease
Myocarditis
Toxin exposure (chemotherapy, cocaine)
Underlying systemic disorders (e.g., thyroid
    disease, hemochromatosis, sarcoidosis,
    amyloidosis)
Nutritional deficiencies
Collagen vascular disease
Peripartum disease
Neuromuscular disorders
Age
Obesity

Risk Factors

Observational and epidemiologic studies have identified multiple risk factors for HF, including systemic hypertension, coronary artery disease, diabetes mellitus, cardiotoxic drug therapy, alcohol abuse, history of rheumatic fever, family history of cardiomyopathy, and obesity [2,11–13]. Although these risk factors are well-recognized, HF does not develop in all patients so exposed. For example, some instances of noncoronary disease related HF may well require more than a single genetic abnormality, epidemiologic or environmental exposure, or coexistent disease condition to evolve [19]. A "multiple hit" hypothesis has been promoted to account for these epidemiological observations in HF pathophysiology analogous to the "multiple hit" hypothesis advanced in cancer pathophysiology [20]. According to this attractive paradigm, the population-attributable risk bequeathed by a single HF risk factor is modified by a unique constellation of individual genetic characteristics, other risk factors, concurrent cardiovascular and noncardiovascular diseases or conditions, environmental exposures, body habitus, physical condition, and medications. Known risk factors for the development of HF appear in Table 2. Of particular interest in clinical research at present are the single or multiple gene defects that may either precipitate HF directly [19, 21–29) or enhance the predisposition to HF given a specific environmental exposure or exposures [30]. The "customization" of both "prophylactic" and chronic pharmacological therapy based upon genotype is the long-term aim of much current HF clinical and translational research (Chapter 7) [31–33].

PATHOPHYSIOLOGY

Normal Integrated Function of the Heart

As a pump, the normal heart is designed to apply circumferential compressive force to the blood pool resident within the heart following diastolic filling [34]. Since blood is a relatively incompressible fluid, the pressure within the blood pool rises steeply as compressive force develops during isovolumic contraction. Eventually the pressure within the relatively noncompressible blood pool exceeds the pressure across the aortic valve, the aortic valve opens, and ventricular ejection ensues. In healthy circumstances, the anatomy and physiology of the heart are carefully construed and maintained so as to perform compressive mechanical work at near-maximal efficiency to deliver an adequate cardiac output over the normal range of rest and exertional pressure-volume conditions, commensurate with the demands of the body's metabolizing tissues.

Heart Failure

Heart failure, systolic or diastolic, may be conceived as a pathophysiological state in which either the delivery of cardiac output is inadequate to meet the metabolic demands of tissues or an adequate cardiac output is delivered only under conditions of abnormally elevated intracardiac pressures, which prematurely precipitate systemic or pulmonary venous congestion [35]. In the latter instance, exertion is curtailed prematurely as the supranormal intracardiac pressures exceed the maximal capacitance of either the systemic or pulmonary venous and lymphatic circulations. An excessive volume of interstitial fluid accumulates in response constitutively elevating systemic or pulmonary hydraulic capillary pressure gradients and resulting in symptoms or signs and exertional limitation.

Although still debated, the primary "locus" of dysfunction in most instances of systolic HF appears to reside largely within the myocyte compartment of the heart. At least in the end-stage human heart, both in vivo and in vitro studies support a marked reduction in "contractility reserve" in response to increasing heart rate of sympathetic stimulation [36]. Whether this reduction in myocardial "contractility reserve" results from intrinsic abnormalities of myocyte contractile function or myocyte response to alterations in the myocardial and extracellular matrix neurohormonally modulated "milieu," is still uncertain.

Normal integrated function of the heart depends upon a host of factors that include normal ultrastructural and gross architecture of the heart, an adequate number of myocytes, normal myocyte contractile and relaxant function, normal structure and function of cardiac valves, normal structure, composition, and metabolism of the myocardial extracellular matrix, adequate myocardial perfusion, and normal myocardial metabolism. Not surprisingly, abnormalities in any of these major anatomic and functional components may result in HF. Among the more common causes of HF are loss of myocytes (ischemic, inflammatory or toxic necrosis, apoptosis), acute or chronic contractile dysfunction of myocytes (inflammation, alcohol, chemotherapeutic agents, sepsis, hypoxia), excessive myofiber architectural disorganization or disarray (hypertrophic cardiomyopathy, infiltrative cardiomyopathy), extracellular matrix structural or functional abnormalities (excessive fibrosis leading to abnormal force transduction, myocyte linkage, and inadequate "compressive force" efficiency), distortion of the three-dimensional shape of the heart itself (aneurysm, infarction, chronic valvular disease), and intractable pressure or volume overload (hypertension, valvular heart disease) (Table 3).

Under the current "neurohormonal" hypothesis, the initial myocardial injury or overload results in a perceived diminution in the rate, pattern or distribution of perfusion to the vital regulatory organs and centers of the circulation [37]. Such alterations in perfusion invoke a complex cascade of initially "homeostatic" responses (positive inotropy and chronotropy, vasoconstriction, sodium retention) mediated largely by multiple interacting and amplifying neurohormonal axes (such as the renin-angiotensin-aldosterone systems and the sympathetic nervous system) that provide initial restoration of perfusion. Over time, however, the constitutive activation of these diverse neurohormonal systems, particularly the ongoing elaboration of high circulating, and tissue levels, of key effector molecules (e.g., angiotensin II, norepinephrine, epinephrine, aldosterone, and the endothelin

Table 3 Causes of Systolic
Heart Failure

Coronary artery disease
Hypertension
Alcohol
Valvular heart disease
Familial/genetic cardiomyopathy
Myocarditis
Toxins (chemotherapy, cocaine)
Collagen vascular disease
Metabolic disorders
Endocrine disorders
Electrolyte disorders
Acidosis
Sepsis
Hypoxia
Severe sleep apnea
Peripartum

---

family of peptides) proves progressively pathological and promotes both: (a) deleterious alterations in circulatory dynamics, which impose greater myocardial load (e.g., volume expansion due to excessive salt and water retention, vasoconstriction); and (b) deleterious changes in myocardial structure and function, which effect adverse ventricular remodeling (e.g., accelerated myocyte loss via apoptosis, increasing myocardial fibrosis). Many instances of adverse myocardial remodeling are accompanied, likely, by an ever-dwindling myocyte mass due to ongoing necrosis, apoptosis, or aging. Although there appears to be a small population of cardiac stem-like cells within myocardial tissue capable of terminal differentiation into functional myocytes, the majority of preexisting terminally differentiated myocytes cannot undergo hyperplasia at a rate sufficient to repopulate a dwindling myocyte mass [38].

Central to the progression of HF, once initiated and the target of current pharmacological management of heart failure, is the process of adverse ventricular remodeling (Chapter 6) [4]. Once exposed to significant injury or unrelieved pressure and volume overload, the heart responds by remodeling itself with, at times, a remarkable degree of plasticity with respect to structure and function [39]. Remodeling is largely mediated by exogenous and endogenous neurohormonal axes activated in response to altered systemic perfusion or chronic myocardial pressure and volume overload itself. The process of remodeling alters ventricular dimensions and shape as well as myocyte and extracellular matrix composition, integration, and function. In addition to the neurohormonal axes previously described, diverse autocrine, paracrine, and endocrine signaling systems are simultaneously activated and play important roles in modulating the pace and outcome of remodeling [40].

Underappreciated is the heterogeneity of the mechanisms, not only initiating HF but also influencing the course of remodeling once HF supervenes. For example, genetic defects underlie up to one-third of cases of idiopathic dilated cardiomyopathy and likely all instances of hypertrophic cardiomyopathy [19]. Undoubtedly, other genetic factors impact the myocardial response to injury or overload and determine, in part, the course of remodeling. These diverse and intersecting pathophysiological mechanisms are often paradoxically "hidden" in individuals by the stereotypical clinical symptoms and signs, and histopathological features of established chronic systolic HF.

Systolic Heart Failure

In addition to the structural and functional considerations previously presented, normal systolic function also depends on a precise sequence of electrical activation of the myocardium (apex to base), a torsional translational motion of the ventricle (a "wringing" out), a precise anatomic array of myofibers that mechanically maximizes force generation (myofibers wrapped in orthogonal layers), an appropriate degree of hypertrophy of myocytes given load, and a suitably deformable and elastic extracellular matrix that maintains myocardial orientation and recoil. Systolic dysfunction, signifying inadequate "compressive force generation" requisite over the normal range of circulatory pressure and volume conditions, may, thus, also result or be exacerbated by diverse alterations in myocardial activation, contractile sequence, macro- or microanatomy, and abnormalities of the extracellular matrix.

Despite evidence for abnormal "contractile reserve" in end-stage human HF, in may instances it is not yet possible in clinical practice to adequately characterize the precise anatomic (submyocyte, myocyte, myofiber, matrix), physiological, molecular, or metabolic "loci" of clinically encountered "failing" myocardial tissue [37,41]. Some important myocardial characteristics are not easily quantifiable in the intact heart, such as the number of viable myocytes, myocyte and myofiber array, the degree of individual myocyte hypertrophy, the integrity, composition, and metabolic activity of the extracellular matrix. Undoubtedly, incomplete "phenotyping" of failing myocardial tissue has hampered not only a more intimate understanding of HF pathophysiology and ventricular remodeling, but also the customization of pharmacological and device therapies to individual patients [42–45]. Several of the most important abnormalities accounting for systolic dysfunction appear in Table 4.

Diastolic Heart Failure

The clinical syndrome of normal or near-normal left ventricular dimension and resting ejection fraction, coupled with the symptoms of dyspnea, exertional limitation, and epi-

Table 4 Abnormalities Resulting in Systolic Dysfunction

Myocyte compartment
  Myocyte loss (necrosis, apoptosis, aging)
  Abnormal force transduction (e.g., dystrophin mutations)
  Abnormal force generation (calcium release, substrate deficiency)
  Abnormal relaxation (abnormal calcium reuptake)
  Excessive myocyte hypertrophy
Myocardial load
  Volume overload (mitral or aortic regurgitation, renal or hepatic failure)
  Pressure overload (hypertension, increased arterial stiffness)
Heart rate and conduction
  Excessive tachycardia (weeks)
  Discoordinate contraction (right ventricular pacing)
Extracellular matrix compartment
  Fibrosis
  Altered metabolism (cardiofibroblast function, protein synthesis and
    degradation, paracrine/autocrine signaling)
Cardiac structure
  Abnormal myocardial fiber "wrapping" or alignment
  Focal infarction or aneurysm
  Advanced remodeling (increased sphericity)

Table 5   Criteria for Diagnosis of Diastolic Heart Failure

European Study Group:
  1. Evidence of CHF
  2. Normal or mildly abnormal LV systolic function
  3. Evidence of abnormal LV relaxation, filling, distensibility or stiffness
Framingham Heart Study:
  1. Definitive diagnosis of CHF (signs and symptoms; CXR; response to diuretics)
  2. LVEF greater than or equal to 50% within 72 hours of episode
  3. Objective evidence of LV diastolic dysfunction (abnormal LV relaxation/filling/
     distensibility indices by catheterization)

Source: From Ref. 46a and Ref. 52.

sodic pulmonary congestion, accounts for up to 40% to 50% of HF diagnosed and treated in the community (Chapter 9) [2,3]. A cause of considerable morbidity, including a high rate of recurrent hospitalization, mortality from diastolic HF is lower than in systolic HF but is increased four-fold compared with age-adjusted baseline mortality [46].

Controversy abounds regarding the existence, definition, diagnosis, and therapy of isolated ''diastolic'' HF (Table 5) [5,47–52]. The incidence and prevalence of diastolic HF are steeply age-dependent due to the confluence of several age-dependent processes including progressive loss of myocytes (by age 80 years, one-third of myocytes have been lost), myocardial fibrosis, arterial stiffening (attrition of elastic fibers, atherosclerosis, calcification and fibrosis, and loss of normal endothelial-dependent vasodilation), and the long-term sequelae of hypertension and atherosclerotic coronary artery and peripheral vascular disease [53]. In the less common instances of diastolic HF in younger patients, myocardial tissue typically exhibits abnormally relaxant, noncompliant, nondistensible, or excessively stiffened characteristics under the normal range of circulatory pressure-volume loads (Table 6) [5]. Cardiac output is maintained in such instances at rest with obligate elevation of ventricular filling pressures. Albeit normal at rest, the cardiac output either fails to rise appropriately with increased demand or does so with an abrupt rise in filling pressures, and the resultant precipitation of systemic or pulmonary venous and lymphatic congestion that causes limitation of exertion or symptoms.

There is increasing evidence that abnormalities of systolic function accompany most if not all instances of apparently ''isolated'' diastolic HF [6,54,55]. In elderly patients, such

Table 6   Abnormalities Resulting in Diastolic Heart Failure

Extreme myocardial overload
  Severe hypertension, aortic stenosis, mitral or aortic regurgitation)
Impaired myocardial relaxation
  Ischemia, hypertrophy, hypothyroidism, aging, cardiomyopathy
Impaired ventricular filling
  Mitral stenosis, endocardial fibroelastosis
Reduced ventricular distensibility
  Constrictive pericarditis, pericardial tamponade, extrinsic compression
Increased ventricular stiffness
  Age, ischemia, myocardial fibrosis or scarring, infiltrative cardiomyopathy,
    myocardial edema, microvascular congestion

Source: Adapted from Ref. 6.

systolic dysfunction not uncommonly results from the increased impedance to ventricular ejection into an increasingly stiffened arterial vascular circuit. Although a lesser degree of neurohormonal activation accompanies diastolic HF than systolic HF, exercise capacity in elderly patients with diastolic HF is comparably diminished as in patients with systolic HF [56]. It is not possible on the basis of symptoms and signs alone to distinguish systolic from diastolic HF. Most patients with a history of HF and preserved ejection fraction at rest, evidence abnormal indexes of diastolic function by echocardiography, although such measures serve to confirm rather than establish the diagnosis of diastolic HF [57].

There have been few trials to date of lifestyle, pharmacological or device therapies in this common clinical syndrome. Pharmacological therapy is largely focused toward control of load, heart rate and rhythm, and symptomatic relief of episodic pulmonary congestion [50]. To date, no therapies have been shown to reduce mortality in this common condition, although data from the recently completed CHARM study, suggest that therapy with angiotensin receptor blockers can reduce hospitalizations (therapy for diastolic heart failure is more extensively discussed in Chapter 17). Although a time-honored therapeutic rubric is to maintain patients "···dry, slow, normotensive and in sinus rhythm···," the clinical efficacy of this intuitively attractive rubric remains unproven. No currently available pharmacological agent consistently or significantly improves intrinsic diastolic function or reliably reduces arterial stiffening. In addition to control of myocardial load and rhythm, many HF experts recommend application of the same stepwise pharmacological therapies designed for systolic HF to patients with diastolic HF. Since over time progressive adverse ventricular remodeling also occurs in patients with predominant diastolic dysfunction, beta-blockers, angiotensin II inhibitors, and aldosterone inhibitors likely play an important role in attenuating disease progression [58].

DIAGNOSIS OF HEART FAILURE

Symptoms and Signs

The clinical syndrome of HF, whether systolic of diastolic, must be differentiated from other conditions resulting in dyspnea, fatigue, and exertional intolerance, including but not limited to pulmonary disease, chronic renal or hepatic failure, and anemia [2,7]. Clinical HF rarely fulfills its classic "textbook" clinical profile in toto, i.e., symptoms of exertional dyspnea, orthopnea, and paroxysmal nocturnal dyspnea, and signs of elevated jugular venous pressure, pulmonary rales, a third heart sound, and peripheral edema [59]. No single symptom or sign is pathognomic for HF [60,61], and as previously stated, clinical parameters alone, including symptoms and signs, do not reliably distinguish patients with systolic HF from patients with diastolic HF [56,61–63].

In most observational studies, the symptoms most sensitive for HF include exertional dyspnea, orthopnea, and paroxysmal nocturnal dyspnea [64–68]. The most specific symptoms include orthopnea and paroxysmal dyspnea. The sensitivity and specificity of common symptoms and signs is tabulated in Table 7. As is apparent, the sensitivity of common symptoms for HF ranges from 23% to 66%, and the specificity from 52% to 81%.

The signs of HF are also inherently nonspecific [69]. Rales are absent in up to 80% of patients with chronic HF due to lymphatic hypertrophy [70]. Edema occurs in only 25% of patients under the age of 70 years with chronic HF [69]. Evidence of right-sided HF is lacking in up to 50% of patients at the time of diagnosis with idiopathic dilated cardiomyopathy [7]. In selected patients with severe HF, hepatojugular reflux [71,72] and the Valsalva maneuver [73,74] may provide ancillary evidence of elevated filling pressures [69]. In a retrospective multivariate analysis of the 2569 participants of the SOLVD treat-

Table 7 Sensitivity, Specificity and Predictive Value of Symptoms and Physical Signs in Diagnosing Chronic Heart Failure

Symptom or sign	Sensitivity (%)	Specificity (%)	Predictive accuracy (%)
Exertional dyspnea	66	52	23
Orthopnea	21	81	2
Paroxysmal nocturnal dyspnea	33	76	26
History of edema	23	80	22
Resting heart rate > 100 bpm	7	99	6
Rales	13	91	21
Third heart sound	31	95	61
Jugular venous distention	10	97	2
Edema (on examination)	10	93	3

Source: Adapted from Ref. 68a.

ment trial, the presence of an elevated jugular venous pressure and third heart sound were both independently associated with increase risk of hospitalization for HF, death, or hospitalization for HF and death from pump failure (Fig. 2) [75]. In an observational study of 1000 patients undergoing transplant evaluation, right atrial pressure at cardiac catheterization correlated reasonably well with pulmonary capillary wedge pressure (r = 0.64) [76]. However, there is only fair interobserver agreement on clinician ascertainment of the jugular venous pressure (kappa statistic 0.3–0.65) [77] and the presence of a third heart sound [78]. A proportional pulse pressure less than 25% has a 91% sensitivity and 83% specificity for cardiac index less than 2.2 L/min/m2 in patients with HF [69].

Given the lack of sensitivity and specificity of symptoms and signs, there exists no substitute for the performance of two-dimensional echocardiography to ascertain cardiac structure and function in all instances of suspected HF [2]. Ascertainment of the presence or absence of depression of left ventricular ejection fraction, left ventricular dimensions and wall thickness, valvular regurgitation, right ventricular dimension and function, and estimated pulmonary artery pressure are all crucial not only to accurate diagnosis but also the selection of appropriate therapy.

As emphasized earlier in this text, a large population of individuals with asymptomatic left ventricular dysfunction and high lifetime risk of evolving symptomatic HF exists [2]. Since echocardiographic screening for asymptomatic ventricular dysfunction is not routinely performed, HF is typically diagnosed only once symptoms or signs supervene [3]. The signs and symptoms of HF represent a quite advanced stage of ventricular dysfunction, appearing usually only after all compensatory hemodynamic, neurohormonal, and peripheral circulatory "counter-regulatory" homeostatic mechanisms have been overwhelmed. Earlier diagnosis of suspected asymptomatic or minimally symptomatic left ventricular dysfunction by echocardiography affords the opportunity to provide therapies that can retard ventricular remodeling and forestall morbidity and likely mortality.

Classification and Interpretation of the Clinical Presentation

The clinical diagnosis of HF remains largely empiric, based on the presence of symptoms, signs, radiographic evidence of pulmonary congestion or cardiomegaly, and echocardiographic evidence of ventricular dilatation and/or dysfunction. Clinical HF scoring systems

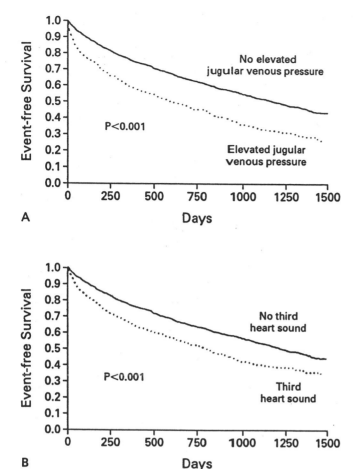

Figure 2 Kaplan-Meier analysis of event-free survival according to the presence or absence of elevated jugular venous pressure (*top panel*) and a third heart sound (*bottom panel*). The end-point was a composite of death or hospitalization for heart failure. (From Ref. 75.)

have been developed for use in population-based epidemiologic studies but are rarely used in clinical practice [79].

Patients with HF present with a constellation of symptoms and signs referable to either a low output state during rest or exercise, systemic or pulmonary venous congestion, or some combination of both [2]. As discussed, symptoms and signs bear an inconstant relationship to resting filling pressures, cardiac index, and ventricular function in individual patients. A clinically useful classification scheme of instances of decompensated HF has been recently proposed (Fig. 3) [70]. In this scheme, patients occupy one of four "quadrants" depending on the presence or absence of symptoms and signs of inadequate cardiac output and systemic venous congestion. This "two-minute" hemodynamic assessment is helpful in the initial triage of patients and institution of initial therapy.

Accurate functional classification remains problematic for individual patients [2]. The NYHA (New York Heart Association) classification scheme is limited by poor reproducibility, and relies exclusively on the presence and severity of symptoms rather than

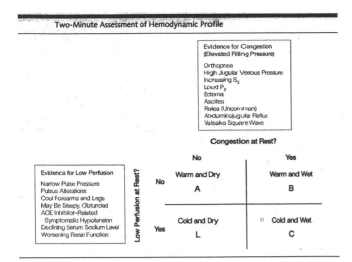

Figure 3 Diagram indicating clinically assessed hemodynamic profiles for patients presenting with heart failure. Most patients can be accurately classified in a 2-minute assessment according to their presenting signs and symptoms. (From Ref. 70.)

any marker of ventricular remodeling [80]. Since the symptoms and signs of HF are inherently mutable and affected by the adequacy of pharmacological therapies, any classification scheme based only on symptoms and signs must suffer from imprecision. Assessment of exercise tolerance (and cardiac reserve) during symptom-limited cardiopulmonary exercise testing, predicts prognosis more accurately than does classification based on symptoms and signs and demarcates disease severity more precisely [81].

Diagnostic Laboratory Modalities

Every patient with suspected or known HF requires an assessment of resting ventricular function and cardiac dimensions by two-dimensional echocardiography [2]. Components of the diagnostic evaluation of newly diagnosed HF in the current ACC/AHA (American College of Cardiology/American Heart Association) guidelines appear in)Table 8. In all patients, the guidelines emphasize: (a) a careful history and physical examination; (b) screening laboratories, including tests of renal and hepatic function, complete blood count, urinalysis, electrocardiogram and chest x-ray; (c) a two-dimensional and Doppler echocardiogram; (d) careful exclusion of coronary artery disease and thyroid disease in all patients; and (e) selective use of other diagnostic modalities, including serologic studies in some patients based upon carefully elicited clinical characteristics, past medical and family history, and risk-factors.

Recently, plasma levels of B-type natriuretic peptides (BNP) [82–84] have been used in the diagnosis of HF [85,86]. Use of the BNP assay has been incorporated into the European Society of Cardiology's guidelines for HF diagnosis [87] and will likely be incorporated in future ACC/AHA/Heart Failure Society of America guidelines. BNP levels have been shown to distinguish between cardiac and noncardiac causes of dyspnea in patients presenting to emergency rooms, and appear to enhance the information provided by clinical assessment alone [88–91]. Declines in BNP in response to beta-blockers are associated with improvements in symptoms and outcome [92,93]. One study showed that

Table 8 Recommendations for the Evaluation of Patients with Heart Failure

Class I

Thorough history and physical examination

Initial and ongoing assessment of ability to perform routine and desired activities of daily living

Initial and ongoing assessment of volume status

Initial measurement of complete blood count, urinalysis, serum electrolytes, blood urea nitrogen, serum creatinine, blood glucose, liver function tests, thyroid-stimulating hormone

Serial monitoring of serum electrolytes and renal function

Initial 12-lead EKG and chest radiograph

Initial 2-dimensional echocardiography with Doppler or radionuclide ventriculography to assess left ventricular systolic function

Cardiac catheterization with coronary angiography in patients with angina who are candidates for revascularization

Class IIa

Cardiac catheterization with coronary angiography in patients who are candidates for revascularization with:

• chest pain who have not had evaluation of their coronary anatomy

• known of suspected CAD but without angina

Noninvasive assessment of ischemia and viability in patients with known CAD without angina

Maximal exercise testing with measurement of respiratory gas exchange to determine:

• cause of exercise limitation

• candidacy for cardiac transplantation

Echocardiography in asymptomatic first-degree relatives of patients with IDCM

Repeat measures of ejection fraction in patients with change in clinical status

Screening for hemochromatosis

Measurement of ANA, RF, urinary VMA and metanephrines in selected patients

Class IIb

Noninvasive imaging to define likelihood of CAD

Maximal exercise testing to prescribe exercise program

Endomyocardial biopsy in patients with known or suspected inflammatory of infiltrative disorder

HIV testing

Class III

Endomyocardial biopsy in routine evaluation

Routine Holter-monitoring or signal-averaged electrocardiography

Repeat coronary angiography or noninvasive testing in patients in whom CAD has been excluded previously as the cause of left ventricular dysfunction

Routine measurement of norepinephrine

CAD: coronary artery disease; IDCM: idiopathic dilated cardiomyopathy; ANA: antinuclear antibody; RF: rheumatoid factor; VMA: vanellylmandelic acid; HIV: human immunodeficiency virus.

titration of chronic pharmacological therapy to BNP levels was superior to titration to global clinical assessment [94]. BNP appears to be more limited as a screening tool for HF in populations [95] because BNP is elevated in diverse cardiovascular conditions (left ventricular hypertrophy, hypertension, acute coronary syndromes [96], and valvular heart disease) and its levels are age- and gender-dependent [97]. BNP also provides prognostic value in chronic symptomatic HF populations [98–101].

Cardiac catheterization remains an important diagnostic tool to exclude significant coronary artery disease and define rest and exercise hemodynamics. Although patients with symptomatic HF may have normal resting hemodynamics, exercise hemodynamics are almost always abnormal, due to either an inadequate rise in cardiac output or an inappropriate rise in filling pressures. Right heart catheterization remains an important, and likely underutilized, diagnostic tool. Given the imprecision in predicting hemodynamics based upon clinical assessment alone, right heart catheterization can be invaluable in fragile patients in instances of uncertain hemodynamics, volume status, or clinical deterioration despite appropriate empiric titration of therapy. The ongoing ESCAPE trial sponsored by the NIH will provide a key insight into the evolving and appropriate role of right heart catheterization as a guide for therapy in chronic, severe HF.

COMMON CLINICAL FEATURES AND COMPLICATIONS

Certain clinical features and complications are common to the course of HF independent of disease etiology.

Arrhythmias

Atrial Fibrillation

Atrial fibrillation (AF) is an increasing public health problem in the United States [102]. AF occurs in approximately 15% to 30% of patients with symptomatic HF [103–105] and in up to 50% of patients with class NYMA IV HF [106]. Mechanisms leading to AF include atrial electrical remodeling, atrial fibrosis, sinus node dysfunction, increased sympathetic activation, and elevated atrial filling pressures [107,108]. The presence of AF is associated with an increased all-cause mortality [103,106,109], including sudden cardiac death [110]. AF with rapid ventricular response (HR > 110 bpm) may also be associated with rate-related but reversible deterioration in ventricular function [111]. While is has not yet been proven that maintenance of normal sinus rhythm improves mortality, [112,113], most practitioners are more aggressive in attempting to restore and maintain normal sinus rhythm in HF patients with AF than in other patient populations. Although atrial pacing may reduce the number of episodes of AF [114], RV (right ventricular) apical pacing in the DDDR mode more than 40% of the time may increase the frequency of HF decompensations and AF by inducing greater mechanical dyssynchrony [115]. Cardiac resynchronization may be beneficial in AF, although studies to date remain few [116]. Atrial defibrillators will be incorporated increasingly into implantable ventricular defibrillator devices in the future [117].

Ventricular Tachycardia

Nonsustained ventricular tachycardia is ubiquitous in symptomatic HF patients occurring in approximately 80% of patients during 24 to 48 hours of continuous ambulatory EKG monitoring [118,119]. The risk of sudden cardiac death is closely related to both the severity of depression of ventricular function and the degree of ventricular enlargement rather than the demonstration of nonsustained ventricular tachycardia. Patients with ischemic cardiomyopathy and left ventricular ejection fractions less than 30% are at particularly high risk of sudden cardiac death, and their mortality can be reduced by empiric implantation of an ICD (implantable cardioverter defibrillator) (Chapter 19).

Functional Limitation and Exercise Capacity

Mechanisms

Exercise limitation in chronic HF is multifactorial [81,120,121]. Hemodynamic (cardiac output, left ventricular systolic and diastolic function, left ventricular filling pressures, and right ventricular systolic function), neurovegetative (degree of sympathetic stimulation, baroreceptor sensitivity), skeletal muscle (muscle mass, perfusion, histochemistry, capillary density, fiber composition, mitochondrial density and oxidative metabolism, and mechanoreceptor function), and pulmonary (respiratory drive and pattern, lung compliance, bronchial reactivity, alveolar-capillary diffusion and ventilatory response to exercise) factors all have varying effects on exercise capacity in individual patients with HF [81].

Cardiac.   During exercise in normal subjects, cardiac output increases four- to six-fold due to a two- to four-fold increase in heart rate from basal levels and 20% to 50% augmentation of stroke volume [120]. Both enhanced contractility and peripheral vasodilation effect greater ventricular emptying. Compared with normal subjects, patients with HF exhibit abnormally low maximal cardiac output due to both more modest increments in stroke volume and heart rate during exercise. The predominant mechanism to augment cardiac output in patients with HF is an increase in heart rate.

Resting indices of ventricular function, such as ejection fraction, correlate poorly with maximal exercise capacity in patients with HF [122]. The most important single factor in limiting exercise capacity in chronic HF is the inability of the left ventricle to augment work appropriately and deliver an adequate volume of oxygenated blood to metabolizing tissues in response to the increasing demand [120]. Not surprisingly, left ventricular stroke work index was the single most potent predictor of prognosis in a study combining measurement of rest and exercise respiratory gas exchange, hemodynamics, and echocardiographic features during symptom-limited exercise testing in patients with advanced HF [123]. In patients with similar ranges of peak oxygen uptake, dobutamine-stimulated left ventricular functional reserve has been shown to be a further discriminator of prognosis [124]. In addition to left ventricular functional reserve, exercise-induced increases in mitral regurgitation limit stroke volume adaptation during exercise and limit exercise capacity as well [125].

Diastolic dysfunction is also exacerbated during exercise and contributes to exercise intolerance in patients with either systolic and diastolic HF [126]. A reduction in cardiac cycle-dependent changes in the thoracic aortic area and distensibility are associated with exercise intolerance in elderly patients with apparently isolated diastolic HF [127].

Peripheral Blood Flow.   Peripheral vasodilatory capacity is impaired in HF patients [128], particularly failure of exercise-induced vasodilation [129]. Upregulation of multiple neurohormonal axes, including the sympathetic nervous, renin-angiotensin, and endothelin systems, likely account for this blunted vasodilatory reserve [120]. There is evidence that at least a component of blunted reactivity results from ''vascular deconditioning'' that is partially reversible with training [130]. Endothelial dysfunction, particularly attenuated nitric oxide mediated endothelial-dependent vasodilation, contributes substantially to the altered distribution of cardiac output in HF patients [131,132]. Exercise training improves endothelial function and may help to restore a more normal pattern of cardiac output distribution [133].

Skeletal Muscle.   Skeletal muscle gross and ultrastructural morphology [134], fiber type [135], innervation, perfusion, and metabolism are abnormal in HF [136,137]. Skeletal muscle mass predicts exercise capacity in noncachectic HF patients [138]. Skeletal muscle adaptations may differ in men and women, with men exhibiting abnormalities not due to deconditioning alone [139]. Apoptosis has been reported in the skeletal muscle of patients with HF, the magnitude of which is associated with the severity of exercise limitation and the degree of muscle atrophy [140]. Metabolic abnormalities also occur in the skeletal muscle unrelated to blood flow [141] and are partly due to decreased levels of mitochondrial oxidative enzymes [142]. The abnormality in skeletal muscle oxidative capacity in HF may also derive from nonmitochondrial abnormalities [143]. Although studies are conflicting, reductions in capillary density are likely not an important mechanism resulting in skeletal muscle dysfunction [120]. Patients with HF exhibit, however, a disproportionate reduction in the distribution of cardiac output to exercising muscle relative to normal subjects [144]. Skeletal muscle training programs may partially offset this disproportionate reduction.

Ergoreflexes. Specific signals arising from exercising muscle may be abnormally enhanced in HF patients and contribute to the resultant abnormal integrated hemodynamic, autonomic, and ventilatory responses to exercise [120]. Ergoreceptors in skeletal muscles are stimulated by metabolic acidosis leading to peripheral vasoconstriction and heart rate acceleration of [145]. Centrally, these ergoreceptors mediate hyperventilation, increase sympathetic outflow, and lead to greater increases in vasoconstriction. Exercise training decreases this hyper-responsiveness [146].

Lungs. Ventilatory efficiency (the rate of increase of minute ventilation per unit of increase carbon dioxide production: VE/VCO_2 slope) is impaired and correlates with exercise limitation and survival [147]. Assessment of ventilatory response to exercise improves risk stratification in patients with chronic HF compared to peak oxygen uptake alone [148], including in patients with preserved exercise capacity [149].

Effects of Gene Polymorphisms on Exercise Capacity. Gene polymorphisms may influence functional capacity in HF patients. Relative to patients with "wild-type" genotypes, exercise capacity is reduced in HF patients with the Gly389 polymorphism of the β_1 allele [150], the Ile64 polymorphism of the β_2 receptor allele [151], and those homozygous for the angiotensin-converting enzyme deletion (DD) genotype [152].

Clinical Assessment of Functional and Exercise Capacity

New York Heart Association

The NYHA functional classification [153] is subject to considerable interobserver variation and is not sensitive to changes in exercise capacity [2]. Correlations between NYHA class, 6-WT (walk test) and peak oxygen uptake have been modest at best in HF populations, and within a given functional class large variations in mortality occur [154]. Despite these limitations, NYHA classification remains a predictor of prognosis in broad HF populations. Specific activity scales have been developed that equate metabolic equivalents to activities of daily living [155]. Other functional status instruments have been developed, but none have been as widely adopted for routine clinical practice as the NYHA classification [10,156–158]. The Minnesota Living with Heart Failure Questionnaire (MLHF) was developed to assess the patient's self-reported perceptions of the effects of heart failure and its treatment on daily life [159]. This 21-question instrument incorporates both a physical domain (dyspnea, fatigue) and an emotional domain. At present, the MLHF is the mostly widely adopted instrument used in most interventional HF studies of pharmacological agents and devices.

6-Walk Test

The 6-Walk Test (6-WT) was developed for use in elderly, frail HF patients [160]. In 898 patients from the SOLVD study, NYHA class and quartiles of 6-WT results were only moderately correlated but the 6-WT results were strongly and independently associated with morbidity and mortality in multivariate modeling [161]. In the RESOLVD pilot study, test-retest reliability of the 6-WT was very good (intraclass correlation coefficient 0.90), but 6-WT results were only weakly inversely correlated to quality of life scores (r =

-0.26) and NYHA class (r $=$ -0.43) [162]. In a study of 315 patients with moderate to severe HF, the 6-WT did not correlate with resting hemodynamics, was only moderately correlated to exercise capacity, and was not selected as an independent predictor of prognosis in multivariate models, including NYHA class and peak oxygen uptake [163]. In a study of severe HF, the 6-WT distance was not a reliable surrogate of peak oxygen uptake or predictor of prognosis [164]. In a separate study of 113 patients with severe HF (mean LVEF [left ventricular ejection fraction] 21%), 6-WT was weakly correlated to right atrial pressure (r $=$ -0.28) and LVEF (r $=$ -033) but not to pulmonary capillary wedge pressure or resting cardiac output, and was not an independent predictor of 1 year survival in multivariate models [165]. Even in elderly frail patients, the 6-WT appears to be reasonably reproducible with an intraclass correlation coefficient of 0.91 reported [166]. Peak oxygen uptake measured during the 6-WT averages 15% lower than peak oxygen uptake measured during formal symptom-limited cardiopulmonary exercise testing in HF patients [167].

Cardiopulmonary ExerciseTesting

Presently, symptom-limited cardiopulmonary exercise testing with simultaneous respiratory gas exchange assessment of peak oxygen uptake remains the most widely used method of determining the maximal exercise capacity and prognosis of patients with advanced HF [81,168,169]. Peak oxygen uptake determination remains critically important in formulating the appropriateness and timing of cardiac transplantation [170]. Accurate determination of peak oxygen uptake requires that patients exceed the anaerobic threshold during exercise. Peak oxygen uptake is 10% to 20% higher by treadmill compared to bicycle exercise protocols. Peak oxygen uptake correlates poorly with resting hemodynamics [123]. Inclusion of additional variables to peak oxygen uptake in multivariate models improves prediction of prognosis in advanced HF [171]. Recently, B-type natriuretic peptide levels were reported to predict exercise capacity in chronic HF [172].

Response to Pharmacological Agents

Multiple therapies improve exercise capacity but are not necessarily associated with improved survival (e.g., enoximone) [173]. Recently, sildenafil has been reported to reduce the Ve-VCO$_2$ slope during the exercise and modestly improve peak oxygen uptake in chronic HF patients [174]. Controlled studies of coenzyme Q$_{10}$ have not shown improvements in exercise capacity [175].

Exercise Training

Published studies suggest that peak oxygen uptake improves 12% to 31% during exercise training in HF patients [120]. There are parallel improvements in 6-WT performance and the ventilatory threshold [176]. Long-term moderate exercise training in patients with HF results in improved quality of life and exercise capacity, and modest attenuation of left ventricular remodeling, including reductions in ventricular volumes [120,177,178]. Improvement in left ventricular ejection fraction is less consistently observed [120,177,178]. Exercise training also improves endothelial function and partially attenuates sympathetic neural overactivity [179]. Limited data suggest that exercise training is effective in older adults with HF [180]. Training programs in carefully selected patients are safe and result in worthwhile improvements in exercise capacity [181]. The duration, supervision, venue of training, volume of working muscle, intensity and mode of training, and concurrent medical therapies all effect the results of exercise training and benefits may not persist without ongoing maintenance [182]. The effects of exercise training on survival are presently unknown and await longer-term trials [120].

Mitral Regurgitation

Mitral regurgitation (MR) frequently accompanies progressive ventricular dilatation without intrinsic pathology of the mitral valve apparatus [183,184]. Such "functional" mitral regurgitation is most commonly due to lateral migration of the papillary muscles and inappropriate "tethering" of the mitral valve leaflets during systole (Chapter 6) [185,186]. Mitral annular dilation, papillary muscle, or subadjacent myocardial hypokinesis may also contribute [187,188]. The regurgitant volume returned to the left ventricle increases preload and adversely affects ventricular remodeling [3]. Not surprisingly, moderate to severe mitral regurgitation is associated with increased morbidity and mortality in chronic HF [189,190]. Careful quantitation of the severity of regurgitation by resting Doppler echocardiography and myocardial "contractile reserve" are both critical in the assessment of the timing and appropriateness of isolated mitral valve repair or replacement in patients with chronic HF and severe mitral regurgitation [191,192]. Increased mitral regurgitant volume during exercise echocardiography correlates well with reduced exercise tolerance [193,194] and higher risk of adverse events [195]. Tailored hemodynamic therapy with optimization of filling pressures and volumes, cardiac resynchronization therapy, and positive inotropic pharmacological agents all reduce the degree of functional mitral regurgitation [196–198]. Encouraging intermediate-term results have been reported from select centers performing mitral valve repair in patients with advanced symptomatic HF and severe mitral regurgitation (Chapter 22) [199–201]. Although moderate MR frequently accompanies ischemic cardiomyopathy and marks a worse prognosis [202], most observational studies to date have been unable to demonstrate improved outcomes when mitral valve repair or replacement is routinely performed in addition to coronary artery bypass grafting [203].

Sleep Apnea

Central sleep apnea (CSA) afflicts approximately 33% to 40% of patients with symptomatic HF [204–208]. In HF patients with CSA, the chronic hyperventilation resulting from pulmonary congestion is exacerbated by increased venous return in the supine position [204]. Apnea is then induced by a greater degree of hyperventilation and further reduction in $PaCO_2$ until terminated by a rise in $PaCO_2$ above the ventilation stimulatory threshold. An enhanced sensitivity to carbon dioxide appears to predispose HF patients to CSA [209]. Risk factors include male sex, hypocapnia, atrial fibrillation, and increasing age, but not obesity [210]. CSA is distinctly less common in women with HF [204]. In HF patients, sleep apnea (central or obstructive) increases blood pressure [211], atrial and ventricular dysrhythmias [212], sympathetic activation [213], filling pressures [214], and the risk of symptomatic deterioration. Since thoracic mechanics remain unaltered, ventricular afterload is not increased, and the effects of CSA on ventricular remodeling are less clear than for obstructive sleep apnea (OSA) [204]. Therapy of OSA with continuous positive airway pressure (CPAP) during sleep improves symptoms and ventricular function [215,216]. Small observational studies have also reported lower mortality in patients with CSA treated with CPAP, but these studies await confirmation in larger trials. Nonetheless, most physicians recommend CPAP for HF patients with documented CSA. Empiric CPAP in the absence of documented CSA has not been studied in HF patients to date. Atrial overdrive pacing may reduce the number of episodes of sleep apnea [217]. OSA afflicts approximately 10% of patients with heart failure [218]. Given the prevalence, morbidity, and ready therapy of either type of sleep apnea in patients with heart failure, it is incumbent on the clinician to screen all patients with symptomatic heart failure for sleep apnea and provide appropriate therapy. Since long-term compliance with CPAP is only 50% to 80% [218], apparent treatment "failures" are commonly encountered in practice.

"Cardiorenal" Phenomena

In chronic HF, deterioration in renal function may result from diminished cardiac output and corresponding reduced glomerular filtration, alterations in the distribution of cardiac output, intrarenal vasoregulation, alterations in circulatory volume, the degree and type of neurohormonal activation, and the multiplicative toxic effects of medications [219]. As a result, patients frequently exhibit altered renal function, including dysregulation of sodium and potassium homeostasis, a greater propensity to azotemia in response to vasodilators or diuretics, reduction in renal clearance of metabolic products or medications, and refractoriness to previously effective doses or schedules of oral or intravenous diuretic therapies [220]. Approximately 25% of hospitalized HF patients exhibit deterioration in renal function despite appropriate medical therapy [221]. In such hospitalized patients, a rise in serum creatinine of 0.1 to 0.5 mg/dL is associated with a longer hospital length of stay and increased in-hospital mortality [222].

This constellation of poorly understood physiological mechanisms and unpredictable clinical responsiveness to appropriate therapies has been termed the "cardiorenal" syndrome [70]. Renal insufficiency is associated with increased mortality in both asymptomatic and symptomatic ambulatory HF patients (Figure 4) [219,223,224]. Patients with advanced HF often exhibit unexpected and unpredictable alterations in renal function, which render management challenging [70]. Hyponatremia is an important prognostic marker in advanced HF and predicts mortality in ambulatory patients with symptomatic HF [225], advanced HF [171], and in patients hospitalized with HF [226].

Cardiac Cachexia

Cardiac cachexia is usually defined as a nonintentional loss of greater than 7.5% of the "usual" weight of the patient [227]. Cardiac cachexia is associated with increased mortal-

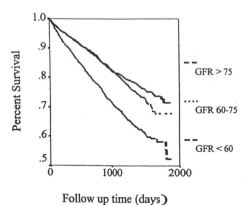

Follow up time (days)

Figure 4 Kaplan-Meier survival analysis by level of glomerular filtration rate at presentation for ambulatory heart failure patients who participated in the Studies of Left Ventricular Dysfunction (SOLVD) trial. (From Ref. 222a.)

ity in chronic HF independent of age, NYHA class, and LVEF and peak oxygen consumption [228]. Compared to noncachectic patients, cachectic HF patients evidence loss of lean muscle, adipose and bone tissue, and raised plasma levels of norepinephrine, epinephrine, cortisol, plasma renin activity, aldosterone, TNF-α (tumor necrosis factor-α) and growth hormone, but reduced levels of insulin-like growth factor 1 and typically high-levels of insulin resistance [227,229–232]. Interestingly, levels of leptin, a hormone secreted in response to TNF-α that decreases food intake and increases energy expenditure, appear to be inappropriately low rather than high in cachectic HF patients [233]. A poorly understood multifactorial process resulting from intersecting neurohormonal and inflammatory mediators, cardiac cachexia forebodes an ominous prognosis and bears appropriate recognition and response by practitioners [230]. No specific therapy to counteract cardiac cachexia yet exists [234].

Anemia

Anemia occurs in up to 17% of patients with HF and is associated with a modest increase in all-cause mortality (Fig. 5) [235–238]. Anemia is less prevalent in recent-onset HF [239]. Potential mechanisms remain speculative but include the effects of chronic disease, excessive cytokine production, malnutrition, and plasma volume overload [240]. Small trials to date have reported that therapy with subcutaneous erythropoietin and iron may not only restore red cell mass but also improve symptoms and exercise capacity in patients with moderate to severe chronic HF [240–242]. There may be little benefit to normalization of the hematocrit via erythropoietin therapy in patients with HF receiving chronic hemodialysis [243]. Elucidation of the role of erythropoietin therapy in patients with HF and anemia awaits larger randomized studies.

Psychiatric

In observational studies to date, approximately 30% to 60% of hospitalized HF patients [244,245] and 10% to 20% of ambulatory HF patients suffer from depression [246–248]. Despite similar measures of objective functional capacity, depressed patients tend to report

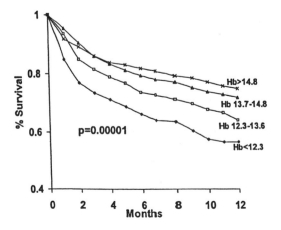

Figure 5 Kaplan-Meier survival analysis for ambulatory heart failure patients enrolled in a comprehensive disease management program stratified by quartile of hemoglobin (Hg) level. (From Ref. 236.)

worse physical functional ability than nondepressed patients [249]. Depression is also associated with reduced survival [247,250,251] and a 26% to 29% increase in the costs of care [252]. Disease management programs for HF may also reduce symptoms of depression and improve quality of life [253]. The prevalence of anxiety does not appear to be increased in HF patients, although studies have been few [244]. A sense of perceived control reduces emotional distress in HF patients, including depression and anxiety [254].

PROGNOSIS

Older studies from the Framingham Heart Study reported in excess of a 50% 5-year mortality for patients with symptomatic HF, and no difference in survival among patients diagnosed between 1948 and 1974 compared with patients diagnosed between 1975 and 1988 [255]. A more recent study from the Framingham group, however, reported a reduction in 30-day, 1-year and 5-year age-adjusted mortality rates in heterogenous cohorts of both men (from 12%, 30%, and 70% to 11%, 28%, and 59%, respectively) and women (from 18%, 28%, and 57% to 10%, 24%, and 45%, respectively) comparing the periods 1950–1969 to 1990–1999 [13].

Observational studies from selected academic centers have reported improved survival in patients with idiopathic dilated cardiomyopathy [256] and advanced HF [154,257]. A large observational study from Scotland noted improved survival in HF patients hospitalized between 1986 and 1995, with declines in case-fatality rates in men and women of 26% and 17% at 30-days; and from 18% and 15% at 1-year, respectively [258]. An observational study of community-dwelling elderly persons found a substantial increase in death from HF with adjusted hazard ratios of 1.25 in patients with no HF and borderline LV function, 1.83 in patients with no HF and impaired LV function, 1.48 in patients with HF and normal LV function, 2.4 in patients with HF and borderline LV function, and 1.88 in patients with HF and impaired LV function [259]. In a population based observational study of 38,702 consecutive unselected community-dwelling patients hospitalized with HF between 1994 and 1997, the crude 30-day and 1-year case-fatality rates after first admission for HF were 11.6% and 33.1%, respectively [260].

The contemporary combination of ''triple'' neurohormonal therapy with ACEI, beta-blockers, and aldosterone antagonists coupled with appropriate implantation of ICDs may reduce the annual mortality of advanced symptomatic heart failure by up to 75% (chronic therapy of heart failure is discussed in more detail in Chapters 12 and 13) In more recent clinical trials, including COPERNICUS, enrolling noninotropic dependent patients with NYHA IV heart failure, the 1-year mortality in the placebo group was 18.5% [261]. However, in a more fragile cohort of inotrope-dependent patients in the REMATCH trial, the mortality in the medical therapy group was 75% at one year [262]. A comprehensive tabulation of the mortality results of recent clinical trials is summarized in Eichorn's comprehensive review [154].

Despite these gratifying results of chronic pharmacological and device therapies, the number of deaths due to HF has increased in the United States, from 19,936 in 1979 to 43,010 in 1995, an increase of 116% [154]. The improved survival reported in interventional pharmacological trials compared to observational population-based studies in HF is likely due to differences in clinical characteristics (age, comorbidities, intensity of pharmacological and device therapies), study exclusion criteria (recent infarction or revascularization, dementia, stroke, life-limiting illness), adherence to prescribed care and process of care (frequent study visits, for example). In particular, factors for improved survival include better dosing of ACI inhibitors, higher penetration of use of beta-blockers and aldosterone antagonists, increased use of aspirin and statin therapy in patients with coronary artery disease, decreased used of calcium channel blockers and type I antiarrhythmics, increasing indications for ICDs and amiodarone, biventricular pacing, ventricular assist devices and cardiac transplantation, specialized physician and nurse practitioners with expertise in heart failure, comprehensive HF centers, and use of HF disease management programs.

PREDICTION OF SURVIVAL

To date, no single study has simultaneously evaluated the more than 50 variables associated with prognosis in chronic HF [154]. In his recent comprehensive review of published studies, Eichhorn identified norepinephrine levels, cardiac norepinephrine spillover, BNP levels, LVEF, peak oxygen uptake, advanced age, history of symptomatic ventricular arrhythmias or sudden cardiac death, and therapy with ACE inhibitors, beta-blockers, aldosterone antagonists, implantation of an ICD and cardiac transplantation as the most important predictors of outcome in chronic HF [154].

Of particular note, LVEF may lose its predictive accuracy in patients with advanced HF symptoms [263,264] or in patients with an LVEF greater than 45% [265]. Among hemodynamic variables measured during symptom-limited cardiopulmonary exercise testing, peak left ventricular stroke work index is the single most informative parameter [123]. Patients admitted to the hospital with simultaneous signs of congestion and hypoperfusion have a higher adjusted hospital mortality [266]. The presence of an S3 gallop and elevated jugular venous pressure upon enrollment into the SOLVD treatment and prevention trials predicted mortality [75,267].

The prediction of sudden cardiac death, which afflicts approximately one-third to one-half of patients with chronic systolic HF, continues to be problematic [118,119]. The prognostic importance of the nearly ubiquitous asymptomatic, nonsustained ventricular tachycardia detected in patients with symptomatic heart failure as a predictor of sudden death remains controversial. In the ATLAS trial, use of beta-blockers or amiodarone was associated with decreased sudden death risk [225]. The clinical prediction of sudden cardiac death and its prophylaxis are discussed in detail in Chapter 19.

CONCLUSION

This chapter has focused on the epidemiology, pathophysiology, and clinical syndrome of HF with particular emphasis on clinical presentation and diagnosis. The last few decades have proved an exciting time in our understanding of the pathophysiology of HF and improvements of therapy. The rather impressive results of ''antiremodeling'' therapy with current ''triple'' neurohormonal antagonists (ACE inhibitors, beta-blockers, and aldosterone antagonists), coupled with that achieved with biventricular pacing and the decease in sudden cardiac death risk with appropriate implantation of ICDs, has ushered in a new era of therapy for chronic heart failure. On the not too distant horizon, a more precise understanding of the pathophysiology and clinical course of HF, based in large part on elucidation of genetic determinants and interactions, may provide an opportunity for a more targeted and customized application of therapy than is now possible. The decades to come will undoubtedly witness a whole new era of mature, durable, and miniaturized devices and novel replacement therapies. It is not only conceivable, but indeed likely, that future therapeutic options will eventually render the all present, all-too-common clinical syndrome of HF a conquered disease of the past.

REFERENCES

1. American Heart Association, Heart Disease and Stroke Statistics-2003 Update. Dallas. TX: American Heart Association, 2002: 2002. page.
2. Hunt SA, et al. ACC/AHA guidelines for the evaluation and management of chronic heart failure in the adult: a report of the American College of Cardiology/American Heart Association Task Force on Practice Guidelines (Committee ro Review the 1995 Guidelines for the Evaluation and Management of Heart Failure). American College of Cardiology Web Site. Available at: htpp://www.acc.org/clinical/guidelines/failure/hf_index.htm, 2001.
3. Jessup M, Brujena S. Heart failure. N Engl J Med 2003; 348:2007–2018.
4. Katz AM. Pathophysiology of heart failure: identifying targets for pharmacotherapy. Med Clinics North Am 2003; 87:303–316.
5. Angeja BG, Grossman W. Evaluation and management of diastolic heart failure. Circulation 2003; 107:659–663.
6. Burkhoff D, Maurer MS, Pacher M. Heart failure with a normal ejection fraction: Is it really a disorder of diastolic function? Circulation 2003; 107:656–658.
7. Dec GW, Foster V. Idiopathic dilated cardiomyopathy. New Engl J Med 1994; 331:1564–1575.
8. Adams KF. New epidemiologic perspectives concerning mild-to-moderate heart failure. Am J Med 2001; 110(7A):6S–13S.
9. Massie BM, Shah NB. Evolving trends in the epidemiology factors of heart failure: rationale for preventive strategies and comprehensive disease management. Am Heart J 1997; 133:703–712.
10. Packer M, et al. Consensus recommendations for the management of heart failure. Am J Cardiol 1999; 83(2A):1A–38A.
11. Ho KKL, et al. The epidemiology of heart failure: the Framingham Study. J Am Coll Cardiol 1993; 22(suppl A):6A–13A.
12. Lloyd-Jones D. The risk of congestive heart failure: sobering lessons from the Framingham Heart Study. Curr Cardiol Rep 2001; 3:184–190.
13. Levy D, et al. Long-term trends in the incidence and survival with heart failure. N Engl J Med 2002; 347:1397–1402.
14. Rich MW. Epidemiology, pathophysiology, and etiology of congestive heart failure in older adults. J Am Geriatr Soc 1997; 45:968–974.
15. Wang TJ, et al. The epidemiology of "asymptomatic" left ventricular systolic dysfunction: implications for screening. Ann Intern Med 2003; 138:907–916.
16. Redfield MM, et al. Burden of systolic and diastolic ventricular dysfunction in the community: appreciating the scope of the heart failure epidemic. JAMA 2003; 289:194–202.
17. O'Connell JB, Bristow MR. Economic impact of heart failure in the United States: time for a different approach. J Heart Lung Transplant 1994; 13:S107–S112.
18. Boccuzzi SJ. Economics and cost-effectiveness in evaluating the value of cardiovascular therapies. Angiotensin-converting enzyme inhibitors in the management of congestive heart failure: a pharmaceutical industry perspective. Am Heart J 1999; 137(5):S120–S122.
19. Towbin JA, Bowles NE. The failing heart. Nature 2002; 415:227–233.
20. Hoshijima M, Chien KR. Mixed signal in heart failure: cancer rules. J Clin Invest 2002; 109:849–855.
21. Fatkin D, et al. Missense mutations in the rod domain of the lamin A/C gene as causes of dilated cardiomyopathy and conduction-system disease. N Engl J Med 1999; 341:1715–1724.
22. Kamisago M, et al. Mutations in sarcomere protein genes as a cause of dilated cardiomyopathy. N Engl J Med 2000; 342:1688–1696.
23. Dalakas MC, et al. Desmin myopathy, a skeletal myopathy with cardiomyopathy caused by mutations in the desmin gene. N Engl J Med 2000; 342:770–80.
24. Franz WM, et al. Association of nonsense mutation of dystrophin gene with disruption of sarcoglycan complex in X-linked dilated cardiomyopathy. Lancet 2000; 355:1781–1785.
25. Mestroni L, et al. Familial dilated cardiomyopathy: evidence for genetic and phenotypic heterogeneity. J Am Coll Cardiol 1999; 34:181–190.

26. Brodsky GL, et al. Lamin A/C gene mutation associated with dilated cardiomyopathy with variable skeletal muscle involvement. Circulation 2000; 101:473–476.

27. Kelly DP, Strauss AW. Inherited cardiomyopathies. N Engl J Med 1994; 330:913–918.

28. Fadic R, et al. Brief report: deficiency of a dystrophin-associated glycoprotein (adhalin) in a patient with muscular dystrophy and cardiomyopathy. N Engl J Med 1996; 334:362–366.

29. Muntoni F, et al. Brief report: deletion of the dystrophin muscle-promoter region associated with X-linked dilated cardiomyopathy. N Engl J Med 1993; 329:921–925.

30. Small KM, et al. Synergistic polymorphisms of beta-one and alpha2C-adrenergic receptors and the risk of congestive heart failure. N Engl J Med 2002; 347:1135–1142.

31. Exner DV, et al. Lesser response to angiotensin-converting-enzyme inhibitor therapy in black as compared with white patients with left ventricular dysfunction. N Engl J Med 2001; 344: 1351–1357.

32. Yancy CW, et al. Race and the response to adrenergic blockade with carvedilol in patients with chronic heart failure. N Engl J Med 2001; 344:1358–1365.

33. Wood AJJ. Racial differences in the response to drugs—pointers to genetic differences. New Engl J Med 2001; 344:1393–1396.

34. Katz AM. Physiology of the Heart. 3rd ed. PA. Lippincott: Philadelphia, 2001.

35. Katz AM. Heart Failure: Pathophysiology, Molecular Biology, and Clinical Management. 1st ed.. PA. Lippincott: Philadelphia, 2000.

36. Houser SR, Margulies KB. Is depressed myocyte contractility centrally involved in heart failure? Circ Res 2003; 92:350–358.

37. Francis GS. Pathophysiology of chronic heart failure. Am J Med 2001; 101(7A):37S–46S.

38. Nadal-Ginard B, et al. Myocyte death, growth, and regeneration in cardiac hypertrophy and failure. Circ Res 2003; 92:139–150.

39. Spinale FG. Matrix metalloproteinases: regulation and dysregulation in the failing heart. Circ Res 2002; 90:520–530.

40. Mann DL. Inflammatory medicators and the failing heart: past, present and the foreseeable future. Circ Res 2002; 91:988–998.

41. Bers DM. Cardiac excitation-contraction coupling. Nature 2002; 415:198–205.

42. Lowes BD, et al. Myocardial gene expression in dilated cardiomyopathy treated with beta-blocking agents. N Engl J Med 2002; 346:1357–1365.

43. Loh E, et al. Common variant in AMPD1 gene predicts improved clinical outcome in patients with heart failure. Circulation 1999; 99:1422–1425.

44. McNamara DM, et al. Pharmacogenetic interactions between beta-blocker therapy and the angiotensin-converting enzyme deletion polymorphism in patients with congestive heart failure. Circulation 2001; 103:1644–1648.

45. McNamara DM, et al. Effect of the Asp298 variant of endothelial nitric oxide synthase on survival for patients with congestive heart failure. Circulation 2003; 107:1598–1602.

46. Vasan RS, et al. Congestive heart failure in subjects with normal versus reduced left ventricular ejection fraction: prevalence and mortality in a population-based cohort. J Am Coll Cardiol 1999; 33:1948–1955.

46a. Working Group Report. How to diagnose diastolic heart failure: European Study Group on Diastolic Heart Failure. Eur Heart J 1998; 19:990–1003.

47. Senni M, R. MM. Heart failure with preserved systolic function: a different natural history?. J Am Coll Cardiol 2001; 38:1277–1282.

48. Petrie MC, Caruana L, Berry C, McMurry JJ. "Diastolic heart failure" or heart failure caused by subtle left ventricular systolic dysfunction?. Heart 2002; 87:29–31.

49. Zile MR, Brutsgert DL. New concepts in diastolic dysfunction and diastolic heart failure: part I diagnosis, prognosis, and measurements of diastolic function. Circulation 2002; 105: 1387–1393.

50. Zile MR, Brutsgert DL. New concepts in diastolic dysfunction and diastolic heart failure: diagnosis, prognosis, and measurements of diastolic function: part II causal mechanisms and treatment. Circulation 2002; 105:1503–1508.

51. Vasan RS, Benjamin EJ, Levy D. Congestive heart failure with normal left ventricular systolic function: clinical approaches to the diagnosis and treatment of diastolic heart failure. Arch Intern Med 1996; 156:146–157.

52. Vasan RS, Levy D. Defining diastolic heart failure: a call for standardized diagnostic criteria. Circulation 2000; 101:2118–2121.

53. Lakatta EG. Arterial and cardiac aging: major shareholders in cardiovascular disease enterprises: part III: cellular and molecular clues to heart and arterial aging. Circulation 2003; 107:490–497.

54. Kawaguchi M, et al. Combined ventricular systolic and arterial stiffening in patients with heart failure and preserved ejection fraction: implications for systolic and diastolic reserve limitations. Circulation 2003; 107:714–720.

55. Yu CM, et al. Progression of systolic abnormalities in patients with "isolated" diastolic heart failure and diastolic dysfunction. Circulation 2002; 105:1195–1201.

56. Kitzman DW, et al. Pathophysiological characterization of isolated diastolic heart failure in comparison to systolic heart failure. JAMA 2002; 288:2144–2150.

57. Zile MR, et al. Heart failure with a normal ejection fraction: is measurement of diastolic function necessary to make the diagnosis of diastolic heart failure?. Circulation 2001; 104: 779–782.

58. Brilla CG, Funck RC, Rupp H. Lisinopril-mediated regression of myocardial fibrosis in patients with hypertensive heart disease. Circulation 2000; 102:1388–1393.

59. Massie BM, Yamani MH. Chronic heart failure: diagnosis and management. In Poole-Wilson PA, et al, Ed. Heart Failure. New York: Churchill Livingstone, 1997:551–566.

60. Cheitlin MD. Can clinical evaluation differentiate diastolic from systolic heart failure? Is so, is it important?. Am J Med 2002; 112:496–497.

61. Badgett RG, Lucey CR, Mulrow CD. Can the clinical examination diagnose left-sided heart failure in adults?. JAMA 1997; 277:1712–1719.

62. Thomas JT, et al. Utility of history, physical examination, electrocardiogram, and chest radiograph for differentiating normal from decreased systolic function in patients with heart failure. Am J Med 2002; 112:437–445.

63. Ghali JK, et al. Bedside diagnosis of preserved versus impaired left ventricular systolic function in heart failure. Am J Cardiol 1991; 67:1002–1006.

64. Harlan WR, et al. Chronic congestive heart failure in coronary artery disease: clinical criteria. Ann Intern Med 1977; 86:133–138.

65. Marantz PR, et al. The relationship between left-ventricular systolic function and congestive heart failure diagnosed by clinical criteria. Circulation 1988; 77:607–612.

66. Mattleman SJ, et al. Reliability of bedside evaluation in determining left ventricular ejection function: correlation with left ventricular ejection fraction determined by radionuclide ventriculography. J Am Coll Cardiol 1983; 1:417–420.

67. Gadsboll N, et al. Symptoms and signs of heart failure in patients with myocardial infarction. reproducibility and relationship to chest x-ray, radionuclide ventriculography, and right heart catheterization. Eur Heart J 1989; 10:1017–1028.

68. Chakko C, et al. Clinical, radiographic, and hemodynamic correlations in chronic heart failure. Conflicting results may lead to inappropriate care. Am J Med 1991; 90:353–359.

68a. Harlan WR, Oberman A, Crimm R, Roseti R. Heart Failure. Ann Int Med 1977; 56:133–8.

69. Stevenson LW, Perloff JK. The limited reliability of physical signs for estimating hemodynamics in chronic heart failure. JAMA 1989; 261:884–888.

70. Nohria A, Lewis E, Stevenson LW. Medical management of advanced heart failure. JAMA 2002; 287:628–640.

71. Ewy GA. The abdominojugular test: technique and hemodynamic correlates. Ann Intern Med 1988; 109:456–460.

72. Butman SM, et al. Bedside cardiovascular examination in patients with severe chronic heart failure: importance of rest of inducible jugular venous distention. J Am Coll Cardiol 1993; 22:968–974.

73. Zema MJ, et al. Left ventricular dysfunction: beside Valsalva manoeuvre. Br Heart J 1980; 44:560–569.

74. Zema MJ, Caccovano M, K. P. Detection of left ventricular dysfunction in ambulatory subjects with the bedside Valsalva maneuver. Am J Med 1983; 75:241–248.

75. Drazner MH, et al. Prognostic importance of elevated jugular venous pressure and a third heart sound in patients with heart failure. New Engl J Med 2001; 345:574–581.

76. Drazner MH, et al. Relationship between right and left-sided filling pressures in 1000 patients with advanced heart failure. J Heart Lung Transplant 1999; 18:1126–1132.

77. McGee SR. Physical examination of venous pressure: a critical review. Am Heart J 1998; 136:10–18.

78. Ishmail AA, et al. Interobserver agreement by auscultation in the presence of a third heart sound in patients with chronic heart failure. Chest 1987; 91:870–873.

79. McKee PA, et al. The natural history of congestive heart failure. The Framingham Study. N Engl J Med 1971; 285:1441–1446.

80. Criteria Committee of the New York Heart Association. Nomenclature and Criteria for Diagnosis of Diseases of the Heart and Great Vessels. 7th ed.. Boston: Little, Brown, 1973.

81. Metra M, et al. Maximal and submaximal exercise testing in heart failure. J Cardiovasc Pharm 1998; 32(I):S36–S45.

82. Wilkins MR, Redondo J, Brown LA. The natriuretic-peptide family. Lancet 1997; 349: 1307–1310.

83. Levin ER, Gardner DG, Stevenson WK. Natriuretic peptides. New Engl J Med 1998; 339: 321–328.

84. Burger MR, de Bold AJ. BNP in decompensated heart failure: diagnostic, prognostic and therapeutic potential. Curr Opinion Invest Drugs 2001; 2:929–935.

85. Shapiro BP, et al. Use of plasma brain natriuretic peptide concentration to aid in the diagnosis of heart failure. Mayo Clin Proc 2003; 78:481–486.

86. Adams KF, Mathur VS, Chengheide M. B-type natriuretic peptide: from bench to bedside. Am Heart J 2003; 145:S34–S46.

87. Remme WJ, Swegberg K. European Society of Cardiology, comprehensive guidelines for the diagnosis and treatment of chronic heart failure: task force for the diagnosis and treatment of chronic heart failure of the European Society of Cardiology. Eur J Heart Fail 2002; 4: 11–22.

88. Maisel AS, et al. Rapid measurement of B-type natriuretic peptide in the emergency diagnosis of heart failure. N Engl J Med 2002; 347:161–167.

89. McCullough PA, Nowak RM, McCord J, Hollander JE, Herrmann HC, Steg PG, Duc P, Westheim A, Omland T, Knudsen CW, Storrow AB, Abraham WT, Lamba S, Wu AH, Perez A, Clopton P, Krishnaswamy P, Kazanegra R, Maisel AS. B-type natriuretic peptide and clinical judgment in emergency diagnosis of heart failure: analysis from Breathing Not Properly (BNP) Multinational Study. Circulation 2002; 106:416–422.

90. Dao Q, et al. Utility of B-type natriuretic peptide in the diagnosis of congestive heart failure in an urgent-care setting. J Am Coll Cardiol 2001; 37:379–385.

91. Collins SP, Ronan-Bentle S, Storrow AB. Diagnostic and prognostic usefulness of natriuretic peptides in emergency department patients with dyspnea. Ann Emerg Med 2003; 41(4): 532–545.

92. Richards AM, et al. Neurohumoral prediction of benefit from carvedilol in ischemic left ventricular dysfunction. Circulation 1999; 99:786.

93. Stanek B, Frey B, Mismann M. Prognostic evaluation of neurohumoral plasma level before and during beta-blocker therapy in advanced left ventricular dysfunction. J Am Coll Cardiol 2001; 38:436–42.

94. Troughton RW, et al. Treatment of heart failure guided by plasma aminoterminal brain natriuretic peptide (N-BNP) concentrations. Lancet 2000; 355:1126–1130.

95. Vasan RS, et al. Plasma natriuretic peptides for community screening for left ventricular hypertrophy and systolic dysfunction: The Framingham Heart Study. JAMA 2002; 288: 1252–1259.

96. de Lemos JA, et al. The prognostic value of B-type natriuretic peptide in patients with acute coronary syndromes. N Engl J Med 2001; 345:1014–1021.

97. Wang TJ, et al. Impact of age and sex on plasma natriuretic peptide levels in healthy adults. Am J Cardiol 2002; 90:254–258.

98. Tsutamoto T, et al. Attenuation of compensation of endogenous cardiac natriuretic peptide system in chronic heart failure: prognostic role of plasma brain natriuretic peptide concentra-

tion in patients with chronic symptomatic left ventricular dysfunction. Circulation 1997; 96: 509–516.

99. Berger R, et al. B-type natriuretic peptide predicts sudden death in patients with chronic heart failure. Circulation 2002; 105:2392–2397.

100. Anand IS, et al. Changes in brain natriuretic peptide and norepinephrine over time and mortality and morbidity in the Valsartan Heart Failure Trial (Val-HeFT). Circulation 2003; 107: 1278.

101. Vrtovec B, et al. Prolonged QTc interval and high B-type natriuretic peptide levels together predict mortality in patients with advanced heart failure. Circulation 2003; 107:1764–1769.

102. Wattingney WA, Mensah GA, Croft JB. Increasing trends in hospitalization for atrial fibrillation in the United States, 1985 through 1999: implications for primary prevention. Circulation 2003; 108:711–716.

103. Wang TJ, Larson MG, Levy D, Vasan RS, Leip EP, Wolf PA, D'Agostino RB, Murabito JM, Kannel WB, Benjamin EJ. Temporal relations of atrial fibrillation and congestive heart failure and their joint influence on mortality: the Framingham Heart Study. Circulation 2003; 107:2920–2925.

104. Hynes BJ, et al. Atrial fibrillation in patients with heart failure. Curr Opinion Cardiol 2003; 18:32–38.

105. Markides V, Prystowsky EN. Mechanisms underlying the development of atrial arrhythmias in heart failure. Heart Fail Rev 2002; 7:243–253.

106. Maisel WH, Stevenson LW. Atrial fibrillation in heart failure: epidemiology, pathophysiology, and rationale for therapy. Amer J Cardiol 2003; 91(6A):2D–8D.

107. Sanders P, et al. Electrical remodeling of the atria in congestive heart failure: Electrophysiological and electroanatomical mapping in humans. Circulation 2003; 108:1461–1468.

108. Falk RH. Atrial fibrillation. N Engl J Med 2001; 344:1067–1078.

109. Dries DL, et al. Atrial fibrillation is associated with an increased risk for mortality and heart failure progression in patients with asymptomatic and symptomatic left ventricular systolic dysfunction: a retrospective analysis of the SOLVD trials. J Am Coll Cardiol 1998; 32: 695–703.

110. Cleland JG, et al. Prevalence and incidence of arrhythmias and sudden death in heart failure. Heart Fail Rev 2002; 7:229–242.

111. Shinbane JS, et al. Tachycardia-associated cardiomyopathy: a review of animal models and clinical studies. J Am Coll Cardiol 1997; 29:709–715.

112. Khand AU, Cleland JG, Deedwania PC. Prevention of and medical therapy for atrial arrhythmias in heart failure. Heart Fail Rev 2002; 7:267–283.

113. Naccarelli GV, et al. Old and new antiarrhythmic drugs for converting and maintaining sinus rhythm in atrial fibrillation: comparative efficacy and results of trials. Amer J Cardiol 2003; 91(6A):15D–26D.

114. Lamas GA, et al. Ventricular pacing or dual-chamber pacing for sinus-node dysfunction. N Engl J Med 2002; 346:1854–1862.

115. Sweeney MO, et al. Adverse effects of ventricular pacing on heart failure and atrial fibrillation among patients with normal baseline QRS duration in a clinical trial of pacemaker therapy for sinus node dysfunction. Circulation 2003; 107:2932–2937.

116. Leon AR, et al. Cardiac resynchronization in patients with congestive heart failure and chronic atrial fibrillation: effect of upgrading to biventricular pacing after chronic right ventricular pacing. J Am Coll Cardiol 2002; 39:1258–1263.

117. Cooper JM, Katcher MS, Oz MV. Implantable devices for the treatment of atrial fibrillation. N Engl J Med 2002; 346:206–268.

118. Stevenson WG, Epstein LM. Predicting sudden death risk for heart failure patients in the implantable cardioverter-defibrillator age. Circulation 2003; 107:514–516.

119. Huikuri HV, et al. Prediction of sudden cardiac death: appraisal of the studies and methods assessing the risk of sudden arrhythmic death. Circulation 2003; 108:110–115.

120. Pina IL, Apstein CS, Balady GJ, Belardinelli R, Chaitman BR, Duscha BD, Fletcher BJ, Fleg JL, Myers JN, Sullivan MJ. American Heart Association Committee on exercise, rehabilitation, and prevention. Exercise and heart failure: a statement from the American Heart Associa-

tion Committee on exercise, rehabilitation and prevention. Circulation 2003; 107(8): 1210–1225.

121. Sullivan MJ, Hawthorne MH. Exercise intolerance in patients with chronic heart failure. Prog Cardiovasc Dis 1995; 38:1–22.

122. Franciosa JA, Park M, Levine TB. Lack of correlation between exercise capacity and indexes of resting left ventricular performance in heart failure. Am J Cardiol 1981; 47:33–39.

123. Metra M, et al. Use of cardiopulmonary exercise testing with hemodynamic monitoring in the prognostic assessment of ambulatory patients with chronic heart failure. J Am Coll Cardiol 1999; 33:943–950.

124. Paraskevaidis IA, Adamopoulos S, Kremastinos DT. Dobutamine echocardiographic study in patients with nonischemic dilated cardiomyopathy and prognostically borderline values of peak exercise oxygen consumption: 18-month follow-up study. J Am Coll Cardiol 2001; 37: 1685–1691.

125. Lapu-Bula R, Robert A, Van Craeynest D, D'Hondt AM, Gerber BL, Pasquet A, Melin JA, De Kock M, Vanoverschelde JL. Contribution of exercise-induced mitral regurgitation to exercise stroke volume and exercise capacity in patients with left ventricular systolic dysfunction. Circulation 2002; 106(11):1342–1348.

126. Little WC, Kitzman DW, Cheng CP. Diastolic dysfunction as a cause of exercise intolerance. Heart Fail Rev 2000; 5:310–316.

127. Hundley WG, et al. Cardiac cycle-dependent changes in aortic area and distensibility are reduced in older patients with isolated diastolic heart failure and correlate with exercise intolerance. J Am Coll Cardiol 2001; 38:796–802.

128. Zelis R, Mason DT, Braunwald E. A comparison of the effects of vasodilator stimuli on peripheral resistance vessels in normal subjects and in patients with congestive heart failure. J Clin Invest 1968; 47:960–970.

129. LeJemtel TH, et al. Failure to augment maximal limb blood flow in response to one-leg versus two-leg exercise in patients with severe heart failure. Circulation 1986; 74:245–251.

130. Sinoway LI, et al. A 30-day forearm work protocol increases maximal forearm blood flow. J Appl Physiol 1987; 62:1063–1067.

131. Kubo SH, et al. Endothelium-dependent vasodilation is attenuated in patients with heart failure. Circulation 1991; 84:1589–1596.

132. Gilligan DM, et al. Contribution of endothelium-derived nitric oxide to exercise-induced vasodilation. Circulation 1994; 90:2853–2858.

133. Hambrecht R, et al. Regular physical exercise corrects endothelial dysfunction and improves exercise capacity in patients with chronic heart failure. Circulation 1998; 98:2709–2715.

134. Sullivan MJ, Green HG, Cobb FR. Skeletal muscle biochemistry and histology in ambulatory patients with long-term heart failure. Circulation 1990; 81:518–527.

135. Drexler H, et al. Alterations of skeletal muscle in chronic heart failure. Circulation 1992; 85: 1751–1759.

136. Minotti J, et al. Impaired skeletal muscle function in patients with congestive heart failure: Relationship to systemic exercise performance. J Clin Invest 1991; 88:2077–2082.

137. Piepoli MF, et al. Skeletal muscle training in chronic heart failure. Acta Physiol Scand 2001; 171:295–303.

138. Cicoira M, et al. Skeletal muscle mass independently predicts peak oxygen consumption and ventilatory response during exercise in noncachectic patients with chronic heart failure. J Am Coll Cardiol 2001; 37:2080–2085.

139. Duscha BD, et al. Deconditioning fails to explain peripheral skeletal alterations in men with chronic heart failure. J Am Coll Cardiol 2002; 39:1170–1174.

140. Vescovo G, Volterrani M, Zennaro R, Sandri M, Ceconi C, Lorusso R, Ferrari R, Ambrosio GB, Libera L. Apoptosis in the skeletal muscle of patients with heart failure: investigation of clinical and biochemical changes. Heart 2000; 84(4):431–437.

141. Massie BM, et al. Skeletal muscle metabolism during exercise under ischemic conditions in congestive heart failure: evidence for abnormalities unrelated to blood flow. Circulation 1988; 78:320–326.

142. Sullivan MJ, Green HJ, Cobb FR. Altered skeletal muscle metabolic responses to exercise in chronic hear failure: relation to skeletal muscle aerobic enzyme activity. Circulation 1991; 84:1597–1607.

143. Mettauer B, et al. Oxidative capacity of skeletal muscle in heart failure patients versus sedentary or active control subjects. J Am Coll Cardiol 2001; 38:947–954.

144. Sullivan MJ, Cobb FR. Central hemodynamic response to exercise in patients with chronic heart failure. Chest 1992; 101(5):340S–346S.

145. McCloskey DI, Mitchell JH. Reflex cardiovascular and respiratory responses originating in exercising muscle. J Physiol 1972; 224:173–186.

146. Piepoli M, Clark AL, Volterrani M, Adamopoulos S, Sleight P, Coats AJS. Contribution of muscle afferent to the hemodynamic, autonomic, and ventilatory responses to exercise in patients with chronic heart failure: effects of physical training. Circulation 1996; 93:940–952.

147. Kleber FX, et al. Impairment of ventilatory efficiency in heart failure: prognostic impact. Circulation 2000; 101:2803–2809.

148. Corra U, et al. Ventilatory response to exercise improves risk stratification in patients with chronic heart failure and intermediate functional capacity. Am Heart J 2002; 143:418–426.

149. Ponikowski P, et al. Enhanced ventilatory response to exercise in patients with chronic heart failure and preserved exercise tolerance: marker of abnormal cardiorespiratory reflex control and predictor of poor prognosis. Circulation 2001; 103:967–972.

150. Wagoner LE, et al. Polymorphisms of the beta-1 adrenergic receptor predict exercise capacity in heart failure. Am Heart J 2002; 144:840–846.

151. Wagoner LE, et al. Polymorphisms of the beta-2 adrenergic receptor determine exercise capacity in patients with heart failure. Circulation 2000; 86:834–840.

152. Abraham MR, Olson LJ, Joyner MJ, Turner ST, Beck KC, Johnson BD. Angiotensin-converting enzyme genotype modulates pulmonary function and exercise capacity in treated patients with congestive stable heart failure. Circulation 2002; 106(14):1794–1799.

153. The Criteria Committee of the New York Heart Association. Nomenclature and Criteria for Diagnosis. 9th ed.. Boston: Little, Brown, 1994.

154. Eichhorn EJ. Prognosis determination in heart failure. Am J Med 2001; 110(7A):14S–35S.

155. Goldman L, Hashimoto B, Cook EF, Luscalzo A. A comparative reproducibility and validity of systems for assessing cardiovascular functional class: advantages of a new specific activity scale. Circulation 1981; 64:1227.

156. Green CP, et al. Development and evaluation of the Kansas City cardiomyopathy questionnaire: a new health status measure for heart failure. J Am Coll Cardiol 2000; 35:1245–1255.

157. Guyatt GH, et al. Development and testing of a new measure of health status for clinical trials in heart failure. J Gen Intern Med 1989; 4:101–107.

158. Feinstein AR, Fisher MB, Pigeon JG. Changes in dyspnea-fatigue ratings as indicators of quality of life in the treatment of congestive heart failure. Am J Cardiol 1989; 64:50–55.

159. Rector TS, Kubo S, Cohn J. Patients self-assessment of their congestive heart failure. Part 2: content, reliability and validity of a new measure: The Minnesota Living with Heart Failure Questionnaire. Heart Fail 1987; 3:198–209.

160. Guyatt GH, et al. The 6-minute walk: a new measure of exercise capacity in patients with chronic heart failure. Can Med Assoc J 1985; 132:919–923.

161. Bittner V, et al. Prediction of mortality and morbidity with a 6-minute walk test in patients with left ventricular dysfunction. JAMA 1993; 270:1702–1707.

162. Demers C, et al. Reliability, validity, and responsiveness of the six-minute walk test in patients with heart failure. Am Heart J 2001; 142:698–703.

163. Opasich C, et al. Six-minute walking performance in patients with moderate-to-severe heart failure: is it s useful indicator in clinical practice?. Eur Heart J 2001; 22:488–496.

164. Lucas C, et al. The 6-min walk and peak oxygen consumption in advanced heart failure: aerobic capacity and survival. Am Heart J 1999; 138:618–624.

165. Woo MA, et al. Six-minute walk test and heart rate variability: lack of association in advanced stages of heart failure. Am J Crit Care 1997; 6:348–354.

166. O'Keeffe ST, et al. Reproducibility and responsiveness of quality of life assessment and six minute walk test in elderly heart failure patients. Heart 1998; 80:377–382.

167. Faggiano P, et al. Assessment of oxygen uptake during the 6-minute walking test in patients with heart failure: preliminary experience with a portable device. Am Heart J 1997; 134: 203–206.

168. Lainchbury JG, Richards AM. Exercise testing in the assessment of chronic congestive heart failure. Heart 2002; 88:538–543.

169. Beniaminovitz A, Mancini DM. The role of exercise-based prognosticating algorithms in the selection of patients for heart transplantation. Curr Opin Cardiol 1999; 14:114–120.

170. Mancini DM, et al. Value of peak exercise oxygen consumption for optimal timing of cardiac transplantation in ambulatory patients with heart failure. Circulation 1991; 83:778–786.

171. Aaronson KD, et al. Development and prospective validation of a clinical index to predict survival in ambulatory patients referred for cardiac transplant evaluation. Circulation 1997; 95:2660–2267.

172. Kruger S, et al. Brain natriuretic peptide levels predict functional capacity in patients with chronic heart failure. J Am Coll Cardiol 2002; 40:718–722.

173. Lowes BD, et al. Low-dose enoximone improves exercise capacity in chronic heart failure. Enoximone Study Group. J Am Coll Cardiol 2000; 36:501–508.

174. Bocchi EA, et al. Sildenafil effects on exercise, neurohormonal activation, and erectile dysfunction in congestive heart failure: A double-blind, placebo-controlled, randomized study followed by a prospective treatment for erectile dysfunction. Circulation 2002; 106: 1097–1103.

175. Khatta M, et al. The effect of coenzyme Q10 in patients with congestive heart failure. Ann Intern Med 2000; 132:636–640.

176. Hambrecht R, et al. Physical training in patients with stable chronic heart failure: effects on cardiorespiratory fitness and ultrastructural abnormalities in leg muscles. J Am Coll Cardiol 1995; 25:1239–1249.

177. Giannuzzi P, et al. Antiremodeling effect of long-term exercise training in patients with stable chronic heart failure: results of the exercise in left ventricular dysfunction and chronic heart failure (ELVD-CHF) trial. Circulation 2003; 108:554–559.

178. Sullivan MF, Higginbotham MB, Cobb FR. Exercise training in patients with severe left ventricular dysfunction: hemodynamic and metabolic effects. Circulation 1988; 78:506–515.

179. Linke A, et al. Endothelial dysfunction in patients with chronic heart failure: systemic effects of lower-limb exercise training. J Am Coll Cardiol 2001; 37:392–397.

180. Fleg JL. Can exercise conditioning be effective in older heart failure patients?. Heart Fail Rev 2002; 7:99–103.

181. Coats AJ. Exercise and heart failure. Cardiol Clin 2001; 19:517–524.

182. Smart N, Fang ZY, Marwick TH. A practical guide to exercise training for heart failure patients. J Card Fail 2003; 9:49–58.

183. Otto CM. Evaluation and management of chronic mitral regurgitation. N Engl J Med 2001; 345:740–746.

184. Robbins JD, et al. Prevalence and severity of mitral regurgitation in chronic systolic heart failure. Am J Cardiol 2003; 91:360–362.

185. He S, et al. Integrated mechanism for functional mitral regurgitation: leaflet restriction versus coapting force: in vitro studies. Circulation 1997; 96:1826–1834.

186. Otsuji Y, et al. Restricted diastolic opening of the mitral leaflets in patients with left ventricular dysfunction: evidence for increased valve tethering. J Am Coll Cardiol 1998; 32:398–404.

187. Enriquez-Sarano M, Schaff HV, Frye RL. Mitral regurgitation: what causes the leakage is fundamental to the outcome of valve repair. Circulation 2003; 108:253–256.

188. Karagiannis SE, et al. Increased distance between mitral valve coaptation point and mitral annular plane: significance and correlations in patients with heart failure. Heart 2003; 89: 1174–1178.

189. Trichon BH, et al. Relation of frequency and severity of mitral regurgitation to survival among patients with left ventricular systolic dysfunction and heart failure. Am J Cardiol 2003; 91:538–543.

190. Koelling TM, et al. Prognostic significance of mitral regurgitation and tricuspid regurgitation in patients with left ventricular systolic dysfunction. Am Heart J 2002; 144:373–376.

191. Thomas JD. Doppler assessment of valvular regurgitation. Heart 2002; 88:651–657.

192. Enriquez-Sarano M. Timing of mitral valve surgery. Heart 2002; 87:79–85.

193. Lebrun F, Lancellotti P, Pierard LA. Quantitation of functional mitral regurgitation during bicycle exercise in patients with heart failure. J Am Coll Cardiol 2001; 38:1685–1692.

194. Lapu-Baul R, et al. Quantitation of functional mitral regurgitation during bicycle exercise in patients with heart failure. Circulation 2002; 38:1685–1692.

195. Lancellotti P, et al. Prognostic importance of exercise-induced changes in mitral regurgitation in patients with chronic ischemic left ventricular dysfunction. Circulation, 2003; 108: 1713–1717.

196. Stevenson LW. Tailored therapy to hemodynamic goals for advanced heart failure. Eur J Heart Fail 1999; 1:251–257.

197. Saxon LA, Ellenbogan KA. Resynchronization therapy for the treatment of heart failure. Circulation 2003; 108:1044–1048.

198. Stevenson LW. Clinical use of inotropic therapy for heart failure: Looking backward or forward?. Circulation 2003; 108:367–372; 492–497.

199. Bolling SF, et al. Intermediate-term outcome of mitral reconstruction in cardiomyopathy. J Thorac Cardiovasc Surg 1998; 115:381–386.

200. Bolling SF. Mitral valve reconstruction in the patients with heart failure. Heart Fail Rev 2001; 6:177–185.

201. Badhwar V, Bolling SF. Mitral valve surgery in the patients with left ventricular dysfunction. Semin Thorac Cardiovasc Surg 2002; 14:133–136.

202. Grigioni F, et al. Ischemic mitral regurgitation: long-term outcome and prognostic implications with quantitative Doppler assessment. Circulation 2001; 103:1759–1764.

203. Trichon BH, et al. Survival after coronary revascularization, with and without mitral valve surgery, in patients with ischemic mitral regurgitation. Circulation 2003; 108(II):II-103–II-110.

204. Bradley TD, Floras JS. Sleep apnea and heart failure: I obstructive sleep apnea; II central sleep apnea. Circulation 2003; 107:1671–1678, 1822–1826.

205. Bradley TD, F. JS. Pathophysiologic and therapeutic implications of sleep apnea in congestive heart failure. J Cardiac Fail 1996; 2:223–240.

206. Wolk R, Kara T, Somers VK. Sleep-disordered breathing and cardiovascular disease. Circulation 2003; 108:9–12.

207. Leung RST, Bradley TD. Sleep apnea and cardiovascular disease. Am J Respir Crit Care Med 2001; 164:2147–2165.

208. Kohnlein T, et al. Central sleep apnea syndrome in patients with chronic heart disease: a critical review of the current literature. Thorax 2002; 57:547–555.

209. Javaheri S. A mechanism of central sleep apnea in patients with heart failure. N Engl J Med 1999; 341:949–954.

210. Sin DD, et al. Risk factors for central and obstructive sleep apnea in 450 men and women with congestive heart failure. Am J Respir Crit Care Med 1999; 160:1101–1106.

211. Sin DD. et al. Relationship of systolic BP to obstructive sleep apnea in patients with heart failure. Chest 2003; 123:1536–1543.

212. Javaheri S, Corbett WS. Association of low PaCO2 with central sleep apnea and ventricular arrhythmias in ambulatory patients with stable heart failure. Ann Intern Med 1998; 128: 204–207.

213. Narkiewicz K, et al. Altered cardiovascular variability in obstructive sleep apnea. Circulation 1998; 98:1071–1077.

214. Naughton MT, et al. Effect of continuous positive airway pressure on intrathoracic and left ventricular transmural pressures in patients with congestive heart failure. Circulation 1995; 91:1725–1731.

215. Sin DD, et al. Effects of continuous positive airway pressure on cardiovascular outcomes in heart failure patients with and without Cheyne-Stokes respiration. Circulation 2000; 102: 61–66.

216. Yan AT, Bradley TD, Lui PP. The role of continuous positive airway pressure in the treatment of congestive heart failure. Chest 2001; 120:1675–1685.

217. Garrigue S, Bordier P, Jais P. Benefit of atrial pacing in sleep apnea syndrome. NEJM 2002; 346:404–412.

218. Flemons WW. Obstructive sleep apnea. N Engl J Med 2002; 347:498–504.

219. Hillege HL, et al. Renal function, neurohormonal activation and survival in patients with chronic heart failure. Circulation 2000; 102:203–210.

220. Shlipak MG. Pharmacotherapy for heart failure in patients with renal insufficiency. Ann Intern Med 2003; 138:917–924.

221. Weinfield MS, Chertow GM, Stevenson LW. Aggravated renal dysfunction during intensive therapy for advanced chronic heart failure. Am Heart J 1999; 138:285–290.

222. Gottlieb SS, et al. The prognostic importance of different definitions of worsening renal function in congestive heart failure. J Cardiac Fail 2002; 8:136–141.

222a. Al-Ahmad A, Rand WM, Manjonath G, Konstam MA, Salem DN, Levey AS, Sarnach MJ. Reduced kidney function and anemia as high factors for mortality in patients with left ventricular dysfunction. J Am Coll Cardiol 2001; 38:958:955–62.

223. Dries DL, et al. The prognostic implications of renal insufficiency in asymptomatic and symptomatic patients with left ventricular dysfunction. J Am Coll Cardiol 2000; 35:681–689.

224. Mahon NG, et al. The prognostic value of estimated creatinine clearance alongside functional capacity in ambulatory patients with chronic congestive heart failure. J Am Coll Cardiol 2002; 40:1106–1113.

225. Poole-Wilson PA, et al. Mode of death in heart failure: findings from the ATLAS trial. Heart 2003; 89:42–48.

226. Chin MH, Goldman L. Correlates of major complications or death in patients admitted to the hospital with congestive heart failure. Arch Intern Med 1996; 156:1814–1820.

227. Anker SD, et al. Hormonal changes and catabolic/anabolic imbalance in chronic heart failure and their importance for cardiac cachexia. Circulation 1997; 96:526–534.

228. Anker SD, et al. Wasting as independent risk factor for mortality in chronic heart failure. Lancet 1997; 349:1050–1053.

229. Anker SD, et al. Tumor necrosis factor and steroid metabolism in chronic heart failure: possible relation to muscle wasting. J Am Coll Cardiol 1997; 30:997–1001.

230. Anker SK, Sharma R. The syndrome of cardiac cachexia. Int J Cardiol 2002; 85:51–66.

231. Neibauer J, et al. Deficient insulin-like growth factor 1 in chronic heart failure predicts altered body composition, anabolic deficiency, cytokine and neurohormonal activation. J Am Coll Cardiol 1998; 32:393–397.

232. Swan JW, et al. Insulin resistance in chronic heart failure: relation to severity and etiology of heart failure. J Am Coll Cardiol 1997; 30:527–532.

233. Murdoch DR, et al. Inappropriately low plasma leptin concentration in the cachexia associated with chronic heart failure. Heart 1999; 82:352–356.

234. Nagaya N, Kangawa K. Ghrelin improves left ventricular dysfunction and cardiac cachexia in heart failure. Curr Opin Pharmacol 2003; 3:146–151.

235. Ezekowitz JA, McAlister FA, Armstrong PW. Anemia is common in heart failure and is associated with poor outcomes: insights from a cohort of 12,065 patients with new-onset heart failure. Circulation 2003; 107:223–225.

236. Horwich TB, et al. Anemia is associated with worse symptoms, greater impairment in functional capacity and a significant increased in mortality in patients with advanced heart failure. J Am Coll Cardiol 2002; 39:1780–1786.

237. Mozaffarian D, Nye R, Levy WC. Anemia predicts mortality in severe heart failure: the prospective randomized amlodipine survival evaluation (PRAISE). J Am Coll Cardiol 2003; 41:1933–1939.

238. Kosiborod M, et al. The prognostic importance of anemia in patients with heart failure. Am J Med 2003; 114:112–119.

239. Kalra PR, et al. Hemoglobin concentration and prognosis in new cases of heart failure. Lancet 2003; 362:211–212.

240. Mancini DM, et al. Effect of erythropoietin on exercise capacity in patients with moderate to severe chronic heart failure. Circulation 2003; 107:294–299.

241. Silverberg DS, et al. The use of subcutaneous erythropoietin and intravenous iron for the treatment of severe, resistant heart failure improves cardiac and renal function, functional cardiac class, and markedly reduces hospitalization. J Am Coll Cardiol 2000; 35:1737–1744.

242. Silverberg DS, et al. The effect of correction of mild anemia in severe, resistant congestive heart failure using subcutaneous erythropoietin and intravenous iron: a randomized controlled study. J Am Coll Cardiol 2001; 37:1775–1780.

243. Besarab A, et al. The effects of normal as compared to low hematocrit values in patients with cardiac disease who are receiving hemodialysis and epoetin. N Engl J Med 1998; 339: 584–590.

244. MacMahon KMA, Lip GYH. Psychological factors in heart failure. Arch Intern Med 2002; 162:509–516.

245. Guck TP, et al. Depression and congestive heart failure. Congest Heart Fail 2003; 9:163–169.

246. Krumholz HM, et al. Prognostic importance of emotional support for elderly patients hospitalized with heart failure. Circulation 1998; 97:958–964.

247. Faris R, et al. Clinical depression is common and significantly associated with reduced survival in patients with non-ischemic heart failure. Eur J Heart Fail 2002; 4:541–551.

248. Turvey CL, et al. Prevalence and correlates of depressive symptoms in a community sample of people suffering from heart failure. J Am Geriatr Soc 2002; 50:2003–2008.

249. Skotzko CE, et al. Depression is common and precludes accurate assessment of functional status in elderly patients with congestive heart failure. J Card Fail 2000; 6:300–305.

250. Rozzini R, et al. Depression and major outcomes in older patients with heart failure. Arch Intern Med 2002; 162:362–364.

251. Jiang W, et al. Relationship to depression to increased risk of mortality and rehospitalization in patients with congestive heart failure. Arch Intern Med 2001; 161:1849–1856.

252. Sullivan M, et al. Depression-related costs in heart failure care. Arch Intern Med 2002; 162: 1860–1866.

253. Benatar D, et al. Outcomes of chronic heart failure. Arch Intern Med 2003; 163:347–352.

254. Dracup K, et al. Perceived control reduces emotional stress in patients with heart failure. J Heart Lung Transplant 2003; 22:90–93.

255. Ho KKL, et al. Survival after the onset of congestive heart failure in Framingham Heart Study subjects. Circulation 1993; 88:107–115.

256. Di Lenarda A, et al. Changing mortality in dilated cardiomyopathy. Br Heart J 1994; 72(suppl): S46–S51.

257. Stevenson WG, et al. Improving survival for patients with advanced heart failure: a study of 737 consecutive patients. J Am Coll Cardiol 1995; 26:1417–1423.

258. MacIntyre K, et al. Evidence of improving prognosis in heart failure: trends in case fatality in 66,547 patients hospitalized between 1986 and 1995. Circulation 2000; 102:1126–1131.

259. Gottdeiner JS, et al. Outcome of congestive heart failure in elderly persons: influence of left ventricular systolic function.. Ann Intern Med 2002; 137:631–639.

260. Jong P, et al. Prognosis and determinants of survival in patients newly hospitalized for heart failure. Arch Intern Med 2002; 162:1689–1694.

261. Packer M, et al. Effect of carvedilol on survival in severe chronic heart failure. N Engl J Med 2001; 344:1651–1658.

262. Rose EA, et al. Long-term use of a left ventricular assist device for end-stage heart failure. N Engl J Med 2001; 345:1435–1443.

263. Kao W, Constanzo MR. Prognosis determination in patients with advanced heart failure. J Heart Lung Transplant 1997; 16:S2–S6.

264. Wilson JR, et al. Prognosis in severe heart failure: relation to hemodynamic measurements and ventricular ectopic activity. J Am Coll Cardiol 1983; 2:403–410.

265. Curtis JP, et al. The association of left ventricular ejection fraction, mortality, and cause of death in stable outpatients with heart failure. J Am Coll Cardiol 2003; 42:736–742.

266. Nohria A, et al. Clinical assessment identifies hemodynamic profiles that predict outcomes in patients admitted with heart failure. J Am Coll Cardiol 2003; 41:1797–1804.

267. Drazner MH, Rame JE, Dris DL. Third heart sound and elevated jugular venous pressure as markers of the subsequent development of heart failure in patients with asymptomatic left ventricular dysfunction. Am J Med 2003; 114:431–437.

11

Clinical Profiles and Prognosis in Heart Failure

Lynne Warner Stevenson and Paul Zei
Cardiovascular Division, Brigham and Women's Hospital
Boston, Massachusetts, USA

Heart failure is often described as a disease with a 50% 5-year mortality. Earlier initiation of therapies that delay progression of heart failure is likely to prolong survival beyond that reported for previous cohorts. Thus, it is rare to discuss a 50% 5-year survival prediction to a patient and family. Current populations of patients with a diagnosis of heart failure include those with less than 10% risk of dying in the next year to those who are more likely to die than survive (Fig. 1) [1]. Although many factors have been proposed and published to refine these predictions, those based on clinical assessment continue to dominate decisions for individual patients. From characterization of trial populations and of individual patients, profiles are emerging that better define short-term outcomes.

PURPOSES OF PROGNOSTIC FACTORS/FEATURES

Prognostic factors proposed for heart failure are best explored by considering the three major purposes for which they may be used (Fig. 2): (a) discovery of a primary characteristic associated with outcome may further our understanding of the pathophysiology of cardiac injury or progression to ventricular dysfunction, leading to development of new therapies. In this case, it is critical to isolate association from causation and to establish independence of this from other factors known to be important. As heart failure reflects a complex path with multiple endogenous and exogenous contributors, there is usually a relatively weak relationship between the proposed primary factor and outcomes for individual patients. (b) a prognostic factor may be useful because it identifies a target population for current therapies. Not all prognostic factors represent such targets, as they may be linked to outcome by hidden association with other causes, thus "bystander factors." Even when factors are causative, therapy to change them is not necessarily associated with better outcome. On the other hand, factors not necessarily causative can be useful to characterize a population with a given likelihood of outcomes that might improve with therapy. Results from trial populations can be interpolated to clinical settings. (c) the most common use of prognostic factors is to advise individual patients. It may be most appropriate to consider these prognostic "features" rather than factors. Use of prognostic features

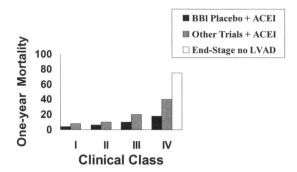

Figure 1 Estimated 1-year mortality on medical therapy including angiotensin converting enzyme inhibitors (without beta-blockers) for heart failure according to New York Heart Association clinical class, demonstrating increasing mortality with worse symptoms, but also demonstrating the variability within class definitions between eras and between trials. For patients receiving angiotensin converting enzyme inhibitors (ACEI), the mortality is lower in the beta-blocker trials than in previous trials, even for the patients not receiving beta-blockers (BBI placebo). The highest mortality for patients considered to have class IV symptoms (at rest or minimal exertion) was seen in the trial of left ventricular assist devices, for which the majority of patients were receiving intravenous inotropic therapy at the time of randomization.

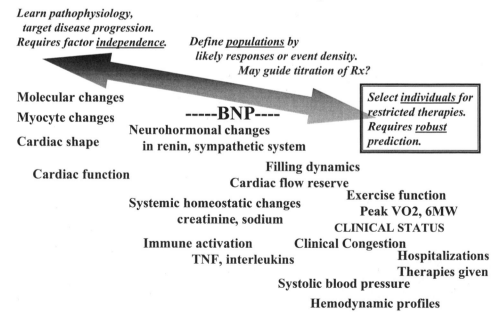

Figure 2 Diagram showing the range of different parameters proposed as prognostic factors. These factors can be arranged from molecular to systemically integrated. The use of prognostic factors varies similarly from understanding of pathophysiology, which is advanced by identification of independent predictive power, to selection of high-risk therapies for individual patients, which requires robust but not independent power.

for individual patients may allow better allocation of further therapies that are restricted by intrinsic risk or limited resource availability. When no specific therapies are available, patients and families may be helped to resume or realign their expectations for the future. These prognostic features for the individual generally represent integrated rather than isolated components, and must carry a high degree of certainty for the individual.

MAJOR OUTCOMES PREDICTED

The most common outcomes predicted are survival or death. For heart failure, most deaths occur suddenly or due to progressive hemodynamic deterioration. (Fig. 3) Defibrillator firing and cardiac arrest are combined with sudden death in some series. For mild heart failure, the proportion of deaths occurring suddenly is higher but the absolute risk is about 5% annually [1–3]. At this stage of disease, sudden death is often described as "unexpected." As heart failure progresses in severity, the absolute risk of sudden death is higher, but increases less than total mortality.

Deaths occurring in patients with refractory symptoms of heart failure are generally attributed to heart failure. In these patients, it is difficult to distinguish between death due to primary arrhythmias and death due to terminal hemodynamic and metabolic derangement, which can also cause dysrhythmias, and the distinction has few therapeutic implications. Heart failure hospitalization is often a component of heart failure endpoints, although open to more interpretation.

Considerable effort has been expended to find risk factors that preferentially predict sudden or heart failure events. Such risk factors could help to identify the patients most likely to benefit from defibrillators, particularly in countries with more restrained use of this technology. As tachyarrhythmias, bradyarrhythmias, recurrent myocardial ischemia, pulmonary emboli, and cerebrovascular events can all cause sudden death, it is not surprising that risk factors specific for sudden death have been difficult to identify. From a practical standpoint, this distinction becomes less important for patients with long QRS complexes and moderate-severe heart failure symptoms, who are now increasingly receiv-

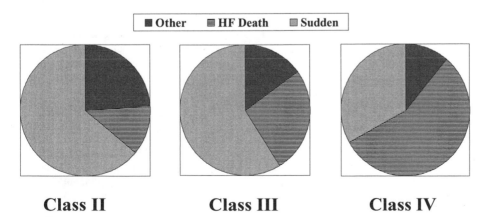

Figure 3 Attributable causes of death in heart failure according to clinical class. Sudden death predominates when symptoms are mild, whereas death is most often attributed to hemodynamic deterioration, "pump failure," when symptoms are severe. Data is adapted from the MERIT trial of extended-release metoprolol in heart failure. (From Ref. 2.)

ing biventricular pacemakers for their hemodynamic effects combined with defibrillation capability on the same device platform.

CLASSIFYING PROGNOSTIC FACTORS AND FEATURES

In addition to clarifying the major role for a given prognostic factor as previously described, it is useful to consider it in terms of the system level described (Table 1) [3]. Considerable overlap exists within a system such that different parameters are interrelated and often fail to provide independent information. With the modest size of most populations studied, it is often difficult to determine which of the related variables carries the most predictive power.

Among the demographic variables, older age consistently predicts higher mortality among adults with chronic heart failure, although teen-agers and young adults are more vulnerable to acute onset cardiomyopathy. Etiology interacts with both gender and race. In most series, women have a better prognosis [4]. In part, this relates to gender differences in etiology and physiology of hypertrophy, as women have more heart failure with preserved left ventricular ejection fraction (LVEF) and hypertrophy, whereas men have more coronary artery disease. The African-American population demonstrates worse prognosis with heart failure than Caucasian populations, after controlling as much as possible for socio-economic factors (Chapter 20) [5]. The etiology for heart failure in blacks includes hypertension in more than 60%, whereas only 30% have coronary artery disease. Although

Table 1 Types of Prognostic Factors

Type of System		Examples
Demographics		Age, gender, race, comorbidity
Etiology		CAD, amyloidosis
Physiology expression	Molecular	Genotype, mRNA, protein
fraction	Microscopic	Myocyte size, degree of fibrosis
	Ventricular structure/function	LV mass, volume, ejection
	Hemodynamics clinical	Filling pressures, CI, SBP, fraction
	Electrical properties	Atrial fibrillation, QT dispersion, nonsustained VT
	Systemic integration	Exercise response: pkVO2, 6MW
		Neurohormonal: BNP, NE
		Serum sodium
		Inflammatory markers: TNF, IL4
	Renal function	Creatinine, BUN, Na
	Metabolic status	Thyroid regulation, nutritional
Patient/Environment	Therapies taken	ACE inhibitors, beta-blockers, Inotropic agents
	Perceived function	NYHA, Minnesota Heart Failure
	Clinical stability	Hospitalization, congestion score
	Referral bias	Transplant evaluation, not eligible for transplant or LVAD
	Events	Hospitalization

Abbreviations: 6 MW, six minute walk distance; BNP, brain natriuretic peptide; BUN, blood urea nitrogen; CAD, coronary artery disease; CI, cardiac index; IL4, interleukin 4; LV, left ventricle; LVAD, left ventricular assist device; Na, serum sodium; NE, norepinephrine; NYHA, New York Heart Association; pkVO2, peak oxygen consumption; SBP, systolic blood pressure; TNF, tumor necrosis factor alpha; VT, ventricular tachycardia.

less effective for hypertension, angiotensin-converting enzyme inhibition is effective for the therapy of heart failure in the African-American population [6], in whom volume retention may be more avid. Diabetes confers a 30% higher risk of poor outcome in both asymptomatic and symptomatic heart failure [7], an effect primarily on patients with coronary artery disease, in whom the risk of progressive heart failure is increased by almost 50% if diabetes is present.

In addition to the classifications in Table 1, prognostic factors can also be classified by the breadth of the population included. Many features prominent in advanced disease are absent in early disease, yielding encouraging correlation coefficients when both are shown on the same graph. Although these features may contribute to understanding the pathophysiology of decompensation, they are unlikely to add useful information beyond that obtained by even a perfunctory clinical assessment. On the other hand, factors that vary widely within a narrow range of disease severity may help to identify individual patients with outcomes different from the average for the group studied. Prognostic features may be constant or variable over time; in the latter case utility may be greater when measured after standardized intervention, or when serial changes are tracked over time.

MICROSCOPIC FEATURES

The explosion of new information regarding genetic differences, gene regulation and expression, and proteomics will soon contribute to our understanding of outcomes and hopefully therapies in heart failure, but is not now generally pertinent for predicting individual outcomes. Notable exceptions are the presence of certain beta-adrenoreceptor polymorphisms that are prevalent in African-American populations [8]. Larger myocyte size and more extensive fibrosis were found to predict outcome in small early experiences with endomyocardial biopsy tissue [9] and fibrosis predicted less response to beta-blocker therapy in dilated cardiomyopathy [9]. The degree of histological change has been used to predict development of subsequent heart failure after doxorubicin hydrochloride (Adriamycin) therapy [10]. The specificity of the identification of viral genomic material in myocardial tissues remains controversial, but may guide testing of new therapies beyond those that failed in previous trials of myocarditis diagnosed by lymphocytic infiltration alone. The invasive nature of endomyocardial biopsy limits its application to prognosis for heart failure outside of specific limited etiologic subsets.

VENTRICULAR STRUCTURE AND FUNCTION

Gross assessment of ventricular structure is predominantly performed with echocardiography. Other than left ventricular mass, most measures of structure are highly dependent on loading conditions and, thus, linked to assessment of function. Widely measured, left ventricular ejection fraction is easily understood and applied for all three purposes related to prognosis. Across a broad spectrum of patients, those with low ejection fraction reliably fare worse than those with normal ejection fraction. However, the clinical utility is greatest in patients with few or no symptoms of heart failure. Once symptoms of heart failure are major (Class III or IV), left ventricular ejection fraction has little additional prognostic value [11]. Patients with left ventricular ejection fractions above 30% (or ''preserved'') have lower mortality in some but not all studies and have equivalent rehospitalization rates. Many of the major prognostic factors, such as clinical severity and renal function indices, apply similarly to patients with low and ''preserved'' ejection fractions. The most notable difference between these two groups is the rarity of hypotension and clinical hypoperfusion in patients with preserved ejection fraction.

It is increasingly questioned whether the left ventricular ejection fraction is as relevant as the left ventricular dimension. This determines wall stress, a major stimulus for ventricular remodeling and a powerful predictor of outcomes in asymptomatic populations, such as those after myocardial infarction or with primary valvular regurgitant lesions. Remodeling toward more spherical shape is associated with worse outcomes. As heart failure progresses, left ventricular dilation remains a robust predictor of outcomes even once severe symptoms have developed. Patients referred with advanced heart failure and left ventricular diastolic dimension over 8 cm, or dimension index over 4 cm/m^2, have mortality that is 50% at 2 years compared with 25% for smaller ventricles [12].

Even when left ventricular ejection fraction is severely reduced, exercise capacity and prognosis are further worsened by development of right ventricular dysfunction [13]. Due to its irregular shape, right ventricular ejection fraction is less often measured, requiring first-pass radionuclide angiography, magnetic resonance imaging, or approximate area measurements from echocardiography. As there are better tools for measurement, right ventricular performance will increasingly be recognized as a determinant of compensation in advanced disease. In biventricular failure, the right ventricle is often the border-forming segment of the chest x-ray, contributing to cardiothoracic (CT) ratio. This ratio was commonly used to assess the severity of heart failure prior to the common use of echocardiography. As right ventricular volumes vary markedly with acute changes in circulating volume status, CT ratio can change significantly over a short period of diuretic therapy.

Mitral and tricuspid regurgitation develop secondarily as a result of distortion of the supporting structures of the left ventricular wall and papillary muscles due to both dilation and regional fibrosis. Even when not audible on physical examination, mitral and/or tricuspid regurgitation are present in almost all patients with severe clinical decompensation [14]. Their presence heralds worse outcome, as seen with other markers of severely elevated filling pressures (see following text). This dynamic regurgitation can account for up to 75% of total stroke volume in severe decompensation, and diminish to 25% acutely after therapy to decrease filling pressures and vascular resistance [15].

CENTRAL HEMODYNAMICS

Many parameters determine and reflect central hemodynamics. There is considerable overlap between hemodynamic variables and the ventricular structure/function relationships previously discussed. Most direct hemodynamic measurements focus on intracardiac or arterial pressures or flows, although they are inextricably related. As indicated by the "dynamic" term, these measurements change from moment to moment. Their use for diagnosis, therapy, and prediction depends on appropriate definition of the circumstances of measurement. They are most commonly measured during quiet supine rest, but additional information may be derived from measurements obtained during supine or upright exercise. As for many other prognostic factors, their relationship to clinical function and outcome may be enhanced by serial measurements after specific therapies.

Filling Pressures

Although heart failure was at one time envisioned as primarily an abnormality of low cardiac output, resting perfusion may be decreased little or not at all in many patients with severe symptoms. The "congestive" picture of heart failure relates instead to the symptoms and signs of elevated filling pressures (Table 2). Elevated left ventricular end-diastolic pressures increase left atrial filling pressures, and both are further increased by

Table 2 Factors Reflecting Filling Pressures

Direct measurement:
LVEDP, LAP, PCW
PAS, PAD
RAP, CVP
Echocardiographic correlates:
Left atrial pressure estimated
Pulmonary artery systolic pressure estimated
Mitral/tricuspid regurgitation
Mitral inflow patterns
Pulmonary venous flow patterns
Inferior vena cava diameter and motion
Radiographic correlates:
"Pulmonary vascular congestion"
Pulmonary vascular redistribution
Cardiothoracic ratio
Laboratory
Natriuretic peptides
(Total blood volume)
Clinical assessment
Jugular venous pressure (JVP) height and waveform
Third heart sound (weakly correlated)
"Wet" profile
Clinical congestion score (1–5 scale)

Abbreviations: CVP, central venous pressure; LAP, left atrial pressure; LVEDP, left ventricular end-diastolic pressure; PAD, pulmonary artery diastolic pressure; PAS, pulmonary artery systolic pressure; PCW, pulmonary capillary wedge pressure; RAP, right atrial pressure.

the development of mitral regurgitation. Using the pulmonary artery catheter, pulmonary capillary wedge pressure is the most common pressure used to describe populations and disease severity. In patients without major intrinsic lung disease, the pulmonary artery diastolic pressure tracks well with wedge pressure. Although pulmonary pressures may be raised with multiple other conditions, such as chronic pulmonary emboli and intrinsic lung disease, pulmonary artery systolic pressure is usually about twice the pulmonary capillary wedge pressure in patients with chronically elevated left-sided filling pressures [16]. Development of right ventricular failure with elevated right atrial pressures and engorgement of the inferior vena cava usually occurs after chronic left-sided pressure elevation, and to some extent indicates chronicity and severity of left-sided failure. The development of right ventricular dysfunction often heralds inexorable decline, with decreased exercise tolerance as cardiac reserve diminishes, and declining nutritional status as hepatosplanchnic congestion ensues. It is not yet possible to establish a hierarchy for the prognostic value of right- or left-sided filling pressures. Some analyses include only one index of filling pressures; in other studies, the close interdependence of the filling pressure measurements precluded their use as independent predictors of outcome. The overall robustness of the relationship between filling pressures and survival may be due to the duality of causal links: (a) high filling pressures cause many of the symptoms leading to severe functional limitation, and (b) the intraventricular filling pressures stimulate changes in gene expression and myocyte function, while worsening the supply-demand imbalance for myocardial oxygen.

There is marked heterogeneity in the degree of filling pressure elevation at a given level of left ventricular dysfunction and a given level of symptoms. Many patients with markedly elevated filling pressures chronically do not show obvious heart failure signs or symptoms [17]. Nonetheless, patients with normal filling pressures have the best prognosis. More important than the hemodynamics at the time of presentation are those that can be achieved during aggressive therapy with vasodilators and diuretics. Among two groups of patients with initial pulmonary wedge pressure 28–30 mm Hg during evaluation for transplantation, those in whom therapy with vasodilators and diuretics tailored to reduce filling pressures achieved pulmonary wedge pressure less than or equal to 16 mm Hg, 1-year survival was 83% compared with 38% in patients in whom final pulmonary wedge pressures remained higher [18].

Echocardiographic parameters have also been shown to predict survival outcomes (Table 2). Radiographic evidence of heart failure offers relatively less information because abnormalities are generally present in the majority of chronic heart failure patients, and there is little quantitation; findings also change unpredictably with variations in clinical status. As previously described, the cardiothoracic ratio in chronic dilated heart failure usually reflects the right ventricle as border-forming element, and right ventricular size changes rapidly with changing volume status. Using a threshold value for CT ratio has some prognostic value in large series [19].

Natriuretic peptides can be elevated by myocardial injury and increased wall stress, both acutely and chronically [20]. Unlike many biochemical markers (see following text), natriuretic peptides may become elevated during the asymptomatic phase of left ventricular dysfunction in unselected community populations and after myocardial infarction. These elevations may reflect acute injury, in the case of acute myocardial infarction, and subsequently increased wall stress due to subtle regional remodeling and/or intermittently increased filling pressures. Once left ventricular dysfunction has become advanced, changes in natriuretic peptides track most closely with changes in left-sided filling pressures [21]. Across both broad and focused spectra of patients, brain natriuretic peptide and the pro-peptide divide patients into groups with better and worse prognosis (Fig. 4) [22]. Compared with other single markers, natriuretic peptides appear more reliable in predicting severity of clinical decompensation and likelihood of early re-hospitalization or death. There is a wide range of values for a given clinical state [23], however, and serial measurements reveal frequent examples in which the levels are inexplicably higher or lower than expected in an individual patient.

Cardiac Output

Understanding the role of cardiac output in outcomes has been complicated by difficulties in its assessment. The "gold standard" is laboratory measurements of arterio-venous oxygen differences with simultaneous measurement of inspired oxygen from the Fick calculation. Estimated Fick outputs using assumed oxygen consumption are reasonable for broad classification, as the mixed-venous oxygen saturation correlates with the adequacy of perfusion except at the extremes. The thermodilution pulmonary artery catheters provide more accessible measurements that stratify populations and can guide therapy. Measurements made more than two decades ago indicate that patients with low cardiac output fair worse than those with preserved cardiac output. Further, patients who can augment their cardiac output from resting levels generally have less impairment in exercise capacity. However, individual degrees of compensation are often not accurately predicted by either cardiac output or filling pressures.

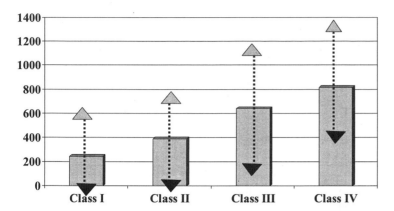

Figure 4   Levels of brain natriuretic peptide (BNP; ng/ml) in relation to estimated New York Heart Association clinical class. Although there is a strong trend for higher BNP levels in more severe class, there is marked variation within each group. The major source for the data is derived from assessment of patients presenting to the Emergency Department with dyspnea. (From Ref. 59.)

Much disillusion regarding the importance of cardiac output resulted from the multiple trials of inotropic therapy. Inotropic therapy reliably provides acute increases in cardiac output. Chronic investigational oral inotropic agents have been associated with increased mortality due to sudden death; further, milrinone has also been shown to increase heart failure deaths [24]. Interestingly, cardiac output when measured during chronic inotropic therapy did not increase over baseline, but deteriorated further when the inotropic agents were discontinued, suggesting intervening deterioration. Increasing reduced cardiac output appears less important than lowering elevated filling pressures, whether assessed by symptomatic response or survival after redesign of standard oral therapies [18].

Clinical Assessment

The most widely employed assessment methods are those that can be performed immediately in the clinical setting with minimal disruption. While some symptoms and physical signs have been associated with objective hemodynamic measurements, the prognostic importance of such physical findings may be greater than abnormalities identified unexpectedly from invasive hemodynamic assessment done for other reasons.

Orthopnea

Orthopnea is one of the most useful symptoms for characterization of filling pressures. Patients with a history of heart failure who develop orthopnea are generally assumed to have elevated filling pressures unless proven otherwise. In patients recently discharged from hospitalization for decompensated heart failure, the persistence of orthopnea at 1 month is associated with a three-fold higher mortality at 1 and 2 years [25].

Jugular Venous Pressure

This physical sign has a direct correlate to measured right atrial pressure, when jugular venous pressure in cm height is 1.3 times the right atrial pressure in mm Hg. There is marked variation in the ability of clinicians to accurately identify the jugular venous pulse and further discrepancy in the quantitative assessment. Nonetheless, even the information of "elevated" or "not elevated" was found to have prognostic implications among patients with asymptomatic or mildly symptomatic heart failure, The identification of elevated jugular venous pressure is associated with a 30% higher risk of death or heart failure hospitalization [26].

Third Heart Sound

The circumstances creating the third heart sound during rapid filling in early diastole are not well understood. Although often considered to be a sign of elevated filling pressures, the third heart sound is much more common in systolic heart failure and ventricular dilatation than when filling pressures are elevated in heart failure with normal ventricular size and ejection fraction. Some patients never develop third heart sounds during periods of heart failure decompensation, while other patients never lose them. Third heart sounds are unquestionably more prevalent in patients with elevated filling pressures. The new appearance or an increased intensity of a third heart sound during serial follow-up usually correlates with increasing volume overload. Among patients who otherwise appear clinically similar, the presence of a third heart sound predicts a substantially higher rate of heart failure events [26].

Blood Pressure

As vasodilator and neurohormonal antagonist therapy for heart failure evolved, it became clear that these therapies led to major benefits despite lowering blood pressures. Patients tolerated systolic blood pressures in the 80 mm range surprisingly well. Thus, the emphasis on blood pressure was minimized, unless patients described symptomatic hypotension.

With the majority of patients now on ACEI and many on beta-adrenergic receptor blockers titrated as tolerated, the baseline conditions are more uniform and the relevance of blood pressure is again becoming apparent. Clinical trial populations stratified by 1-year mortality demonstrate an inverse relationship between outcome and baseline systolic blood pressure (Figure 5). Blood pressure is a complex function of cardiac output, large

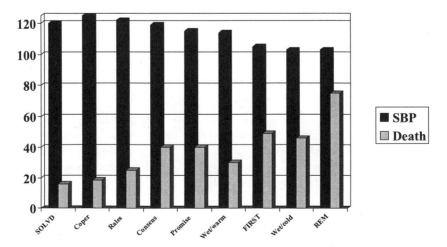

Figure 5 Relationship of baseline systolic blood pressure (mm Hg) to 1-year mortality in clinical trials and the wet-warm and wet-cold populations. (From Ref. 27.)

vessel and small vessel compliance, and vascular responsiveness. For instance, lower blood pressure may indicate a lower baseline cardiac output, which would be adverse, or less intense peripheral vasoconstriction, which may be salutary. Hypotension often limits uptitration of ACEI and beta-blockers that may improve subsequent outcome. Whenever included in multivariate analysis of advanced heart failure patients, systolic blood pressure has been found to be highly correlated with early outcomes.

Hemodynamic Profiles

In practice, multiple components of the clinical assessment are generally integrated to characterize patients. These profiles are used to guide therapy and also provide general information regarding subsequent prognosis. Four basic hemodynamic profiles accurately and readily divide patients according to evidence of congestion and hypoperfusion at rest [27] (Figures 6 and 7). Evidence of congestion include jugular venous distention, positive hepato-jugular reflex, and a square wave Valsalva maneuver response. Peripheral edema is also included but is present in fewer than 30% of patients younger than 70 years with chronic heart failure and evidence of congestion. Further, its presence in older patients frequently reflects peripheral venous insufficiency rather than elevation in right-sided filling pressures. Rales are uncommon despite severely elevated filling pressures if heart failure is chronic, due to the compensatory hypertrophy of pulmonary lymphatics to maintain clear airspaces. Evidence of hypoperfusion is often based on the difference between systolic and diastolic blood pressure, which must be auscultated carefully by a trained clinician. Cool extremities, particularly calves and forearms also suggest hypoperfusion.

The majority of ambulatory patients with NYHA (New York Heart Association) class I–II symptoms have hemodynamic profile A (warm and dry). Within groups of patients with limiting daily symptoms (Class III–IV), the hemodynamic profiles provide further characterization: patients with profile B (warm and wet) have a 1.8-fold higher risk of death or transplantation within the next year than patients with the warm and dry Profile A (Figure 6). Patients with profile C (cold and wet) have the worst prognosis, with 2.5-fold higher mortality than profile A. Most patients who initially appear to be profile L (cold and dry) are actually profile C, but the few patients with true profile L usually have exercise intolerance with few symptoms at rest and prognosis that may be better but certainly not worse than profile B.

Although the criteria used to classify patients are based on hemodynamic considerations, the profiles may carry more information than the measured hemodynamic parameters. For instance, a given elevation in left-sided filling pressures may be more deleterious when it causes orthopnea, perhaps as a result of low net oncotic pressures in the pulmonary circulation, or an adverse impact through disordered sleep. A given reduction in cardiac output may be more deleterious when associated with peripheral vasoconstriction causing cool extremities. Even more important, assessment of clinical profiles can be done within 2 minutes in any setting and repeated serially to follow clinical changes over time [27].

Biochemical Markers

The biochemical markers that reflect neurohormonal activation are of particular interest because they clarify pathophysiology and represent targets for therapy. *Plasma norepinephrine* levels have been shown by Chidsey with Braunwald and colleagues in 1964 [28] to be elevated in experimental heart failure. Their importance in clinical heart failure was demonstrated by Cohn to be greater than the contribution of mean arterial pressure, heart rate, serum sodium, and measured hemodynamics [29]. Of more than 700 patients from

Two Minute Assessment of Hemodynamic Profile

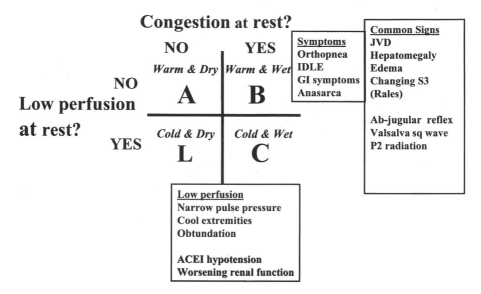

Figure 6 Two minute assessment of clinical hemodynamic profile from simple clinical information [60]. The four profiles are defined as described by Nohria and colleagues [27]. The letter L is used for cold and dry rather than D to avoid the incorrect implication that the cold-dry profile occurs after the cold-wet C or denotes more severe disease. In fact, patients usually feel much better with the cold-dry than the cold-wet and the prognosis appears to be better, although this group is too small to analyze extensively. The symptoms that weigh into the diagnosis of "wet" are orthopnea, immediate dyspnea on light exertion (IDLE), gastrointestinal complaints of fullness, early satiety, anorexia, or right upper quadrant tenderness. Peripheral fluid retention can lead to edema, when severe to anasarca, which can be either symptoms or signs. Jugular venous distention is the most sensitive and specific sign of volume overload. The abdomino-jugular reflex, the Valsalva square wave, and a P2 that radiates beyond the left lower sternal border are helpful signs for the experienced examiner. Low perfusion is more difficult to identify accurately, but is suggested by a narrow pulse pressure and cool extremities. It is one cause of obtundation and one of many causes of worsening renal function. Patients who develop symptomatic hypotension even to low doses of ACE inhibitors in the presence of clinical congestion, often have critically low cardiac output that is dependent on intrinsic neurohormonal activation.

the Veterans Administration Heart Failure trials, dominated by New York Heart Association Class II patients, the median plasma norepinephrine level was 490 pg/ml [30] compared with normals showing less than 200 pg/ml. For levels below 600 pg/ml, 1-year mortality was approximately 7%, for levels between 600 and 900 pg/ml it was 15%, and for levels greater than 900 pg/ml it was 25%. Although increased norepinephrine levels trended with increased mortality at all levels, the striking increase occurred when levels exceeded 900 pg/ml, in which case mortality annualized from over more than 4 years doubled from approximately 14% to 30%.

Plasma renin levels have been related to prognosis with left ventricular dysfunction even in populations with few or no symptoms of heart failure. For patients with symptomatic heart failure, the median level was 7 ng/ml. The 25% of patients in that study with

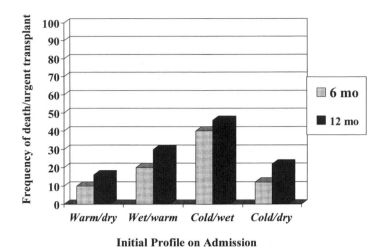

Figure 7 Relationship of subsequent outcomes to initial profile obtained at the time of hospitalization [27]. Event rates of death + urgent transplantation are shown for patients discharged after hospitalization with heart failure.

renin activity greater than 16 ng/ml had higher mortality throughout the trial [30]. Interestingly, there was little relationship between elevation in norepinephrine and elevation in plasma renin activity. Both, however, identified the groups in which enalapril was clearly superior to the hydralazine-isosorbide combination. The use of plasma renin activity as a prognostic factor has little value in this era because the routine use of renin-angiotensin system antagonist leads to increased plasma renin levels.

Multiple other response systems are affected by advancing heart failure. Unlike the sympathetic and renin angiotensin system, this activation has not been clearly implicated as a cause rather than as an effect of disease severity. For example, serum endothelin levels are high in decompensated disease and reduced with therapy. Inflammatory activation is progressively increased with worsening heart failure severity. Circulating cytokines, of which the best studied is tumor necrosis factor alpha, are generally elevated in advanced disease [31]. However, variability in binding and fate of circulating cytokines limits their utility as prognostic markers within an advanced disease population.

In contrast to norepinephrine, plasma renin and cytokine activity, *serum sodium concentration* is measured routinely and serially during the course of disease. As heart failure progresses, serum sodium levels are inversely correlated with activation of the renin-angiotensin system, but may reflect other factors as well, such as the stimulation of antidiuretic hormone (vasopressin) and excessive thirst. Serum sodium appears as a continuous variable, predicting worse outcome throughout the range from normal to severe hyponatremia. Its impact on prognosis is most evident in the late stages of disease. In one study of advanced heart failure (mean LVEF 17%, creatinine 1.8 mg/dL, cardiac index < 2.0 L/min/m^2, left ventricular end-diastolic pressure of 26 mmHg) performed prior to the routine use of neurohormonal antagonist therapy, patients with serum sodium greater than 137 mEq/L had a 1-year survival of 50%, whereas those with serum sodium between 133 and 137 mEq/L had 1-year survival of 35%, and those below 133mEq/L had less than 20% 1-year survival [32]. Low serum sodium appears to identify patients less likely to tolerate angiotensin converting enzyme inhibitors, but also more likely to benefit if they can be tolerated. In a more recent study of patients referred for transplantation with

NYHA class IV symptoms and left ventricular ejection fraction less than 25%, those patients who had a serum sodium greater than or equal to 136mEq/: had 1-year survival of 70%, whereas those with serum sodium less than 134 mEq/L had 1-year survival of only 50% [11].

Serum creatinine is increasingly recognized as an important prognostic factor. Although it was once assumed that higher serum creatinine in heart failure reflected worse renal function due to progressive disease, worse renal function itself contributes to heart failure progression and worse outcome, as shown in both the asymptomatic and symptomatic heart failure populations in the Studies of Left Ventricular Dysfunction [33]. This relationship persists even when patients with serum creatinine above 2.0 mg/dl are excluded. An estimated creatinine clearance less than 60 cc/min predicted 1.7 times higher risk of heart failure death in the asymptomatic population, and 1.5-fold higher in the symptomatic population. Although often not reported in earlier trials, every recent trial of heart failure has found serum creatinine to predict higher rate of hospitalization and death, which is particularly dramatic when the baseline serum creatinine level exceeds 2.0 mg/dl.

Plasma natriuretic factors are elevated progressively from the asymptomatic stage through end-stage disease. Elevation in both the atrial and brain (B-type) natriuretic peptides predicts worse outcome after myocardial infarction, emergency room visit, and in the setting of chronic heart failure. The most useful measure appears to be B-type natriuretic peptide (BNP), which is released predominantly from the left ventricle under conditions of stress (Figure 4). BNP levels correlate in large heart failure populations with NYHA heart failure symptoms (Class I: 244 $\pm$ 286 ng/ml; Class II: 389 $\pm$ 374 ng/ml; Class III 640 $\pm$ 447 ng/ml; and Class IV: 817 $\pm$ 435 ng/ml) [23]. For any given severity of symptoms, BNP levels tend to be lower in heart failure with preserved LVEF than in heart failure with ventricular dilatation.

Metabolic parameters change late in the disease process. At this stage, changes in nutrition and related functions can contribute to further deterioration [34]. Markedly elevated right-sided filling pressures and tricuspid regurgitation can result in anorexia, impaired absorption of nutrients (and medications), and decreased hepatic function. Serum prealbumin levels fall before serum albumin. Intrahepatic conversion of T4 shifts away from T3 to reverse T3; thus, the declining ratio of T3 to reverse T3 identifies more severe disease and predicts worse outcome in advanced disease [35] (note: this relationship does not apply in the presence of amiodarone therapy, which also affects T4 to T3 conversion).

Markers of Dysrhythmia Risk

Electrical markers of prognosis vary from clinical arrhythmias to baseline QRS morphology to specialized invasive and surface recordings. The presence of atrial fibrillation confers a worse prognosis in both asymptomatic left ventricular dysfunction and mild-moderate heart failure. In the combined populations, the risk of death attributed to pump failure was 34% vs. 23% over the four years, an independent risk of 1.42, without significant increase in unexpected death [36]. This excess risk appears to have decreased as use of type I anti-arrhythmic therapy decreased and the use of amiodarone increased [37].

Asymptomatic nonsustained ventricular tachycardia is increasingly frequent as the disease severity worsens, runs greater than or equal to 3 beats were observed in half of patients with Class II and III heart failure in the V-HeFT trial [38]. The presence of couplets or nonsustained ventricular tachycardia predicted increased overall mortality of 25% vs. 15% at 2 years, suggesting that asymptomatic ventricular ectopy serves more as a marker for disease severity rather than a specific one for arrhythmic substrate. It may be more specific for predicting sudden death in patients with a history of prior myocardial infarction. A history of sustained ventricular tachycardia or cardiac arrest is well known to predict subsequent arrhythmic events and is now an indication for placement of an implantable defibrillator, which successfully aborts most recurrences. Syncope in heart failure also predicts increased risk of sudden death regardless of etiology, whether or not a precipitating cause for the syncope can be identified [39].

Prolonged QRS duration is increasingly prevalent with increasing severity of heart failure. The prognostic significance in future populations will be confounded by the increasing use of biventricular pacemakers, with or without defibrillation capability, to improve ventricular synchrony in patients with long QRS.

QT interval prolongation has been shown to predict worse outcome in patients without cardiac diagnoses, those with diabetes mellitus, and patients with history of myocardial infarction. Interactions may be important, as a shorter resting QT interval predicted lower mortality during dofetilide therapy in patients with heart failure after myocardial infarction [40]. The maximum QT interval predicted overall mortality, sudden death, and heart failure death in a United Kingdom study of ambulatory heart failure patients, but was no longer predictive when other clinical variables were included [41]. A recent study of patients selected for BNP levels greater than 400 pg/ml demonstrated over a three-fold higher event rate at 6 months in patients whose average baseline corrected QT interval exceeded 440 msec, after excluding patients with paced or irregular rhythms [42]. Most of the events in that study were attributed to pump failure rather than arrhythmias.

The signal-averaged ECG (SAECG) is influenced by heterogeneity of ventricular repolarization [43] but is also affected by prolonged QRS duration and has not been shown to be a sufficiently strong predictor of sudden death risk to guide therapy [44]. The degree of QT dispersion on the resting ECG may also reflect heterogeneity of repolarization, but is not sufficiently predictive to identify either high- or low-risk populations at baseline [45], or during therapy with dofetilide [46]. Another potential marker of electrical instability, T-wave alternans during exercise testing, is currently undergoing evaluation as a predictor of increased risk for life-threatening ventricular tachyarrhythmias [47].

CLINICAL INTEGRATORS

Clinical Class

Despite the multiplicity of single predictors of outcome and objective scales of functional capacity, the NYHA clinical class, and minor variations continue to be useful descriptors of overall mortality (Figure 1). The annual mortality of patients in NYHA Class I, without recent index events, such as a myocardial infarction or hospitalization for heart failure, is less than 10%, probably closer to 4% to 5% depending more on the likelihood of other cardiovascular conditions than the left ventricular dysfunction itself. For Class II, mortality is estimated at 5% to 15%; Class III is 15% to 30%; and Class IV is 30% to 70%, depending on responses to therapy and evidence of systemic decompensation [1]. Data from many clinical trials tend to underestimate this mortality, as the trial populations are younger (mean ages 55–65 years) and selected for absence of comorbidities. Further, there has emerged the phenomenon of "class creep" in order to meet enrollment benchmarks. The recent COPERNICUS trial describing the benefits of beta-blocking agents in the elusive population of patients considered to be functional class IV with normal volume status showed a 1-year mortality of only 18.5% in the placebo arm [48]. The MERIT trial of extended release metoprolol described 1-year mortality of 6% in Class II, 10% in Class III, and 19% in class IV [2]. On the other hand, the 1-year mortality of patients with refractory Class IV symptoms on standard medical therapy, left ventricular ejection fraction less than or equal to 25%, and mean peak oxygen consumption less than 12 ml/kg, in the REMATCH trial of left ventricular assist devices was 60% [49]. The persistence of this inexact and subjective classification offered by the New York Heart Association classification testifies to the importance of both clinical integration and simplicity of predictors of outcome.

More quantitative approaches to integration have been developed. Heart failure scoring systems have been proposed that summate points for many of the individual prognostic factors in order to assign an overall risk factor score. This approach has been complicated by inclusion of some continuous variables, such as sodium and creatinine, which must either be reduced to arbitrary threshold levels or given a range of values that is hard to validate in combination with other variables. The Aaronson heart failure score is currently the best validated approach to patients referred for cardiac transplantation, as it was developed from one dataset and confirmed in another later set [50]. The noninvasive model included presence of ischemic heart disease, resting heart rate, left ventricular ejection fraction, mean blood pressure, intraventricular conduction delay, peak oxygen consumption, and serum sodium, while the invasive model added pulmonary capillary wedge pressure as a variable. Application of such risk scores to contemporary heart failure populations has been limited, however, by the rapid evolution of new medical and device-based therapies. For instance, much of the earlier data has been rendered less relevant by the increasing prevalence of implantable defibrillators, which decrease the sudden death component of mortality. Similarly, the rapid growth in the use of biventricular pacing now frequently obscures variables related to the native QRS complex. Heart rate may also be less predictive as beta-blocking agents have become standard therapy for most patients. The contribution of serum sodium concentration may now be altered by wider use of aldosterone antagonists.

While providing sophisticated integration, the clinical scores lack not only generalizability but also simplicity. Scores from multiple variables are feasible for study populations or institutional case-mix adjustments. They remain impractical for calculation for routine use during daily clinical practice for individual patient decisions.

FUNCTIONAL ASSESSMENT

The four clinical classes of heart failure in the New York Heart Association system are intended to reflect the global limitation of daily activity. More objective measurement can be made of exercise capacity. This is actually an integrative assessment, as multiple physiological factors determine exercise capacity. Oxygen delivery is a function of heart rate, stroke volume, and oxygen carrying capacity. Although rarely limiting in the absence of intrinsic pulmonary disease, adequate pulmonary gas exchange is also necessary. Even if peripheral oxygen delivery is adequate, the peripheral circulation must respond to distribute the additional blood flow to exercising muscles. The state of the peripheral muscles is the last major physiological determinant of oxygen consumption, which can be markedly effected by deconditioning. Peak oxygen consumption during symptom-limited exercise is considered the gold standard for assessment of exercise capacity, as the level of anaerobic metabolism helps to indicate the degree of effort expended and the role of cardiac limitation in the overall exercise performance.

The prognostic value of measured peak oxygen consumption depends on the population being studied. Like most measures of prognosis, the highest and lowest values are most widely separated, but these are also the clinical profiles easiest to identify without formal exercise testing. The landmark work by Mancini established the peak oxygen consumption measurement as part of evaluation of ambulatory patients undergoing consideration for cardiac transplantation [51]. One-year survival was more than 90% for patients when peak oxygen consumption exceeded 18 ml/kg/min (correlates approximately with NYHA II functional class). The widely used threshold for transplant eligibility is 14–15 mk/kg/min, or less than 50% predicted maximum. However, most of the predictive power of this threshold derives from the dismal prognosis of patients with peak oxygen consumption less than 10 ml/kg/min, about the amount of oxygen uptake required for easy walking. In the initial study, survival at 1 year was less than 50% when peak oxygen consumption was below 10 ml/kg/min. The majority of patients had peak oxygen consumption between 10 and 18 ml/kg/min, a broad range in which peak oxygen consumption had less power to correctly identify patients with high early mortality risk. Pulmonary capillary wedge pressure measurements can provide additional information to peak oxygen consumption [51]. A later study by Lucas and colleagues of 307 patients showed 2-year survival of 85% with peak oxygen consumption greater than 16 ml/kg/min, and 2-year survival of 50% with initial peak oxygen consumption below 10 ml/kg/min [52].

The 6-minute walk test is an easier physiological measurement than peak oxygen consumption. As with other measures, the highest and lowest values identify patients most and least likely to survive. Lucas and colleagues have reported that patients walking more than 425 meters in 6 minutes had 2-year survival of 80%, whereas those walking fewer than 300 meters had 2-year survival of 65%. The 6-minute walk distance has been used in a mild-moderate heart failure population to discriminate the highest risk patients, who still had a mortality of only 10% during extended follow-up [53]. Therefore, the 6-minute walk distance appears less able to predicted adverse outcomes than peak oxygen consumption among more active patients with mild-moderate heart failure symptoms [52]. It may be more sensitive to changes in therapy when baseline values are very low in advanced stage disease.

Multiple questionnaires have been used to summarize patient-perceived limitations. These correlate in a general way with functional status and exercise capacity. The additional important psychological inputs of belief systems, depression, and anxiety may add to the power of these questionnaires to predict outcomes.

RESPONSES AFTER THERAPY

Heart failure is a chronic disease with the potential for dips and plateaus. Although the disease is slowly progressive, many of the troughs are transient and can be followed by prolonged periods of clinical stability. The duration of the plateaus seems to be extending with earlier and broader use of angiotensin-converting enzyme inhibitors and beta-blocking agents. A patient profile at any one point in time may provide misleading information about the overall course of disease, particularly as patients are most likely to be assessed during a trough period of clinical instability.

There is increasing interest toward identifying disease markers that can be assessed over time and for which a change would be more important than the initial baseline value. During therapy with vasodilators in the Veterans Administration Heart Failure trials (predominantly NYHA class II, average initial ejection fraction 30%), a five point fall in left ventricular ejection fraction during the first 6 months identified patients twice as likely to die during the next year as those whose ejection fraction rose by 5 to 10 points [54]. More recently, improvement in left ventricular ejection fraction has also correlated with better survival during therapy with beta-adrenergic blocking agents. Left ventricular dimension may prove more sensitive and useful as a marker of changing prognosis during therapy, because those nonsurgical therapies with long-term benefits have been shown to be those that decrease left ventricular volumes. The current difficulty of measuring small changes in ventricular dimensions and volumes has, thus far, limited this parameter for routine clinical monitoring. Changes in neurohormonal measurements over time closely correlate with clinical status and outcomes for populations. Norepinephrine (NE) levels increase less dramatically over time during more intense inhibition of the renin-angiotensin system. Absolute differences in mortality stratified by norepinephrine levels remain significant when examining large numbers of patients, but are not as striking for an individual patient. In the V-HeFT trial, mortality in the highest quartile of NE increase is approximately 20% higher than in the lowest quartile, but the prognostic value of changes is not sufficiently robust to predict outcomes reliably for individual patients.

ACE inhibitors and beta-adrenergic blocking agents are cornerstones of heart failure therapy, increasingly emphasized in guidelines and performance measures. Earlier studies indicating worse prognosis for patients not receiving these medications reflected not only their therapeutic benefit but also the inexperience of their treating physicians. Contemporary studies now include more subtle physiological risk stratification of patients unable to tolerate these life-saving medications. Intolerance can result from idiosyncratic side effects, but also from dependence upon higher levels of neurohormonal activation, triggered by need for acute neurohormonal support during progressive heart failure decompensation.

SELECTION FOR END-STAGE THERAPIES

Most of the prognostic factors discussed above have been useful to describe large groups of patients, and in some cases to understand disease progression. Populations with more abnormal parameters are more likely to have subsequent clinical events. However, as the disease progresses, population averages become less meaningful. Therapies need to be individualized according to the relative weights of risks and benefits and after adjusting for immediate versus delayed risk. Surgical therapies often bring a front-loaded risk with anticipated better outcomes later. When considering current replacement therapies with transplantation or assist devices, a critical inflexion point may be whether a given patient is more likely to be dead than alive at the end of the next 12 months (Fig. 8).

Patients considering end-stage therapies are generally those with limiting symptoms of heart failure during daily life, a NYHA class "IIIB" or IV, most of the time. Many patients presenting with these symptoms can nonetheless return to a comfortable quality of life with better prognosis if aggressive therapy can render them free of congestion and stability can be maintained, usually including intensive heart failure disease management (Fig. 9). During follow-up after hospitalization with class IV symptoms of failure, more than half of patients had no evidence of congestion at 1 month, and had a 2-year survival of 87%, compared with 67% for patients with one to two points for congestion, and 41% for patients with three to five points for congestion using a simple five-point congestion score including elevated jugular venous pressure, orthopnea, edema, recent weight gain, or need for diuretic increase [25]. Interestingly, much of the information from this score was contained in the orthopnea component alone.

As the disease progresses, therapeutic regimens must also change. Patients may become intolerant to medications that they previously tolerated. Renal function and hypotension pose more substantial limitations than during earlier stages of heart failure. The "cardiorenal syndrome" has been defined as renal function deterioration during diuresis, despite persistently severe volume overload [55]. This seems more common with longer

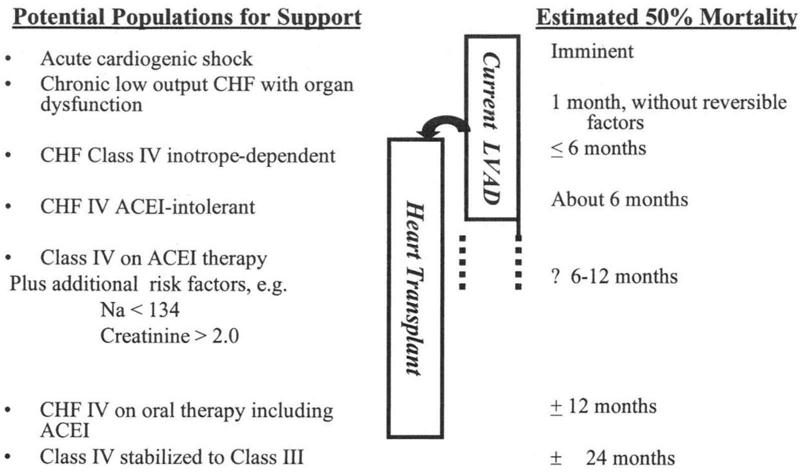

Potential Populations for Support
Acute cardiogenic shock
Chronic low output CHF with organ dysfunction
CHF Class IV inotrope-dependent
CHF IV ACEI-intolerant
Class IV on ACEI therapy
Plus additional risk factors, e.g.
Na < 134
Creatinine > 2.0
CHF IV on oral therapy including ACEI
Class IV stabilized to Class III
Current LVAD
Heart Transplant
Estimated 50% Mortality
Imminent
1 month, without reversible factors
≤ 6 months
About 6 months
? 6-12 months
± 12 months
± 24 months

Figure 8 Bar graph comparing 1-year mortality from two trials of advanced heart failure to mortality for escalating severity of disease defined after adjustment of medical therapy. The COPERNICUS trial describes class IV patients after excluding patients with fluid retention or recent inotropic therapy [61]. The RALES trial describes patients with current or recent class IV symptoms [62]. The reevaluation of patients in terms of clinical congestion score showed that those patients discharged from a hospitalization for Class IV symptoms had better survival if they had 0 on a congestion score 1 month later, than if they have persistent evidence of clinical congestion [25]. Patients receiving intravenous inotropes have less than 50% 1-year survival, with the worst outcome in those patients truly demonstrated to be dependent after repeated weaning attempts [49,63,64].

Mortality in first year
100
80
60
40
20
0
COPERN
RALES
IV to III
IV no congestion
IV still wet
ACE - Intolerant
IV Inotropes
"Ino-Dependent"
REMATCH Med

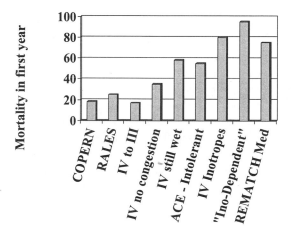

Figure 9 Potential populations for transplantation or mechanical support, demonstrating the importance of knowing prognosis with current therapies in order to select patients likely to have better prognosis with high-risk therapies, such as transplantation or mechanical support. (Adapted from Ref. 65.)

duration of disease and more severe right ventricular dysfunction, but may also be exacerbated by underlying hypertensive, diabetic, or atherosclerotic renal disease. The blood urea nitrogen is usually disproportionately elevated. Few studies have included patients with severely impaired renal function, so it is only recently that the vital importance of cardiorenal interactions have begun to be reemphasized. As previously discussed, declining systolic blood pressure also identifies higher risk cohorts, assuming institution of standard medications without unacceptable symptoms of hypotension.

The ability to tolerate ACE inhibitors seems to be a strong predictor of better outcomes, once heart failure has progressed. In one study of patients hospitalized with NYHA class IV heart failure symptoms, ACEI were discontinued due to progressive renal dysfunction or hypotension in 23% of patients who had previously tolerated them at standard doses. The average disease duration was 5 years vs. 2 years in patients who remained on ACEI [56]. One-year survival for those patients discharged on oral medications without ACEI was 45% compared with 77% for those on continued long-term ACE inhibitor treatment (Fig. 9).

Ambulatory patients at highest risk for morbid or fatal events during the next year are those felt to need outpatient inotropic therapy. These patients have had a mortality of approximately 50% by 6 months, 80% to 95% by 12 months [57]. The evaluation and declaration of "inotrope dependence" remains vague and contentious. The poor outcome of this group likely reflects both the severity of illness triggering inotropic therapy, and the risks added by inotropic therapy itself [57].

Current information is accumulating from disparate experiences regarding patients sick enough to be considered for replacement therapy but well enough from the noncardiac standpoint to recover from a major cardiovascular procedure. Increasingly precise outcome data will help these patients make decisions according to the fundamental principle that

BENEFIT = Outcome (product of quality X length of survival) with intervention
minus Outcome (quality X length) without intervention

Experience with more than 60,000 patients after cardiac transplantation now indicates a 1-year survival in the range of 85%, with 10-year survival of almost 50%.[58]. Many patients with heart failure have a predicted natural history worse than this, so selection for the very limited number of donor hearts is based largely on the relative risk of early death without transplantation, and the potential comorbidities that could compromise long-term outcome.

Conversely, the current outcome data for left ventricular assist devices as "destination" therapy for permanent support is derived from only 129 patients who were ineligible for transplantation. The 1-year survival with the left ventricular assist device was in the range of 50% [49]. Even though outcomes are improving rapidly with mechanical support, the appropriate candidate population at the present time would need to have an expected 1-year mortality substantially higher than 50% on medical therapy in order to expect a survival benefit from a ventricular assist device. Increasing depth of data about this population with and without devices will refine our ability to select patients for these newer therapies (Figure 8).

THE PROGNOSIS FOR CHANGE

Our current approach to predicting outcomes in heart failure is rapidly becoming obsolete as broader understanding about the genetic basis for disease and the molecular events central to disease progression are elucidated. The complexity of adaptive and maladaptive reflex responses to cardiac and circulatory compromise are being better defined. At the same time, our ability to image and measure pathological processes already exceeds our wisdom to apply this new information in order to individualize therapy.

The success of current therapies has created a new population of survivors for which baseline characteristics and modes of risk differ from the classic studies that defined our earlier prognostic risk models. Even the mode of death is evolving away from the tragically unexpected ''sudden death'' to the more expected progressive form of advanced heart failure for which palliative therapies no longer remain adequate to maintain a comfortable life.

The mosaic of previous prognostic factors turns in a kaleidoscope with newer factors that may soon dominate. Regardless of the specific factors found, it remains vital to classify them as to their purpose: to understand pathophysiology, to identify targets for design of therapy, to compare populations, or to provide individual patients with the best information on which to plan the remainder of their lives.

REFERENCES

1. Uretsky BF, Sheahan RG. Primary prevention of sudden cardiac death in heart failure: will the solution be shocking? J Am Coll Cardiol 1997; 30:1589–1597.
2. Effect of metoprolol CR/XL in chronic heart failure: Metoprolol CR/XL Randomized Intervention Trial in Congestive Heart Failure (MERIT-HF). Lancet 1999; 353:2001–2007.
3. Deedwania PC. The key to unraveling the mystery of mortality in heart failure: an integrated approach. Circulation 2003; 107:1719–1721.
4. Kimmelstiel CD, Konstam MA. Heart failure in women. Cardiology 1995; 86:304–309.
5. Yancy CW. Heart failure in blacks: etiologic and epidemiologic differences. Curr Cardiol Rep 2001; 3:191–197.
6. Shekelle PG, Rich MW, Morton SC, et al. Efficacy of angiotensin-converting enzyme inhibitors and beta-blockers in the management of left ventricular systolic dysfunction according to race, gender, and diabetic status: a meta-analysis of major clinical trials. J Am Coll Cardiol 2003; 41:1529–1538.
7. Dries DL, Sweitzer NK, Drazner MH, et al. Prognostic impact of diabetes mellitus in patients with heart failure according to the etiology of left ventricular systolic dysfunction. J Am Coll Cardiol 2001; 38:421–428.
8. Rathz DA, Gregory KN, Fang Y, et al. Hierarchy of polymorphic variation and desensitization permutations relative to beta 1- and beta 2-adrenergic receptor signaling. J Biol Chem 2003; 278:10784–10789.
9. Yamada T, Fukunami M, Ohmori M, et al. Which subgroup of patients with dilated cardiomyopathy would benefit from long-term beta-blocker therapy? A histologic viewpoint. J Am Coll Cardiol 1993; 21:628–633.
10. Mason JW, Bristow MR, Billingham ME, et al. Invasive and noninvasive methods of assessing Adriamycin cardiotoxic effects in man: superiority of histopathologic assessment using endomyocardial biopsy. Cancer Treat Rep 1978; 62:857–864.
11. Stevenson LW, Couper G, Natterson B, et al. Target heart failure populations for newer therapies. Circulation 1995; 92:II174–II181.
12. Lee TH, Hamilton MA, Stevenson LW, et al. Impact of left ventricular cavity size on survival in advanced heart failure. Am J Cardiol 1993; 72:672–676.
13. Di Salvo TG, Mathier M, Semigran MJ, et al. Preserved right ventricular ejection fraction predicts exercise capacity and survival in advanced heart failure. J Am Coll Cardiol 1995; 25:1143–1153.
14. Strauss RH, Stevenson LW, Dadourian BA, et al. Predictability of mitral regurgitation detected by Doppler echocardiography in patients referred for cardiac transplantation. Am J Cardiol 1987; 59:892–894.

15. Stevenson LW, Brunken RC, Belil D, et al. Afterload reduction with vasodilators and diuretics decreases mitral regurgitation during upright exercise in advanced heart failure [see comments]. J Am Coll Cardiol 1990; 15:174–180.

16. Drazner MH, Hamilton MA, Fonarow G, et al. Relationship between right and left-sided filling pressures in 1000 patients with advanced heart failure. J Heart Lung Transplant 1999; 18: 1126–1132.

17. Stevenson LW, Perloff JK. The limited reliability of physical signs for estimating hemodynamics in chronic heart failure. JAMA 1989; 261:884–888.

18. Stevenson LW, Tillisch JH, Hamilton M, et al. Importance of hemodynamic response to therapy in predicting survival with ejection fraction less than or equal to 20% secondary to ischemic or nonischemic dilated cardiomyopathy. Am J Cardiol 1990; 66:1348–1354.

19. Cohn JN, Johnson GR, Shabetai R, et al. Ejection fraction, peak exercise oxygen consumption, cardiothoracic ratio, ventricular arrhythmias, and plasma norepinephrine as determinants of prognosis in heart failure. The V-HeFT VA Cooperative Studies Group. Circulation 1993; 87: VI5–V16.

20. Clerico A, Iervasi G, Del Chicca MG, et al. Circulating levels of cardiac natriuretic peptides (ANP and BNP) measured by highly sensitive and specific immunoradiometric assays in normal subjects and in patients with different degrees of heart failure. J Endocrinol Invest 1998; 21:170–179.

21. Johnson W, Omland T, Hall C, et al. Neurohormonal activation rapidly decreases after intravenous therapy with diuretics and vasodilators for class IV heart failure. J Am Coll Cardiol 2002; 39:1623–1629.

22. Cheng V, Kazanagra R, Garcia A, et al. A rapid bedside test for B- type peptide predicts treatment outcomes in patients admitted for decompensated heart failure: a pilot study. J Am Coll Cardiol 2001; 37:386–391.

23. Maisel AS, Krishnaswamy P, Nowak RM, et al. Rapid measurement of B-type natriuretic peptide in the emergency diagnosis of heart failure. N Engl J Med 2002; 347:161–167.

24. Packer M, Carver JR, Rodeheffer RJ, et al. Effect of oral milrinone on mortality in severe chronic heart failure. The PROMISE Study Research Group. N Engl J Med 1991; 325: 1468–1475.

25. Lucas C, Johnson W, Hamilton MA, et al. Freedom from congestion predicts good survival despite previous class IV symptoms of heart failure. Am Heart J 2000; 140:840–7.

26. Drazner MH, Rame JE, Stevenson LW, et al. Prognostic importance of elevated jugular venous pressure and a third heart sound in patients with heart failure. N Engl J Med 2001; 345:574–81.

27. Nohria A, Tsang S, Fang J, et al. Clinical assessment identifies hemodynamic profiles that predict outcomes in patients admitted with heart failure. Journal Am Coll Cardiol 2003; 41: 1797–1804.

28. Chidsey CA, Kaiser GA, Sonnenblick EH, et al. Cardiac norepipherine stores in experimental heart failure in the dog. J Clin Invest 1964; 43:2386–2393.

29. Cohn JN, Levine TB, Olivari MT, et al. Plasma norepinephrine as a guide to prognosis in patients with chronic congestive heart failure. N Engl J Med 1984; 311:819–823.

30. Francis GS, Cohn JN, Johnson G, et al. Plasma norepinephrine, plasma renin activity, and congestive heart failure. Relations to survival and the effects of therapy in V-HeFT II. The V-HeFT VA Cooperative Studies Group. Circulation 1993; 87:VI40–V148.

31. Torré-Amione G, Kapadia S, Benedict C, et al. Proinflammatory cytokine levels in patients with depressed left ventricular ejection fraction: a report from the Studies of Left Ventricular Dysfunction (SOLVD). J Am Coll Cardiol 1996; 27:1201–1206.

32. Packer M, Lee WH, Kessler PD, et al. Role of neurohormonal mechanisms in determining survival in patients with severe chronic heart failure. Circulation 1987; 75:IV80–IV92.

33. Dries DL, Exner DV, Domanski MJ, et al. The prognostic implications of renal insufficiency in asymptomatic and symptomatic patients with left ventricular systolic dysfunction. J Am Coll Cardiol 2000; 35:681–689.

34. Carr JG, Stevenson LW, Walden JA, et al. Prevalence and hemodynamic correlates of malnutrition in severe congestive heart failure secondary to ischemic or idiopathic dilated cardiomyopathy. Am J Cardiol 1989; 63:709–713.

35. Hamilton MA, Stevenson LW, Luu M, et al. Altered thyroid hormone metabolism in advanced heart failure. J Am Coll Cardiol 1990; 16:91–95.

36. Dries DL, Exner DV, Gersh BJ, et al. Atrial fibrillation is associated with an increased risk for mortality and heart failure progression in patients with asymptomatic and symptomatic left ventricular systolic dysfunction: a retrospective analysis of the SOLVD trials. Studies of Left Ventricular Dysfunction. J Am Coll Cardiol 1998; 32:695–703.

37. Stevenson WG, Stevenson LW, Middlekauff HR, et al. Improving survival for patients with atrial fibrillation and advanced heart failure. J Am Coll Cardiol 1996; 28:1458–1463.

38. Fletcher RD, Cintron GB, Johnson G, et al. Enalapril decreases prevalence of ventricular tachycardia in patients with chronic congestive heart failure. The V-HeFT II VA Cooperative Studies Group. Circulation 1993; 87:VI49–VI55.

39. Middlekauff HR, Stevenson WG, Stevenson LW, et al. Syncope in advanced heart failure: high risk of sudden death regardless of origin of syncope. J Am Coll Cardiol 1993; 21:110–116.

40. Brendorp B, Elming H, Jun L, et al. QTc interval as a guide to select those patients with congestive heart failure and reduced left ventricular systolic function who will benefit from antiarrhythmic treatment with dofetilide. Circulation 2001; 103:1422–1427.

41. Brooksby P, Batin PD, Nolan J, et al. The relationship between QT intervals and mortality in ambulant patients with chronic heart failure. The United Kingdom heart failure evaluation and assessment of risk trial (UK-HEART). Eur Heart J 1999; 20:1335–1341.

42. Vrtovec B, Delgado R, Zewail A, et al. Prolonged QTc interval and high B-type natriuretic peptide levels together predict mortality in patients with advanced heart failure. Circulation 2003; 107:1764–1769.

43. Silverman ME, Pressel MD, Brackett JC, et al. Prognostic value of the signal-averaged electrocardiogram and a prolonged QRS in ischemic and nonischemic cardiomyopathy. Am J Cardiol 1995; 75:460–464.

44. Bigger JT. Prophylactic use of implanted cardiac defibrillators in patients at high risk for ventricular arrhythmias after coronary-artery bypass graft surgery. Coronary Artery Bypass Graft (CABG) Patch Trial Investigators. N Engl J Med 1997; 337:1569–1575.

45. Somberg JC, Molnar J. Usefulness of QT dispersion as an electrocardiographically derived index. Am J Cardiol 2002; 89:291–294.

46. Brendorp B, Elming H, Jun L, et al. QT dispersion has no prognostic information for patients with advanced congestive heart failure and reduced left ventricular systolic function. Circulation 2001; 103:831–835.

47. Armoundas AA, Tomaselli GF, Esperer HD. Pathophysiological basis and clinical application of T-wave alternans. J Am Coll Cardiol 2002; 40:207–217.

48. Packer M, Coats AJ, Fowler MB, et al. Effect of carvedilol on survival in severe chronic heart failure. N Engl J Med 2001; 344:1651–1658.

49. Gelijns AC, Moskowitz AJ, Heitjan DF, Stevenson LW, Dembitsky W, Long JW, Ascheim DD, Tierney AR, Levitan RG, Watson JT, Meier P, et al. Long-term use of a left ventricular assist device for end-stage heart failure. N Engl J Med 2001; 345:1435–1443.

50. Aaronson KD, Schwartz JS, Chen TM, et al. Development and prospective validation of a clinical index to predict survival in ambulatory patients referred for cardiac transplant evaluation. Circulation 1997; 95:2660–2667.

51. Mancini DM, Eisen H, Kussmaul W, et al. Value of peak exercise oxygen consumption for optimal timing of cardiac transplantation in ambulatory patients with heart failure. Circulation 1991; 83:778–786.

52. Lucas C, Stevenson LW, Johnson W, et al. The 6-min walk and peak oxygen consumption in advanced heart failure: aerobic capacity and survival [see comments]. Am Heart J 1999; 138: 618–624.

53. Bittner V, Weiner DH, Yusuf S, et al. Prediction of mortality and morbidity with a 6-minute walk test in patients with left ventricular dysfunction. SOLVD Investigators [see comments]. JAMA 1993; 270:1702–1707.

54. Cintron G, Johnson G, Francis G, et al. Prognostic significance of serial changes in left ventricular ejection fraction in patients with congestive heart failure. The V-HeFT VA Cooperative Studies Group. Circulation 1993; 87:VI17–VI23.

55. Weinfeld MS, Chertow GM, Stevenson LW. Aggravated renal dysfunction during intensive therapy for advanced chronic heart failure. Am Heart J 1999; 138:285–290.
56. Kittleson M, Hurwitz S, Shah MR, et al. Development of circulatory-renal limitations to angiotensin-converting enzyme inhibitors identifies patients with severe heart failure and early mortality. J Am Coll Cardiol 2003; 41:2029–2035.
57. Stevenson LW. Clinical use of inotropic therapy for heart failure: looking backward or forward? Part I: inotropic infusions during hospitalization. Circulation 2003; 108:367–372.
58. Taylor DO, Edwards LB, Mohacsi RJ, et al. The Registry of the International Society for Heart and Lung Transplantation: twentieth official report-2003. J Heart Lung Transplant 2003; 22:616–24.
59. Harrison A, Morrison LK, Krishnaswamy P, et al. B-type natriuretic peptide predicts future cardiac events in patients presenting to the emergency department with dyspnea. Ann Emerg Med 2002; 39:131–138.
60. Nohria A, Lewis E, Stevenson LW. Medical management of advanced heart failure. JAMA 2002; 287:628–640.
61. Packer M, Fowler MB, Roecker EB, et al. Effect of carvedilol on the morbidity of patients with severe chronic heart failure: results of the carvedilol prospective randomized cumulative survival (COPERNICUS) study. Circulation 2002; 106:2194–2199.
62. Pitt B, Zannad F, Remme WJ, et al. The effect of spironolactone on morbidity and mortality in patients with severe heart failure. Randomized Aldactone Evaluation Study Investigators. N Engl J Med 1999; 341:709–717.
63. Stevenson LW. The cul-de-sac at the end of the road. J Card Fail 2003; 9:188–191.
64. Hershberger R, Nauman D, Walker T, et al. Care processes and clinical outcomes of continuous outpatient inotropic therapy in patients with refractory endstage heart failure. J Cardiac Failure 2003; 9:180–187.
65. Stevenson LW, Rose E. Left ventricular assist devices: bridges to transplant, recovery, or destination for whom. Circulation 2003; 108:3059–63.

12

Conventional Therapy of Chronic Heart Failure: Diuretics, Angiotensin-Converting Enzyme Inhibitors, and Digoxin

G. William Dec
*Heart Failure and Transplantation Unit, Massachusetts General Hospital
Boston, Massachusetts, USA*

TREATMENT GOALS

Heart failure treatment goals should include improvement in symptoms, increased functional capacity, prevention or partial amelioration of left ventricular dilatation, and improvement in survival. Although never prospectively validated in clinical trials, several general measures are advisable for most heart failure patients because they are not harmful and generally improve functional capacity. Obese patients should lose weight, smokers should discontinue tobacco use, and low-level aerobic physical activity should be encouraged. Every effort should be made to identify and correct reversible causes for heart failure. Specific treatment should be initiated for anemia, thyrotoxicosis, or other causes of high cardiac output failure. Systemic hypertension should be aggressively treated, and surgical correction of significant valvular, congenital or cardiac lesions should be considered. Withdrawal of any cardiac depressants, such as alcohol, should be encouraged.

Heart failure that persists, after correction of reversible causes, should be treated with dietary sodium restriction, diuretics for volume overload, vasodilator therapy (particularly ACE [angiotensin-converting enzyme] inhibitors), digitalis, and β-adrenergic blockers (Fig. 1). Sodium restriction is generally not necessary for patients with mild (New York Heart Association [NYHA] class I or II) heart failure symptoms. However, a restriction below 4 g per day is generally indicated for patients with more advanced heart failure symptoms [1].

PHARMACOLOGIC THERAPY FOR SYSTOLIC HEART FAILURE

Diuretics

Diuretics remain the mainstay of treatment for "congestive" symptoms, but have not been shown to improve survival. Diuretics interfere with sodium retention by inhibiting the resorption of sodium or chloride in the renal tubules. Most agents produce further chronic activation of a renin-angiotensin system in heart failure patients by lowering

THERAPY FOR CHF

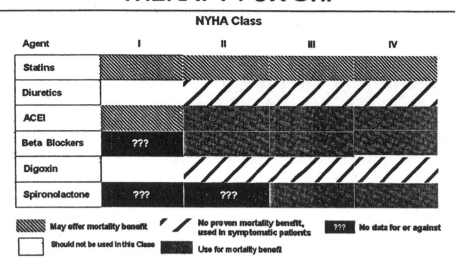

Figure 1 Standard pharmacological approach to heart failure based upon agent and severity of clinical heart failure symptoms. (From Ref. 1a.)

afferent glomerular renal blood flow. However, neurohormonal activation (renin, angiotensin, endothelin-1 and BNP [brain natriuretic peptides]) have been shown to acutely decrease after short-term diuretic therapy designed to decrease markedly elevated filling pressures among patients with decompensated heart failure [2]. All diuretics except spironolactone reach luminal transport sites within the kidney through the tubular fluid. A high degree of protein binding (> 95%) limits glomerular filtration, even among patients who are hypoalbuminemia. Binding to serum proteins traps the diuretic in the vascular space so it can be effectively delivered to the secretory sites of the proximal tubular cells. The plasma half-life of a diuretic determines the frequency of administration. Two pharmacological classes of agents are available: loop diuretics and agents that act in the distal tubule [3] (Table 1). Dyazides and distal diuretics have sufficiently long half-lives that they can be administered once or twice daily. Loop diuretics have shorter half-lives that range from 1 hour for bumetanide to 3 to 4 hours for torsemide. The half-life of furosemide is 1.5 to 2 hours [3].

The relationship between the arrival of a diuretic at its site of action in the kidney, and the natriuretic response determines the pharmacodynamics of the drug (Fig. 2). This pharmacodynamic relationship holds for all loop diuretics, although the curve may be shifted to the right or left. This response means that in a given patient, the maximum response to each loop diuretic is the same. The same type of dose-response also holds true for thiazide diuretics. This relationship indicates that a threshold quantity of drug must be achieved at the site of action in order to produce a diuretic response. Thus, diuretic dosing must be individualized in order to determine the dose that will be sufficient to achieve this steep portion of the curve, as shown in Figure 2 (i.e., the effective dose).

Loop Diuretics

The loop diuretics include ethacrynic acid, furosemide, torsemide, and bumetanide. These are the most potent diuretics currently available and inhibit tubular reabsorption of sodium

Table 1 Characteristics and Dosages of Commonly Used Diuretic Agents

	Diuretic	Brand Name	Principal Site and Mechanism of Action	Effect on Electrolytes		Usual Dosage	Action		
				In Urine	In Blood		Onset (hr)	Peak (hr)	Duration (hr)
	Chlorothiazide	Diuril	Distal tubule: inhibition of NaCl reabsorption			500–1,000 mg/day p.o. / 500 mg q. 12 hr I.V.	1 / –	4 / –	6–12 / 2
Thiazides	Hydrochlorothiazide	HydroDIURIL		↑Na, ↑Cl, ↑K	↓Cl, ↓K, ↑HCO$_3$	50–100 mg/day	2	4	6–12
	Trichlormethiazide	Methahydrin, Naqua				4–8 mg/day	2	6	24
	Chlorthalidone[a]	Hygroton	Distal tubule (cortical diluting segment) and proximal tubule			100 mg/day	2	6	24
	Metolazone	Zaroxolyn, Diulo				2.5–20 mg/day p.o.	1	2	12–24
	Furosemide	Lasix				40–160 mg/day p.o. / 10–80 mg I.V.	1 / 5 min	1–2 / –	6–8 / 4–6
Loop Diuretics	Torsemide	Demadex	Ascending limb of loop of Henle: inhibition of Cl reabsorption	↑Na, ↑Cl, ↑HCO$_3$, ↑K, ↑H	↓Cl, ↑HCO$_3$, ↓K, ↓Na	5–200 mg/day p.o. / 5–20 mg I.V.	1 / 10 min	1–2 / 1	6–8 / 4–6
	Ethacrynic acid	Edecrin				50–150 mg/day p.o. / 20–100 mg I.V.	– / 5 min	2 / –	6–8 / 3
	Bumetanide	Bumex				0.5–2.0mg b.i.d., p.o. / 0.25–2.0 mg I.V.	–1 / –	1–2 / –	4–6 / –1
Potassium-Sparing Diuretics	Spironolactone	Aldactone	Distal tubule: aldosterone antagonism	↓K, ↓H; slight ↑Na, ↑Cl, and ↑HCO$_3$	↑K	25 mg q.i.d.	Gradual	2–3 days after starting therapy	2–3 days after starting therapy
	Triamterene	Dyrenium	Distal tubule: membrane effect		↑K	100–300 mg/day	2–4	3	12–16
	Amiloride	Midamor	Proximal and distal tubules: inhibition of Na$^+$, K$^+$-ATPase		↑K	5–10 mg/day p.o.	2	6–10	24

[a]Chlorthalidone is chemically different from, but pharmacologically similar to, the thiazides.
Source: From Ref. 41.

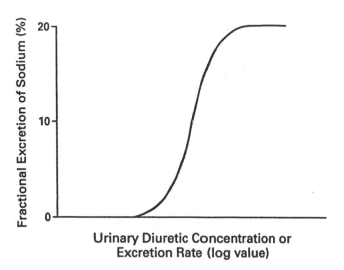

Figure 2 Pharmacodynamic effect of a loop diuretic. The relationship between the natri-uretic response and the amount of diuretic reaching the site of action is represented by a sigmoid-shaped curve. (From Ref. 3.)

chloride in the ascending limb of the loop of Henle (the diluting segment). Up to 30% of the filtered load of sodium chloride is excreted in the urine after intravenous administration of furosemide. Recent data suggest that torsemide and bumetanide may be more effective than furosemide in advanced heart failure [3,4]. Although the oral availability of furose-mide varies widely (10% to 100%), absorption of torsemide and bumetanide is nearly complete (ranging from 80% to 100%) [3]. These newer drugs are particularly effective in the presence of right-sided heart failure, which impairs absorption of the agent from the gastrointestinal tract. Once a day dosing of a loop diuretic is usually effective, but patients with persistent fluid retention may require twice daily dosing.

Long-term oral administration of loop diuretics may lead to hypokalemia, hypomag-nesemia, extracellular volume contraction, orthostatic hypotension, azotemia, and hypo-chloremic, hypokalemic alkalosis. Nonetheless, loop diuretics remain effective, even in the presence of metabolic alkalosis, or substantially impaired renal function.

Thiazide Diuretics

Thiazides act mainly by inhibiting reabsorption of sodium and chloride in the distal convo-luted tubules of the kidney. They also increase potassium secretion in the distal convoluted tubules and collecting ducts, resulting in potassium depletion. Thiazide-induced diuresis is generally relatively modest; these agents are ineffective when the glomerular filtration rate falls below 40 mL per minute [3]. Chlorothiazide and hydrochlorothiazide are the most commonly prescribed agents. Undesirable side effects include hypokalemia and hypo-magnesemia. Drug fever and allergic dermatitis may also occur. Thrombocytopenia, leuko-penia, and vasculitis are all rare complications of these agents. Thiazides often precipitate or exacerbate hyperglycemia, worsen hyperuricemia, and may decrease sexual function. Further, thiazides can adversely affect lipid metabolism, producing up to an 8% elevation of low density lipoprotein (LDL) cholesterol and a 15% to 20% increase in triglyceride levels. Fortunately, many of these adverse effects on lipids may be short-term; serum cholesterol levels have been reported to decline back to baseline within 12 to 24 months of therapy.

Metolazone is a member of the quinazoline-sulfonamide group; it exerts its effects primarily by inhibiting sodium reabsorption at the cortical diluting site, and in the proximal convoluting tubule. The drug's prolonged duration of action is generally believe attributed to protein binding and entero-hepatic recycling.

Potassium Sparing Diuretics

Spironolactone, triamterene, and amiloride are relatively weak diuretics on their own, but enhance the action and counteract the kaliuretic effects of the more potent loop diuretics. The spironolactones are steroid analogs of the mineralocorticoids, and work by inhibiting the effects of aldosterone on the distal tubule. These agents should be employed only in patients with advanced heart failure whose creatinine is below 2.5 mg/dL, and potassium level is below 5.0 mEq/L. Both spironolactone and eplerenone have been shown to improve survival in advanced heart failure and following acute myocardial infarction, respectively (Chapter 15). Ongoing trials should address the important therapeutic question whether aldosterone-inhibiting agents will benefit patients with mild heart failure or asymptomatic left ventricular dysfunction.

Triamterene has a site of action similar to that of spironolactone, and causes similar urinary changes. Amiloride acts at the proximal and distal tubules, principally by inhibiting Na^+-K^+-ATPase. These potassium sparing agents should also be used cautiously in patients with renal dysfunction as they may precipitate significant hyperkalemia.

Diuretic Tolerance

Lack of response to diuretic therapy may be cause by excessive sodium intake, use of agents that antagonize their effects (e.g., nonsteroidal anti-inflammatory drugs, including cyclooxygenase-2 [COX-2] inhibitors), worsening renal dysfunction, or compromised renal blood flow due to worsening cardiac function. Further, long-term administration of a loop diuretic is associated with hypertrophy of the distal nephron segments, with concomitant increases in reabsorption of sodium [5]. Sodium that escapes from the loop of Henle is, therefore, actively reabsorbed at more distal sites, decreasing overall diuresis. This phenomenon results in long-term tolerance to loop diuretics. Thiazide diuretics block the nephron sites at which this hypertrophy occurs. Thus, the combination of a loop diuretic plus a thiazide may create a synergistic response and should be considered for patients who do not have an adequate response to an optimal dose of a loop diuretic. Metolazone exacts a markedly additive response when administered with furosemide; this combination may offer an alternative to intravenous therapy for patients with significant edema. High-dose furosemide when administered as a continuous infusion may also be more effective than given as bolus administration for hospitalized patients with acutely decompensated heart failure [6]. In cases of advanced (NYHA class III–IV) heart failure, patients should be instructed to follow a flexible diuretic program, whereby they adjust their daily diuretic dose to maintain a desired prespecified body weight, ascertained to minimize their symptoms of venous congestion. This ''ideal'' body weight should be periodically reevaluated during office visits.

Vasodilator Therapy

Vasodilator therapy remains one of the two cornerstones of heart failure treatment (Fig. 1, Table 2). The mechanisms of action of different vasodilators vary and include a direct

Table 2 Effects and Dosages of Major Vasodilators Used in Heart Failure Management

Agent	Mechanism of Action	Venous Dilating Effect	Arteriolar Dilating Effect	Usual Dosage
Nitroglycerin	Direct	+++	+	25–500 μg/min I.V.
Isosorbide dinitrate	Direct	+++	+	5–20 mg q. 2 hr s.l. or 10–60 mg q. 4 hr p.o.
Hydralazine	Direct	–	+++	10–100 mg q. 6 hr p.o.
Sodium nitroprusside	Direct	+++	+++	5–150 μg/min I.V.
Epoprostenol (prostacyclin)	Direct	+++	+++	5–15 ng/kg/min I.V.
Captopril	Inhibition of angiotensin-converting enzyme	+++	++	6.25–50.0 mg q. 6–8 hr p.o.
Enalapril	Inhibition of angiotensin-converting enzyme	+++	+++	5–20 mg b.i.d., p.o.
Lisinopril	Inhibition of angiotensin-converting enzyme	+++	++	10–40 mg/day p.o.
Quinapril	Inhibition of angiotensin-converting enzyme	+++	++	10–40 mg/day p.o.
Ramipril	Inhibition of angiotensin-converting enzyme	+++	++	1.25–5 mg/day p.o.
Losartan	Angiotensin II receptor blockade	+++	++	25–100 mg/day p.o.
Valsartan	Angiotensin II receptor blocade	+++	++	80–320 mg/day p.o.
Candesartan	Angiotensin II receptor blockade	+++	++	16–32 mg/day p.o.
Irbesartan	Angiotensin II receptor blockade	+++	++	75–300 mg/day p.o.

Source: From Ref. 41.

effect primarily on venous capacitance vessels (nitrates), arterioles (hydralazine), or a direct balanced effect on the venous and arterial systems (sodium nitroprusside, α-adrenergic blocking agents, angiotensin-converting enzyme (ACE) inhibitors, and angiotensin II receptor blockers).

Agents that are primarily venodilators reduce elevated cardiac filling pressures. Thus, nitrates can effectively reduce pulmonary congestion, while having little effect on systemic blood pressure. Conversely, agents that primarily dilate the arterioles (true afterload reducing agents) reduce systemic vascular resistance and improve cardiac output, but produce little change in ventricular filling pressures. If the rise in cardiac output leads to improvement in renal perfusion, however, diuresis may ensue with a secondary decrease in cardiac filling pressures. Drugs that produce balanced venous and arteriolar dilation should generally be chosen as first-line therapy because most heart failure patients have elevated preload and afterload that require pharmacologic modulation.

The ACE inhibitors play a crucial initial role in the treatment of heart failure by altering the vicious cycle of hemodynamic abnormalities and neurohormonal activation.

The renin angiotensin aldosterone system is known to exert a crucial pathophysiological role in the production of both heart failure symptoms and disease progression [7]. Enhanced sympathetic neural activity also leads to further renal-mediated renin production through vasoconstriction of efferent renal arterioles. These elevated levels of angiotensin II and sympathetic neural activity produce clinically important vasoconstriction and increased renal production of aldosterone. Angiotensin II exerts its actions in target organs and tissues by binding to both angiotensin II, type 1, and 2 (AT_1 and AT_2) receptors. Most adverse effects in humans are mediated primarily by the AT_1 receptor [7]. ACE inhibitors decrease the formation of angiotensin II that inhibit the breakdown of bradykinin. In turn, increased bradykinin levels result in the formation of nitric oxide and other important endogenous vasodilators. Most ACE inhibitors are formulated as prodrugs, requiring esterification in the liver, and are cleared by renal mechanisms. Although tissue affinities differ between drugs, this property has not been shown to impact clinical outcomes.

Randomized, controlled clinical trials have demonstrated the beneficial effects of ACE inhibitors on functional status, neurohormonal activation, quality of life, and survival in patients with chronic heart failure due to left ventricular systolic dysfunction [8,9]. ACE inhibitors reduce the risk of death due to heart failure, sudden cardiac death, and myocardial infarction; similar mortality benefits have been demonstrated with multiple agents in a broad range of patients [8] (Table 3). Although randomized trials in patients with NYHA class II or III heart failure symptoms have shown that survival is improved by either an ACE inhibitor or the combination of hydralazine and isosorbide dinitrate, a review of more than 30 randomized trials indicates that only the ACE inhibitors are associated with both enhanced survival and improved functional status [8]. In patients with NYHA class III or IV heart failure symptoms, captopril increases survival to a greater extent than hydralazine when doses are titrated to achieve the same hemodynamic goals, and when nitrates are included in both regimens; this beneficial effect is presumably due to captopril's additional actions on neurohormonal activation [10].

There is clear and compelling evidence that ACE inhibitor therapy should be used whenever feasible in all symptomatic heart failure patients (Fig. 2). A variety of well-designed prospective, placebo-controlled studies, particularly CONSENSUS I (Cooperative New Scandinavian Enalapril Study I), V-HeFT II (Vasodilator Heart Failure Trial II), SOLVD (Studies of Left Ventricular Dysfunction) trials, and the MHFT (Munich Mild Heart Failure Trial) have shown improvement in symptoms and survival in patients with

Table 3   Effect of ACE Inhibitors on Mortality in Patients with Heart Failure

Trial	Mortality		RR (95% CI)
	ACEI	Controls	
Chronic CHF			
CONSENSUS I	39%	54%	0.56 (0.34–0.91)
SOLVD (Treatment)	35%	40%	0.82 (0.70–0.97)
SOLVD (Prevention)	15%	19%	0.92 (0.79–1.08)
POST MI			
SAVE	20%	25%	0.81 (0.68–0.97)
AIRE	17%	23%	0.73 (0.60–0.89)
TRACE	35%	42%	0.78 (0.67–0.91)
SMILE	10%	14%	0.71 (0.49–0.94)

heart failure symptoms, ranging from NYHA class I–IV [9]. The benefits are far-reaching with a survival benefit evident for up to 12 years among patients who participated in the SOLVD trial [11] (Fig. 3).

Despite the unequivocal benefits of ACE inhibitor therapy, only 60% to 75% of all symptomatic patients take these agents [12]. Lack of treatment in the elderly remains problematic. Initiating treatment in this population often causes the clinician greatest concern; yet, this is the cohort in whom heart failure is most prevalent, and that includes the largest number of patients who may benefit from therapy. The dose of ACE inhibitors should be slowly uptitrated in the elderly to avoid orthostatic hypotension, but fully effective doses can usually be achieved.

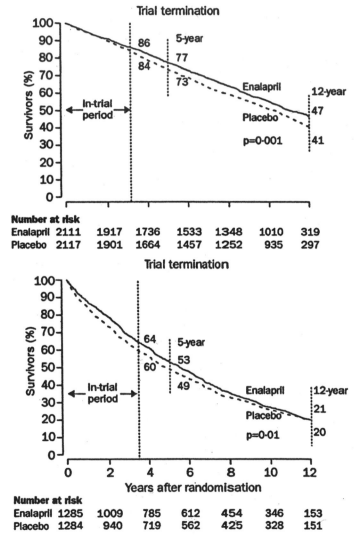

Figure 3   Long-term survival for patient who participated in the Studies of Left Ventricular Dysfunction (SOLVD) Prevention (*upper panel*) and Treatment (*lower panel*) trials. Survival analysis extends to 12 years. Numbers beside the curves denote the percentage of survival at trial termination, 5 years, and 12 years after randomization, calculated by the Kaplan-Meier method. (From Ref. 11.)

Important racial differences may also exist in pharmacological responsiveness to different vasodilator agents. Retrospective analyses of both the V-HeFT and SOLVD populations have confirmed that although enalapril was effective in decreasing mortality and hospitalizations among white patients, it was less effective in black patients with heart failure of comparable severity [13,14] (Fig. 4). In contrast, conventional therapy utilizing hydralazine and isosorbide dinitrate appears effective in lowering all-cause mortality in blacks [13] (Chapter 20). Whether these differences are related to genetic polymorphisms in key genes, such as the angiotensin-converting enzyme, is currently unknown.

Dosing

Controlled trials have generally targeted high doses regardless of the patient's therapeutic response. The Assessment of Treatment with Lisinopril And Survival (ATLAS) trial dem-

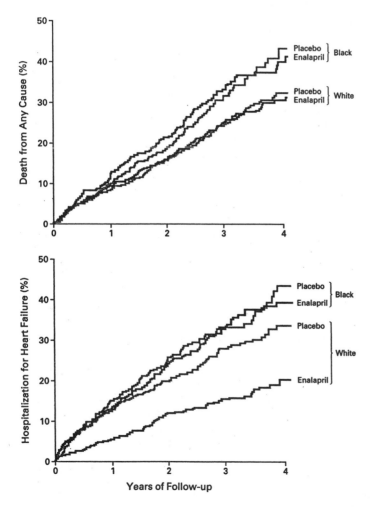

Figure 4   All-cause mortality (*top panel*) and hospitalizations (*bottom panel*) for heart failure among black patients and white patients randomly assigned to enalapril or placebo. The rate of hospitalization for heart failure among black patients receiving enalapril was significantly higher than among white patients receiving enalapril (p< .001). Mortality was similar among black and white patients regardless of treatment. (From Ref. 13.)

onstrated that high doses of lisinopril (32.5 to 35 mg daily) were better than low dosages (2.5 to 5 mg daily) in reducing the risk of hospitalization, but the two dosages had *similar* effects on symptoms and mortality [15]. Nanes and colleagues found no significant difference in survival, and clinical or hemodynamic variables, between patients who received standard dose enalapril (mean dose 18 ± 4 mg daily) or high dose enalapril (42 ± 19 mg daily) [16]. Further, a recent study by Tang and colleagues could not demonstrate any difference between high- and low-dose enalapril on serum aldosterone or plasma angiotensin II suppression, despite a dose-dependent reduction in serum ACE activity [17]. Thus, dosing should be guided by the higher doses used in randomized clinical trials. However, even low doses confer a significant benefit, and dose adjustments may be necessary in order to permit the use of other agents, particularly β-blockers, in patients when marginal blood pressure (e.g., < 85 mm Hg) is present.

ACE Inhibitors in Postmyocardial Infarction Management

ACE inhibitor therapy has become the standard of care among patients with asymptomatic or minimally symptomatic left ventricular dysfunction to slow disease progression and is also indicated to reduce mortality after acute myocardial infarction. Postinfarction trials have now randomized more than 100,000 patients, and have demonstrated that ACE inhibitor treatment results in a 10% to 27% reduction in all-cause mortality, and a 20% to 50% reduction in the risk of developing symptomatic heart failure [18] (Table 3).

The largest randomized clinical trials have included the Survival And Ventricular Enlargement (SAVE} trial, the Acute Infarction Ramipril Efficacy (AIRE) trial, the Survival of Myocardial Infarction Long-Term Evaluation (SMILE) trial, the Gruppo Italiano per lo Studio Della Sopravvivenza Nell'Infarto Miocardico-3 (GISSI-3) trial, and the Fourth International Study of Infarct Survival (ISIS-4). Pooled mortality data from the SAVE, AIRE, and TRACE studies found an odds ratio for ACE inhibitor therapy vs. placebo of 0.74 (95% confident intervals, 0.66–0.83), p<001 [19] (Fig. 5). The absolute event-rate difference was 5.7% between treatment groups. For every 1000 patients treated, approximately 60 deaths would be avoided (or, to avoid one death, about 15 patients would need to be treated for about 30 months). Oral ACE inhibitors, begun within 24 hours of acute myocardial infarction, are safe and appear most beneficial for patients whose left ventricular ejection fractions are reduced below 40% to 45%.

ACE Inhibitor-Aspirin Interaction

Aspirin is frequently prescribed when heart failure results from ischemic heart disease. Two retrospective analyses of large-scale clinical trials have suggested that aspirin lessens the beneficial effects of ACE inhibitors on survival and cardiovascular morbidity [20]. Despite these concerning post-hoc findings, no prospective studies have evaluated the possible adverse interaction between these two commonly prescribed agents.

There is some evidence that the potential interaction between aspirin and ACE inhibitors may be dose-related. A recent meta-analysis of all hypertension and heart failure patients who had received both agents suggest that aspirin at doses less than or equal to 100 mg showed no interaction with ACE inhibitors [21].

A potential mechanism for the hypothesized adverse interaction between aspirin and ACE inhibitors in heart failure patients involve prostaglandin synthesis. ACE inhibitors are known to augment bradykinin, which in turn stimulates synthesis of key prostaglandins that may contribute to vasodilatation. In the presence of aspirin, the bradykinin-induced increases in prostaglandins may be attenuated, thereby potentially reducing the benefits

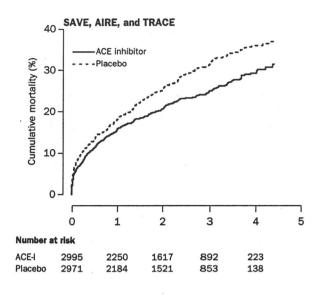

Number at risk

ACE-I	2995	2250	1617	892	223
Placebo	2971	2184	1521	853	138

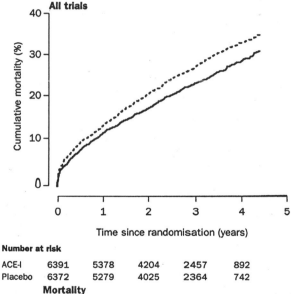

Number at risk

ACE-I	6391	5378	4204	2457	892
Placebo	6372	5279	4025	2364	742

Figure 5 Cumulative mortality for patients who participated in the SAVE (Survival and Ventricular Enlargement), AIRE (Acute Infarction Ramipril Efficacy), and TRACE (Trandolapril in patients with reduced left ventricular function after acute myocardial infarction) trials. Number of patients at risk at each of the first 5 years of observation following myocardial infarction are indicated along the horizontal axis. (From Ref. 19.)

of ACE inhibition. No data are available on the potential interaction between adenosine diphosphate (ADP) antagonists, such as clopidogrel and ACE inhibitors. Current Heart Failure Society of America practice guidelines recommend that each medication be considered on its own merits. These guidelines indicate that there is currently insufficient evidence concerning the potential negative therapeutic interaction between aspirin and ACE inhibitors to warrant withholding either of these medications when an indication exists for their administration [22].

Digitalis

Cardiac glycosides have played an important role in the treatment of heart failure for over three centuries. Withering described in stunning detail, clinically important aspects of the therapeutic properties and toxicity of the common foxglove plant (*digitalis purpurea*) in 1785 [23]. Throughout most of the 20th century, controversy existed about whether the risks of digitalis outweighed its therapeutic benefits, particularly among patients with heart failure who remained in sinus rhythm. During the past 15 years, a variety of clinical trials have carefully examined this issue in heart failure patients. Digoxin is a semi-synthetic derivative made from the leaves of the plant *digitalis lanata*. At the cellular level, digitalis acts by inhibiting sarcolemmal Na^+-K^+-ATPase activity, thereby restricting the transport of sodium and potassium across the plasma membrane [24]. This enzymatic inhibitor property leads to an increase in the intracellular sodium and an efflux of potassium from the cell. Coupled with the influx of sodium is an increase in calcium uptake, which is then made available to the contractile elements of the myofibrils. Diastolic calcium levels are minimally increased because of rapid sequestration of intracellular calcium by the sarcoplasmic reticulum.

In addition to its positive inotropic effects on cardiac muscle, digitalis also reduces activation of the sympathetic nervous system and the renin-angiotensin system [25]. Abnormalities of carotid baroreceptor function and excess sympathetic nervous system activity are both important components of chronic heart failure. Digitalis can partially restore the inhibitory effects of the cardiac baroreceptor system on sympathetic efferent outflow from the central nervous system [25]. Digoxin also partially restores the impaired circadian pattern of heart rate variability that is prominent in heart failure patients [26]. Van Veldhuisen and colleagues found digoxin to be more effective than placebo in reducing plasma norepinephrine and renin activity and improving exercise duration when administered as monotherapy in mild heart failure patients [26] (Fig. 6). Thus, chronic digoxin usage exhibits favorable inhibitory effects on the sympathetic nervous system and enhanced parasympathetic effects [26–28].

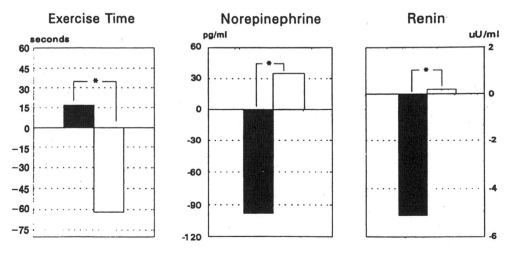

Figure 6   Effect of 6-months of treatment with digoxin (n = 22; solid bars) or placebo (n = 20; open bars) on exercise time, plasma norepinephrine and plasma renin in patients with mild heart failure (p<0.05) (From Ref. 26a.)

Clinical Trials of Digoxin Efficacy in Chronic Heart Failure

A variety of short- and long-term controlled and uncontrolled clinical trials have provided unequivocal evidence that chronic digoxin administration can increase left ventricular ejection fraction, improve exercise capacity, decrease heart failure symptoms, and reduce heart failure-associated hospitalizations and emergency room visits [28]. The first well-designed trial was reported by Dobbs and colleagues in 1977 [29]. These investigators completed a double-blind, placebo-controlled, single-crossover study of chronic digoxin treatment in 46 patients: 34% of patients deteriorated while receiving placebo, 8 of whom improved following reinstitution of digoxin. Interpretation of the study is complicated by the inclusion of almost one-third of patients with atrial fibrillation whose outcomes were not distinguished from those who remain in sinus rhythm. Flag and colleagues performed a double-blind, placebo-controlled crossover study in 30 NYHA class II–III patients over a 3-month period [30]. Digoxin discontinuation resulted in a significant decline in ejection fraction, though was not associated with changes in orthopnea, paroxysmal nocturnal dyspnea, or exercise tolerance. An elegant study by Lee and colleagues reported beneficial effects of chronic digoxin therapy as assessed by a summated clinical heart failure score that consisted of a dyspnea index, presence or absence of pulmonary rales, heart rate, signs of right-sided congestion, and chest x-ray findings of left-sided heart failure [31]. Patients who demonstrated a favorable response had more chronic and severe heart failure symptoms, greater left ventricular dilatation, and more markedly impaired ventricular function. Multivariate analysis showed that the presence of a third heart sound was the strongest predictor of improvement during digoxin treatment in that study [31].

The Captopril Multicenter Research Group trial was the first randomized, placebo-controlled prospective trial of sufficient power to address the true efficacy of digoxin therapy. This study evaluated the outcome of captopril, digoxin, or placebo treatment in 300 patients maintained on chronic diuretic therapy [32]. More than 85% of patients had mild NYHA class I or II symptoms, and all patients had left ventricular ejection fractions below 40%. Ejection fraction rose by 4.1% in the digoxin group vs. 1.3% in the placebo group ($p < 0.05$), and a nonsignificant improvement in exercise duration was observed. Importantly, there were eight hospitalizations for decompensated heart failure among digoxin-treated patients, compared with 19 for those who received placebo.

The Prospective Randomized Study of Ventricular Function and Efficacy of Digoxin (PROVED) and Randomized Assessment of Digoxin on Inhibitors of Angiotensin Converting Enzyme (RADIANCE) examined the outcome of digoxin withdrawal in patients with stable mild to moderate heart failure (NYHA functional class II or III), and systolic dysfunction (LVEF < 35%), [33,34]. These studies were double-blind and target digoxin levels during the baseline run-in phase averaged 0.9 to 2.0 ng/ml. Following digoxin withdrawal, 40% of patients demonstrated worsening of heart failure symptoms (defined as increased diuretic requirement, need for emergency room visit, or hospital treatment) (Fig. 7). Treadmill exercise tolerance and quality of life measures also worsened (Fig. 8). Selection bias may have resulted, however, from the study design that included patients who had been successfully maintained on digoxin and, therefore, may have been responders to this form of therapy [28]. When the results from the PROVED and RADIANCE trials are combined, patients who continue digoxin as part of triple therapy with a diuretic and ACE inhibitor were less likely to develop worsening heart failure (4.7%) compared with those treated with a diuretic alone (39%, $p < 0.001$), or a diuretic plus digoxin (19%, $p = 0.009$) [35] (Fig. 9). Although there are no clinical trials that have specifically examined the digoxin efficacy in patients with NYHA class IV symptoms, there is evidence that the agent works across the spectrum of left ventricular systolic dysfunction. A prespecified

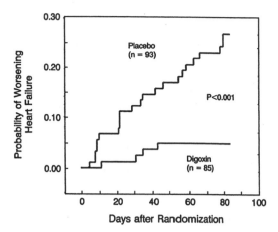

Figure 7 Kaplan-Meier plot analysis of the cumulative probability of worsening heart failure in patients continuing digoxin compared with those switched to placebo. (From Ref. 34.)

subgroup analysis of patients enrolled in the Digitalis Investigation Group (DIG) Trial, with evidence of severe heart failure (LVEF < 25% or cardiothoracic ratio > 0.55) showed significant benefit of digoxin [22]. Reductions in the combined endpoint of all-cause mortality or hospitalization were observed for digoxin compared to placebo that included: 16% reduction (95% CI, 7% to 24%) in patients with LVEF less than 25% and 15% reduction (95% CI, 6% to 23%) in patients with cardiothoracic ratio greater than 0.55 [32].

Effects on Mortality

The Digitalis Investigator's Group (DIG) Trial addressed the effect of digoxin on survival in over 6500 patients with mild to moderate heart failure. Importantly, the majority of

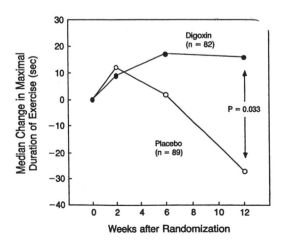

Figure 8 Median changes in maximal duration of exercise after 2 to 12 weeks in patients who continued digoxin compared with those randomized to placebo. Changes were assessed during treadmill testing using a modified Naughton protocol. (From Ref. 34.)

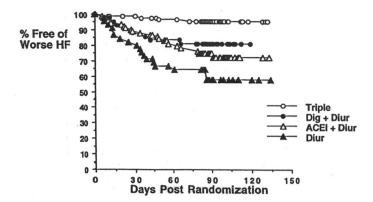

Figure 9 Likelihood of deterioration in heart failure (HF) status in four treatment groups. Patients receiving triple therapy were less likely to experience treatment failure compared with any of the other three groups. Triple: digoxin, ACE inhibitor, and diuretic; Dig plus Diur: digoxin and diuretic; ACEI plus Diur: angiotensin-converting enzyme inhibitor and diuretic; Diur: diuretic alone. (From Ref. 35.)

patients had not been previously receiving digoxin prior to trial randomization. Baseline characteristics did not differ significantly between digoxin and placebo groups, particularly demographics, heart failure etiology, baseline ejection fraction, percent use of ACE inhibitors, nitrates, or diuretics. At a mean follow-up of 37 months, no differences were noted in all-cause or cardiovascular mortality [36] (Fig. 10). There was a nonsignificant trend

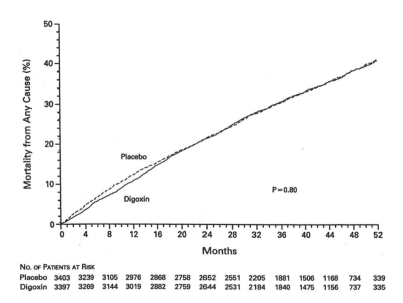

Figure 10 Long-term mortality for the digoxin and placebo treatment groups in the Digitalis Investigation Group (DIG) trial. The number of patients at risk at each 4-month interval is shown below the figure. (From Ref. 36.)

toward reduction in deaths from heart failure, with a relative risk ratio of 0.88 (95% CI, 0.77–1.01). However, substantially fewer patients who received digoxin were hospitalized for worsening heart failure (26.8% vs. 34.7%; risk ratio, 0.72; 95% CI, 0.66–0.79; p<0.001) [36] (Fig. 11). As in earlier smaller studies, the reduction in relative risk for adverse events was greatest among patients with more advanced heart failure symptoms, particularly those whose left ventricular ejection fractions were below 25% at study entry [36]. One cautionary note has arisen since publication of this trial. Retrospective subgroup analysis has suggested an increased risk of all-cause mortality among women who received digoxin during the DIG Trial [37]. It has been speculated that this increased risk may have been related to higher mean digoxin levels among women compared to men. Whether this represents a true increased risk or simply an aberrant finding during post-hoc analysis remains uncertain. Nonetheless, digoxin dosing should be carefully monitored among women during initiation of the drug.

Digoxin Dosing

Digoxin is excreted predominantly by the kidney, and its clearance is closely related to creatinine clearance. A patient with normal renal function excretes approximately 37% of the digoxin that has been administered; maintenance therapy should replace this amount each day. The blood level of digoxin plateaus at approximately 7 days after initiation of therapy. Poor renal perfusion, as indicated by an elevated BUN, small lean body mass, or elderly patients are at greater risk for developing toxic digoxin levels if a standard maintenance dose is utilized. In addition, a number of commonly used drugs, including quinidine, verapamil, flecainide, propafenone, spironolactone, and amiodarone will significantly increase serum digoxin levels.

   Recent data suggests that the target dose of digoxin should be lower than traditionally assumed. Although higher doses may be necessary for maximum hemodynamic improvement, beneficial neurohormonal and functional effects appear to be achieved at a relatively

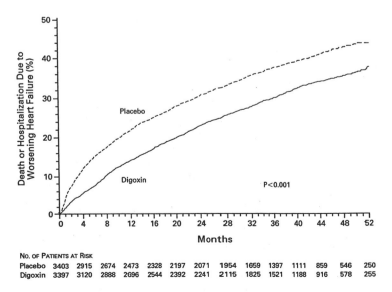

No. of Patients at Risk													
Placebo	3403	2915	2674	2473	2328	2197	2071	1954	1659	1397	1111	859	546	250
Digoxin	3397	3120	2888	2696	2544	2392	2241	2115	1825	1521	1188	916	578	255

Figure 11   Incidence of death or hospitalization for worsening heart failure for the digoxin and placebo treatment groups in the Digitalis Investigation Group (DIG) trial. The number of patients at risk at each 4-month interval is shown below the figure. (From Ref. 36.)

low serum digoxin concentration, typically that associated with a dose of 0.125–0.25 mg daily [34,35,37]. In particular, the serum digoxin concentration achieved in the RADI-ANCE Trial was 1.2 ng/mL and in the DIG Trial it was 0.8 ng/dL [34,36]. For patients with normal renal function, dosage of digoxin of 0.25 mg per day is appropriate [22]. For patients with reduced renal function, the elderly, those small in stature, or those with substantial conduction defects on ECG, the initial starting dose should be 0.125 mg daily, and can be uptitrated as necessary to achieve a trough level less than 1.0 ng/dL.

Consensus Guidelines on Digoxin Use

Consensus guidelines from the Heart Failure Society of America and the American College of Cardiology/ American Heart Association provide the following recommendations on digoxin administration [22,39]:

1. Digoxin should be considered for outpatient treatment of all patients who have persistent heart failure symptoms (NYHA class III to IV) despite standard pharmacologic therapy with diuretics, an ACE inhibitor, and a beta-blocker, when the heart failure is caused by systolic dysfunction (strength of evidence: A for NYHA class II–III; C for NYHA class IV).
2. Digoxin should not be used for primary treatment of acutely decompensated heart failure (strength of evidence: B), rather it should be initiated prior to discharge as part of a long-term maintenance program.
3. Digoxin should not be administered to patients who have significant sinus or atrial ventricular block, unless the block has been treated with a permanent pacemaker (strength of evidence: B). Further, it should be used cautiously among patients who are receiving other agents known to depress sinus or atrioventricular nodal function (such as amiodarone or beta-blocker) (strength of evidence: B).
4. The dosage of digoxin should be 0.125 to 0.25 mg daily in the majority of patients (strength of evidence: C).
5. Serial assessment of serum digoxin levels is unnecessary in most patients. Levels should be reassessed if renal function deteriorates or drug-drug interactions are suspected.
6. Higher doses of digoxin (> 0.25 mg daily) are not indicated for purposes of rate control among patients with heart failure and rapid atrial fibrillation. When necessary, additional rate control should be achieved by addition of a beta-blocker or amiodarone (strength of evidence: C). If amiodarone is added, the dose of digoxin should be reduced.

REFERENCES

1. Konstam MA, Mann DL. Contemporary medical therapy for treating patients with heart failure. Circulation 2002; 105:2244–2246.
1a. Eichhorn E. Current pharmacologic treatment of heart failure. Clin Cardiol 1999; 22:V21-29.
2. Johnson W, Omland T, Hall C, Lucas C, Myking GL, Collins C, Pfeffer M, Roulegu JL, Stevenson LW. Neurohormonal activation rapidly decreases after intravenous therapy with diuretics and vasodilators for class IV heart failure. J Am Coll Cardiol 2002; 39:1623–1629.
3. Brater DC. Diuretic therapy. N Eng J Med 1998; 339:397–395.
4. Hariman RT, Bremmer S, Louie EM, Rogers WJ, Koshs JB, Nocero MA, Jones JP. Dose-response study of intravenous torsemide in congestive heart failure. Am Heart J 1994; 128:352–357.

5. Loon NR, Wilcox CS, Unswin RJ. Mechanism of impaired natriuretic response to furosemide during prolonged therapy. Kidney Int 1989; 83:113–116.

6. Dormans TPJ, VanMeyel JJM, Gerlag DGG, Tan Y, Russel PGM, Smits P. Diuretic efficacy of high dose furosemide in severe heart failure: bolus infusion versus continuous infusion. J Am Coll Cardiol 1996; 28:376–382.

7. Givertz MM. Manipulation of the renin-angiotensin system. Circulation 2001; 104:e14–e18.

8. Garg R, Yusuf S. Overview of randomized trials of angiotensin-converting-enzyme inhibitors on mortality and morbidity in patients with heart failure: Collaborative Group on ACE Inhibitor trials. JAMA 1995; 273:1450–1456.

9. Packer M, Cohn JN. on behalf of the Steering Committee and Membership of the Advisory Council to Improve Outcomes Nationwide in Heart Failure. Consensus recommendations for management of chronic heart failure. Am J Cardiol 1999; 83:1A–38A.

10. Fonarow GC, Chelimsky-Fallich C, Stevenson LW. Effect of direct vasodilation with hydralazine versus angiotensin-converting-enzyme inhibition with captopril on mortality in advanced heart failure. J Am Coll Cardiol 1992; 19:842–850.

11. Jong P, Yusuf S, Rousseau MF, Ahn SA, Bangdiwala SI. Effect of enalapril on 12-year survival and life-expectancy in patients with left ventricular systolic dysfunction: a follow-up study. Lancet 2003; 361:1843–1848.

12. Stafford RS, Radley DC. The underutilization of cardiac medicines of proven benefit, 1990 to 2002. J Am Coll Cardiol 2003; 41:56–61.

13. Exner DV, Dries DL, Domanski MJ, Cohn J. Lesser response to angiotensin-converting enzyme inhibitor therapy in black compared to white patients with left ventricular dysfunction. N Eng J Med 2001; 344:1351–1357.

14. Shekelle PG, Rich MW, Morton SC, Atkinson SW, Tu W, Maglione M, Rhodes S, Barrett M, Fonarow GC, Greenberg B, Neindenreich PA, Knable T, Kunstum MA, Steinle A, Stevenson LW. Efficacy of angiotensin-converting enzyme inhibitors and beta-blockers in the management of left ventricular systolic dysfunction according to race, gender, and diabetic status. A meta-analysis of major clinical trials. J Am Coll Cardiol 2003; 41:1529–1538.

15. Packer M, Poole-Wilson PA, Armstrong PW, Cleland JGF, Horowitz JD, Massie BM, Rydan L, Thygenson F, Uretsky BF on behalf of the ATLAS study group. Comparative effects of low and high doses of the angiotensin-converting-enzyme inhibitor, lisinopril, on morbidity and mortality in chronic heart failure: the ATLAS study group. Circulation 1999; 100: 2312–2318.

16. Nanas JK, Alexopoulos G, Anastansiou-Nana MI, Karids K, Tirologos A, Zobolo SS, Pirgako V, Anthopoulos L, Sideris D, Stamatelopoulos SF, Moulopoulos SD for the High Enabapril Study Group. Outcome of patients with congestive heart failure treated with standard versus high doses of enalapril: a multi-center study. J Am Coll Cardiol 2000; 36:2090–2095.

17. Tang WHW, Vagelos RH, Yee YG, Benedict CR, Wilson K, Liss CL, LaBelle P, Fowler M. Neurohormonal and clinical responses to high- versus low-dose enalapril therapy in chronic heart failure. J Am Coll Cardiol 2002; 39:70–78.

18. ACE Inhibitor Myocardial Infarction Collaborative Group. Indications for ACE inhibitors in the early treatment of acute myocardial infarction: systematic overview of individual data from 100,000 patients in randomized trials. Circulation 1991; 97:2202–2212.

19. Flather MD, Yusuf S, Kuber L, et al. for the ACE Inhibitor Collaborative Group. Long-term ACE inhibitor therapy in patients with heart failure or left ventricular dysfunction: a systemic overview of data from individual patients. Lancet 2000; 355:1575–1581.

20. Al-Khadra SS, Salem DN, Rand WM, Udelson JE, Sniple JJ, Konstam MA. Anti-platelet agents and survival: a cohort analysis of the Studies of Left Ventricular Dysfunction (SOLVD) trial. J Am Coll Cardiol 1998; 31:419–425.

21. Nawarskas JJ, Spinler AS. Does aspirin interfere with the therapeutic efficacy of angiotensin-converting enzyme inhibitors in hypertension or heart failure?. Pharmacotherapy 1998; 18: 1041–1052.

22. Adams K, Baughman KL, Dec GW, Elkayam U, Forbes AD, Gharghiade M, Hermann D, Kunstum MA, Liu P, Massie BM, Pattersen JM, Silver MA, Stevenson LW. Heart Failure

Society of America (HFSA) guidelines for management of patients with heart failure caused by left ventricular systolic dysfunction-pharmacological approaches. J Card Fail 1999; 5: 357–362.

23. Withering W. An account of the foxglove and some of its medical uses, with practical remarks on dropsy, and other diseases. In: Willius FA , Keys TE, Eds. Classics of Cardiology. New York: Dover Publications, Inc., 1941:231–252.

24. Smith TW. Digitalis. Mechanisms of action and clinical uses. N Eng J Med 1988; 318: 358–365.

25. Hauptman PJ, Kelly RA. Digitalis. Circulation 1999; 99:1265–1270.

26. Gheorghiade M, Ferguson D. Digoxin. A neurohormonal modulator in heart failure? Circulation 1991; 84:2181–2186.

26a. Van Velduisen DK, Graff PA, Remme WJ, Lie KI. Value of digoxin in heart failure and sinus rhythm: new features of an old drug? J Am Coll Cardiol 1996; 28:813-9.

27. Newton GE, Tong JH, Schofield AM, Baines AD, Floras JS, Parker JD. Digoxin reduces cardiac sympathetic activity in severe heart failure. J Am Coll Cardiol 1996; 28:155–161.

28. Dec GW. Digoxin is useful in the management of chronic heart failure. In: Baglia R, Narula J, Eds. Med Clin N Am, 2003;87:317–337.

29. Dobbs SN, Kenyon WI, Dobbs RJ. Maintenance digoxin after an episode of heart failure. Placebo controlled trial in outpatients. Br Heart J 1977; 1:749–755.

30. Fleg L, Gottlieb SH, Lakatta EG. Is digoxin really important in compensated heart failure? Am J Med 1982; 73:244–250.

31. Lee DCS, Johnson RA, Bingham JB, Leahy M, Dinsmore RE, Goroll AM, Newell JB, Strauss WH, Kaber E. Heart failure in outpatients. A randomized trial of digoxin versus placebo. N Eng J Med 1988; 306:699–705.

32. Captopril Digoxin Multicenter Research Group: Comparative effects of therapy with captopril and digoxin in patients with mild to moderate heart failure. JAMA 1988; 259:539–544.

33. Uretsky BF, Young JB, Shahidis J, Yellen LG, Harrison MC, Jolly MTC on behalf of the PROVED Investigative group. Randomized study assessing the effect of digoxin withdrawal in patients with mild to moderate chronic congestive heart failure. Results of the PROVED trial. J Am Coll Cardiol 1993; 22:955–962.

34. Packer M, Gheorghiade M, Young JB, Costantini PJ, Adams F, Cody RJ, Smith LR, Van Voorhees L, Gourley LA, Jolly MK for the RADIANCE study. Withdrawal of digoxin from patients with chronic heart failure treated with angiotensin-converting-enzyme inhibitors. N Eng J Med 1993; 329:1–7.

35. Young JB, Gheorghiade M, Uretsky BF, Patterson JH, Adams KF. Superiority of ''triple' drug therapy in heart failure: insights from the PROVED and RADIANCE trials. J Am Coll Cardiol 1998; 32:686–692.

36. The Digitalis Investigation Group. The effect of digoxin on mortality and morbidity in patients with heart failure. N Eng J Med 1997; 336:525–533.

37. Rathorne SS, Wang Y, Krumholz HM. Sex-based differences in the effect of digoxin for the treatment of heart failure. N Eng J Med 2002; 347:1403–1411.

38. Gheorghiade M, Hall VB, Jacobsen G, Alam M, Rosman H, Goldstein H. Effects of increasing maintenance dose of digoxin on left ventricular function and neurohormones in patients with chronic heart failure treated with diuretics and angiotensin-converting enzyme inhibitors. Circulation 1995; 92:1801–1817.

39. Hunt SA, Baker DW, Chin WH, Cinquegrani MP, Feldman AM, Francis GF, Ganiats TG, Goldstein S, Gregoratos G, Jessup ML, Nobel RJ, Pacher M, Silver MA, Stevenson LW. ACC/AHA guidelines for the evaluation and management of chronic heart failure in the adult. Circulation 2001; 104:2996–3007.

13

Conventional Therapy of Chronic Heart Failure: Beta-Adrenergic Blockers

G. William Dec

Heart Failure and Transplantation Unit, Massachusetts General Hospital
Boston, Massachusetts, USA

The failing human heart is adrenergically activated, which helps to maintain cardiac performance during the short-term through increased contractility and heart rate [1,2]. In contrast, there is no adrenergic support present in the normally functioning human left ventricle [3]. A variety of studies indicate that it is the increased cardiac adrenergic tone, rather than an increased circulating plasma norepinephrine level that is ultimately detrimental to the failing human myocardium [1,4,5].

In the failing heart, beta-adrenergic signal transduction is reduced, secondary to desensitization of both the β_1 and β_2 receptors, to increases in the inhibitory G protein (G_i), an enzyme responsible for modulating receptor activity by phosphoroiyization of β–adrenergic receptor kinase (BARK), and to changes in expression of adenyl cyclase activity itself [6]. In end-stage heart failure, 50% to 60% of the total signal transducing potential of the myocardium is lost; nonetheless, substantial signaling capacity remains present [6] (Chapter 5) Data from experimental models suggest that the beta-adrenergic receptor pathway desensitization in the failing heart represents adaptive changes, and that potentially effective therapy might add to this endogenous antiadrenergic strategy by inhibiting receptor signal transduction [1,8–10]. Thus, the continuously increased adrenergic drive present in chronic heart failures delivers adverse biological signals to the cardiac myocytes via β_1, β_2, and α_1 adrenergic receptors. Beta blocker therapy helps to partially restore the efficacy of this all important adrenergic signaling pathway. Long-term therapy results in improvement in cellular, hemodynamic, and clinical parameters.

BENEFICIAL EFFECTS OF BETA ADRENERGIC BLOCKERS

The long-term effects of beta blockade on myocardial function are diametrically opposite to their short-term negative inotropic effects [2,11]. Tables 1 and 2 summarize potential cellular and hemodynamic beneficial effects of these agents. Virtually every placebo-controlled clinical trial of greater than 3 months treatment duration has demonstrated improvement in systolic function despite initial short-term negative hemodynamic effects [11]. Improvement in ventricular ejection fraction has been one of the most consistent

Table 1 Potential Beneficial Cellular Effects of β-adrenergic
Blocker Therapy in Heart Failure

Upregulation of β_1-receptors
Correction of G_s and G_i abnormalities
Protection against cytosolic calcium overload
Shift in metabolic substrate utilization from fatty acids to glucose
Decrease in renin release
Prevention of myocyte hypertrophy
Antioxidant effects
Decrease in apoptosis
Antiarrhythmic effects

long-term effects of these agents, seen with both cardioselective and nonselective agents
(see following text). Although an initial drop in LVEF (left ventricular ejection fraction)
is observed at the start of treatment with beta blockers due to acute effects on inotropic
and chronotropic function, a clinically significant rise in ejection fraction (generally 5 to
8 EF units) is consistently observed during long-term treatment (Fig. 1). The observed
rise in ejection fraction has been shown to be dose-related in at least some studies [12]
(Fig. 2).

Treatment with beta blockers generally leads to improvement in heart failure symptoms, as manifested by a decrease in NYHA (New York Heart Association) functional
class and Minnesota Living with Heart Failure scores [11]. As with ejection fraction, there
is frequently an initial worsening of symptoms before the more sustained beneficial effects
become apparent. It is for this reason that the recommended strategy for initiation of these
agents is to begin at the lowest effective dose, and then slowly uptitrate the dose as
tolerated.

Exercise Tolerance

It is logical to assume that improvements in ejection fractions in heart failure patients
would lead to improvement in exercise capacity as well. Interestingly, data from a variety
of clinical trials suggest only modest favorable results for cardioselective agents, in contrast
to predominantly neutral effects for the nonselective beta blockers. The likely explanation
for this apparent paradox is the blunted maximum heart rate response during exercise
under the influence of full beta-adrenergic blockade. This effect may offset the favorable
hemodynamic improvements achieved by enhanced contractility.

Ventricular Remodeling

By preventing excessive adrenergic exposure, beta blockers retard the effects of norepinephrine on myocardial necrosis and apoptosis, alter genetic expression, and promote

Table 2 Potential Hemodynamic Benefits of
Chronic β-adrenergic Blockade in Heart Failure

Alterations in loading conditions of the ventricles
Negative chronotropic effects
Improved myocardial contractility
Improved lusitropy

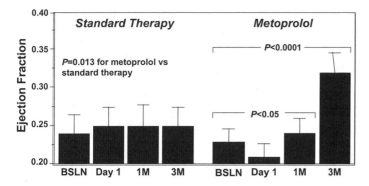

Figure 1 Time course of changes in left ventricular function during beta-blocker therapy. A transient fall in ejection fraction was observed on day 1 of treatment with metoprolol but was not observed in the control group. Ejection fraction had risen by month 3 in the metoprolol group. BSLN, baseline measurement; M, month. (From Ref. 12.)

reverse ventricular remodeling. Treatment for 4 to 12 months has been shown to favorably affect left ventricular mass and geometry [11,13]. Hall and colleagues have convincingly shown regression of left ventricular hypertrophy, a decrease in left ventricular mass, and partial restoration of the elliptical ventricular shape, as quantified by an increased sphericity index [13] (Fig. 3). These time-dependent biological effects of beta blockers are class effects and are observed after treatment with both second- and third-generation compounds (see following text) [1]. Reverse remodeling and the effects on systolic function are unique to beta blocker therapy. Although inhibitors of the renin angiotensin system can attenuate

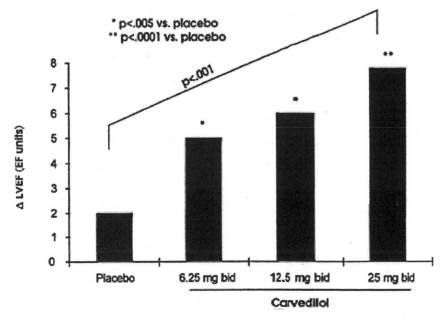

Figure 2 Dose-related changes in left ventricular ejection fraction during treatment with carvedilol. LVEF, left ventricular ejection fraction. (From Ref. 11.)

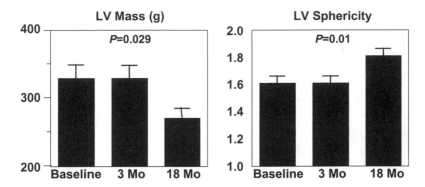

Figure 3 Time course for changes in left ventricular mass and sphericity during beta-blocker therapy. A fall in left ventricular mass was evident at 18 months of treatment with metoprolol; no such change was observed for the control group (data not shown). Likewise, an improvement in left ventricular sphericity was evident at 18 months of metoprolol therapy but was not seen for the control population (data not shown). LV, left ventricular; Mo, months. (From Ref. 12.)

the remodeling process, these agents do not typically reverse it and do not produce improvements in intrinsic systolic function [1,13,14].

DRUG CLASSES OF BETA BLOCKERS: ARE THESE DRUGS INTERCHANGEABLE?

There are now three distinct classes of beta blockers available for clinical use (Table 3). Propranolol is the prototype nonselective agent, introduced into clinical use in 1968. Propranolol and other "first-generation" compounds, such as timolol, are nonselective agents with equal affinity for blocking the β_1 and β_2 receptors; they have no pharmacologic properties beyond beta-adrenergic blockade [1]. Second-generation agents, particularly metoprolol and bisoprolol, are "cardioselective" compounds that block the β_1 receptor to a much greater extent than the β_2 receptor. Metoprolol is approximately 75-fold more selective for β_1 vs. β_2 receptors [1]. Bisoprolol is 120-fold more selective for β_1 receptors than β_2 receptors. Third-generation compounds, principally labetalol, carvedilol, and bucindolol, block both the β_1 and β_2 receptors with almost equal affinity [1]. These agents also have ancillary effects, including α_1 blockade (labetalol and carvedilol), antioxidant

Table 3 Antiadrenergic Profile of the Commonly Used β-Blockers

		Receptor Blocked		
Generation	Compound	β_1	β_2	α_1
First/Nonselective	Propranolol, timolol	+	+	−
Second/Cardioselective	Metoprolol	+ + +	+	−
	Bisoprolol	+ + +	+	−
Third/β-blocker-Vasodilator	Carvedilol	+ + +	+ +	+
	Bucindolol	+ + +	+ +	−

properties (carvedilol), and intrinsic sympathomimetic (ISA) (bucindolol) activity. Labetalol has been studied extensively in hypertensive heart disease, but has not been prospectively validated for use in heart failure populations. Carvedilol is a slightly β_1 selective agent (approximately 7-fold) that becomes nonselective at higher target doses [1]. Carvedilol has a 2- to 3-fold selectivity for β_1 vs. α_1 receptors. This degree of α_1 blockade is responsible for its moderate vasodilator properties. Third-generation compounds provide more comprehensive antiadrenergic effects than do first or second degeneration drugs [15].

Effects on Mortality

The most persuasive outcome measure in heart failure therapy remains all-cause mortality. Combined clinical endpoints, including mortality or hospitalization, or mortality and hospitalization for heart failure, have also emerged as key measures. These latter combined endpoints represent a more comprehensive assessment of the influence of therapy on disease progression, and are assuming more importance as mortality rates decline with treatment. A substantial beneficial effect of beta blocker therapy on both mortality and combined endpoints has been demonstrated in randomized clinical trials of patients with NYHA class II to IV symptoms who received treatment with metoprolol controlled release/extended release (CR/XL), bisoprolol, and carvedilol. Large-scale, well-designed clinical trials with these agents represent the combined worldwide experience with beta blocker therapy in patients with chronic heart failure, and were generally performed on stable patients receiving background therapy that included ACE inhibitors ($>90\%$) and diuretics ($>90\%$) [16].

Metoprolol

The first placebo-controlled multicenter trial with a beta blocker was the Metoprolol and Dilated Cardiomyopathy (MDC) trial that compared metoprolol tartrate to placebo in 383 patients with heart failure due to idiopathic dilated cardiomyopathy [17]. All patients had NYHA class II–III symptoms, and left ventricular ejection fractions below 40%. The trial was powered based on an expected 50% reduction by metoprolol on the combined endpoint of all-cause mortality and clinical deterioration requiring listing for cardiac transplantation. Metoprolol (mean dose: 108 mg daily) reduced the primary composite endpoint by 34%, a finding of marginal significance ($p = 0.058$) [17]. The benefit was entirely due to a reduction by metoprolol in the morbidity endpoint. In fact, the absolute number of deaths in the metoprolol group was slightly higher than that observed in the placebo group (23 vs. 19, $p = 0.69$) [17]. Importantly, metoprolol did improve ventricular function, quality of life, decreased hospitalizations, and improved exercise tolerance at 12 months [17]. These results were viewed as nondefinitive but quite promising, and led to the organization of large scale clinical trials.

The Metoprolol CR/XL Randomized Intervention Trial in Congestive Heart Failure (MERIT-HF) was the first large-scale, randomized, placebo-controlled beta-blocker mortality trial. The trial included 3991 patients with NYHA functional class II–IV heart failure; 96% of study patients were functional class II or III [18]. Both ischemic and nonischemic heart failure etiologies were included. The average dose of metoprolol achieved in the MERIT-HF trial was larger than in MDC (159 mg vs. 108 mg daily). The study was prematurely discontinued by the Data Safety Monitoring Board when interim analysis revealed a 34% reduction in mortality in the metoprolol group (relative risk of 0.66; 95% confidence interval, 0.53 to 0.81, $p = 0.006$) (Fig. 4). Significantly, mortality resulting

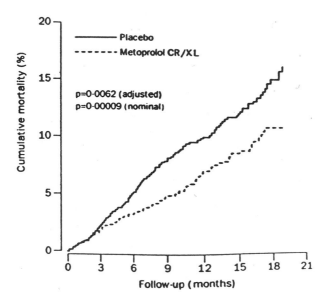

Figure 4 Kaplan-Meier analysis of all-cause mortality for patients enrolled in the MERIT-HT trial. (From Ref. 17.)

from either sudden death or progressive heart failure was reduced (Fig. 5) [18]. Further, the mortality reductions were observed across most demographic groups, including older vs. younger patients, nonischemic vs. ischemic etiologies for heart failure, and lower vs. higher ejection fractions [18]. However, there was almost no mortality reduction in the relatively small number of female patients enrolled (23% of the total trial population), suggesting that sex may influence response to beta blocker therapy in heart failure populations.

Bisoprolol

Two clinical trials have been performed using this β_1 selective agent (Table 4). The Cardiac Insufficiency Bisoprolol Study (CIBIS-I) randomized 641 patients with left ventricular

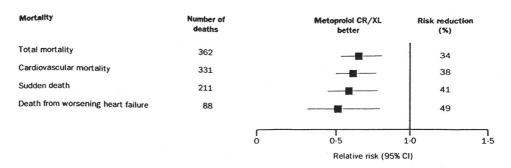

Figure 5 Relative risk ratios (and 95% confidence limits [CI] for total mortality, cardiovascular mortality, sudden death, and worsening heart failure for patients enrolled in the MERIT-HF trial. (From Ref. 17.)

Table 4 Overview of Major β-Blocker Clinical Trials

Feature	USCS	CIBIS-II	MERIT-HF	BEST	COPERNICUS	COMET		
						carvedilol	vs.	metoprolol[b]
Drug	carvedilol	bisoprolol	metoprolol[a]	bucindolol	carvedilol	carvedilol		metoprolol[b]
Starting dose (mg)	6.25 b.i.d.	1.25 q.d.	12.5 q.d.	3 q.d. 100–200	3.125 b.i.d.	3.125 b.i.d.		5 b.i.d.
Target dose (mg)	25–50 b.i.d.	10 q.d.	200	q.d.	25 b.i.d.	25 b.i.d.		50 b.i.d.
No. of patients	1094	2647	3991	2708	2289	1511		1518
Mean age (yrs)	58	61	64	60	64	62		62
Mean LVEF (%)	22	27	28	23	20	26		26
NYHA class	II–IV	III–IV	III–IV	III–IV	IV	II–IV		II–IV
RR in mortality (%)	65	34	34	10	35	CRV 17% relative to MET		
P value	0.0001	0.0005	0.00009	0.11	0.00014	0.0017		

RR, relative reduction; CRV, carvedilol; MET, metoprolol; USCS, United States Carvedilol Studies.
[a] metoprolol succinate
[b] metoprolol tartarate

systolic dysfunction and NYHA class III to IV symptoms [19]. The primary endpoint was all-cause mortality. Bisoprolol was initially dosed at 1.25 mg daily and was increased to a maximum of 5 mg daily. The trial was powered based on an unrealistically high expected event rate in the control group, and demonstrated a significantly insignificant 20% mortality reduction [1,19]. The risk of hospitalization was significantly reduced by 34% (28% placebo group vs. 19% bisoprolol group, p < 0.01) [19].

The favorable trends observed in the initial CIBIS-I trial led investigators to undertake the larger CIBIS-II Study. CIBIS-II enrolled 2647 patients with NYHA class III or IV heart failure symptoms [20]. Both ischemic and nonischemic heart failure etiologies were included with a median follow-up of 1.3 years. The trial was terminated prematurely by the Data Safety Monitoring Committee. Treatment with bisoprolol reduced annual mortality by 34% (13.2% placebo vs. 8.8% bisoprolol; hazard ratio 0.66; 95% competence interval 0.54 to 0.81, p < 0.001) [20]. Hospitalizations for worsening heart failure were also decreased by 32%. Although both trials started with the same initial dose of bisoprolol (1.25 mg daily), CIBIS-II aimed for a higher target dose of 10 mg daily. Post-hoc analysis from CIBIS-I had suggested benefit might be greater in patients with nonischemic cardiomyopathy; this finding was not confirmed in the larger CIBIS-II trial [20].

Carvedilol

Carvedilol, a nonselective third-generation beta blocker and alpha blocker, has been extensively studied for heart failure therapy. Four separate study populations were examined and the data from 1094 patients were combined to evaluate the effect of carvedilol on disease progression [21]. Clinical progression was defined as worsening heart failure leading to death, hospitalization, or in one study, a sustained increase in background medications [21]. The patients included had left ejection fractions of 35% or less, NYHA class II to IV symptoms, and had tolerated a 6.25 mg b.i.d. run-in open label 2-week treatment period. The target doses for the studies ranged from 50 to 100 mg daily. Patients completing the run-in phase were randomized, based on the results of a 6-minute walk test into mild, moderate, or severe trials. The overall trial was prematurely terminated (mean follow-up: 6.5 months), by the Data Safety Monitoring Board, based on a reduction in mortality across the four combined trials for patients treated with carvedilol [21].

The combined trials demonstrated an all-cause mortality risk reduction of 65% compared with placebo (p < 0.0001) [21,22]. Further, the combined risk of hospitalization or death was also reduced by 38% (20% for placebo vs. 14% for carvedilol; (p < 0.001) [21] (Table 4, Fig. 6). Two component trials, the MOCHA [23] and PRECISE [24] trials were completed before the entire program was stopped; however, the mild [25] and severe [26] trials were terminated prematurely. Although neither MOCHA or PRECISE demonstrated an improvement in their primary endpoint of submaximal exercise capacity, both found that carvedilol reduced the risk of the combined endpoint of mortality or heart failure hospitalizations by 39% to 49% [23,24]. The MOCHA Study provided strong evidence for increased benefit from higher doses (25 mg b.i.d.) vs. lower doses (6.25 mg b.i.d.) of carvedilol; thus, uptitration of the drug to 25 mg b.i.d. is generally recommended. Nonetheless, favorable effects were noted even at the 6.25 mg b.i.d. dose. The MOCHA trial did demonstrate a highly significant, dose-dependent reduction in all-cause mortality of 73% [23]. The mild trial demonstrated a significant reduction in the primary combined endpoint of total mortality, cardiovascular hospitalizations, or increasing heart failure medications [25].

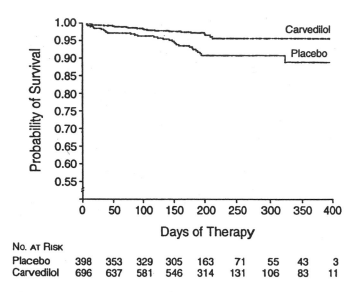

Figure 6 Kaplan-Meier analysis of survival among patients with chronic heart failure in the placebo and carvedilol treatment groups. (From Ref. 21.)

The Australia-New Zealand carvedilol trial enrolled 415 patients with ischemic cardiomyopathy and left ventricular ejection fractions of less than 45% [27]. The majority of patients enrolled were NYHA class I (30%) or II (54%) during an average follow-up of 19 months, Carvedilol reduced the combined risk of all-cause mortality or any hospitalization by 26% (relative risk 0.74; 95% confidence interval 0.57 to 0.95, p = 0.02). Based upon the United States carvedilol trials and the Australian-New Zealand trial, the Food and Drug Administration (FDA) approved carvedilol for heart failure treatment in 1997. Its indications were for delaying the progression of myocardial disease and lowering the combined risk of morbidity and mortality.

The mortality benefits of beta blocker therapy in patients with advanced (NYHA class IV) heart failure symptoms has only recently been established. Prior trials have generally included only a small minority of patients with advanced heart failure [22] (Table 5). The Carvedilol Prospective Randomized Cumulative Survival (COPERNICUS) trial randomized 2289 patients with heart failure symptoms at rest or on minimal exertion, and an ejection fraction below 25% to treatment with either carvedilol or placebo, in addition to conventional therapy, including diuretics and ACE inhibitors [28]. Carvedilol therapy reduced all-cause mortality by 35% (Fig. 6). In addition, carvedilol reduced the combined

Table 5 Frequency of Beta-Adrenergic Blocker Use in Patients with NYHA Class IV Heart Failure Symptoms Enrolled in Clinical Trials

Trial	% Enrolled
U.S. Carvedilol Program	3%
MERIT-HF	4%
CIBIS II	16%
BEST	8%

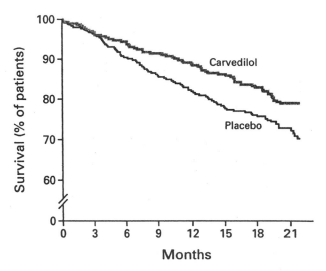

No. of Patients at Risk

Placebo	1133	937	703	580	446	286	183	114
Carvedilol	1156	947	733	620	479	321	208	142

Figure 7 Kaplan-Meier analysis of time to death in the placebo and carvedilol treatment groups. (From Ref. 28)

risk of death or hospitalization for cardiovascular causes by 27% (p < 0.001), and the combined risk of death or hospitalization for heart failure by 31% (p < 0.001) [29]. Further, patients who received carvedilol treatment spent 40% fewer days in the hospital for heart failure decompensation (p < 0.001) [29]. This key study validated the use of beta blocker therapy for patients with severe heart failure, provided they are euvolemic at the time of instituting treatment.

Bucindolol

Bucindolol is a third-generation nonselective beta blocker with ISA properties. The Beta Blocker Evaluation of Survival Trial (BEST) randomized 2708 patients with advanced heart failure (class III and IV) to placebo or bucindolol (Table 4) [30]. Bucindolol produced a nonsignificant 10% reduction in total mortality (p = 0.10) and a favorable reduction in most secondary endpoints [30] (Fig. 8). Retrospective analysis of the BEST trial indicated that the majority of the study population (non-black patients with NYHA class III symptoms) experienced a mortality reduction consistent with results of other major beta blocker trials in similar populations [30]. The overall efficacy was statistically insignificant, as mortality reductions were not observed among patients with NYHA class IV symptoms or blacks in this trial. Whether the lack of overall mortality benefit was due to the population demographics or the effect of the drug's intrinsic sympathomimetic activity is uncertain.

BETA BLOCKER USE IN SPECIAL POPULATIONS

The vast majority of patients enrolled in heart failure clinical trials have been Caucasian males with ischemic heart disease. Although the benefit of beta blockers have been demon-

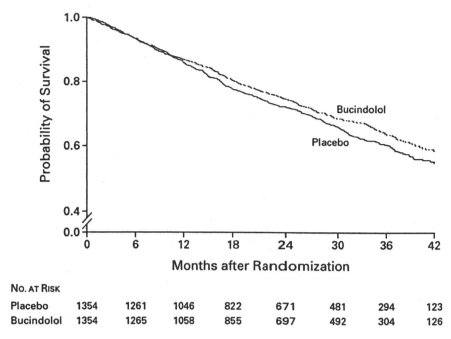

No. at Risk

Placebo	1354	1261	1046	822	671	481	294	123
Bucindolol	1354	1265	1058	855	697	492	304	126

Figure 8 Survival among patients with chronic heart failure randomized to receive either placebo or bucindolol treatment. (From Ref. 30.)

strated to be robust regardless of disease etiology, less clear evidence exists for the benefits of these agents among women and minorities (Chapter 20). Recently, Ghali and colleagues performed a retrospective analysis of female patients enrolled in the MERIT-HF trial [31]. Women comprised 22.5% of patients included in the study. Treatment with Metoprolol CR/XL resulted in a 21% reduction in the primary combined endpoint of all-cause mortality and hospitalizations (p = 0.04) [31]. Further, the number of cardiovascular hospitalizations was reduced by 29% and hospitalizations for heart failure was reduced by 42%. Shekelle and colleagues recently performed a meta-analysis that included the effects of gender on response to beta blocker therapy in major clinical trials [32]. Pooling data from CIBIS-II, U.S. Carvedilol trials, MERIT-HF, and COPERNICUS yielded a total of 2134 female patients enrolled in these trials. The relative risk reduction for females receiving beta blockers averaged 0.63 (95% confidence interval 0.44 to 0.91). These findings were virtually identical to the results seen in males randomized in these trials who experienced a risk reduction of 0.66 (95% confidence interval 0.59 to 0.75) [32]. Thus, the effectiveness of beta blockers appears unequivocal among females with moderate to advanced heart failure symptoms.

The lack of efficacy of bucindolol among black heart failure patients has raised the question of whether differences in racial background may influence the response to specific agents. Shekelle and colleagues examined this issue by pooling data from the MERIT-HF, U.S. Carvedilol, COPERNICUS and BEST trials [32]. In aggregate, the four studies included 1172 blacks and more than 8000 white heart failure patients. The risk reduction among black patients was only 0.97 (95% confidence interval 0.68 to 1.37), whereas for white patients, it was 0.69 (95% confidence interval 0.55 to 0.85) (Fig. 9) [32]. However, when the results from the BEST trial were excluded from ad-hoc analysis, the risk reduction on mortality for black patients was 0.67 (95% confidence interval 0.38 to 1.16), similar

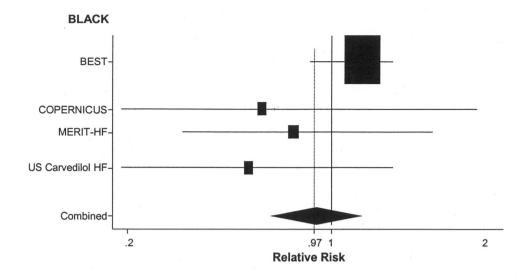

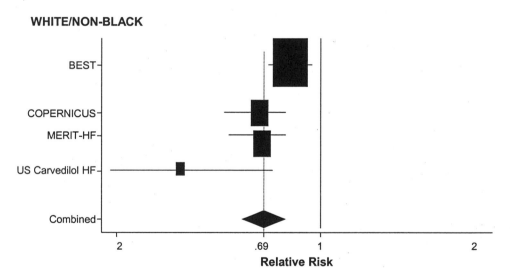

Figure 9   Effect of beta-blockers on mortality in patients with heart failure. For each study, the *size of the box* is proportional to the sample size, and the lines denote the 95% confidence interval. For the combined results, the *ends of the diamond shape* denotes the 95% confidence interval. (From Ref. 32.)

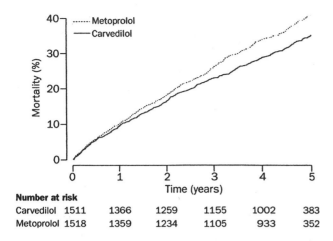

Figure 10 All-cause mortality for patients enrolled in the Carvedilol or Metoprolol European Trial (COMET) by type of beta-blocker. (From Ref. 43.)

to that observed for non-black patients. The authors of this meta-analysis conclude that black patients may experience the same risk reduction as white patients when treated with currently approved beta blockers–bisoprolol, metoprolol, or carvedilol. However, other investigators remain less convinced.

Recent data on differences in genetic polymorphisms in α- and β-adrenergic receptors among races may have clinical relevance to therapeutic response to beta blockade. Small and colleagues recently reported that a double adrenergic receptor polymorphism, specifically an α_{2c} deletion-loss of function genotype (α_{2c} del 322 to 325), combined with a high functioning β_1 receptor genotype (β_1 Arg 389), conferred a 10-fold increased risk for the development of heart failure [33]. Importantly, this α_{2c} polymorphism is enriched in black populations and may provide a partial explanation for the poorer cardiac function and prognosis observed among black heart failure patients [33]. It is conceivable that the α_{2c} polymorphism may have predisposed black patients who received bucindolol to the adverse effects of enhanced sympatholysis [34]. Recent data from McNamara and colleagues also confirm pharmacogenetic interactions between beta blocker therapy and polymorphisms in the angiotensin converting enzyme (ACE) gene among heart failure recipients (Chapter 7) [35]. Ultimately, more precise pharmacogenetic profiling may be used to predict response to specific beta-blocking agents; this more careful profiling should allow selection of the optimum drug based on age, gender, and racial background.

CLINICAL CONSIDERATIONS IN SELECTION OF A SPECIFIC BETA BLOCKER

Given the beneficial effects of metoprolol, bisoprolol, and carvedilol, clinicians are often confronted with selecting the most appropriate beta blocker for their patients. A variety of small physiological studies have compared the hemodynamic and clinical effects of metoprolol to carvedilol [36–42]. Similar comparative studies have not been performed for bisoprolol. Both drugs improve NYHA functional class, decreased heart rate, and improved submaximal exercise capacity [37–40]. Studies by DiLenarda and colleagues and a recent meta-analysis by Packer and colleagues demonstrated that carvedilol produces greater increases in left ventricular ejection fraction than metoprolol [36,40]. Conversely, some, but not all, studies show that metoprolol improves maximum exercise capacity to a greater degree than carvedilol [38–40]. It is postulated that these differences may be partially explained by carvedilol's ability to improve postreceptor events, most notably by downregulation of BARK, which leads to presensitization of the beta receptors. The Carvedilol Or Metoprolol European Trial (COMET) was the first large-scale study to *directly* compare the effects of carvedilol to metoprolol on mortality and morbidity in patients with mild to severe heart failure [43]. This multicenter, double-blind study enrolled 3029 patients with chronic heart failure (NYHA class II to IV) and ejection fractions below 35%, who were receiving optimal therapy with diuretics and an angiotensin-converting enzyme inhibitor (unless not tolerated). The mean study duration was quite long at 58 months. The all-cause mortality was 34% for carvedilol compared with 40% for metoprolol (hazard ratio 0.83) (95% confidence interval 0.74 to 0.93, p = 0.0017) [43] (Fig. 9). However, the composite endpoint of mortality or all-cause hospitalizations did not differ between treatment groups (74% for carvedilol, 76% for metoprolol, p = 0.122). Likewise, the incidence of side effects and drug withdrawals did not differ between treatment groups. Although this pivotal trial suggests that nonselective third-generation beta blockers may be preferable to β_1 elective agents such as metoprolol, several methodological questions have been raised about this conclusion [44]. One key question is whether the doses of the two agents were equivalent. The drug dosing in COMET aimed for a comparable reduction in resting heart rate between the two groups. While the resting heart rate reduction for patients who receive carvedilol was 13 beats per minute (identical to that achieved in the U.S. Carvedilol trials), the heart rate reduction in the metoprolol group was 11.7 beats per minute (compared to 15 beats per minute in the MDC trial) [17,44]. Further, the preparation used in MERIT-HF was metoprolol succinate in a controlled release/extended release formula (Metoprolol CR/XL). In that study, the target dose was 200 mg daily, the mean dose actually taken was equivalent to approximately 106 mg of metoprolol tartrate [18]. Thus, the specific drug formulation, the lower achieved average daily dose, and the more modest effects on resting heart rate confound comparison of the two drugs. Hence, it is difficult to be sure that in COMET, metoprolol exerted a similar degree of β_1 blockade to carvedilol. Nonetheless, it is hard to argue that carvedilol was not found to be superior to metoprolol in the COMET trial despite these methodological concerns. At present, clinicians should consider initiating carvedilol as first-line therapy, given its broader antiadrenergic effects. For patients with marginal blood pressure in whom α blockade may be deleterious, metoprolol XL/CR should be the drug of choice.

UNANSWERED QUESTIONS REGARDING BETA BLOCKER ADMINISTRATION

Asymptomatic Left Ventricular Dysfunction

Data from the SOLVD Prevention trial demonstrated the efficacy of ACE inhibitor therapy in delaying the onset of heart failure symptoms and the need for treatment or hospitalization for heart failure in asymptomatic patients with left ventricular dysfunction (LVEF ≤ 35%). Unfortunately, similar controlled trial data supporting the use of beta blocker treatment for asymptomatic left ventricular dysfunction are lacking. Significant support can be inferred from clinical trials in coronary artery disease and hypertension. Previous data indicate that beta blocker therapy should be used in patients after myocardial infarction, and in patients with myocardial revascularization who have residual left ventricular dysfunction. Given the impressive ability of beta blockers to retard disease progression and improve ventricular function in patients with symptomatic disease, the current Heart Failure Society of America Practice Guidelines indicate that beta blocker therapy should be considered for patients with left ventricular systolic dysfunction (LVEF ≤ 40%) who are asymptomatic (NYHA class I), and are receiving ACE inhibitor therapy [45]. Likewise, the new ACC/AHA Practice Guidelines also recommend the use of beta blockers in Stage B (asymptomatic left ventricular dysfunction) [46].

Cardiac Pacemaker Implantation

Some physicians are now considering pacemaker implantation when symptomatic bradycardia or heart block prevents the initiation of beta blocker therapy. Consideration should be given to withdrawal of other drugs that may have bradycardic effects (e.g., calcium channel blockers or digoxin), so that beta blocker therapy may be started. Currently, no data exist to support this therapeutic approach. Further, the role of ventricular pacing in worsening cardiac dyssynchrony argues against a strategy that would promote predominant ventricular pacing, rather than utilize the patient's intrinsic ventricular activation sequence when QRS duration is < 130 milliseconds. Beta blocker therapy should be considered following initiation of biventricular pacing if clinically indicated.

Concomitant Use with Inotropic Therapy

The results of the COPERNICUS trial indicate that even patients with advanced (NYHA class IV) heart failure benefit from chronic beta blocker therapy. Unfortunately, this group often is unable to tolerate even the smallest doses during initial attempts at drug initiation. Some investigators are now combining phosphodiesterase (PDE)-III inhibitors (particularly enoximone or intravenous milrinone) with a beta blocker. Phosphodiesterase inhibitors improve hemodynamics and can increase exercise performance; however, this enhanced inotropic effect often occurs at an increased risk of exacerbating myocardial ischemia and promoting ventricular arrhythmias. Theoretically, beta blockers should be able to cancel the ischemic and the arrhythmic properties of the PDE inhibitors and provide synergistic benefits. Several small uncontrolled short-term studies suggest that this approach may be beneficial for patients with refractory heart failure [47,48]. A randomized clinical trial is now evaluating the safety and efficacy of this combination therapy.

CONCLUSION

Beta-adrenergic receptor blockers remain the single most important addition to the pharmacologic management of heart failure during the past decade. Although advocated for use since the mid-1970s, it is only during the past 5 years that they have become a standard part of the recommended consensus practice guidelines. Current recommendations suggest that beta blocker therapy should be routinely administered to clinically stable patients with left ventricular systolic dysfunction (LVEF ≤ 40%) and mild, moderate, or severe heart failure symptoms who are on standard therapy, typically including ACE inhibitors, diuretics as needed to control fluid retention, and digoxin (class I, strength of evidence: A) [46]. Most clinicians also advocate their use in asymptomatic left ventricular dysfunction. Treatment should be initiated at very low doses and gradually uptitrated every 2 to 3 weeks as tolerated. Usual starting doses are 3.125 mg twice daily for carvedilol, or 6.25 mg twice daily for metoprolol. "Target" doses must be individualized. The most recent ACC/AHA guidelines do not recommend specific doses or specific heart rate thresholds as surrogates for the level of beta blockade [46]. However, it is recommended that efforts be made to achieve a dose that has been proven effective in major clinical trials (i.e., carvedilol 25 to 50 mg b.i.d., metoprolol succinate 200 mg daily or metoprolol tartrate 50 mg b.i.d.). When properly initiated, more than 90% of heart failure patients will be able to tolerate this cornerstone of pharmacologic therapy.

REFERENCES

1. Bristow MR. Beta-adrenergic receptor blockade in chronic heart failure. Circulation 2000; 101:558–569.
2. Hasking GJ, Esler MD, Jennings GL, Burton K, Korner PI. Norepinephrine spillover into plasma in patients with chronic congestive heart failure: evidence of increased overall and cardiorenal sympathetic nervous activity. Circulation 1986; 73:615–621.
3. Haber HL, Christopher LS, Gimple LW, Bergin JD, Subbiah F, Jayaweera AR, Powers ER, Feldmann MD. Why do patients with congestive heart failure tolerate the initiation of beta-blocker therapy? Circulation 1993; 88:1610–1619.
4. Bristow MR, Binobe W, Rasmussen R, Larrabee P, Skerl L, Klein JW, Anderson FL, Murry J, Mesteni L, Faward SV. Beta-adrenergic neuroeffector abnormalities in the failing human heart are produced by local rather than systemic mechanisms. J Clin Invest 1992; 89:803–815.
5. Kay DM, Lefkovits J, Jennings GL, Bergin P, Broughton A, Esler D. Adverse consequences of high sympathetic nervous activity in the failing human heart. J Am Coll Cardiol 1995; 26: 1257–1263.
6. Bristow MR. Changes in myocardial and vascular receptors in heart failure. J Am Coll Cardiol 1993(Suppl A):61A–71A.
7. Tan LB, Benjamin IJ, Clark WA. Beta-adrenergic receptor desensitization may serve a cardio-protective role. Cardiovasc Res 1992; 26:608–614.
8. Bristow MR. The adrenergic nervous system in heart failure. N Eng J Med 1984; 311:850–851.
9. Bristow MR, Kantrowitz NE, Ginsburg R, Fowler MB. Beta-adrenergic function in heart muscle disease and heart failure. J Mol Cell Cardiol 1985; 17(Suppl 2):41–52.
10. Fowler MB, Bristow MR. Rationale for beta-adrenergic blocking drugs in cardiomyopathy. Am J Cardiol 1985; 55:D120–D124.
11. Eichhorn EJ, Bristow MR. Medical therapy can improve the biologic properties of the chroni-cally failing heart: a new era in the treatment of heart failure. Circulation 1996; 94:2285–2296.
12. Bristow MR, Gilbert EM, Abraham WT, Adams RF, Fowler MB, Hershberger RE, Rubu S, Narahara RA, Ingersoll M, Krueger S, Young S, Shusterman N. Carvedilol produces dose-related improvements in left ventricular function and survival in subjects with chronic heart failure. Circulation 1996; 94:2807–2816.
13. Hall SA, Cigarroa CG, Marcoux L, Risser RC, Grayburn PA, Eichhorn EJ. Time course of improvement in left ventricular function, mass, and geometry in patients with congestive heart failure treated with beta-adrenergic blockade. J Am Coll Cardiol 1995; 25:1154–1161.
14. Cohn JN. Structural basis for heart failure: ventricular remodeling and its pharmacological inhibition. Circulation 1995; 91:2504–2507.
15. Bristow MR. Mechanism of action of beta-blocking agents in heart failure. Am J Cardiol 1997; 80:26L–40L.
16. Lechat P, Packer M, Charlton S, Cucherat M, Arab T, Bulssel JP. Clinical effects of beta-adrenergic blockade in chronic heart failure: a meta-analysis of double-blind, placebo-con-trolled, randomized trials. Circulation 1998; 98:1184–1191.
17. Waagstein JP, Bristow MR, Swedberg K, Camerini F, Fowler MB, Johnson M, Silver MA, Gilbert EM, Hjalmarson Å. Beneficial effects of metoprolol in idiopathic dilated cardiomyopa-thy. Lancet 1993; 342:1441–1446.
18. MERIT-HF Study Group. Effect of metoprolol CR/XL in chronic heart failure: metoprolol CR/XL randomized intervention trial in congestive heart failure (MERIT-HF). Lancet 1999; 353:2001–2007.

19. CIBIS Investigators and Committees, A randomized trial of beta-blockade in heart failure: The Cardiac Insufficiency Bisoprolol Study (CIBIS). Circulation 1994; 90:1765–1773.

20. CIBIS II Investigators and Committees. The Cardiac Insufficiency Bisoprolol Study II (CIBIS II): a randomized trial. Lancet 1999; 353:9–13.

21. Packer M, Bristow MR, Cohn JN, et al, for the US. Carvedilol Heart Failure Study Group. The effect of carvedilol on morbidity and mortality in patients with chronic heart failure. N Engl J Med 1996; 334:1349–1355.

22. Dumanski MJ, Krause-Steinrauf M, Massie BM, Deedwania P, Fellmann D, Kovar D, Murray D, Oren R, Rosenberg Y, Young J, Ziler M, Eichorn E, for the BEST Investigators. A Comparative analysis of the resultss from 4 treats of B-Blockers therapy for heart failure: BEST, CIBIS-TC, MERIT-MF, and CoPernicus J Cardiac Failure. 2003; 19:354.

23. Bristow MR, Gilbert EM, Abraham WT, Adams KF, Fowler MB, Hershberger RE, Kubo SH, Narahara RA, Ingersoll M, Krueger S, Yung S, Shusterman N for the MOCHA Investigators. Multicenter Oral Carvedilol Heart Failure Assessment (MOCHA): A six-month dose response evaluation in class II–IV patients. Circulation 1995; 92(Suppl I):I142–I146.

24. Packer M, Colucci WS, Sackner-Bernstein JD, Gregory JJ, Kantrowitz NE, LeJemtel TR, Young ST, Lucas MA, Shusterman NR. for the PRECISE Study Group. Double-blind, placebo-controlled study of the effects of carvedilol in patients with moderate to severe heart failure: the PRECISE trial. Circulation 1996; 94:2793–2799.

25. Colucci WS, Packer M, Bristow MR, et al, for the US. Carvedilol Study Group. Carvedilol inhibits clinical progression in patients with mild symptoms of heart failure. Circulation 1996; 94:2800–2806.

26. Cohn JN, Fowler MB, Bristow MR, et al, for the Carvedilol Heart Failure Study Group. Effect of carvedilol in severe chronic heart failure. J Am Coll Cardiol 1996; 27:169A.

27. Australia-New Zealand Heart Failure Research Collaborative Group. Effects of carvedilol, a vasodilator-β-blocker, in patients with congestive heart failure due to ischemic heart disease. Circulation 1995; 92:212–218.

28. Packer M, Coats AJ, Fowler MB, Kalus HA, Krum M, Mohacsi P, Rouleau JL, Tendera M, Castalgue A, Roecker EB, Schultz MK, Demets DL for the concluded perspective randomized cumulative survival study group. Effect of carvedilol on survival in severe chronic heart failure. N Eng J Med 2001; 344:1651–1658.

29. Packer M, Fowler MB, Roecker EB, Ratus MA, Krum H, Mohacsi P, Rouleau JL, Tendera M, Stulger C, Nolcslew TL, Amann-Falan I, Demets DL for the COPERNICUS study group. Effect of carvedilol on the morbidity of patients with severe heart failure. Results of the carvedilol Prospective randomized cumulative survival (COPERNICUS) study. Circulation 2002; 106:2194–2149.

30. BEST Trial Investigators. A trial of the β-adrenergic blocker bucindolol in patients with advanced heart failure. N Eng J Med 2001; 344:1659–1667.

31. Ghali JK, Pina IL, Gottlieb SS, Deedwania PC, Wihshaund JC on behalf of the MERIT-HF study group. Metoprolol CR/XL in female patients with heart failure. Analysis of the experience in Metoprolol Extended-release Randomized Intervention Trial in Heart Failure (MERIT-HF). Circulation 2002; 105:1585–1591.

32. Shekelle PG, Rich MW, Morton SC, Athinson SW, Tu W, Maglione M, Rhodes S, Burrett M, Finarow GC, Greenbery R, Heusdenreich PA, Knable T, Kinstrum MA, Steimle A, Stevenson LW. Efficacy of angiotensin-converting enzyme inhibitors and beta-blockers in the management of left ventricular systolic dysfunction according to race, gender, and diabetes status. A meta-analysis of major clinical trials. J Am Coll Cardiol 2003; 41:1529–1538.

33. Small KM, Wagoner LE, Levin AM, Kardia SLR, Liggett SB. Synergistic polymorphisms of the β_1 and α_{2c} adrenergic receptors and the risk of congestive heart failure. N Eng J Med 2002; 347:1135–1142.

34. Bristow MR. Antiadrenergic therapy of chronic heart failure. Surprises and new opportunities. Circulation 2003; 107:1100–1102.

35. McNamara DM, Holubkov R, Janosko K, Palmer A, Wang JJ, Macbouvan GA, Morali S, Rosenblum WD, London B, Feldum AM. Pharmacogenetic interactions between β-blocker

therapy and the angiotensin-converting enzyme deletion polymorphism in patients with congestive heart failure. Circulation 2001; 103:1644–1648.

36. Packer M, Antonopoulos GV, Berlin JA, Chittams J, Konstam MA, Udelson JE. Comparative effects of carvedilol and metoprolol on left ventricular ejection fraction in heart failure: results of a meta-analysis. Am Heart J 2001; 141:899–907.

37. Maack C, Elter T, Nickenig GT, La Rosse K, Crivaro M, Stablein A, Wutthe H, Bohm M. Prospective crossover comparison of carvedilol and metoprolol in patients with chronic heart failure. J Am Coll Cardiol 2001; 38:939–946.

38. Metra M, Giubbini R, Nodari S, Boldi E, Nodena MG, Deicas L. Differential effects of beta-blockers in patients with heart failure. A prospective, randomized, double-blind comparison of the long-term effects of metoprolol vs. carvedilol. Circulation 2000; 102:546–551.

39. Gilbert EM, Abraham WT, Olsen S, Matler B, White M, Megly P, Larrabee P, Bristow M. Comparative hemodynamic, left ventricular functional and antiadrenergic effects of chronic treatment with metoprolol versus carvedilol in the failing heart. Circulation 1996; 94: 2817–2825.

40. Di Lenarda A, Sabbadini G, Salvatore L, Sinagra G, Mestoni L, Plamanto B, Gregori DL, Clani F, Muzzi A, Rlugmann S, Cumerini F, and the heart-muscle disease study group. Long-term effects of carvedilol in idiopathic dilated cardiomyopathy with persistent left ventricular dysfunction despite chronic metoprolol. The Heart-Muscle Disease Study Group. J Am Coll Cardiol 1999; 33:1926–1934.

41. Sanderson JE, Chan SK, Yip G, Yeung LYC, Chan RW, Raymond R, Woo RS. Beta-blockade in heart failure: a comparison of carvedilol with metoprolol. J Am Coll Cardiol 1999; 34: 1522–1528.

42. Kukin ML, Charney RH, Levy DK, Levy DR, Bucholz-Varley C, Ocampo ON, Ang C. Prospective, randomized comparison of effect of long-term treatment with metoprolol or carvedilol on symptoms, exercise, ejection fraction, and oxidative stress in heart failure. Circulation 1999; 99:2645–2651.

43. Poole-Wilson PA, Swedberg K, Cleland JCF, Di Lenarda A, Kahraple P, Romajda M, Lubsen J, Glutiger B, Metra M, Demme WJ, Torpe-Dedasson C, Scherhag A, Shene A for COMET Investigators. Comparison of carvedilol and metoprolol on clinical outcomes in patients with chronic heart failure in the Carvedilol Or Metoprolol European Trial (COMET): randomized controlled trial. Lancet 2003; 362:7–13.

44. Dargie HJ. Beta-blockers in heart failure. Lancet 2003; 362:2–3 (editorial).

45. Adams K, Baughman KL, Dec GW, Alkayam U, Forbes AD, Ghearghigde M, Hermann D, Konstum MA, Liu P, Massie BM, Parthgen JM, Silver MA, Stevenson LW. Heart Failure Society of America Guidelines for management of patients with heart failure caused by left ventricular systolic dysfunction-pharmacological approaches. J Cardiac Fail 1999; 5:357–382.

46. Hunt S, Baker DW, Chin MH, Cinquearani MP, Feldman AM, Francis GF, Ganiats TG, Goldstein S, Gregorators G, Jessup M, Nobel RJ, Pucher M, Silver MA, Stevenson LW. ACC/AHA guidelines for the evaluation and management of chronic heart failure in the adult: executive summary. A report of the American College of Cardiology/American Heart Association Task Force on Practice Guidelines (Committee to Revise the 1995 Guidelines for the Evaluation and Management of Heart Failure) developed in collaboration with the International Society for Heart and Lung Transplantation endorsed by the Heart Failure Society of America. J Am Coll Cardiol 2001; 38:2101–2113.

47. Metra M, Nodari S, D'Aloia A, Muneretto C, Roberston AD, Brotow MR, Deicas L. Beta-blocker therapy influences the hemodynamic response to inotropic agents in patients with heart failure: a randomized comparison of dobutamine and enoximone before and after chronic treatment with metoprolol or carvedilol. J Am Coll Cardiol 2002; 40:1248–1258.

48. Shakar SF, Abraham WT, Gilbert EM, Robertson AX, Lowes BD, Osman LS, Ferguson DA, Brestow MR. Combined oral positive inotropic and beta-blocker therapy for treatment of refractory class IV heart failure. J Am Coll Cardiol 1998; 31:1336–1340.

14

Angiotensin Receptor Blockers for Heart Failure

John G. F. Cleland, Nikolay Nikitin, Justin Ghosh, Alison P. Coletta, Anwar Memon, and Andrew Clark
Department of Cardiology, University of Hull
Hull, UK

INTRODUCTION

Angiotensin receptor blockers (ARBs) are already established as an important class of antihypertensive agent that alter blood pressure and clinical outcomes favorably [1]. These agents have a good safety and tolerability profile making them easy to use and highly acceptable to patients [2]. For instance, 9193 patients with hypertension and left ventricular hypertrophy were randomized in the LIFE trial [1] to atenolol, a beta-1-selective blocker, or losartan, an ARB. Losartan exerted a greater reduction in stroke, with a strong trend to lower overall mortality. The effect in diabetics appeared especially favorable [3]. Whether losartan would have proved as effective against other beta-blockers that have shown benefit more consistently than atenolol [4] or against ACE inhibitors [5] is unclear. Also, despite expectations, ACE inhibitors have not proved consistently superior to other agents in reducing mortality and morbidity when used for the management of hypertension [6,7].

ARBs are also widely used in patients with heart failure. The purpose of this chapter is to examine the clinically important potential and/or established roles of this class of agent in such patients. Improving symptoms and quality of life, reducing morbidity and disability, and prolonging life are the key markers of efficacy that will be reviewed. Safety and tolerability are also of concern, but only if efficacy is proven first.

Important clinical questions include:

1. Are ARBs more effective than placebo in patients not taking an ACE inhibitor?
2. Are ARBs and ACE inhibitors more effective when used in combination rather than as single agents?
3. Are ARBs as or more effective than an ACE inhibitor?
4. Are the benefits and side effects of ARBs dose related?
5. Are there clinically relevant differences between ARBs?
6. Are there important interactions between ARBs and other classes of drug used in heart failure, (including aspirin, beta-blockers, and aldosterone antagonists)?

An important additional dimension to all of the above questions is whether or not the patient has left ventricular systolic dysfunction (LVSD). Up to 50% of patients who are reported to have heart failure do not have LVSD [8,9]. However, heart failure without LVSD cannot easily be equated with diastolic heart failure [10,11]. This group of patients is likely to be diagnostically heterogeneous and include a substantial number of patients who have been misdiagnosed and whose symptoms are not cardiac in origin [10]. It is becoming clear that, overall, this group of patients has a lower mortality and probably a lower morbidity than do patients with heart failure and LVSD. There is little evidence that any treatment can alter the natural history of this condition, although treatment of concomitant hypertension and atrial fibrillation may alter prognosis, and diuretics will relieve edema and symptoms of fluid overload. ACE inhibitors are not, as yet, known to be effective in this rather ill-defined group of patients [11,12]. If ARBs can show benefits in this setting they could become the first treatment to be recommended for the management of heart failure in patients with preserved left ventricular systolic function. If ARBs fail to show an overall benefit in this broad category of patients, it will not preclude the possibility that some types of heart failure with preserved left ventricular function, such as those with long-axis systolic dysfunction [13] or diastolic heart failure due to impaired myocardial relaxation might benefit.

Most of the evidence on which the clinical role of ARBs for the management of patients with major cardiac dysfunction has been obtained from seven (ELITE, ELITE II, RESOLVD, Val-HeFT, CHARM-Alternative, CHARM-Added and CHARM-Preserved) major trials of heart failure [14–18] [19–23], two meta-analyses of smaller trials (one of losartan [24] and the other of candesartan [25]) and two trials in the postinfarction setting (OPTIMAAL [26,27] and VALIANT [28,29]). Altogether, more than 30,000 patients have been included in these randomized controlled trials. A further trial investigating the role of an ARB in patients with heart failure and preserved LVSD (I-PRESERVE) and another comparing 50 mg vs. 150 mg of losartan (HEAL) will not report for some years. Undoubtedly, more trials will follow.

A brief report of the rationale for the use of ARBs in heart failure is followed by a description of each of the main trials and the two-meta-analyses of small trials, and finally by a discussion on how data from these trials can be applied to provide some answers to clinically important questions. Other trials that help fill gaps in our knowledge are mentioned briefly.

RATIONALE FOR THE USE OF ARBS IN HEART FAILURE

The organization of the RAAS (renin-angiotensin-aldosterone system) is outlined in Figure 1. Angiotensin-converting enzyme is responsible not only for the production of angiotensin II (AII) but also the degradation of bradykinin [30,31]. Other possible substrates for ACE include erythropoietin and the enkephalins.

Angiotensin II has numerous actions. The acute effects of AII include arterial and, probably, venous constriction, reduced parasympathetic and increased sympathetic nervous activity and, possibly, direct effects on the kidney resulting in salt and water retention [32–38]. Chronic effects include cardiac and vascular remodeling and a potential role in the genesis of atheroma [39,40].

Less is known about bradykinin because it is difficult to measure accurately, it acts very close to its site of synthesis with little spill-over into the circulation, and because pharmacologic tools for manipulating its actions on its receptor site have only recently become available [30]. In general the actions of bradykinin are opposite to those of AII and include vasodilatation, stimulation of nitric oxide and vasodilator prostaglandin production, the latter being a potential mechanism for the interaction

Renin-Angiotensin-Aldosterone System

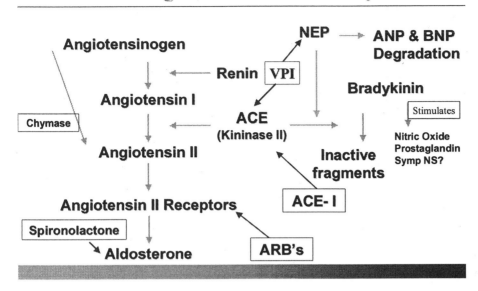

Figure 1 Activation pathways of the renin-angiotensin system in heart failure. ANP, atrial natriuretic peptide; BNP, brain natriuretic peptide; Symp NS, sympathetic nervous system; ACE-I, angiotensin-converting enzyme inhibitor; ARBs, angiotensin receptor blockers; NEP, neutral endopeptidase; VPI, vasopeptidase inhibitor.

between ACE inhibitors and aspirin [30]. Bradykinin may also have favorable effects on left ventricular remodeling, endothelial function, and the development of atheroma. However, bradykinin has also been purported to activate the sympathetic nervous system, a potentially undesirable effect [41], and may be responsible for ACE inhibitor-induced cough and angioneurotic edema.

There are alternative pathways for the generation of AII. Chymase can convert angiotensin I to II by an ACE independent pathway [42–44]. Whether it is present in sufficient quantity to generate significant amounts of AII either systemically or at a local (tissue) level in humans is uncertain. Chymotrypsin, angiotensin generating enzyme, and cathepsin D are other pathways for AII production that are not blocked by ACE inhibitors.

The current principal classification of angiotensin receptors in humans is into AT_1 and AT_2 receptors but it is likely that the number of receptor subtypes described will increase. AT_1 receptors are widely distributed in the heart, on the luminal surface of the vascular endothelium, noradrenergic nerve terminals, adrenal cortex, and kidneys [45,46]. AT_2 receptor expression is high in fetal tissues and in healing wounds. In the human heart the AT_2 receptor predominates and the concentration is maintained or increased, compared with that of AT_1 receptors as CHF (chronic heart failure) develops [47–49].

The AT_1 receptor appears responsible for the mediation of all the classic effects of AII [42,43]. Stimulation of the AT_2 receptor may cause vasodilatation and have antiproliferative effects but may also stimulate apoptosis, which could have adverse effects on cardiovascular remodeling [50,51]. Thus, the clinical effects of selective AT_1 receptor blockade could be superior, inferior, or identical to those of nonselective blockade AT receptor blockade.

WHY MIGHT THE EFFECTS OF ARBs AND ACE INHIBITORS DIFFER?

ACE "Breakthrough"

Although acute administration of an ACE inhibitor reduces plasma AII to about the limit of detection, plasma angiotensin II and aldosterone are often not suppressed after several months of treatment [52,53]. Poor compliance might be responsible in some instances for the apparent loss of ACE inhibition, but the problem appears too prevalent to be accounted for by poor compliance alone [54]. ACE inhibition leads to an accumulation of the precursor for AII, angiotensin I. Although 80% ACE inhibition may be enough to suppress AII formation at normal levels of angiotensin I, much more intense inhibition may be required in the presence of increased substrate. Small doses (e.g., 5 mg of enalapril or lisinopril) of an ACE inhibitor may be adequate to suppress AII initially, but much larger doses (e.g., 35 mg lisinopril or 40 mg of enalapril) may be required for long-term inhibition. Increasing levels of angiotensin I may also be converted to AII through ACE independent pathways and, therefore, even intense ACE inhibition may not be adequate to suppress AII production in the long-term [42–44]. ARBs block the downstream effects of AII and, therefore, it does not matter which route generates AII.

AT2 Receptor Stimulation

Activation of the RAAS is normally limited by negative feedback of AII on the AT_1 receptor. ARBs block the AT_1 receptor and, therefore, release the RAAS from negative feedback. Accordingly plasma concentrations of AII rise and consequently stimulation of the unblocked AT_2 receptor may increase. Therefore, unlike ACE inhibitors, ARBs may increase stimulation of the AT_2 receptor, which may, or may not, be beneficial (see previous text).

Bradykinin-Prostaglandin and Other Pathways

ACE inhibitors, unlike ARBs, increase bradykinin [30] and hence, nitric oxide and vasodilator and antiaggregatory prostaglandins. This could confer additional vasodilator, antithrombotic, and antiatherogenic effects on ACE inhibitors as well as having favorable effects on cardiovascular remodeling. Neutralization of the prostaglandin-mediated effects of ACE inhibition could account for the adverse interaction between aspirin and ACE inhibitors [55–61]. The lack of effect of ARBs on the bradykinin/prostaglandin pathway suggests that they might not reduce vascular events, especially coronary events, as effectively as ACE inhibitors. Although no adverse interaction between ARBs and aspirin would be expected, this reflects the lack of a beneficial ancillary effect of ARBs on prostaglandin metabolism.

ACE inhibitors may also inhibit other enzymes that could have beneficial (e.g. neutral endopeptidase or matrix metalloproteinases) or possibly deleterious effects on symptoms or cardiovascular remodeling.

Effects on Hematocrit

ACE inhibitors cause hematocrit to fall, either because of hemodilution or because of a fall in red cell volume due to a decline in erythropoietin, an effect either mediated directly or through an improvement in renal blood flow [38,62]. Hemodilution could reduce oxygen uptake and transport, and detract from the benefits of ACE inhibitors on symptoms and functional capacity. However, reducing hematocrit could also reduce the risk of thrombotic events. There are data to suggest that ARBs may also reduce hematocrit [63].

Electrophysiological and Autonomic Effects

Compared with captopril, losartan may exert a greater effect on progressive electrical remodeling and QT dispersion [64]. However, ARBs (losartan 50 mg/day), unlike ACE inhibitors [33,35,65] may not cause a beneficial increase in parasympathetic mediated tone as assessed by heart rate variability [66]. This suggests that ACE inhibitors might have a greater effect on arrhythmias, at least compared with modest doses of ARBs.

Uricosuric Effect

The apparently specific uricosuric effect of losartan [67,68] could do more than just protect against gout. Plasma concentrations of uric acid may be a marker of oxidant stress [69] that, in turn, may have adverse effects on cardiac and vascular function. Whether these properties are shared by other ARBs is not clear as yet.

Tolerability

ARBs may be better tolerated than, at least, some ACE inhibitors [2]. Only if a drug is taken can it be effective and, therefore, greater tolerability may translate into greater efficacy. ARBs have generally been better tolerated than placebo in studies of hypertension, although it should be pointed out that fewer patients have generally been withdrawn from ACE inhibitors than placebo in studies of CHF.

Will the Combination of ACE inhibitors and ARBs Prove Superior to Either Class Used Alone?

Renin secretion is suppressed by AII, and AT_1 receptor antagonists increase plasma renin by releasing it from this negative feedback loop. As renin rises so do angiotensin I and II levels [2,70]. Just as the effects of ACE inhibition may be overcome by competition from rising concentrations of angiotensin I, so AT_1 inhibition may be overcome by rising concentrations of AII, either by displacing ARBs that bind reversibly to the AT_1 receptor or by stimulating unblocked receptors more powerfully. Also, it is possible that excessive stimulation of unblocked AT_2 receptors could be harmful.

Rather than being alternatives, it is possible that the actions of ARBs and ACE inhibitors are complimentary. ACE inhibition could prevent the rise in AII associated with ARBs, thereby reducing competition for binding of the ARB to the AT_1 receptor and protecting unblocked AT_1 receptors, whereas ARBs could block the effects of any residual AII formed despite ACE inhibition. Studies show that the rise in AII induced by an ARB can be attenuated by ACE inhibition, at least in the short term, whereas addition of an ARB to an ACE inhibitor results in a further decline in aldosterone, indicating better renin-angiotensin system blockade [16,71].

The Question of Dose

Surprisingly, despite 15 years of research we still know comparatively little about the optimal dose of any ACE inhibitor for CHF [72–74]. This is a very important issue because when comparing the effects of two classes of drugs, it is important to know that merely changing the dose of one or other drug would not have replicated any difference observed, or if no difference was observed then this did not reflect the use of an inadequate dose of one or the other drug. The NETWORK study showed no difference in outcome from 2.5 mg, 5 mg, or 10 mg b.i.d. of enalapril over 6 months, whereas the ATLAS study suggested a greater morbidity/mortality benefit with 35 mg compared with 5 mg/day of lisinopril over 46 months [72,73]. However, these studies still do not define the optimal long-term dose of an ACE inhibitor.

LANDMARK TRIALS AND META-ANALYSES PRINCIPALLY DESIGNED TO COMPARE ARBS WITH PLACEBO IN THE ABSENCE OF AN ACE INHIBITOR

This section includes two landmark trials addressing this question, CHARM-Alternative [19] and CHARM-Preserved [20,23], and two meta-analyses of smaller trials, one of losartan [24] and the other of candesartan [25]. The VAL-HeFT study included a subgroup of patients who were not taking ACE inhibitors [75]. This study is addressed in the section focusing on ARBs added to ACE inhibitors. (Table 1)Apart from the CHARM-Preserved trial, comparing candesartan and placebo in patients with heart failure and preserved left ventricular systolic function, these trials all focused on heart failure due to left ventricular systolic dysfunction. The I-PRESERVE trial [10] is also investigating the effects of an ARB, irbesartan, in patients with heart failure and preserved left ventricular systolic function and, as in CHARM-Preserved, some use of ACE inhibitors is allowed.

The Losartan Meta-Analysis

This meta-analysis [24] consisted of six randomized, double-blind trials in patients with heart failure due to LVSD; three comparing losartan (mostly 50 mg/day) with placebo, two comparing losartan (25–50 mg/day) with enalapril (10 mg b.i.d.) and one (the ELITE trial, see following text) comparing losartan and captopril. The three trials comparing losartan with placebo included 890 patients with 12 weeks of follow-up. One was a dose-ranging hemodynamic study and the others had exercise capacity as their primary endpoint. Approximately 50% of patients had previously received an ACE inhibitor, but this treatment had been discontinued either because of side effects or to qualify for study entry. These trials were conducted prior to widespread use of beta-blockers. The mean age of the patients was 62 years, about 70% were men, and coronary disease was the predominant etiology of their left ventricular dysfunction.

The meta-analysis showed a significant reduction in mortality with losartan compared with placebo (1.8% vs. 4.7%; p = 0.014).

The hemodynamic study showed that after 3 months therapy and 12 hours following a further dose, 25 mg of losartan reduced systemic vascular resistance by about 20%, pulmonary capillary wedge pressure (PCWP) by 5 mmHg, blood pressure by 6 mmHg, and heart rate by 6 bpm (all placebo-corrected), and increased cardiac index by about 0.4 L/min/m [70]. The 50-mg dose exerted similar, but no greater effect. Other doses exerted less consistent effects. Only the 50-mg dose reduced cardiothoracic ratio significantly over 3 months. Thus, as with ACE inhibitors, the long-term hemodynamic benefits were generally modest. Reductions in aldosterone were observed after 12 weeks of the 10-mg, 25-mg and 50-mg doses of losartan. Increases in renin and angiotensin II that appeared after acute dosing were not present after 12 weeks. Norepinephrine changed little if at all.

Table 1 Study Design of and Baseline Characteristics of Patients Included in Landmark Trials of Heart Failure Comparing ARB with Placebo in the Absence (Mainly) of an ACE Inhibitor

	CHARM-Alternative (19,20)	Val-HeFT (subgroup) (75)	CHARM-Preserved (20,23)
Comparison	Candesartan vs. Placebo	Valsartan vs. Placebo	Candesartan vs. Placebo
N =	2028	366	3023
Follow-up (months)	33.7	23	36.6
Mean age (years)	67	67	67
≥ 75 years (%)	23	63[a]	27
Women (%)	32	29	40
NYHA (II/III/IV shown as %)	47/49/4	53/47[b]	61/37/2
Mean LVEF (entry criterion in brackets)	30 (≤40%)	28 (<40%)	54 (>40%)
Mean systolic blood pressure (mmHg)	130	126	136
Main Cause of Heart Failure			
Ischemic heart disease	68	68	56
Idiopathic	20	–	9
Hypertension	6	–	23
Other	6	–	2
Medical History			
Diabetes	27	–	28
Atrial fibrillation	25	–	29
Hypertension	50	–	64
Current angina	23	–	28
Pacemaker	9	–	7
Implantable defibrillator	3	–	1
CABG	25	–	22
Treatment			
Diuretic	85	–	75
ACE inhibitors	Excluded	Excluded	19
Beta–blockers	55	38	56
Spironolactone	24	–	12
Calcium channel blocker	16	–	31
Digoxin	46	–	28
Anticoagulant	31	–	25
Aspirin	58	–	58
Statin	42	–	42

– = data not reported
[a] ≥65 years rather than ≥75 years.
[b] data for NYHA III/IV combined.

The 25-mg and 50-mg doses of losartan reduced plasma concentrations of N-terminal proatrial natriuretic peptide and this correlated with the decline in PCWP [76].

The hemodynamic study, but not the exercise testing studies, showed an improvement in symptoms. Neither exercise testing study showed an improvement in exercise capacity but a prespecified combined analysis showed a reduction in mortality and heart-failure–related hospitalization [24]. It is difficult to show improvement in exercise capacity with cardiovascular drugs in patients who have few symptoms or only minor exercise limitation. It is possible that patients with more severe symptoms were not enrolled by investigators due to concerns about placing them on placebo for 3 months.

In summary, these trials suggested that losartan might improve morbidity and mortality, and possibly symptoms, in patients with heart failure when used instead of an ACE inhibitor. Although the hemodynamic study suggested that 50 mg/day of losartan was at the top of the dose response, fewer than 30 patients were studied at each dose.

The Candesartan Meta-Analysis

This meta-analysis [25] consisted of five randomized, double-blind trials (including STRETCH [77] and SPICE [78]) in patients with heart failure due to left ventricular systolic dysfunction. Four trials, including 1189 patients, compared candesartan in doses ranging from 2 to 16 mg/day against placebo without background ACE inhibitor. One trial, including only 98 patients, compared candesartan (dose 8 to 32 mg/day) and placebo on top of background ACE inhibitors. The mean age of the patients was 63 years, most were men with coronary disease and predominantly mild symptoms. The largest trial (STRETCH; n = 844), lasted 12 weeks and the longest trial lasted 52 weeks (n = 463). Two trials included only ACE inhibitor intolerant patients.

The meta-analysis showed no effect of candesartan on mortality, which was low overall (1.8% on placebo vs. 1.6% of candesartan). All-cause hospitalization was also unaffected, but candesartan appeared effective in reducing the number of patients requiring hospitalization for acute decompensation of heart failure (3.5% vs. 1.1%; p = 0.002).

Compared with placebo, candesartan improved symptoms and exercise capacity significantly in the STRETCH study [77], with the highest does (16 mg/day) having the greatest effect. Adverse effects were no more common even with the highest dose of candesartan compared with placebo, and only two patients required treatment to be withdrawn for an adverse effect.

The SPICE study [78] screened 9580 patients with CHF and ejection fraction 35% or less to identify ACE intolerant patients. A total of 9% of patients was found to be intolerant of ACE inhibitors, mainly due to cough or hypotension. Overall, 179 patients were randomized to candesartan (uptitrated to 16 mg/day) or placebo and followed for 12 to 14 weeks. Trends in favor of candesartan on morbidity outcomes were not statistically significant. Trends to an improvement in symptoms with candesartan were not significant.

Detailed reports on the other component studies have not been published. A subsequent long-term study, not included in this meta-analysis [79–81], compared placebo and candesartan (8 mg/day) in 305 Japanese patients with predominantly mild heart failure. Candesartan was associated with a reduction in worsening heart failure.

In summary, these trials suggested that candesartan *might* improve morbidity and possibly symptoms in patients with heart failure when used instead of an ACE inhibitor. The low event rate precludes any comment on mortality.

CHARM-Alternative

The CHARM program consisted of three separate randomized, double-blind clinical trials that were also designed to be analyzed as a single outcome trial [22,82]. However, as each component study asks a different, clinically relevant question, the trials are probably best interpreted individually rather than as a whole. Also, all-cause mortality, the primary endpoint of the overall analysis [22], was not reduced significantly by candesartan using the principal preplanned analysis that was not adjusted for covariates.

CHARM-Alternative [19,20] included patients with symptomatic heart failure due to LVSD who had a history of ACE inhibitor intolerance, predominantly ACE inhibitor-induced cough (72%). Candesartan was initiated at 4 mg/day (81% of patients) or 8 mg/

day according to the discretion of the investigator, and then titrated at not more than 2-week intervals to 32 mg/day. Monitoring of serum potassium and creatinine was recommended during titration. Patients were monitored long-term at 4 monthly intervals. The primary end-point was cardiovascular death or unplanned admission to hospital for the management of worsening heart failure, defined as worsening symptoms or signs and requiring treatment with intravenous diuretics.

A total of 2028 patients was randomized and followed for a mean of 33.7 months. The mean age of the patients was 66 years; 23% were aged 75 years or more. Most patients were men and had coronary disease. Of those randomized to candesartan, 55% were taking a beta-blocker (rising to 64% during the course of the study), and 25% were receiving spironolactone (unchanged during the study on candesartan but increasing to 29% on placebo). The target dose was achieved in 59% of patients randomized to candesartan vs. 73% randomized to placebo at 6 months. Adverse events led to withdrawal of study medication in 22% and 19% of patients randomized to candesartan and placebo, respectively. However, patients who had previously withdrawn from ACE inhibitors because of cough or angio-edema rarely discontinued study medication because of adverse events. In each group, 6% of patients started an open-label ACE inhibitor and 9% an open-label ARB. Patients randomized to candesartan were more likely to withdraw for hypotension (3.7% vs. 0.9%), renal dysfunction (6.1% vs. 2.7%) and hyperkaliemia (1.9% vs. 0.3%) and these events were most likely to occur in patients who had previously discontinued ACE inhibitors for these problems (Fig. 2). Serum creatinine more than doubled in 5.5% of patients (vs. 1.6% on placebo) and serum potassium increased to 6 mmol/L or more in 3% of patients (vs. 1.3% on placebo). Candesartan reduced systolic blood pressure by a mean of 4 mmHg.

The absolute risk reduction (ARR) in the primary end-point with candesartan was 7.0% or a relative risk reduction (RRR) of 23% (p = 0.004), increasing to 30% after adjusting for imbalances between randomized groups in patients' baseline characteristics (Fig. 3A, Table 2a). This effect was brought about by a somewhat greater effect on heart failure hospitalizations (ARR 7.8%; RRR 39%; p<0.0001 adjusted for covariates) and a slightly lesser effect on cardiovascular death (ARR 3.2%; RRR 20%; p = 0.02 adjusted). The total number of investigator-defined hospital admissions for heart failure was reduced by 56 events (from 211 to 155) per thousand patients per year (p = 0.0001) (Fig. 4), which is very similar to the effect of enalapril compared with placebo in SOLVD-trial treatment (reduced by 65 events from 219 to 154 events per thousand patients per year) [83].

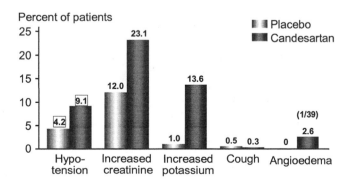

Figure 2   Reasons for permanent discontinuation of treatment with either placebo or candesartan for patients enrolled in the CHARM-Alternative trial. All patients had a prior history of intolerance to an ACE inhibitor.

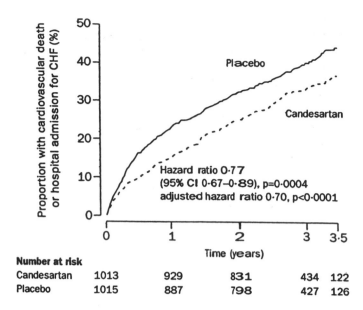

Figure 3 (**A**) Composite end-point of cardiovascular death or hospitalization for heart failure among patients participating in the CHARM-Alternative trial. Candesartan was associated with a 23% reduction in events (From Ref. 19.)

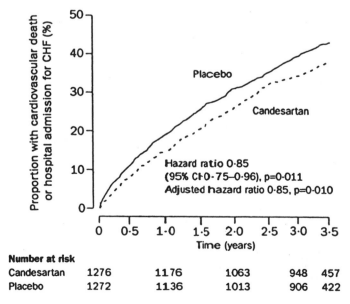

Figure 3 (**B**) Composite end-point of cardiovascular deaths or hospitalizations for heart failure among patients enrolled in the CHARM-Added trial. The addition of candesartan to an ACE inhibitor was associated with a 15% reduction in overall events. [From Ref. 21.)

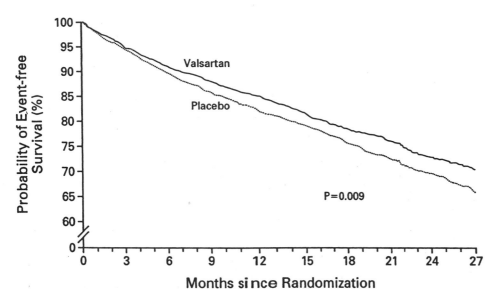

Figure 3 (**C**) Kaplan-Meier analysis of event-free survival for patients randomized to valsartan or placebo in the Val-HeFT trial. (From Ref. 17.)

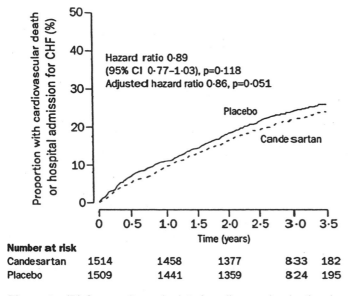

Figure 3 (**D**) Composite endpoint of cardiovascular death or hospitalization for heart failure for patients with heart failure and preserved left ventricular systolic function who participated in the CHARM-Preserved trial. Candesartan therapy was associated with a nonsignificant reduction in events. (From Ref. 23.)

Table 2a Summary of Outcome of Landmark Trials of Heart Failure Comparing ARB with Placebo in the Absence of an ACE Inhibitor in Patients with Left Ventricular Systolic Dysfunction

	Patients		Follow-up (months)	Mortality		Total Number of Hospitalizations		Death or HF Hospitalization Number and % of Patients		Total HF Hospitalizations	
	Placebo	ARB		Placebo	ARB	Placebo	ARB	Placebo	ARB	Placebo	ARB
Losartan Meta-analysis (24)	274	616	3	13 (4.7%)	11 (1.8%)	–	–	–	–	–	–
Candesartan Meta-analysis (25)	606	1287	3	11 (1.8%)	20 (1.6%)	–	–	43 (7.1%)	56 (4.4%)	–	–
Val-HeFT subset (75)	181	185	23	49 (27.1%)	32 (17.3%)	262	199	77 (42.5%)	46 (24.9%)	117	51
CHARM-Alternative (19)	1015	1013	34	296 (29.2%)	265 (26.2%)	1835	1718	433 (42.7%)	371 (36.6%)	608	445
Japanese Candesartan Study (79)	144	148	5	3 (2.1%)	2 (1.4%)	–	–	13 (9.0%)	31 (20.9%)	–	–
Total	**2220**	**3249**		**372 (16.8%)**	**330 (10.2%)**	**2097**	**1917**	**566 (29.1%)**	**504 (19.1%)**	**725**	**496**

Table 2b Summary of Outcome of Landmark Trials of Heart Failure Comparing ARB with Placebo in Patients with Preserved Left Ventricular Systolic Dysfunction

	Patients		Follow-up (months)	Mortality		Total Number of Hospitalizations		Death or HF Hospitalization Number and % of Patients		Total HF Hospitalizations	
	Placebo	ARB		Placebo	ARB	Placebo	ARB	Placebo	ARB	Placebo	ARB
CHARM-Preserved (23)	1509	1514	36	237 (15.7%)	244 (16.1%)	2545	2510	366 (24.3%)	333 (22.0%)	566	402

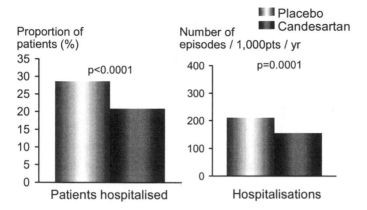

Figure 4 (**A**) Summary of hospitalizations (percentage of patients and episodes/1000/year) for heart failure among patients randomized to candesartan or placebo who participated in the CHARM-Alternative trial. All patients had a documented prior intolerance to an ACE inhibitor.

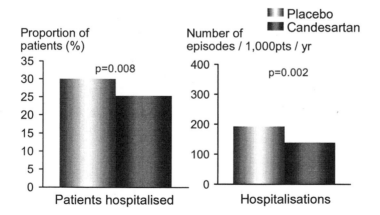

Figure 4 (**B**) Summary of hospitalizations (overall percentage of patients and episodes/1000/year) for heart failure among patients who participated in the CHARM-Added trial. Patients were randomized to receive either candesartan or placebo in addition to an ACE inhibitor.

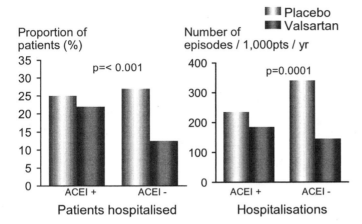

Figure 4 (**C**) Summary of hospitalizations for heart failure for patient who participated in the Valsartan Heart Failure trial (Val-HeFT), *left panel:* percentage of patient hospitalized while receiving valsartan or placebo by presence or absence of chronic ACE inhibitor therapy, *right panel:* hospitalizations (episodes/1000/year) for patients receiving valsartan or placebo with or without concomitant ACE inhibitor therapy;

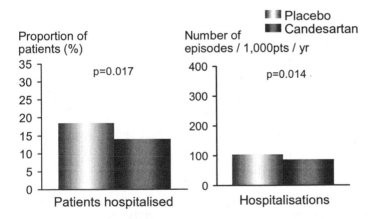

Figure 4 (**D**) Summary of hospitalizations (overall percentage of patients and episodes/1000/year) for heart failure among patients who participated in the CHARM-Preserved trial. Patients were randomized to receive either candesartan or placebo.

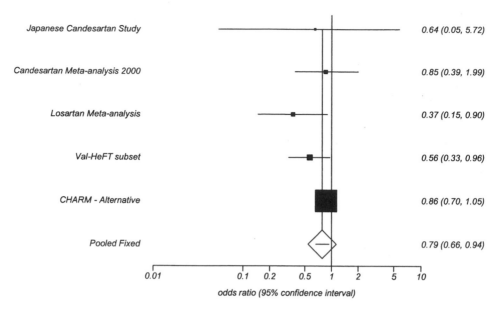

Figure 5 Meta-analysis of randomized, controlled trials comparing an angiotensin receptor blocker to placebo in patients with advanced left ventricular systolic dysfunction and not receiving an ACE inhibitor on mortality.

Candesartan was associated with slightly more myocardial infarctions (n = 75 vs. 48; p = 0.025) but not strokes (n = 36 vs. 42), although few patients suffered either event. This might suggest that candesartan, unlike ACE inhibitors [40,84,85], does not reduce vascular events in this setting but as candesartan was associated with somewhat fewer cardiovascular deaths these data need to be interpreted with caution.

All-cause mortality was reduced, however, this was significant only after adjusting for covariates (ARR 3.1%; RRR 17% adjusted; p = 0.033). The reduction in heart failure admissions was reflected in a strong trend for a reduction in all-cause hospitalization (p = 0.06). Patients randomized to candesartan also had a symptom benefit.

In summary, this trial suggests that candesartan at a dose of 32 mg/day is well tolerated, substantially more effective than placebo and, at this dose, as effective as an ACE inhibitor would have been had it been tolerated [80,81]. Caution is required in extrapolating these results to patients who have been withdrawn from ACE inhibitors because of hypotension or renal dysfunction, or in extrapolating these data to infer that ARBs may be used in preference to an ACE inhibitor in a patient who does not exhibit ACE inhibitor intolerance. As the trial was analyzed on an intention-to-treat basis and a substantial number of patients randomized to placebo subsequently received treatment with an ACE inhibitor or ARB, the trial underestimates the true magnitude of benefit that should be observed in clinical practice.

Overall, this group of trials suggest that, compared with placebo, ARBs improve symptoms, reduce hospitalizations (Fig. 4) and lower mortality (Fig. 5) [80,81].

CHARM-Preserved

This is the first substantial trial [20,23] to assess the effects of treatment in patients with a clinical syndrome suggestive of heart failure but in whom heart failure due to LVSD or major valve disease has been excluded. Epidemiological studies suggest that up to half of patients with heart failure belong to this category and predict that this group should be older and predominantly female [8]. Follow-up studies have suggested that this group of patients has a better short-term survival but that longer-term survival may be as poor as for patients with LVSD, and that they have a high rate of hospitalization for heart failure [10,11]. However, it is likely that the patients enrolled in this study are a highly heterogeneous group of patients including misdiagnosis of heart failure, patients with forme fruste systolic dysfunction, and perhaps some patients with isolated diastolic dysfunction [10].

CHARM-Preserved included patients with symptomatic heart failure who had been hospitalized at some time in the past for a cardiac problem (69% had a previous admission with heart failure) and who had a left ventricular ejection fraction greater than 40%. Candesartan was initiated at 4 mg/day (75% of patients) or 8 mg/day according to the discretion of the investigator, and then titrated at not more than 2-week intervals to 32 mg/day. The primary end-point was cardiovascular death or unplanned admission to hospital for the management of worsening heart failure.

A total of 3205 patients was randomized and followed for a mean of 36.6 months. The mean age of the patients was 67 years; 27% were aged 75 years or more; 60% of patients were men and 44% had had a myocardial infarction. Of those randomized to candesartan, 56% were taking a beta-blocker at baseline and 11% were taking spironolactone. Nineteen percent of patients were taking an ACE inhibitor at baseline, which increased to about 24% during the study in both groups. In each group, 3% of patients started an open-label ARB. Target doses were achieved in 67% of patients randomized to candesartan vs. 79% randomized to placebo at 6 months. Overall, 18% of those randomized to candesartan vs. 14% of those randomized to placebo discontinued trial medication because of an adverse event. Patients randomized to candesartan were more likely to withdraw for hypotension (2.4% vs. 1.1%), renal dysfunction (4.8% vs. 2.4%) and hyperkalemia (1.5% vs. 0.6%). Serum creatinine more than doubled in 6% of patients (vs. 3% on placebo) and serum potassium increased to 6 mmol/L or more in 2% of patients (vs. 1% on placebo).

The annual event rate for the primary endpoint in the placebo group was 9.1%, half that observed in CHARM-Alternative (Fig. 3D). The absolute reduction in the primary end-point with candesartan was just 2.0%, or a relative reduction of 11% (p = ns), increasing to 14% (p = 0.051) after adjusting for imbalances between randomized groups in patients' baseline characteristics. There was no effect on mortality but a trend for a favorable effect on heart failure hospitalizations (ARR 2.4%; RRR 16% adjusted; p = 0.047) (Table 2b). The total number of investigator-defined hospital admissions for heart failure was reduced by 36 (123 vs. 87) events per thousand patients per year (p = 0.014) (Fig. 4D). No effect of candesartan on vascular events, such as myocardial infraction or stroke, was observed. All-cause mortality and all-cause hospitalization were both unchanged by candesartan. The proportion of deaths and hospitalizations that were noncardiovascular were substantially greater in this study than in CHARM-Alternative.

In summary, this trial suggests that candesartan may have some modest effect on altering the natural history of heart failure with preserved left ventricular systolic function but further information on symptoms is required to gauge whether the treatment is really worthwhile. It is possible that stricter entry criteria that required more substantial evidence of cardiac dysfunction would have identified patients with greater benefit. An analysis of the data including only patients who were not receiving an ACE inhibitor would also be valuable.

I-PRESERVE

This is a randomized, double-blind study comparing irbesartan (target dose 300 mg/day) with placebo in patients with heart failure but without LVSD. It is similar in design to

CHARM-Preserved. It is difficult to see why the outcome of this trial would be substantially different to CHARM-Preserved, however, the size and the duration of the trial could make a difference to the confidence intervals around the effect.

LANDMARK TRIALS PRINCIPALLY DESIGNED TO COMPARE ARBS WITH PLACEBO IN THE PRESENCE OF AN ACE INHIBITOR

The Val-HeFT [17,18,75,86–90] and CHARM-Added [20,21] trials are included here. The RESOLVD [16,29] and VALIANT studies [28,91,92] have complex designs including a comparison of combined ACE inhibitor/ARB against each agent used alone and these trials will also be discussed. (Tables 3 and 4)

Table 3 Study Design of and Baseline Characteristics of Patients included in Landmark Trials of Heart Failure Comparing ARB with Placebo in Addition to an ACE Inhibitor

	Val-HeFT (Main) (17)	CHARM-Alternative (20,21)	RESOLVD[a] (16)
Comparison	Valsartan vs. Placebo	Candesartan vs. Placebo	Candesartan vs. Placebo
N =	5010	2548	441
Mean follow-up (months)	23	41	10
Mean age (years)	63	64	63
≥75 years (%)	–	18	–
Women (%)	20	21	13
NYHA (II/III/IV shown as %)	62/36/2	24/73/3	63/35/2
Mean LVEF (entry criterion in brackets)	27 (<40%)	28 (≤40%)	28 (<40%)
Mean systolic blood pressure (mmHg)	124	125	120
Cause of Heart Failure			
Ischemic heart disease	57	62	72
Idiopathic	31	26	17
Hypertension	7	7	–
Other	5	5	11
Medical History			
Diabetes	26	30	–
Atrial fibrillation	12	27	–
Hypertension	–	48	–
Current angina	–	20	–
Pacemaker	–	9	–
Implantable defibrillator	–	4	–
CABG	–	25	–
Treatment			
Diuretic	86	90	85
ACE inhibitors	93	100	Excluded at baseline
Beta-blockers	35	55	13% on combination vs. 23% on enalapril (p<0.05)
Spironolactone	–	17	–
Calcium channel blocker	–	10	15
Digoxin	67	58	69
Anticoagulant	–	38	31
Aspirin	–	51	53
Statin	–	41	–

[a] Includes only patients randomized to combination or enalapril.

Table 4 Summary of Outcome of Landmark Trials of Heart Failure Comparing ARB with Placebo or Control When Added to an ACE Inhibitor

	Patients		Follow-up (Months)	Mortality		Total Number of Hospitalizations		Death or HF Hospitalization Number and % of Patients		Total HF Hospitalizations	
	Placebo	ARB		Placebo	ARB	Placebo	ARB	Placebo	ARB	Placebo	ARB
RESOLVD (16)	109	332	11	4 (3.7%)	29 (8.7%)	–	–	10 (9.2%)	58 (17.5%)	–	–
Val-HeFT–main[a] (17)	2318	2326	23	435 (18.8%)	463 (19.9%)	2844	2657	724 (31.2%)	677 (29.1%)	1072	872
CHARM-Added (21)	1272	1276	41	412 (32.4%)	377 (29.5%)	2798	2462	587 (46.1%)	539 (42.2%)	836	607
Total for Heart Failure	**3699**	**3934**		**851 (23.0%)**	**869 (22.1%)**	**5642**	**5119**	**1321 (35.7%)**	**1274 (32.4%)**	**1908**	**1479**
VALIANT (28,91)	4909	4885	25	958 (19.5%)	941 (19.3%)	–	–	1335 (27.2%)	1331 (27.2%)	–	–
Overall Total	**8608**	**8819**		**1809 (21.0%)**	**1810 (20.5%)**	**5642**	**5119**	**2656 (30.9%)**	**2605 (29.5%)**	**1908**	**1479**

[a] patients not on ACE inhibitors have been excluded.

RESOLVD

RESOLVD [16,29] was a complex randomized, double-blind, dose-ranging study comparing enalapril (10 mg bid) to three doses of candesartan (4 mg, 8 mg and 16 mg/day) in the absence of an ACE inhibitor, and two doses of candesartan (4 mg and 8 mg/day) in addition to enalapril (10 mg bid). The comparison of combination with either agent used alone is the focus of this section. The starting dose of candesartan was 2 mg/day and of enalapril 2.5 mg b.i.d.. Patients with symptomatic heart failure and a LVEF less than 40% were eligible. The primary end-points included exercise distance (6-minute corridor walk), cardiac function, neuroendocrine measures, symptoms, and quality of life. Morbidity and mortality were safety outcomes. After 17 weeks, patients not taking beta-blockers were eligible for rerandomization to placebo or metoprolol in addition to their initial study medication [93].

A total of 436 patients was randomized to either enalapril or candesartan alone and an additional 332 patients to combination therapy. Patients were followed for 43 weeks. Patients were predominantly men; most had few symptoms (63% in NYHA class II), and more than 90% of patients had been withdrawn from ACE inhibitors to enter the study.

Compared with either candesartan or enalapril alone, the combination did not improve exercise distance, LVEF, norepinephrine levels, endothelin levels, symptoms, or quality of life. The latter may reflect the mild severity of symptoms at baseline. However, compared with either agent alone, the combination did inhibit progressive ventricular dilatation, and this was associated with a greater and more sustained reduction in brain natriuretic peptide; similar trends were observed for aldosterone. The highest dose of candesartan exerted the greatest effect. These effects were associated with about a 5 mmHg greater reduction in systolic blood pressure.

RESOLVD was stopped prematurely due to a higher incidence of death in the candesartan (6.1%) and combination groups (8.7%) than in the enalapril group (3.7%). No similar trend was noted for hospitalization.

In summary, the mechanistic data from this study suggested that combination therapy *might* be superior to either agent used alone. The excess mortality with combination therapy, in hindsight, probably reflects a spuriously low mortality in the small number (n = 107) of patients randomized to enalapril alone and a somewhat higher than expected mortality in the group randomized to enalapril in combination with 8 mg/day of candesartan. At the time, it caused considerable concern.

Val-HeFT

The Val-HeFT study [17,18,75,86–90] compared valsartan (target dose 160 mg b.i.d.) to placebo predominantly in patients who were taking substantial doses (e.g., a mean of 17 mg/day of enalapril) of ACE inhibitors (93%) in patients with treated symptomatic heart failure due to LVSD. Only 7% of patients were not receiving an ACE inhibitor at baseline, mainly because of previous intolerance.

Valsartan was initiated at 40 mg b.i.d. and then titrated at 2-week intervals to a target of 160 mg b.i.d. provided the patient had no hypotensive symptoms, the standing systolic blood pressure was greater than 90 mmHg, and renal function had not deteriorated substantially (e.g., 50% increase in creatinine). The coprimary end-points were all-cause mortality and the composite of death, hospitalization for heart failure, resuscitated cardiac arrest, or the administration of intravenous inotropic or vasodilator agents for more than 4 hours without hospitalization. The latter two components of the composite contributed little.

Overall, 5010 patients were randomized and followed for a mean of 23 months. The mean age of the patients was 63 years; 47% were aged 65 years or more, and most patients were men who had coronary artery disease. Of those randomized to valsartan, 35% were taking a beta-blocker, and only 5% were taking spironolactone. A target dose was achieved in 84% of patients randomized to valsartan vs. 93% of those randomized to placebo. Adverse events led to withdrawal of study medication in 9.9% and 7.2% of patients randomized to valsartan and placebo, respectively. Patients randomized to valsartan were more likely to withdraw for hypotension (1.3% vs. 0.8%) and renal dysfunction (1.1% vs. 0.2%). Serum creatinine and serum potassium increased by an average of only 7 μmol/L and 0.05mmol/L, respectively, compared with placebo.

Valsartan had no overall effect on mortality but a statistically significant reduction (p = 0.017 by log-rank test) was noted in the small subgroup of patients who were not receiving an ACE inhibitor at baseline [75] (Table 2a). The corollary of accepting this observation as true is that there was a slight, nonsignificant trend to an excess mortality with valsartan in those patients who were taking an ACE inhibitor at baseline.

Valsartan did reduce the composite morbidity/mortality outcome (ARR 4.4%; RRR 13%; p = 0.009) almost entirely due to a reduction in hospitalizations for heart failure (RRR 24%; p = 0.001) (Fig. 3C). The total number of investigator-defined hospital admissions for heart failure was reduced by 55 (from 241 to 196) events per thousand patients per year (p = 0.002) (Fig. 4C). A slightly greater effect was observed in patients not taking ACE inhibitors. Non– heart-failure admissions were unaffected, but this was enough to dilute the effect on heart failure admissions so that the trend to a reduction in all-cause hospitalization was not significant [87].

Patients taking a combination of beta-blockers and ACE inhibitors at baseline had a higher mortality if randomized to valsartan. However, it is likely that many patients had beta-blockers initiated during the study and so interaction with baseline therapy should be interpreted cautiously. In the light of subsequent data, it is almost certain that this was a chance finding. Other subgroup analyses revealed no significant heterogeneity in the effect of valsartan. Patients with higher NYHA class, lower LVEF, and more dilated left ventricles tended to have more benefit, perhaps reflecting the fact that they were sicker and had more cardiovascular events to prevent. Patients with ischemic heart disease and those with diabetes tended to have less benefit, perhaps suggesting that ARBs have a limited effect on vascular protection or an adverse effect of excessive blood pressure reduction in patients with severe coronary disease.

Valsartan improved symptoms using a variety of measures and quality of life. The effect on symptoms was equivalent to improving one in every twenty patients by one full NYHA class (p<0.001) (Fig. 6). Progressive increases in plasma concentrations of brain

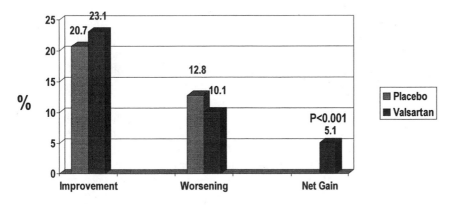

Figure 6 Change in New York Heart Association (NYHA) functional class for patients who received valsartan or placebo in the Valsartan Heart Failure Trial (Val-HeFT).

natriuretic peptide (BNP) and norepinephrine, markers of a worse prognosis, were noted on placebo [86,88]. Valsartan produced a sustained reduction in BNP and attenuated the increase in norepinephrine. These effects were most prominent in patients who were not taking ACE inhibitors but were also observed in the presence of ACE inhibitors and beta-blockers. Most patients in the study had serial echocardiographic measurements of left ventricular function. These showed that valsartan increased left ventricular ejection fraction by about 1.3% placebo-subtracted (i.e., from about 26.6% to 31.1% on valsartan compared with 26.9% to 30.1% on placebo) (p<0.0001)[17,89]. Again, effects were greatest in the absence of an ACE inhibitor and absent in patients taking both a beta-blocker and an ACE inhibitor. Similarly, valsartan reduced left ventricular diastolic dimension by 7 mm/m^2 with the effect being greatest in those not taking ACE inhibitors and least in those taking ACE inhibitors and beta-blockers [89].

In summary, this trial shows that valsartan at a dose of 160 mg b.i.d. is well tolerated, safe, improves symptoms and reduces hospitalization for heart failure when added to an ACE inhibitor, but raised concerns about triple therapy in combination with beta-blockers.

CHARM-Added

The CHARM-added study [20,21] compared candesartan (target dose 32 mg/day) to placebo in patients who were taking substantial doses (e.g., a mean of 17 mg/day of enalapril) of ACE inhibitors for symptomatic heart failure due to LVSD. To exclude patients at a low risk of events, patients who were in NYHA class II were required to have had an admission for a cardiac problem in the previous 6 months

Candesartan was initiated at 4 mg/day (86% of patients) or 8 mg/day according to the discretion of the investigator, and then titrated at not more than 2-week intervals to 32 mg/day. The primary end-point was cardiovascular death or unplanned hospitalization for the management of worsening heart failure.

A total of 2548 patients was randomized and followed for a mean of 41 months. The mean age of the patients was 64 years;18% were older than 75 years, and most patients were men who had coronary disease. Of those randomized to candesartan, 55% were taking a beta-blocker (rising to 64% during the course of the study) and 17% were taking spironolactone. The target dose was achieved in 61% of patients randomized to candesartan vs. 73% randomized to placebo at 6 months. Adverse events led to withdrawal of study medication in 24% and 18% of patients randomized to candesartan and placebo, respectively. In each group, 6% of patients started an open-label ACE inhibitor and 9% an open-label ARB. Patients randomized to candesartan were more likely to withdraw for hypotension (4.5% vs. 3.1%), renal dysfunction (7.8% vs. 4.1%) and hyperkaliemia (3.4% vs. 0.7%). Serum creatinine more than doubled in 7% of patients (vs. 6% on placebo) and serum potassium increased to 6mmol/L or more in 3% of patients (vs. 1% on placebo). These effects were not substantially different in the presence of spironolactone. Candesartan reduced systolic blood pressure by a mean of 5 mmHg by 6 months with no greater effect observed in those patients taking beta-blockers.

The absolute reduction in the primary end-point with candesartan was 4.4% or a relative reduction of 15% (p=0.011) (Fig. 3B). This effect was brought about by very similar effects on heart failure hospitalizations and cardiovascular death. Benefits tended to be greater in patients receiving beta-blockers and higher doses of ACE inhibitors. The total number of investigator-defined hospital admissions for heart failure was reduced by 53 (from 192 to 139) events per thousand patients per year (p=0.002) (Fig. 4B). Candesartan was associated with slightly fewer myocardial infarctions (n = 44 vs. 69; p=0.012) but not strokes (n = 47 vs. 41), although few patients suffered either event. The total number of admissions was reduced (p = 0.023). A trend to a reduction in all-cause mortality was not significant. The trend was identical in the presence or absence of a beta-blocker.

In summary, this trial suggests that candesartan at a dose of 32 mg/day is well tolerated, safe, improves symptoms and reduces hospitalizations when added to ACE inhibitors with or without beta-blockers. This trial provides no definitive evidence of a mortality benefit with ARBs in this clinical setting.

VALIANT

This trial [80,92] compared valsartan (160 mg bid) with captopril (50 mg t.i.d.) and the combination (captopril 50 mg b.i.d. and valsartan 80 mg b.i.d.) in patients with a recent myocardial infarction (12 hours to 10 days) who exhibited clinical (70%) or radiological (39%) evidence of heart failure or who had major LVSD (52%). Overall, 50% fulfilled at least two sets of entry criteria. Patients with a systolic blood pressure less than 100 mmHg or serum creatinine greater than 221 μmol/L were excluded. The focus in this section is on the outcome of combination therapy compared to either agent used alone. (Tables 4, 6 and 7) [28,29,91]

Captopril was initiated at 6.25 mg b.i.d. and valsartan at 20 mg b.i.d. and rapid titration was encouraged prior to discharge. The primary end-point was all-cause mortality and the principal secondary endpoint was a composite time-to-first event analysis of cardiovascular mortality, recurrent myocardial infarction or hospitalization for heart failure.

Overall, 14,703 patients were randomized and followed for a median of 24.7 months. The mean age of the patients was 65 years, 25% were aged 75 years or more, and most patients were men. Approximately 70% were taking a beta-blocker at baseline but few were taking potassium sparing diuretics; 60% had an anterior myocardial infarction, and 67% had a Q-wave infarction. 75% of patients were enrolled within 7-days of infarction. During this period, 46% underwent acute reperfusion therapy (thrombolysis or percutaneous intervention), 25% underwent revascularization, and 17% had significant arrhythmias or conduction disturbances (mostly atrial fibrillation). Diuretics were prescribed in 50% of patients. Of those randomized to valsartan alone, captopril, or the combination, 15.3%, 16.8% and 19.0% had withdrawn from therapy by 12 months, and the proportions taking target doses of therapy were 56%, 56% and 47%. During the whole of course of the study, 5.8%, 7.7% and 9.0% of patients withdrew respectively from valsartan, captopril, or combination therapy for an adverse events. Overall, 20.5%, 21.6% and 23.4% withdrew from therapy for any reason, most commonly patient-choice for unspecified reasons. In each group, at 1 year 7% to 8% were taking an open-label ACE inhibitor, and 2% to 3% were taking an open-label ARB. Patients randomized to the combination were more likely to withdraw for hypotension (1.9% vs. 0.8%) and renal dysfunction (1.3% vs. 0.8%). Comparison of the adverse effect profile of valsartan alone vs. captopril is discussed in the following text. Blood pressure rose during follow-up to a mean of 125/76 mmHg on captopril alone. Treatment with valsartan alone and in combination was associated with reductions in this rise of systolic blood pressures of 0.9 mmHg and 2.2 mmHg (both p<0.001), respectively.

Mortality on combination therapy (19.3%) was similar to that on captopril alone (19.5%). The hazard ratio was 0.98 (95% confidence intervals of 0.89 to 1.09), which provided sufficient evidence to say that combination therapy was not inferior to captopril monotherapy. The proportions of patients reaching the principal secondary endpoint were also similar at 31.1% on combination therapy and 31.9% on captopril alone. There was no interaction with beta-blocker therapy. There was a trend for a reduction in the total number of investigator-defined hospital admissions for myocardial infarction or heart failure (estimated reduction of 15 [from 147 to 132] events per thousand patients per year [p = ns]).

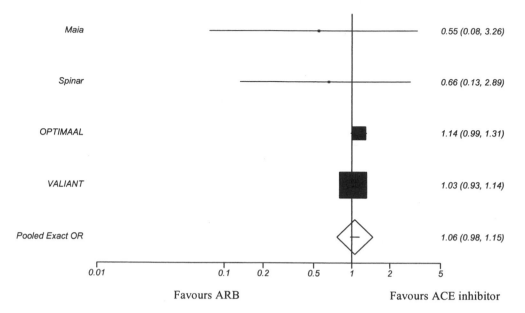

Figure 7 Meta-analysis of outcomes for patients receiving angiotensin receptor blockers (ARBs) compared with angiotensin-converting enzyme (ACE) inhibitors following acute myocardial infarction.

In summary, this trial suggests that there is little advantage to using valsartan and captopril in combination compared to captopril alone. Combination therapy is associated with more adverse events but no obvious health gain. However, data on symptoms and all-cause hospitalization have not yet been reported and could change the perceptions of the outcome of this study. Consistent with data from Val-HeFT and CHARM-Added, VALIANT shows a trend to a reduction in the total number of hospitalizations.

Overall, this group of trials suggest no effect of adding an ARB to an ACE inhibitor on mortality [80,81] (Fig. 7). The trials do suggest a symptomatic benefit leading to a reduction in heart failure hospitalizations, which translates into an overall significant reduction in all-cause hospitalization [80,81]. These effects have been achieved despite the use of high background doses of ACE inhibitors. Although the benefits of adding an ARB to an ACE inhibitor might have been replicated by a substantial increase in the dose of the ACE inhibitor there are few data to support this contention [92].

LANDMARK TRIALS PRINCIPALLY DESIGNED TO COMPARE ARBS WITH ACE INHIBITORS

This section includes the ELITE [14], ELITE-II [15,94] and OPTIMAAL studies [26,27]. The RESOLVD [16] and VALIANT [28,29,80,91,92] studies have complex designs including a comparison of ARB against ACE inhibitor. (Fig. 8) Only a small amount of additional data can be gleaned from the meta-analyses of losartan and candesartan previously mentioned and these are not dealt with further. (Tables 5,6 and 7).

ELITE (Evaluation of Losartan in the Elderly Study)

The ELITE trial [14] randomized 722 patients with heart failure and LVSD to captopril 50 mg t.i.d. or losartan 50 mg once daily in a double-blind study of 48 weeks duration.

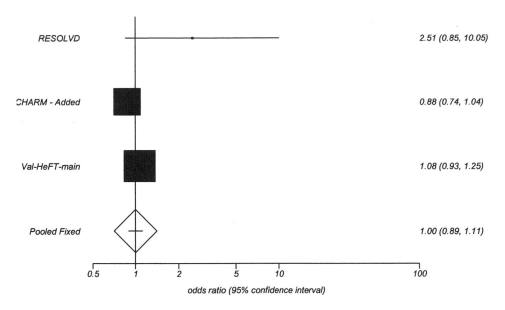

RESOLVD   2.51 (0.85, 10.05)

CHARM - Added   0.88 (0.74, 1.04)

Val-HeFT-main   1.08 (0.93, 1.25)

Pooled Fixed   1.00 (0.89, 1.11)

0.5   1   2   5   10   100

odds ratio (95% confidence interval)

Figure 8 Meta-analysis of randomized, controlled trials comparing an angiotensin receptor blocker to placebo in patients with advanced left ventricular systolic dysfunction and receiving background therapy with an ACE inhibitor on mortality.

The primary end-point was an increase of serum creatinine of 26.5 umol/L (0.3 mg/dL) or more, which, as an index of an important adverse effect on renal function, appears arbitrary and unlikely to make most clinicians withdraw ACE inhibitor therapy or take any other action. The secondary end-point, death and/or admission for CHF, was formulated after patient recruitment was complete and after the results of other smaller studies contained in the losartan meta-analysis had become known. Analyses of all-cause mortality and hospital admission for CHF were other prespecified outcomes of interest, and an analysis of all-cause hospital admission was conducted as a further exploratory analysis.

Patients had to be 65 years of age or older; two-thirds were 70 years of age or older, and most patients were in NYHA class II. Only 74% of patients were receiving diuretics, a powerful stimulus to neuroendocrine activation in heart failure, the substrate upon which ARBs and ACE inhibitors probably work. More than 80% of patients were in NYHA class I or II by the study end in both groups. The mean ejection fraction was 30%. Patients with renal dysfunction (serum creatinine 221 μmol/L [2.5 mg/dL] or greater) were excluded and, thus, a population at low risk of developing serious adverse renal events was identified. The mean baseline serum creatinine was 106 μmol/L (1.2 mg/dL). Compared with the SOLVD-Treatment trial [83], the ELITE population was about a decade older but appeared to have milder heart failure, as the ejection fraction was considerably higher and diuretic use was lower.

There was no difference in outcome with respect to changes in serum creatinine–10.5% of patients in each group having an increase of 26.5 umol/L or more. There was a trend to a greater increase in serum potassium with captopril, but it is not clear if this should be considered beneficial or not.

Losartan reduced overall mortality by 46% (RRR) (p<0.04), largely due to a reduction in sudden deaths (RRR 64%; p<0.05) and death due to myocardial infarction (RRR 76%; p = ns). Death due to progressive CHF occurred in only one patient in each group. Only 5.7% of patients in each group were hospitalized for CHF over 48 weeks, suggesting

Table 5 Study Design of and Baseline Characteristics of Patients Included in Landmark Trials of Heart Failure Comparing ARB with ACE Inhibitors

	ELITE-1 (14)	ELITE-II (15,94)
Comparison	Losartan vs. Captopril	Losartan vs. Captopril
N =	722	3152
Mean follow-up (months)	11	18
Mean age (years)	74	71
≥ 70 years (%) (entry criterion in brackets)	70 (≥65years)	(≥60 years)
Women (%)	33	30
NYHA (II/III/IV shown as %)	65/34/1	52/43/5
Mean LVEF (entry criterion in brackets)	31 (≤40%)	31 (≤40%)
Mean systolic blood pressure (mmHg) (entry criterion in brackets)	137 (>90 mmHg)	134 (>90 mmHg)
Cause of Heart Failure		
Ischemic heart disease	68	79
Other	32	21
Medical History		
Diabetes	25	24
Atrial fibrillation	23	30
Hypertension	57	49
Current angina	–	–
Pacemaker	–	–
Implantable defibrillator	–	–
CABG	–	–
Treatment		
Diuretic	74	78
ACE inhibitors	–	(prior to study 24%)
Beta-blockers	16	22
Potassium sparing diuretic	–	22
Calcium channel blocker	34	23
Digoxin	57	50
Anticoagulant	18	–
Aspirin	48	59
Statin	–	–

–; not provided.

that the patients in ELITE had relatively mild CHF. Losartan and captopril exerted similar benefits on symptoms. Changes in plasma norepinephrine, a potential marker of progressive ventricular dysfunction, were not significantly different between groups.

Despite reducing mortality, which leaves more people at risk of hospitalization, losartan reduced all-cause hospitalization rates by 26% over captopril treatment. This could have reflected the lower side effect profile and better tolerability of losartan. More than 70% of patients were maintained on the target dose of both losartan and captopril, whereas 85% achieved the target dose at some time in the study. Overall, 20.8% of captopril-treated patients withdrew because of side effects vs. 12.2% of losartan treated patients (p<0.002). This difference was largely due to a lower risk of cough, taste disturbance, angioedema, and worsening heart failure. A total of 3.8% of patients discontinued captopril due to cough vs. none on losartan (p<0.002). There was no difference in the rate of hypotensive symptoms (24%).

Table 6 Summary of Outcome of Landmark Trials of Heart Failure Comparing ARB with an ACE Inhibitor

	Patients		Follow-up (Months)	Mortality		Total Number of Hospitalizations		Death or HF Hospitalization Number and % of Patients		Total HF Hospitalizations	
	ACE Inhibitor	ARB		ACE Inhibitor	ARB	ACE Inhibitor	ARB	ACE Inhibitor	ARB	ACE Inhibitor	ARB
ELITE-1 (14)	370	352	11	32	17	–	–	49 (13.2%)	33 (9.4%)	–	–
ELITE-II (15)	1574	1578	18	250	280	–	–	–	–	–	–
Total for Heart Failure	**1944**	**1930**		**282 (14.5%)**	**297 (15.4%)**	–	–	–	–	–	–
OPTIMAAL (26,27)	2733	2744	32	447	499	Mean of 13.6 days	Mean of 13.1 days	–	–	–	–
VALIANT (28,91)	4909	4909	25	958	979	–	–	1335 (27.2%)	1326 (27.0%)	–	–
Total for Myocardial Infarction	**7642**	**7653**		**1405 (18.4%)**	**1478 (19.3%)**	–	–	–	–	–	–
Overall Total	**9,586**	**9,583**		**1,687 (17.6%)**	**1,775 (18.5%)**	–	–	–	–	–	–

Table 7 Study Design and Baseline Characteristics of Patients Included in Landmark Trials of ARBs in the Setting of Post Myocardial Infarction Left Ventricular Systolic Dysfunction and/or Heart Failure

	OPTIMAAL (26,27)	VALIANT (28,29,91)
Comparison	Losartan vs. Captopril	Valsartan vs. Captopril
N =	5477	14,703
Mean follow-up (months)	32	25
Mean age (years)	67	65
> 75 years (%)	–	–
Women (%)	29	31
Killip Class (I/II/III/IV shown as %)	32/57/9/2	29/48/17/6
Mean LVEF (entry criterion in brackets)	(<35% or new anterior Q-waves or heart failure)	35 (see text)
Mean systolic blood pressure (mmHg)	123 (>100 mmHg)	123 (>100 mmHg)
Time from infarction to randomization (median days)	3	5
Anterior site of infarction (%)	51	59
Medical History		
Prior myocardial infarction	18	28
Diabetes	17	23
Atrial fibrillation	10	
Hypertension	36	55
Any angioplasty/CABG[a]	14/3	35/7
Treatment		
Thrombolysis	54	35
Primary angioplasty	–	15
Diuretic	64	50
ACE inhibitors	Excluded	(40% prior to randomization)
Beta-blockers	79	70
Potassium sparing diuretic	–	9
Calcium channel blocker	22	–
Digoxin	11	–
Anticoagulant	–	–
Aspirin	96	91
Statin	31	34

[a] Includes acute revascularization prior to randomization; –, not provided.

Only when an effective drug is ingested can its benefits be realized. Thus, losartan could have proved superior to an ACE inhibitor not because it was more effective but because it was more likely to be taken. Excluding deaths, 18.2% of patients discontinued losartan for any reason vs. 28.6% of those on captopril (p<0.001), but this did not account for the difference in survival (3.7% vs. 8.5% for those remaining on therapy with losartan or captopril, respectively; p = 0.013).

A substudy on 29 patients suggested that captopril and losartan exerted equal effects on ventricular function during treatment but that the effect of captopril may persist for longer after drug withdrawal [95]. A total of 278 patients was enrolled in a quality of life substudy of which 203 completed questionnaires before and after treatment (Sickness Impact Profile, Minnesota Living with Heart Failure). Trends in favor of losartan were not significant after adjustment for multiple analyses [96] but significantly fewer patients withdrew from losartan for adverse events. Patients who withdrew for adverse events were unavailable for the second questionnaire, which biased this substudy against losartan.

ELITE II

The ELITE-II trial [15,94] compared losartan (target dose 50 mg/day) with captopril (target dose 50 mg t.i.d.) in patients older than 60 years with symptomatic heart failure and LVSD. By design, most patients had not previously received an ACE inhibitor or ARB. Patients with a systolic blood pressure less than 90 mmHg, or serum creatinine greater than 220umol/L were excluded. The primary end-point was all-cause mortality. Losartan was initiated at 12.5 mg/day and captopril at 12.5 mg t.i.d. Both were titrated at weekly intervals to target doses.

Overall, 3152 patients were randomized and followed for a mean of 18 months. The mean age of the patients was 72 years, 85% were aged 65years or more, and most were men who had coronary artery disease. Of those randomized to losartan, 23% were taking a beta-blocker and 22% were receiving a potassium sparing diuretic. Adverse events led to withdrawal of study medication in about 15% and 10% of patients randomized to losartan and captopril, respectively. A large proportion of this difference was due to ACE inhibitor induced cough.

There were slightly more deaths (absolute excess risk 1.8%; relative excess risk 13%; p = ns) on losartan compared with captopril. The confidence intervals around this effect were sufficiently large that it is not safe to draw the conclusion that these drugs at these doses had equivalent effects. No significant differences were observed in rates of hospitalization for heart failure or other reasons. Patients taking beta-blockers tended to fare better on captopril, although the statistical test for interaction (which is not a very powerful test) was not significant.

In summary, this trial does *not* support the *substitution* of an ACE inhibitor with losartan 50 mg/day in patients with heart failure. The previous ELITE study result appeared to have occurred by chance.

RESOLVD

This section focuses on the comparison of ACE inhibitor and ARB portion of the trial in which 327 patients were randomized to candesartan (4 mg, 8 mg or 16 mg/day) or enalapril 20 m/day [16]. No differences in symptoms, cardiac function or neuroendocrine activation were observed. Patients on the two lower doses of candesartan tended to have higher mortality than patients on enalapril or the highest dose of candesartan. Differences in heart failure hospitalization favored enalapril. In summary, this trial is compatible with the ELITE-II trial result but hints at the possibility that higher doses of ARBs may produce benefits similar to ACE inhibitors.

OPTIMAAL

The OPTIMAAL trial [26,27] compared losartan (target dose 50 mg/day) with captopril (target dose 50 mg t.i.d.) in patients aged 50 years or older with acute myocardial infarction and evidence of heart failure (81%), or systolic dysfunction (LVEF <35% or end-diastolic dimension >65 mm [14%] or anterior Q-waves [51%]). Patients with a supine systolic blood pressure greater than 100 mmHg or receiving an ACE inhibitor or ARB were excluded. The primary end-point was all-cause mortality. Losartan was initiated at 12.5 mg/day and captopril at 6.25 mg (single-dose) then 12.5 mg t.i.d. (Tables 6 and 7)

A total of 5477 patients was randomized and followed for a mean of 32 months. The mean age of the patients was 67 years, most patients were men who had coronary disease. Of those randomized to losartan, 79% were taking a beta-blocker, and 63% were taking a diuretic. More than 70% of patients had reached target doses of each drug at 1 month, rising to greater than 80% by the end of the study. Adverse events led to withdrawal of study medication in 17% and 23% of patients randomized to losartan and captopril, respectively. A large proportion of this difference was due to ACE inhibitor induced cough but skin rashes, taste disturbances, and angio-edema also made significant contributions. Losartan and captopril had similar effects on blood pressure in the long-term, but captopril exerted a greater reduction after the first dose.

There were slightly more deaths (absolute excess risk 1.8%; relative excess risk 13%; p = ns) on losartan compared to captopril. Despite the larger trial size and greater number of events, the confidence intervals around this effect were still sufficiently large that a difference in mortality of up to 25% could not be excluded. No significant differences were observed in the risk of sudden death, resuscitated cardiac arrest, or myocardial infarction. There was no evidence of an interaction with beta-blockers. Patients in both groups spent a similar number of days in hospital (about 13 days) and had similar severity of symptoms.

In summary, this trial does *not* support the substitution of an ACE inhibitor with losartan 50mg/day in patients with post-infarction heart failure or ventricular dysfunction. These data are very similar to those observed in the ELITE-II trial except that they do not support a beta-blocker interaction.

VALIANT

This section focuses on the comparison of ACE inhibitor and ARB that included 4909 patients randomized to valsartan (160 mg b.i.d.) vs. 4909 randomized to captopril (50 mg t.i.d.) [28,29,80,91,92]. Thus, the study had about twice as many patients compared with the OPTIMAAL trial. Similar numbers of patients developed adverse events on captopril (28.4%) and valsartan (29.4%), however, significantly fewer patients withdrew from valsartan because of side effects (7.7% vs. 5.8%). Overall withdrawals for any reason did not differ (21.6% vs. 20.5%). Hypotension (15.1% vs. 11.9%) and renal dysfunction (4.9% vs. 3.0%) were more common with valsartan but only withdrawal for hypotension (1.4% vs. 0.8%) was statistically significant. Cough (5.0% vs. 1.7%), rash (1.3% vs. 0.7%) and taste disturbance (0.6% vs. 0.3%) were all more common with captopril and more commonly led to withdrawal of therapy. Blood pressure rose during follow-up to a mean of 125/76 mmHg on captopril alone. Treatment with valsartan was associated with a reduction in this rise in systolic blood pressures of 0.9 mmHg (p<0.001).

Mortality on valsartan (19.9%) was similar to that on captopril alone (19.5%). The hazard ratio was 1.00 (97.5% confidence intervals of 0.90 to 1.11), which provided sufficient evidence to say that valsartan was not inferior to captopril. The proportions of patients reaching the principal secondary endpoint were also similar on valsartan and captopril (31.1% vs. 31.9%). There was no interaction with beta-blocker therapy. There was no difference in the total number of investigator-defined hospital admissions for myocardial infarction or heart failure. (Tables 6 and 7)

In summary, the reported data on this trial suggests that valsartan and captopril provide similar benefits but that valsartan is associated with slightly fewer adverse events. This provides an argument for using an ARB in preference to an ACE inhibitor in this clinical setting assuming that the cost of therapy, a very small fraction of overall healthcare, is not important.

These comparative trials suggest that the benefits of treatment with an ACE inhibitor and an ARB, when prescribed in an adequate dose, are similar (Table 6, Fig. 7) [80,81]. However, ARBs are associated with fewer adverse effects and, therefore, they could be considered the treatment of first choice. Although there are concerns that ARBs may exert less effect on reducing vascular events, this could reflect the use of inadequate doses. However, it is also possible that the full benefits of ACE inhibitors are not being observed due to the widespread use of aspirin, a treatment that has not been shown to be effective either in patients with heart failure nor long-term in patients who have had a myocardial infarction [56,60]. As it is clear that aspirin reduces the benefits of ACE inhibitors [60,97] but probably does not reduce the benefits of ARBs, this implies that in patients not treated with aspirin ACE inhibitors remain the drug of choice.

WHY USE AN ARB?

To Improve Symptoms of Heart Failure

There is good evidence that, compared with placebo, ARBs improve the symptoms of heart failure in patients with LVSD when used instead of ACE inhibitors [70,77,79,98]. There is also strong evidence that ARBs and ACE inhibitors improve symptoms to a similar extent [99,100]. ARBs also appear to improve symptoms compared with placebo when added to an ACE inhibitor [17], although the latter effect appears modest, requiring treatment of about 20 patients to improve one patient by one NYHA class compared with placebo. However, when the placebo effect is included, which corresponds better to the patient's experience, the effect may represent a substantial symptomatic benefit for one patient in five.

The excess in adverse events should be set against the benefit on symptoms. Although the placebo-subtracted rate of withdrawal for adverse events is relatively low (2% to 5%) the absolute adverse event rate (more equivalent to the patient experience) may be 10% to 20%.

However, these assumptions do not account for the fact that patients were being closely monitored in clinical trials and knew that the treatment might be ineffective. Assuming that treatment is being recommended, the true benefits may be larger and adverse effects fewer than reported in a controlled trial. Conversely, the inclusion of patients with more comorbidity may increase the adverse event rate.

There are insufficient data to evaluate the possible symptomatic benefits of ARBs in patients with heart failure and preserved left ventricular systolic function.

To Reduce Hospitalization

There is compelling evidence that, compared with placebo, ARBs reduce hospitalizations for worsening heart failure when used instead of ACE inhibitors and that this translates into a reduction in all-cause hospitalization [19,75,80,81]. There is fairly good evidence that ARBs and ACE inhibitors reduce hospitalizations to a similar extent [15,26,94]. There is also good evidence that ARBs reduce heart-failure–related and all-cause hospitalization compared with placebo when added on top of an ACE inhibitor and that the size of this effect is also similar to the effect observed in ACE inhibitor naïve patients, suggesting that the benefits of treatment with this combination is additive [21,80,81,87]. In a recent meta-analysis, combination therapy reduced all-cause mortality or hospitalization for heart failure (odds ratio 0.90 [0.82–0.99]) and heart failure hospitalizations by about 20%, an effect robust enough to reduce all-cause hospitalization [80,81].

The effects of ARBs on heart failure related hospitalization in patients with preserved left ventricular systolic function were smaller and did not translate into a reduction in all-cause hospitalization, leaving some uncertainty about the true effect in this subset of patients [23].

To Reduce Major Vascular Events

Unlike ACE inhibitors [40,84,85,101] there is little evidence that ARBs reduce the risk of myocardial infarction. This conclusion must be viewed with caution in view of the ability of ARBs to reduce death in patients with heart failure, some of which are likely to have been vascular in origin. It is possible that ARBs and ACE inhibitors exert similar effects on vascular events but that the effects are not additive. However, in CHARM-Alternative there was no hint of a reduction in vascular events [19]. In studies of hypertension, ARBs appear effective in reducing stroke but have not reduced the risk of myocardial infarction so far [1]. In studies of heart failure, ARBs have not reduced the risk of stroke.

To Reduce Mortality

There is conclusive evidence that ARBs reduce mortality in patients with heart failure and LVSD in the absence of an ACE inhibitor [19,75,80,81]. In a recent meta-analysis of heart failure trials, ARBs reduced mortality by 20% compared with placebo (exact pooled odds ratio 0.79 [95% CI 0.66–0.94], without evidence of heterogeneity in outcome) [80,81]. This is similar to the effect of ACE inhibitors compared with placebo in a recent meta-analysis (odds ratio 0.83 [0.76–0.90]) [102]. Most but not all of these data are derived from studies of patients who have been intolerant of ACE inhibitors. However, it is rational to assume that patients who can tolerate an ACE inhibitor might obtain similar benefits, although caution is still warranted due to the lack of evidence of an effect on coronary vascular events in trials of heart failure or hypertension. The magnitude of the effect is only similar to that observed with an ACE inhibitor when high doses of an ARB are used. When lower doses of ARB are used there is evidence that they may be somewhat inferior to high-dose ACE inhibition, although dose-ranging studies of ACE inhibitors themselves have not shown a clear dose-response against mortality. Also, ACE inhibitors appear to be disadvantaged by non–evidence-based therapy with aspirin and their benefits may be greater if such treatment is eliminated [56,60,97].

In the presence of an ACE inhibitor, the overall data suggest no mortality benefit from combination therapy compared with an ACE inhibitor only (odds ratio 1.08 [0.62–2.60] in trials of heart failure) [17,21,80,81]. There is no evidence of a mortality benefit in patients with heart failure and preserved LV systolic function. (Figs. 3D,4D)

Adverse Effects

Cough

A persistent dry cough is undoubtedly a side effect of ACE inhibitors, especially among women [19,20,103]. However, the amount of disability it causes is unclear. Cough is reported spontaneously as an adverse effect in studies of ACE inhibitors in about 3% to 5% of cases, little higher than with placebo [101,104]. Some patients have a severe cough due to ACE inhibitors but surprisingly, even if severe, do not report it spontaneously, believing the side effect to be part of their illness. Cough can be disabling, physically tiring the patient, and disrupting sleep; undoubtedly some patients ''cough themselves to death.'' Cough does not appear to be a side effect of ARBs. Recurrence of cough when patients are switched from an ACE inhibitor to an ARB is low. Cough was reported as a side effect of ACE inhibitors in 5% of patients in VALIANT and 18.7% in OPTIMAAL. Respective data for ARBs were 1.7% and 9.3%. Patients were rarely withdrawn for cough on an ARB compared with an ACE inhibitor (2.5% vs. 0.6% in VALIANT; 4.1% vs. 1.0% in OPTIMAAL).

The mechanism underlying ACE inhibitor-induced cough is unclear but may include effects on pulmonary bradykinin or on mast cells [105,106]. Nonsteroidal antiinflammatory drugs have enjoyed mixed success for the relief of cough but are strongly contraindicated in patients with CHF due to their adverse renal effects. Sodium cromoglycate, a mast cell stabilizer, may help [107,108]. Switching ACE inhibitors occasionally helps but this may have more to do with the interruption of therapy than real differences between ACE inhibitors. Anecdotally, ACE inhibitors may perpetuate cough due to a respiratory tract infection; a drug-free interval may be all that is necessary to stop the cough, the patient then being able to resume the same treatment. Switching patients who cough from ACE inhibitors to ARBs seems a reliable way to avoid cough, and there is more evidence to show that ARBs are safe and beneficial in CHF as there is evidence of safety for other strategies for managing ACE inhibitor cough.

Angioneurotic Edema

Clinical trials of CHF have suggested that this side effect of ACE inhibitors is rare; certainly less than 1% [19,20,101,104]. The mechanisms underlying this reaction are also unclear but may be mediated by bradykinin and mast cells. Patients on renal dialysis are at greater risk of angioneurotic reactions [109]. ARBs have not been shown to precipitate more angioneurotic reactions than a placebo.

Hypotension

Serious hypotension was generally no more common with ARB than ACE inhibitor monotherapy. Patients who do not tolerate an ACE inhibitor because of hypotension will commonly not tolerate an ARB [20,98]. Initial doses of either may precipitate acute hypotension indicating that patients should be started on small doses and that patients on large doses of diuretic or with a low arterial pressure, should be observed for a few hours after dosing [35,70,110–112]. The existing data provided in the studies need to be interpreted with caution because they generally fail to distinguish clearly between syncope, a hemodynamic crisis, and symptomless hypotension.

Renal Dysfunction

Renal dysfunction is most likely to occur when ACE inhibitors are given to very elderly patients (older than 75 years), patients with severe CHF and those with preexisting renal disease. No differences in the effects of ACE inhibitors and ARBs on renal function in heart failure have been noted so far [14]. However, it is likely that patient selection excluded many at increased risk for renal dysfunction. Addition of an ARB to an ACE inhibitor may double the risk of the need to withdraw therapy due to worsening renal function (from 4.1% to 7.8% in CHARM-Added; 0.2% to 1.1% in Val-HeFT) [17,21]. ARBs, like ACE inhibitors, appear to reduce proteinuria and retard the long-term decline in renal function in non–heart-failure patients [113–115]. The significance of the uricosuric effect of losartan, an effect that may not be shared with other ARBs, is uncertain [67].

Are the benefits and side effects of ARBs dose related?

Studies investigating a dose-response in hemodynamics, neuroendocrine effects, effects on ventricular function and remodeling, and on symptoms and exercise capacity all suggest a dose-response but have not convincingly shown where the top of the dose response lies [16,70,116]. It is notable that in CHARM, the most successful ARB study so far, the target dose was double the highest dose used in any published dose-response study with this

Table 8 Dose Response Studies with ARBs in Chronic Heart Failure and Clinical Outcome[a]

Drug	Outcome	Placebo	2.5 mg	10 mg	25 mg	50 mg
Losartan (70)	Worsening	26%	NR	20%	10%	9%
n = 134	Improvement	NR	NR	NR	48%	52%
Drug						
Irbesartan (116)		Not Studied	12.5 mg	37.5 mg	75 mg	150 mg
n = 218	Discontinuation for worsening	Not Studied	9.3%	11.1%	3.6%	1.8%
Drug						
Candesartan (RESOLVD) (16)		Enalapril	4 mg	8 mg	16 mg	Combination
N = 768	Death	3.7%	6.3%	7.4%	4.6%	8.7%
	Death or CHF hospitalization	9.2%	15.3%	20.4%	14.8%	17.5%
Candesartan (STRETCH) (77)		Placebo	–	4 mg	8 mg	16 mg
n = 926	Symptoms and exercise capacity		–	Improvement in symptoms with all doses of candesartan compared to placebo. Dose-related improvement in exercise capacity		

NR, not reported.

[a] Trends to prevention of worsening with higher doses were not statistically significant in the studies with losartan and irbesartan.

agent. In contrast, there is no evidence of a dose-response in terms of death or hospitalization in dose-response studies. However, the failure of lower doses of losartan to have equivalent effects to high-dose captopril [15,26,115] and the magnitude of the effect of high-dose candesartan in CHARM, implies that larger doses may be more effective. The HEAL study, comparing losartan 50 mg/day with 150 mg/day in patients with heart failure who are ACE intolerant, may provide some insights. Studies of hypertension suggest that there is also an important dose-response in this setting [117]. (Table 8)

Are There Clinically Relevant Differences Between ARBs?

The current evidence is consistent with a class-effect. Possible differences in outcome appear to owe more to differences in dose. Pharmacokinetic differences may dictate how often the treatment should be given. The possible different effect of losartan on uricosuria is of uncertain significance. Studies of hypertension suggest that there may be differences in potency between ARBs [117] with the maximum blood pressure reduction that can be achieved with losartan being about 3 mmHg less than that achieved with candesartan.

Are There Important Interactions Between ARBs and Other Classes of Drug Used in Heart Failure?

The CHARM-Program suggested no interaction with background therapy [22]. Of note, earlier concerns about a potential interaction with beta-blockers were laid to rest [21,22]. However, a potential synergistic interaction between beta-blockers and ACE inhibitors that is absent with ARBs cannot be discounted.

ARBs increase the risk of hyperkalemia and, therefore, there is a potential for an adverse interaction with aldosterone antagonists. Relatively few patients (n = 1272) were taking spironolactone in CHARM and only 437 patients were in the CHARM-Added trial

[22]. Trends to less effect in this subgroup of patients were not significant in the overall analysis, but data on the safety and utility of quadruple therapy with ACE inhibitors, beta-blockers, aldosterone antagonists, and ARBs are unclear.

There is strong evidence for an adverse interaction on mortality between ACE inhibitors, but not ARBs, and aspirin [56–61,97]. In addition, one small (n = 16) cross-over study with 3 week treatment periods suggested that the improvement in exercise capacity with losartan but not enalapril could be inhibited by aspirin [118].

Heart Failure in the Absence of Left Ventricular Systolic Dysfunction

The CHARM-Preserved study provides weak support for the use of an ARB in patients with heart failure and preserved LVSD. The small observed benefit may be due to improved control of blood pressure. Metzger and colleagues [119] performed a randomized, double-blind, placebo-controlled, crossover study of 2 weeks of losartan (50 mg/day) with a 2-week washout period on 20 patients with normal LV systolic function (EF >55%), no evidence of ischemia, a mitral flow velocity E/A less than 1, normal resting SBP (<150 mmHg), but a hypertensive response to exercise (SBP >200 mmHg). The primary outcome measures were exercise tolerance and quality of life. After 2 weeks of losartan, peak SBP during exercise decreased by 30 mmHg (p<0.01), and exercise time increased by about 60 seconds compared with placebo. Quality of life improved with losartan compared to baseline and placebo.

CONCLUSIONS

ARBs are a substantial step forward in the treatment of heart failure. ARBs are superior to placebo in improving symptoms, morbidity and mortality in patients with CHF who are intolerant of ACE inhibitors or who have contraindications to them. It seems likely that adequate doses of ARBs are as effective as ACE inhibitors and their tolerability profile is impressive. In women, in whom the incidence of ACE inhibitor cough is high, and in patients with a history of multiple allergies or on renal dialysis that could predispose to angioedema, some might consider ARBs as the initial treatment of choice. However, the lack of an effect on vascular events raises the possibility that all the benefits of ACE inhibitors are not replicated by ARBs and that activation of the bradykinin/prostaglandin pathway is an important mechanism of ACE inhibitor benefit, although potentially attenuated by the use of aspirin.

ARBs do not reduce mortality when added to an ACE inhibitor but do improve symptoms and reduce hospitalizations. The benefits appear sufficiently large that such treatment can be advised in many patients, especially those at highest risk of such events. Health economic analyses of cost-effectiveness are awaited.

The data on heart failure with preserved LV systolic function are insufficient to make any strong recommendation. The trends observed are encouraging. Greater understanding of this population and focus on subgroups with increased risk (for instance those with increased brain natriuretic peptide) or that have a substrate upon which ARBs are likely to work (hypertension) may increase the benefits obtained.

REFERENCES

1. Dahlof B, Devereux RB, Kjeldsen SE, Julius S, Beevers G, De Faire U, Fyhrquist F, Ibsen H, Kristiansson K, Lederballe-Pedersen O, Lendholm LH, Nieminen MS, Omuik P, Oparil S, Wedel H; LIFE Study Group. Cardiovascular morbidity and mortality in the losartan

intervention for endpoint reduction in hypertension study (LIFE): a randomized trial against atenolol. Lancet 2002; 359:995–1003.

2. Bloom BS. Continuation of anti-hypertensive medication after 1 year of therapy. Clin Ther 1998; 20:671–681.

3. Lindholm LH, Ibsen H, Dahlof B, Devereux RB, Beevers G, De Faire U, Fyhrquist F, Julius S, Kjeldsen SE, Kristiansson K, Lederballe-Pedersen O, Nieminen MS, Omuik P, Oparil S, Wedel H, Aurup P, Edelman J, Snapinn S; LIFE Study Group. Cardiovascular morbidity and mortality in patients with diabetes in the losartan intervention for endpoint reduction in hypertension study (LIFE): a randomized study against atenolol. Lancet 2002; 359: 1004–1010.

4. Freemantle N, Cleland JGF, Young S, Mason J, Harrison J. Beta blockade after myocardial infarction:systematic review and meta regression analysis. Br Med J 1999; 318:1730–1737.

5. Mason J, Young P, Freemantle N, Hobbs FDR. Safety and costs of initiating angiotensin converting enzyme inhibitors for heart failure in primary care: analysis of individual patient data from studies of left ventricular dysfunction. Br Med J 2000; 321(7269):1113–1116.

6. Wing LM, Reid CM, Ryan P, Beilin LJ, Brown MA, Jennings GL, Johnson CI, McNeil JJ, Macdonald GJ, Marley JE, Morgan TO, West MJ. Second Australian National Blood Pressure Study Group. A comparison of outcomes with angiotensin-converting-enzyme inhibitors and diuretics for hypertension in the elderly. N Engl J Med 2003; 348(7):583–592.

7. The ALLHAT Officers and Coordinators for the ALLHAT Collaborative Research Group. Major outcomes in high-risk hypertensive patients randomized to angiotensin-converting enzyme inhibitor or calcium channel blocker versus diuretic (ALLHAT). JAMA 2002; 288: 2981–2997.

8. Cleland JGF, Swedberg K, Follath F, Komajda M, Cohen-Solal A, Aguilar JC, Dietz R, Gavazzi A, Hobbs R, Korewicki J, Madeira HC, Moiseyev VS, Preda I, Van Gilst WH, Widimsky J. for the Study Group on Diagnosis of the Working Group on Heart Failure of the European Society of Cardiology Freemantle N , Eastaugh J , Mason J, Eds. The Euro heart failure survey programme: survey on the quality of care among patients with heart failure in Europe. Part 1: patient characteristics and diagnosis. Eur Heart J, 2003.

9. Cleland JGF, Cohen-Solal A, Cosin-Aguilar J, Dietz R, Eastaugh J, Follath F, Freemantle N, Gavazzi A, Hobbs FDR, Korewicki J, Madeira HC, Preda I, Swedberg K, van Gilst W, Widimsky J. for the IMPROVEMENT of Heart Failure Programme Committees and Investigators and the Study Group on Diagnosis of the Working Group on Heart Failure of the European Society of Cardiology. An international survey of the management of heart failure in primary care. The IMPROVEMENT of heart failure programme. Lancet 2002; 360: 1631–1639.

10. Banerjee P, Banerjee T, Khand A, Clark AL, Cleland JGF. Diastolic heart failure - neglected or misdiagnosed? J Am Coll Cardiol 2002; 39(1):138–141.

11. Cleland JGF, Tendera M, Adamus J, Freemantle N, Gray CS, Lye M, O'Mahony D, Polonski L, Taylor J. on behalf of the PEP-CHF investigators. Perindopril for elderly people with chronic heart failure: the PEP-CHF study. Eur J Heart Fail 1999; 1:211–217.

12. Cleland JGF. ACE inhibitors for 'diastolic' heart failure? Reasons not to jump to premature conclusions about the efficacy of ACE inhibitors among older patients with heart failure. Eur J Heart Fail 2001; 3:637–639.

13. Nikitin NP, Witte KKA, Clark AL, Cleland JGF. Color tissue Doppler-derived long-axis left ventricular function in heart failure with preserved global systolic function. Am J Cardiol 2003; 90:1174–1177.

14. Pitt B, Segal R, Martinez FA, Meurers G, Cowley AJ, Thomas I, Deedwania PC, Ney DE, Snavely DB, Chang PI. on behalf of the ELITE study group. Randomized trial of losartan versus captopril in patients over 65 with heart failure (Evaluation of losartan in the elderly study, ELITE). The Lancet 1997; 349:747–752.

15. Pitt B, Poole Wilson PA, Segal R, Martinez FA, Dickstein K, Camm AJ, Konstam MA, Riegger G, Klinger GH, Neaton J, Sharma D, Thiyagarajan B. on behalf of the ELITE II investigators. Effect of losartan compared with captopril on mortality in patients with symptomatic heart failure: randomized trial–the losartan heart failure survival study ELITE II. Lancet 2000; 355(May 6):1582–1587.

16. McKelvie RS, Yusuf S, Pericak D, Math M, Avezum A, Burns RJ, Probstfield J, Tsuyuki RT, White M, Rouleau J, Latini R, Maggioni A, Young J, Pogue J. Comparison of candesartan, enalapril and their combination in congestive heart failure. Randomized evaluation of strategies for left ventricular dysfunction (RESOLVD) Pilot Study. Circulation 1999; 100(10): 1056–1064.

17. Cohn JN, Tognoni G. for the Valsartan Heart Failure Trial Investigators. A randomized trial of the angiotensin-receptor blocker Valsartan in chronic heart failure. N Engl J Med 2001; 345(23):1667–1675.

18. Cohn JN, Tognoni G, Glazer RD, Spormann D. Baseline demographics of the valsartan heart failure trial. Eur J Heart Fail 2000; 2:439–446.

19. Granger CB, McMurray JJV, Yusuf S, Held P, Michelson EL, Olofsson B, Ostergren J, Pfeffer MA, Swedberg K. for the CHARM Investigators and Committees. Effects of candesartan in patients with chronic heart failure and reduced left-ventricular systolic function intolerant to angiotensin-converting-enzyme inhibitors: the CHARM-Alternative trial. Lancet 2003; 362: 772–776.

20. McMurray J, Ostergren J, Pfeffer M, Swedberg K, Granger C, Yusuf S, Held P, Michelson E, Olofsson B. on behalf of the CHARM committees and investigators. Clinical features and contemporary management of patients with low and preserved ejection fraction heart failure: baseline characteristics of patients in the candesartan in heart failure–assessment of reduction in mortality and morbidity (CHARM) programme. Eur J Heart Fail 2003; 5:261–270.

21. McMurray JJV, Ostergren J, Swedberg K, Granger CB, Held P, Michelson EL, Olofsson B, Yusuf S, Pfeffer MA. for the CHARM Investigators and Committees. Effects of candesartan in patients with chronic heart failure and reduced left-ventricular systolic function taking angiotensin-converting-enzyme inhibitors: the CHARM-Added trial. Lancet 2003; 362: 767–771.

22. Pfeffer MA, Swedberg K, Granger CB, Held P, McMurray JJV, Michelson EL, Olofsson B, Ostergren J, Yusuf S. for the CHARM Investigators and Committees. Effects of candesartan on mortality and morbidity in patients with chronic heart failure; the CHARM-Overall programme. Lancet 2003; 362:759–766.

23. Yusuf S, Pfeffer MA, Swedberg K, Granger CB, Held P, McMurray JJV, Michelson EL, Olofsson B, Ostergren J. for the CHARM Investigators and Committees. Effects of candesartan in patients with chronic heart failure and preserved left-ventricular ejection fraction: the CHARM-Preserved Trial. Lancet 2003; 362:771–781.

24. Sharma D, Buyse M, Pitt B, Rucinska EJ. and the Losartan Heart Failure Morbidity Meta-analysis Study Group. Meta-analysis of observed mortality data from all controlled, double-blind multiple-dose studies of losartan in heart failure. Am J Cardiol 2000; 85:187–192.

25. Erdmann E, George M, Voet B, Belcher G, Kolb D, Hiemstra S, Pietrek M, Held P. The safety and tolerability of candesartan cilexetil in CHF. JRAAS 2000; 1(Supplement 1):31–36.

26. Dickstein K, Kjekshus J. and the OPTIMAAL steering committee for the OPTIMAAL study group. Effects of losartan and captopril on mortality and morbidity in high-risk patients after acute myocardial infarction: the OPTIMAAL randomized trial. Lancet 2002; 360:752–760.

27. Dickstein K, Kjekshus J. for the OPTIMAAL trial steering committee and investigators. comparison of baseline data, initial course and management: losartan versus captopril following acute myocardial infarction (The OPTIMAAL Trial). Am J Cardiol 2001; 87:766–771.

28. Pfeffer MA, McMurray JJV, Velazquez EJ, Rouleau JL, Kober L, Maggioni AP, Solomon SD, Swedberg K, Van De Werf F, White H, Leimberger JD, Henis M, Edwards S, Zelenkofske S, Sellers MA, Califf RM. for the Valsartan in Acute Myocardial Infarction Trial Investigators. Valsartan, captopril, or both in myocardial infarction complicated by heart failure, left ventricular dysfunction, or both. N Engl J Med 2003; 349:1893–1906.

29. Velazquez EJ, Pfeffer MA, McMurray JJV, Maggioni AP, Rouleau JL, Van De Werf F, Kober L, White HD, Swedberg K, Leimberger JD, Gallo P, Sellers MA, Edwards S, Henis M, Califf RM. Valsartan in acute myocardial infarction (VALIANT) trial: baseline characteristics in context. Eur J Heart Fail 2003; 5:537–544.

30. Cleland JGF, Witte K, Thackray S. Bradykinin and ventricular function. Eur Heart J 2000; Suppl H(2):H20–H29.

31. Zusman RM. Effects of converting-enzyme inhibitors on the renin-angiotensin-aldosterone, bradykinin, and arachidonic acid-prostaglandin systems: correlation of chemical structure and biological activity. Am J Kidney Dis 1987; 10:13–23.

32. Cleland JGF, Dargie HJ, Hodsman GP, Ball SG, Robertson JI, Morton JJ, East BW, Robertson I, Murray GD, Gillen G. Captopril in heart failure. A double blind controlled trial. Br Heart J 1984; 52(530):535.

33. Cleland JGF, Semple P, Hodsman GP, Ball SG, Ford I, Dargie HJ. Angiotensin II levels, hemodynamics and sympathoadrenal function after low-dose captopril in heart failure. Am J Med 1984; 77:880–886.

34. Cleland JGF, Dargie HJ, Ball SG, Gillen G, Hodsman GP, Morton JJ, East BW, Robertson I, Ford I, Robertson JL. Effects of enalapril in heart failure: a double blind study of effects on exercise performance, renal function, hormones and metabolic state. Br Heart J 1985; 54: 305–312.

35. Cleland JGF, Dargie HJ, McAlpine H, Ball SG, Morton JJ, Robertson JL, Ford I. Severe hypotension after first dose of enalapril in heart failure. Br Med J 1985; 291:1309–1312.

36. Cleland JGF, Dargie HJ, East BW, Robertson I, Hodsman GP, Ball SG, Gillen G, Robertson JI, Morton JJ. Total body and serum electrolyte composition in heart failure: the effects of captopril. Eur Heart J 1985; 6:681–688.

37. Cleland JGF, Dargie HJ. Heart failure, renal function, and angiotensin converting enzyme inhibitors. Kidney Int 1987; 31:S220–S228.

38. Cleland JGF, Gillen G, Dargie HJ. The effects of frusemide and angiotensin-converting enzyme inhibitors and their combination on cardiac and renal haemodynamics in heart failure. Eur Heart J 1988; 9(2):132–141.

39. Cleland JGF, Krikler D. Modification of atherosclerosis by agents that do not lower cholesterol. Br Heart J 1993; 69:54–62.

40. Lonn EM, Yusuf S, Jha P, Montague TJ, Teo KK, Benedict CR, Pitt B. Emerging role of angiotensin converting enzyme inhibitors in cardiac and vascular protection. Circulation 1994; 90:2056–2069.

41. Minisi AJ, Thames MD. Distribution of left ventricular sympathetic afferents demonstrated by reflex responses to transmural myocardial ischemia and to intracoronary and epicardial bradykinin. Circulation 1993; 87:240–246.

42. Morgan K, Wharton J, Webb JC, Keogh BE, Smith PLC, Taylor KM, Oakley CM, Polak JM, Cleland JGF. Co-expression of renin-angiotensin system component genes in human atrial tissue. Journal of Hypertension 1994; 12(suppl 4):S11–S19.

43. Cleland JGF, Cowburn PJ, Morgan K. Neuroendocrine activation after myocardial infarction: causes and consequences. Heart 1996; 76(suppl 3):53–59.

44. Johnston CI, Risvanis J. Preclinical pharmacology of angiotensin II receptor antagonists. Am J Hypertens 1997; 10:306S–310S.

45. Smith RD, Timmermans C. Human angiotensin receptor subtypes. Curr Opinion Nephrol Hypertens 1994; 3:112–122.

46. Timmermans PBM, Benfield P, Chiu AT, Herblin WF, Wong PC, Smith RD. Angiotensin II receptors and functional correlates. Am J Hypertens 1992; 5:2215–2355.

47. Asano K, Dutcher DL, Port JD, Minobe WA, Tremmel KD, Roden RL, Bohlmeyer TJ, Bush EW, Jenkin MJ, Abraham WT, Raynolds MV, Zisman LS, Bristow MR, Perryman MB. Selective downregulation of the angiotensin II AT-1-receptor subtype in failing human ventricular myocardium. Circulation 1997; 95:1193–1200.

48. Haywood GA, Gullestad L, Katsuya T, Hutchinson HG, Pratt RE, Horiuchi M, Fowler MB. AT-1 and AT-2 angiotensin receptor gene expression in human heart failure. Circulation 1997; 95:1201–1206.

49. Regitz-Zagrosek V, Friedel N, Heymann A, Bauer P, Neuss M, Rolfs A, Steffen C, Hildebrandt A, Fleck E. Regulation of the angiotensin receptor subtypes in cell cultures, animal models and human diseases. Circulation 1995; 91:1461–1471.

50. Stoll M, Stecklings UM, Paul M, Bottari SP, Metzeger R, Unger T. The angiotensin AT2-receptor mediates inhibition of cell proliferation in coronary endothelial cells. J Clin Invest 1995; 95:651–657.

51. Yamada T, Akishita M, Pollman MJ, Gibbons GH, Dzau VJ, Horiuchi M. Angiotensin II type 2 receptor mediates vascular smooth muscle cell apoptosis and antagonizes angiotensin II type I receptor action: an in vitro gene transfer study. Life Sci 1998; 63:PL289–PL295.

52. Pitt B. 'Escape' of aldosterone production in patients with left ventricular dysfunction treated with an angiotensin converting enzyme inhibitor: Implications for therapy. Cardiovasc Drugs Ther 1995; 9(1):145–149.

53. MacFadyen RJ, Lee AFC, Morton JJ, Pringle SD, Struthers AD. How often are angiotensin II and aldosterone concentrations raised during chronic ACE inhibitor treatment in cardiac failure?. Heart 1999; 82(1):57–61.

54. Struthers AD, Anderson G, MacFadyen RJ, Fraser C, MacDonald TM. Non-adherence with ACE inhibitor treatment is common in heart failure and can be detected by routine serum ACE activity assays. Heart 1999; 82:584–588.

55. Teo K, Yusuf S, Pfeffer M, Kober L, Hall A, Pogue J, Latini R, Collins R. for the ACE Inhibitors Collaborative Group. Effects of long-term treatment with angiotensin-converting-enzyme inhibitors in the presence or absence of aspirin: a systematic review. Lancet 2002; 360:1037–1043.

56. Cleland JGF, Bulpitt CJ, Falk RH, Findlay IN, Oakley CM, Murray G, Poole-Wilson PA, Prentice CRM, Sutton GC. Is aspirin safe for patients with heart failure? Br Heart J 1995; 74(3):215–219.

57. Cleland JGF, John J, Houghton T. Does aspirin attenuate the effect of angiotensin-converting enzyme inhibitors in hypertension or heart failure?. Curr Opin Nephrol Hypertens 2001; 10: 625–631.

58. Cleland JGF. No reduction in cardiovascular risk with NSAIDs–including aspirin? Lancet 2002; 359(9301):92–93.

59. Cleland JGF. For Debate: Preventing atherosclerotic events with aspirin. Br Med J 2002; 324(7329):103–105.

60. Cleland JGF. Is aspirin 'the weakest link' in cardiovascular prophylaxis. The surprising lack of evidence supporting the use of aspirin for cardiovascular disease. Prog Cardiovasc Dis 2002; 44:275–292.

61. Cleland JGF. Anticoagulant and antiplatelet therapy in heart failure. Curr Opinion Cardiol 1997; 12:276–287.

62. Herrlin B, Nyquist O, Sylven C. Induction of a reduction in haemoglobin concentration by enalapril in stable, moderate heart failure: A double blind study. Br Heart J 1991; 66(3): 199–205.

63. Belcher G, Hubner R, George M, Elmfeldt D, Lunde H. Candesartan cilexetil: safety and tolerability in healthy volunteers and patients with hypertension. J Hum Hypertens 1997; 11(suppl 2):S-85–S-89.

64. Brooksby P, Robinson PJ, Segal R, Klinger G, Pitt B, Cowley AJ. Effects of losartan and captopril on QT-dispersion in elderly patients with heart failure. ELITE study group. Lancet 1999; 354:395–396.

65. Binkley PF, Haas GJ, Starling RC, Nunziata E, Hatton PA, Leier C, Cody RJ. Sustained augmentation of parasympathetic tone with angiotensin-converting enzyme inhibition in patients with congestive heart failure. J An Cell Cardiol 1993; 21:655–661.

66. Binkley PF, Nunziata E, Leier CV. Selective AT-1 blockade with losartan does not restore autonomic balance in patients with heart failure. J Am Coll Cardiol 1998; 31(suppl A):250A.

67. Wurzner G, Gerster JC, Chiolero A, Maillard M, Fallab-Stubi CL, Brunner HR, Burnier M. Comparative effects of losartan and irbesartan on serum uric acid in hypertensive patients with hyperuricemia and gout. J Hypertens 2001; 19:1855–1860.

68. Puig JG, Torres R, Ruilope LM. AT1 blockers and uric acid metabolism: are there relevant differences? J Hypertens 2002; 20(suppl 5):S29–S31.

69. Leyva F, Anker S, Swan JW, Godsland IF, Wingrove CS, Chua TP, Stevenson JC, Coats AJS. Serum uric acid as an index of impaired oxidative metabolism in chronic heart failure. Eur Heart J 1997; 18:858–865.

70. Crozier I, Ikram H, Awan N, Cleland JGF, Stephen N, Dickstein K, Frey M, Young J, Klinger G, Makris L, Rucinska E. Losartan in heart failure: hemodynamic effects and tolerability. Circulation 1995; 91:691–697.

71. Pitt B, Dickstein K, Benedict C, Packer R, Willenheimer R, Murali S, Denlay MC, Change PI, Grossman W for the RAAS Investigators. The randomized angiotensin receptor antagonist – ACE inhibitor study (RAAS) – pilot study. Circulation 1996; 94(suppl):I-428.

72. Packer M, Poole Wilson PA, Armstrong PW, Cleland JGF, Horowitz JD, Massie B, Ryden L, Thygesen K, Uretsky B. on behalf of the ATLAS investigators. Comparative effects of low and high doses of the angiotensin-converting enzyme inhibitor, lisinopril, on morbidity and mortality in chronic heart failure. Circulation 1999; 100:2312-2-318.

73. The NETWORK Investigators. Clinical outcome with enalapril in symptomatic chronic heart failure; a dose comparison. Eur Heart J 1998; 19:481–489.

74. Cleland JGF, Poole Wilson PA. ACE inhibitors for heart failure: a question of dose. Br Heart J 1994; 72:106–110.

75. Maggioni A, Anand I, Gottlieb SO, Latini R, Tognoni G, Cohn JN. for the Valsartan Heart Failure Trial Investigators. Effects of valsartan on morbidity and mortality in patients with heart failure not receiving angiotensin converting enzyme inhibitors. J Am Coll Cardiol 2002; 40:1414–1421.

76. Klinge R, Polis A, Dickstein K, Hall C. Effects of angiotensin II receptor blockade on N-terminal proatrial natriuretic factor plasma levels in chronic heart failure. J Cardiac Fail 1997; 3:75–81.

77. Riegger GAJ, Bouzo H, Petr P, Munz J, Spacek R, Pethig H, von Brehen V, George M, Arens H-J. for the STRETCH Investigators. Improvement in exercise tolerance and symptoms of congestive heart failure during treatment with candesartan cilexetil. Circulation 1999; 100: 2224–2230.

78. Bart BA, Ertl G, Held P, Kuch J, Maggioni AP, McMurray J, Michelson EL, Rouleau JL, Warner-Stevenson L, Swedberg K, Young JB, Yusuf S, Sellers MA, Granger CB, Califf RM, Pfeffer MA. Contemporary management of patients with left ventricular systolic dysfunction. Results from the study of patients intolerant of converting enzyme inhibitors (SPICE) registry. Eur Heart J 1999; 20(16):1182–1190.

79. Matsumori A. Assessment of Response to Candesartan in Heart Failure in Japan (ARCH-J) Study Investigators. Efficacy and safety of oral candesartan cilexetil in patients with congestive heart failure. Eur J Heart Failure 2003; 5:669–77.

80. Cleland JGF, Freemantle N, Kaye GC, Nasir M, Velavan P, Lalukota K, Mudawi T, Shelton R, Clark AL, Coletta AP. Clinical trials update from the American Heart Association: omega-3 fatty acids and arrhythmia risk in patients with an implantable defibrillators, ACTIV in CHF, VALIANT, the Hanover autologous bone marrow transplantation study, SPORTIF V, ORBIT and PAD and DEFINITE. Eur J Heart Fail 2004; 6:109–15.

81. Coletta AP, Cleland JGF, Freemantle N, Loh H, Memon A, Clark AL. Clinical trials update from the European Society of Cardiology: CHARM, BASEL, EUROPA and ESTEEM. Eur J Heart Fail 2003; 5:697–704.

82. Swedberg K, Pfeffer M, Granger C, Held P, McMurray J, Ohlin G, Olofsson B, Ostergren J, Yusuf S. for the CHARM-Programmed Investigators. Candesartan in heart failure – assessment of reduction in mortality and morbidity (CHARM): rationale and design. J Card Fail 1999; 5(3):276–282.

83. Yusuf S, et al. Effect of enalapril on survival in patients with reduced left ventricular ejection fractions and congestive heart failure the SOLVD Investigators. New Engl J Med 1991; 325: 293–302.

84. The Heart Outcomes Prevention Evaluation Study Investigators. Effects of angiotensin-converting-enzyme inhibitor, ramipril, on cardiovascular events in high risk patients. New Engl J Med 2000; 342:145–153.

85. The European trial on reduction of cardiac events with perindopril in stable coronary artery disease investigators. Efficacy of perindopril in reduction of cardiovascular events among patients with stable coronary artery disease: randomized, double-blind, placebo-controlled, multicentre trial (the EUROPA study). Lancet 2003; 362:782–788.

86. Anand IS, Fisher LD, Chiang YT, Latini R, Masson S, Maggioni AP, Glazer RD, Tognoni G, Cohn JN. for the Val-HeFT Investigators. Changes in brain natriuretic peptide and norepinephrine over time and mortality and morbidity in the valsartan heart failure trial (Val-HeFT). Circulation 2003; 107:1278–1283.

87. Carson P, Tognoni G, Cohn JN. Effect of valsartan on hospitalization: results from Val-HeFT. J Card Fail 2003; 9:164–171.

88. Latini R, Masson S, Anand I, Judd D, Maggioni AP, Chiang YT, Bevilacqua M, Salio M, Cardano P, Dunselman PHJM, Holwerda NJ, Tognoni G, Cohn JN. for the Val-HeFT Investigators. Effects of valsartan on circulating brain natriuretic peptide and norepinephrine in symptomatic chronic heart failure: the valsartan heart failure trial (Val-HeFT). Circulation 2002; 106:2454–2458.

89. Wong M, Staszewsky L, Latini R, Barlera S, Volpi A, Chiang YT, Benza R, Gottlieb SO, Kleemann TD, Rosconi F, Vandervoort PM, Cohn JN. Valsartan benefits left ventricular structure and function in heart failure: Val-HeFT echocardiographic study. J Am Coll Cardiol 2002; 40(5):970–975.

90. Cohn JN, Tognoni G, Glazer RD, Spormann D, Hester A. Rationale and design of the valsartan heart failure trial: a large multinational trial to assess the effects of valsartan, an angiotensin-receptor blocker, on morbidity and mortality in chronic congestive heart failure. J Card Fail 1999; 5:155–160.

91. Pfeffer MA, McMurray JJV, Velazquex EJ, Rouleau JL, Kobel L, Maggioni HP, Solomon SD, Swedberg K, Van de Werf F, White H, Leimberger JD, Henis M, Edwards S, Zelenkofske S, Sellers MA, Califf RM; Valsartain in Acute Myocardial Infarction Trial Investigators. Valsartan, captopril, or both in myocardial infarction complicated by heart failure, left ventricular dysfunction, or both. N Eng J Med 2003; 349:1893–1906.

92. Velazquez EJ, Pfeffer MA, McMurray JV, Maggioni AP, Rouleau JL, Van de Werf F, Kober L, White HD, Swedberg K, Leimberger JD, Gallo P, Sellers MA, Edwards S, Henis M, Califf RM; VALIANT Investigators. Related Article Links VALSartan In Acute myocardial iNfarCtion (VALIANT) trial: baseline characteristics in context. Eur J Heart Fail 2003 Aug; 5(4): 537–44.

93. The RESOLVD Investigators. Effects of metoprolol CR in patients with ischemic and dilated cardiomyopathy. The randomized evaluation of strategies for left ventricular dysfunction pilot study. Circulation 2000; 101:378–384.

94. Pitt B, Poole-Wilson PA, Segal R, Martinez FA, Dickstein K, Camm AJ, Konstam MA, Riegger G, Klinger GH, Neaton J, Sharma D. Effects of losartan versus captopril on mortality in patients with symptomatic heart failure: rationale, design and baseline characteristics of patients in the losartan heart failure survival study–ELITE II. J Card Fail 1999; 5:146–154.

95. Konstam M, Patten RD, Thomas I, Ramahi T, La Bresh K, Goldman S, Lewis W, Gradman A, Self KS, Bittner V, Rand W, Kinan D, Smith JJ, Ford T, Segal R, Udelson JE. Effects of losartan and captopril on left ventricular volumes in elderly patients with heart failure; results of the ELITE ventricular function substudy. Am Heart J 2000; 139(6):1081–1087.

96. Cowley AJ, Wiens BL, Segal R, Rich MW, Santanello NC, Dasbach EJ, Pitt B. ELITE Investigators. Randomised comparison of losartan vs captopril on quality of life in elderly patients with symptomatic heart failure: the losartan heart failure ELITE quality of life substudy. Qual Life Res 2000; 9(4):377–384.

97. Teo KK, Yusuf S, Pfeffer M, Torp-Pedersen C, Kober L, Hall A, Pogue J, Latini R, Collins R. ACE inhibitors Collaborative Group. Effects of long-term treatment with ACE inhibitors in the presence or absence of aspirin: a systematic review. Lancet 2002; 360:1037–1043.

98. Granger CB, Ertl G, Kuch J, Maggioni AP, McMurray J, Rouleau JL, Stevenson LW, Swedberg K, Young J, Yusuf S, Califf RM, Bart BA, Held P, Michelson EL, Sellers MA, Ohlin G, Sparapani R, Pfeffer MA. Randomized trial of candesartan cilexetil in the treatment of patients with congestive heart failure and a history of intolerance to angiotensin-converting enzyme inhibitors. Am Heart J 2000; 139(4):609–617.

99. Dickstein K, Chang P, Willenheimer R, Haunso S, Remes J, Hall C, Kjekshus J. Comparison of the effects of losartan and enalapril on clinical status and exercise performance in patients with moderate or severe chronic heart failure. J Am Coll Cardiol 1995; 26(2):438–445.

100. Lang RM, Elkayam U, Yellen LG, Krauss D, McKelvie RS, Vaughan DE, Ney DE, Makris L, Chang PI. on behalf of the Losartan Pilot Exercise Study Investigators. Comparative effects of losartan and enalapril on exercise capacity and clinical status in patients with heart failure. J Am Coll Cardiol 1997; 30:983–991.

101. Yusuf S. Effect of enalapril on survival in patients with reduced left ventricular ejection fractions and congestive heart failure. New Engl J Med 1991; 325:293–302.

102. Eccles M, Freemantle N, Mason JM. for the North of England Evidence Based Guideline Development Project. Evidence based clinical practice guideline: ACE inhibitors in the primary care management of adults with symptomatic heart failure. Br Med J 1998; 316:1369–1375.

103. Os I, Bratland B, Dahlof B, Gisholt K, Syvertsen JO, Tretli S. Female sex as an important determinant of lisinopril-induced cough. Lancet 1992; 339:303–310.

104. Kostis JB, Shelton B, Gosselin G, Goulet C, Hood WB, Kohn RM, Kubo SH, Schron E, Weiss MB, Willis III PW, Young JB, Probstfield J. Adverse effects of enalapril in the studies of left ventricular dysfunction (SOLVD). Am Heart J 1996; 131:350–355.

105. Israili ZH, Hall WD. Cough and angioneurotic edema associated with angiotensin-converting enzyme inhibitor therapy. A review of the literature and pathophysiology. Ann Intern Med 1992; 117:234–242.

106. Malini PL, Strocchi E, Zanardi M, Milani M, Ambrosioni E. Thromboxane antagonism and cough induced by angiotensin-converting enzyme inhibitor. Lancet 1997; 350:15–18.

107. Cleland JGF. Lack of effect of nedocromil sodium in ACE inhibitor-induced cough. Lancet 1995; 345:394.

108. Hargreaves MR, Benson MK. Inhaled sodium cromoglycate in angiotensin converting enzyme inhibitor induced cough. Lancet 1995; 345:13–16.

109. Schulman G, Hakim R, Arias R, Silverberg M, Kaplan AP, Arbeit L. Bradykinin generation by dialysis membranes: possible role in anaphylactic reaction. J Am Soc Nephrol 1993; 3: 1563–1569.

110. Gottleib SS, Dickstein K, Fleck E, Kostis J, Levine TB, LeJemtel T, DeKock M. Hemodynamic and neurohormonal effects of the angiotensin II antagonist Losartan in patients with congestive heart failure. Circulation 1993; 88:1602–1609.

111. Cleland J, Semple P, Hodsman P, Ball S, Ford I, Dargie H. Angiotensin II levels, hemodynamics, and sympathoadrenal function after low dose captopril in heart failure. Am J Med 1984; 77: 880–886.

112. Kostis J, Shelton BJ, Yusuf S, Weiss MB, Capone RJ, Pepine CJ, Gosselin G, Delahaye F, Probstfield JL, Cahill L, Dutton D. Tolerability of enalapril by patients with left ventricular dysfunction: results of the medication challenge phase of the studies of left ventricular dysfunction. Am Heart J 1994; 128:358–364.

113. Mogensen CE, Neldam S, Tikkanen I, Oren S, Viskoper R, Watts RW, Cooper ME. for the CALM Study Group. Randomised controlled trial of dual blockade of renin-angiotensin system in patients with hypertension, microalbuminuria and non-insulin dependent diabetes: the candesartan and lisinopril microalbuminuria (CALM) study. Br Med J 2000; 321(7274):1440–1444.

114. Lewis EJ, Hunsicker LG, Clarke WR, Berl T, Poke MA, Lewis JB, Ritz E, Atkins RC, Rohde R, Raz I; Collaborative Study Group. Related Articles, Links Renoprotective effect of the angiotensin-receptor antagonist irbesartan in patients with nephropathy due to type 2 diabetes. N Engl J Med. 2001 Sep 20; 345(12):851–60.

115. Brenner BM, Cooper ME, de Zeeuw D, Keane WF, Mitch WE, Parving HH, Remuzzi G, Snapinn SM, Zhang Z, Shahinfar S; RENAAL Study Investigators. Related Articles, Links effects of losartan on renal and cardiovascular outcomes in patients with type 2 diabetes and nephropathy. N Engl J Med Sep 20; 345(12):861–9.

116. Havranek EP, Thomas I, Smith WB, Ponce GA, Bilsker M, Munger MA, Wolf RA. Dose-related beneficial long-term hemodynamic and clinical efficacy of Irbesartan in heart failure. J Am Coll Cardiol 1999; 33(5):1174–1181.

117. Elmfeldt D, George M, Hubner R, Olofsson B. Candesartan cilexetil, a new generation angiotensin II antagonist, provides dose dependent antihypertensive effect. J Hum Hypertens 1997; 11(suppl 2):S49–S53.

118. Guazzi M, Melzi G, Agostoni P. Comparison of changes in respiratory function and exercise oxygen uptake with losartan versus enalapril in congestive heart failure secondary to ischemic or idiopathic dilated cardiomyopathy. Am J Cardiol 1997; 80:1572–1576.

119. Warner JGJ, Metzger DC, Kitzman DW, Wesley DJ, Little WC. Losartan improves exercise tolerance and quality of life in patients with diastolic dysfunction. J Am Coll Cardiol 1999; 33: 1567–1572.

15

Role of Mineralocorticoid Antagonists in Patients with Heart Failure

Bertram Pitt and Sanjay Rajagopalan
University of Michigan School of Medicine
Ann Arbor, Michigan, USA

SYNOPSIS

Circulating aldosterone levels are elevated in relation to heart failure severity and affect left ventricular remodeling following acute myocardial infarction. Potential deleterious effects include endothelial dysfunction, increased oxidative stress, enhanced platelet activation, activation of matrix metalloproteinases, and increased sympathetic neuronal activation. The mineralocorticoid receptor (MR) antagonist, spironolactone, has been shown to reduce all-cause mortality and sudden cardiac death risk in patients with advanced chronic heart failure by 30%. Similarly, eplerenone can attenuate adverse post-MI (myocardial infarction) ventricular remodeling and has been shown to reduce all-cause mortality and sudden cardiac death following myocardial infarction. Future controlled clinical trials will test the hypothesis that MR antagonists will have beneficial effects on cardiovascular mortality and ventricular function among patients with asymptomatic left ventricular dysfunction or mild to moderate heart failure symptoms.

INTRODUCTION

The outlook for patients with chronic heart failure secondary to systolic left ventricular systolic dysfunction (SLVD) has improved significantly over the past two decades through the routine use of ACE inhibitors, beta-blockers, ± diuretics, and digoxin. Although ACE inhibitors alone or in conjunction with β-blockers have been shown to result in a significant reduction in cardiovascular morbidity and mortality in these patients [1,2], the mortality in this patient population remains relatively high. Recent attempts to further reduce morbidity and mortality in these patients beyond traditional approaches have been disappointing. For example, endothelin antagonists [3], TNFα antibodies [4,5], angiotensin II type I receptor antagonists [6], and angiotension converting enzyme-neutral endopeptidase inhibitors [7] have all failed to significantly reduce mortality. In contrast, targeting the aldosterone axis with the mineralocorticoid receptor (MR) antagonist spironolactone has been shown to reduce mortality in patients with severe heart failure treated with an ACE-inhibitor with or without a beta-blocker by 30%.[8] (Fig.1) The application of this strategy to patients with mild-to-moderate heart failure is currently limited by the lack of evidence that MR antagonists are effective in reducing mortality in these patients. The patients

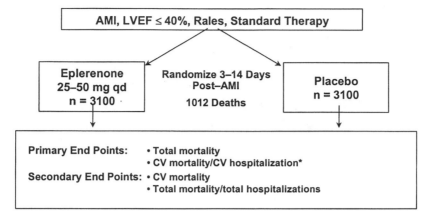

Figure 1   The study design of EPHESUS (Eplerenone Post-AMI Heart Failure Efficacy and Survival Study).

randomized in the RALES trial had severe heart failure as evidenced by a greater than 20% per year mortality rate in the placebo group. The use of β-blocking agents was relatively low in this study (10% to 11%) and can be attributed to the fact that at the time this study was initiated, definitive evidence for the effectiveness of β-blocking agents in reducing mortality was not yet available, especially in patients with severe heart failure [2]. The results of the recently concluded EPHESUS study [9] in patients with evidence of systolic left ventricular dysfunction and heart failure post–myocardial infarction, (the majority of whom were treated with both an ACE-inhibitor and a beta-adrenergic-blocking agent,) suggest, however, that mineralocorticoid antagonists will have a beneficial effect on cardiovascular mortality in patients with mild-to-moderate congestive heart failure. (Fig. 2) It is also likely that patients with asymptomatic systolic left ventricular dysfunction, treated with both an ACE-inhibitor and a β-blocker will benefit from this approach. The application of this therapeutic strategy to patients with mild-to-moderate heart failure and

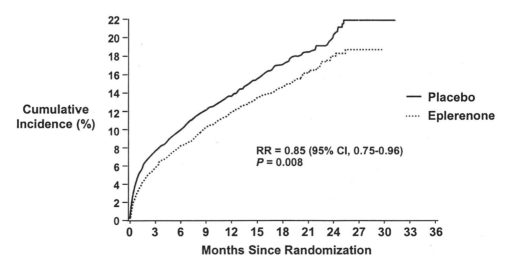

Figure 2   Risk of total mortality during follow-up in the EPHESUS study (Ref 9).

asymptomatic systolic left ventricular dysfunction, however, must await well-designed, prospective, randomized clinical trials. As a framework for the potential applicability of MR antagonists in these situations, we will discuss pertinent mechanisms by which MR antagonists reduce mortality. These mechanisms should be viewed as providing a basis for the design of future large-scale randomized studies in situations other than systolic heart failure, rather than as a call for immediate therapeutic application. Although the focus of this discussion will be on patients with chronic heart failure due to systolic left ventricular dysfunction and those with systolic left ventricular dysfunction following myocardial infarction, it must be acknowledged that many of the mechanisms are common to heart failure patients in general and occur in chronic heart failure due to preserved systolic function as well (diastolic dysfunction). Thus, although clinical evidence from large-scale prospective randomized trials is lacking in patients with heart failure due to diastolic heart failure, it can be speculated that MR antagonists may have a major role in these patients as well.

THE EFFECT OF ALDOSTERONE RECEPTOR ANTAGONISTS ON SODIUM EXCRETION AND DIURESIS

The effects of aldosterone on the renal MR have been appreciated for several decades. Aldosterone antagonists have an important natriuretic and diuretic effect and high doses of spironolactone have been shown to be effective in inducing diuresis in patients with chronic heart failure who become resistant to loop diuretics [10–12]. Although in experimental animal models, subhemodynamic doses of spironolactone seem to exert a significant diuretic effect when combined with an ACE-inhibitor [13], it is unlikely that the beneficial effects of spironolactone in RALES can be attributed to its diuretic effect alone. In the RALES study, patients in New York Heart Association (NYHA) class IV were shown to have a significantly greater sodium retention score than those in NYHA class III heart failure [14]. However, there was no significant difference in the sodium retention score either in NYHA class III or class IV patients randomized to spironolactone or placebo. It should also be emphasized that patients in the RALES trial were on standard doses of a loop diuretic and that clinicians could increase the dose of loop diuretic at any time during the trial. Previous studies by Sharpe and his colleagues [15] have shown that loop diuretics do not prevent ventricular remodeling in patients with chronic heart failure due to systolic left ventricular dysfunction. In a retrospective analysis of the SOLVD trials, Cooper and his colleagues [16] have suggested that loop diuretics are not effective in reducing death due to progressive heart failure, whereas potassium sparing diuretics, mainly spironolactone, were shown to reduce death due to progressive heart failure. In the EPHESUS trial [9], although only a minority of the deaths could be attributed to progressive heart failure, there was also a trend for a reduction in death due to progressive heart failure in patients randomized to eplerenone in comparison to placebo. The number of deaths attributed to progressive heart failure in the EPHESUS trial was rather small (n = 231; 3.5%), however, there was no evidence of a major diuretic effect of eplerenone at a mean of 43 mg daily in comparison to placebo. Thus, although MR antagonists reduce death due to progressive heart failure in patients with severe chronic heart failure due to systolic left ventricular dysfunction and in patients with systolic left ventricular dysfunction post–myocardial infarction, their natriuretic and diuretic effects do not appear to be major factors. It is, however, possible that both spironolactone (25 mg) and eplerenone (50 mg) when used in combination with an ACE inhibitor may induce diuretic effect, as evidenced by an increase in serum potassium [9]. At higher doses, both of these agents can be expected to have important diuretic effects and may be useful in patients with volume overload who become resistant to loop diuretics [10–12]. When used at these higher doses, serum potassium should be monitored frequently and the dose reduced to that recommended in the RALES [14] and EPHESUS [9] trials as soon as possible. Serum potassium should also be monitored at least 1, 2, and 4 weeks after initiating therapy with either of these agents or after increasing their dose, and then every 3 months thereafter. Although there is a potential risk of serious hyperkalemia (potassium ≥ 6.0 meql) when on an MR antagonist, especially when used in conjunction with an ACE inhibitor or an angiotensin-receptor-blocking agent and a β-blocker, this risk is low (< 2 %) in patients with preserved renal function. For example in the RALES [14] and EPHESUS [9] trials in which patients with a serum creatinine greater than 2.5 mg/dL or a potassium greater than 5.0 mEq/L were excluded, there were no deaths attributable to hyperkalemia in almost 4000 patients exposed to these drugs. There was a small but statistically significant increase in serum potassium in patients randomized to spironolactone in comparison to placebo; however, serum potassium levels remained within the normal therapeutic range in both these trials. The fact that there were no deaths attributable to hyperkalemia in these trials can, in part, be attributed to the fact that serum potassium in these trials was closely monitored and the dose of aldosterone blockade adjusted according to serum potassium levels. In clinical practice, where patients may not be as closely monitored as in a randomized trial, it may be prudent to further define the extent of renal dysfunction that would contraindicate the use of this agent, such as a calculated creatinine clearance cut off of less than 30 ml/min rather than a serum creatinine of greater than 2.5mg/dL. If one attempts to use MR antagonists in patients with compromised renal function, such as those with a creatinine clearance greater than 30 ml/min but less than 50 ml/min, serum potassium should be closely monitored, especially in those patients with concomitant diabetes mellitus.

EFFECTS OF MR ANTAGONISTS ON VENTRICULAR REMODELING

Ventricular remodeling with a progressive increase in left ventricular end-systolic volume and end-diastolic volume has been suggested to be of importance in the morbidity as well as mortality associated with chronic heart failure. Several mechanisms, including myocyte apoptosis and alterations in the myocardial cytoskeleton–including progressive collagen formation with a resultant stiffening, and diastolic dysfunction have been implicated in this process. In experimental studies, aldosterone appears to be a key determinant of fibrosis. (Fig. 3) The mechanism by which aldosterone induces these effects is a topic of active investigation, but sodium appears to be an important determinant [17]. Among other potentially important mechanisms, aldosterone may independently induce collagen synthesis at a transcriptional level, although this finding has not always been reproduced [18–20]. Also, aldosterone either alone or in conjunction with glucocorticoids, appears to upregulate AT-1 receptor density [21,22]. Increased PAI-1 expression and activity could exert independent profibrotic effects as well, perhaps through reduction in plasmin levels and reduced activation of matrix metalloproteinases [23,24] Recently, it has been postulated that inflammation could underlie the excessive collagen deposition noted with aldosterone. Rocha and colleagues have shown that aldosterone administration is associated with activation of osteopontin and MCP-1 with subsequent diffuse microvascular inflammation. It appears, at least in this animal model, that the perivascular fibrosis occurs subsequent to this microvascular inflammation, with damage especially in the heart, kidneys, and brain [25]. In concordance with the insights gained in experimental animal models, in which aldosterone exerts positive effects on collagen deposition, these profi-

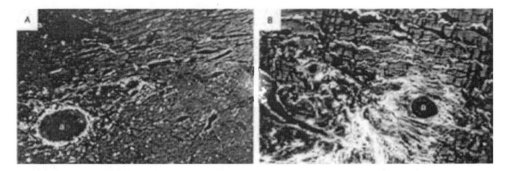

Figure 3 Photomicrographs of coronary vascular remodeling in hyperaldosteronism rats. (**A**) Panel shows a section from a normal heart with evidence of a normal intramural coronary artery surrounded by a small amount of fibrillar collagen. (**B**) Panel shows a section of myocardium from a rat administered aldosterone and sodium. It shows marked perivascular fibrosis of coronary vessels and of the interstitial space between myofibrils. (Sirus red staining and polarized light, X 40.) (Ref 25a)

brotic effects can be prevented by the administration of an MR antagonist. MR antagonists have been shown to prevent progressive ventricular remodeling and collagen formation in patients with chronic heart failure [15,26]. In a canine model of chronic heart failure, Suzuki and colleagues have shown that eplerenone prevents ventricular remodeling, and collagen formation [27]. In a rat model of heart failure after myocardial infarction, Wang and colleagues have shown that the combination of eplerenone and an ACE inhibitor is better than either agent alone in preserving ventricular function and in preventing ventricular remodeling [28]. There is increasing data to show that aldosterone antagonists are effective in patients with chronic heart failure in reducing progressive collagen formation [29–31]. Collagen formation, a fundamental determinant of myocardial stiffness correlates with diastolic ventricular dysfunction and may be an important predictor of subsequent heart failure [32]. Progressive collagen formation as evidenced by an increase in the circulating levels of fragments of procollagen type III (amino-terminal peptide [PIIINP]) and procollagen type I (carboxy-terminal peptide [PICP], procollagen type I amino-terminal peptide [PINP]) was measured in a RALES substudy [30]. In this study, the survival benefit was most predominant in subgroups with PICP, PINP, and PIIINP baseline levels above median, reflecting on-going collagen formation. Patients with baseline PIIINP greater than.85 μg/L, compared with patients with PIIINP less than 3.85 μg/L, had a relative risk of death of 2.36 (95% CI 1.34 to 4.18, P = 0.003) and a relative risk of death and/or CHF hospitalization of 1.83 (95% CI 1.18 to 2.83, P = 0.007). Spironolactone was shown to significantly reduce levels of PIIINP in this study [30].

An increase in serum potassium as a consequence of MR antagonism may also underlie some of the effects of MR antagonism in preventing myocardial fibrosis, at least in experimental models [33]. However, Martinez and co-workers have shown that modulating potassium levels through supplementation is not as effective as eplerenone in preventing vascular damage and fibrosis [34]. Similarly, Struthers and colleagues have compared the potassium sparing diuretic amiloride to spironolactone in patients with heart failure due to systolic left ventricle dysfunction [35]. At relatively similar potassium levels, spironolactone but not amiloride was effective in improving endothelial function and decreasing serum markers of collagen formation. This suggests that the beneficial effects of MR antagonists are not entirely due to an increase in serum potassium.

MR antagonists have also been shown to be effective in preventing the progression of left ventricular hypertrophy [36]. Left ventricular hypertrophy has been shown to be an important marker of cardiovascular risk and subsequent heart failure. In the 4E study, eplerenone 200 mg daily was compared with enalapril 40 mg daily and the combination of eplerenone 200 plus enalapril 10 mg daily in patients with hypertension and baseline evidence of left ventricular hypertrophy by magnetic resonance imaging (MRI) [37]. Eplerenone was found to be equally effective to enalapril in reducing blood pressure, left ventricular hypertrophy, and microalbuminuria in these patients. However, the effect of eplerenone/enalapril in reducing LVH by MRI (-27.2 g) was significantly better than eplerenone alone (-14.5 g, p $= 0.007$) and trended strongly positively in comparison to enalapril alone (-19.7 g).

ALDOSTERONE AS AN INFLAMMATORY MEDIATOR

An emerging paradigm is that of aldosterone as an inflammatory mediator. In the genetically hypertensive animal model, the stroke-prone hypertensive rat (SHR), exogenous aldosterone in the presence of an ACE inhibitor accentuates end-organ damage in the heart and the kidney through proinflammatory effects [38]. (Fig. 4) Conversely, the usage of spironolactone in this animal model in subhemodynamic doses decreased proteinuria, histologic evidence of inflammatory injury, and improved survival in comparison to control animals [39]. These effects may relate to the ability of aldosterone to increase free radical production. Recent data from Virdis and colleagues support the ability of aldosterone to

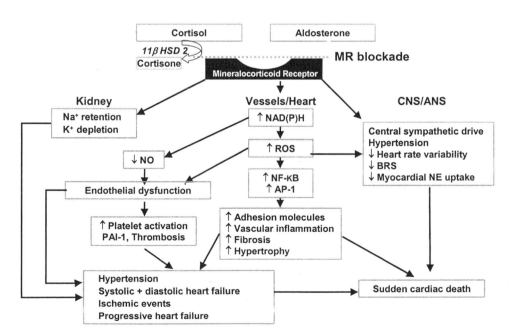

Figure 4   A role for the mineralocorticoid receptor (MR) in maladaptive adaptations in the cardiovascular system. NO, nitric oxide; ROS, reactive oxygen species; NO, nitric oxide; HRV, heart-rate variability; NAD(P)H, Nicotinamide adenine dinucleotide phosphate; PAI-1, plasminogen activator inhibitor-1; NF-kB, Nuclear factor kappa B; AP-1, Activator protein −1; BRS, Baroreflex sensitivity; NE, Norepinephrine.

drive free radical production, independent of angiotensin II [40]. As such, these observations confirm the ability of aldosterone to activate free radical mediated transcription pathways such as NF-κB and AP-1 signaling pathways [41]. The inflammatory pathways activated by aldosterone may be compounded in a positive feedback manner by the effect of aldosterone on the expression of ACE expression[42,43]. These effects of aldosterone are completely abolished by MR antagonists suggesting an MR mediated effect and lend credence to the concept that antagonizing the MR may exert powerful antiinflammatory effects. These effects of MR antagonists collectively may have important implications for the therapy of heart failure and other cardiovascular disease, such as atherosclerosis.

EFFECTS OF MR ANTAGONISTS ON VASCULAR TONE

Individuals with heart failure demonstrate marked abnormalities in endothelial function and this may underlie some of the counter-regulatory mechanisms that potentiate heart failure [44,45]. Therapies that modulate endothelial function may, thus, be applicable for the treatment of heart failure. An important effect of MR antagonists that may be relevant in patients with heart failure is their favorable effects on the nitric oxide pathway and endothelial function. In a double-blind, crossover study of patients with mild-to-moderate heart failure maintained on an ACE inhibitor, spironolactone was found to significantly improve endothelial function in comparison to placebo as assessed by venous occlusion plethysmography [46]. This effect was associated with evidence of a significant decrease in serum ACE activity [46]. Studies in rats with experimental heart failure have shown that MR antagonists prevent the free radical scavenging of nitric oxide by superoxide and markedly synergize with ACE inhibitors in improving aortic endothelial function [13]. Experimental studies in the lipid fed rabbit model have shown that eplerenone significantly decreases vascular NADPH-NADH oxidase activity and oxygen free radical production in atherosclerosis with a resultant increase in endothelial function [47]. Thus, there are a number of potential mechanisms whereby aldosterone antagonists may prevent the progression of heart failure and/or to prevent its occurrence. Although it is difficult to be certain which (if any) of these mechanisms are most important in a particular patient, there is clear evidence that MR antagonists are effective in preventing the progression of severe heart failure and reducing death in progressive heart failure as well as hospitalization due to heart failure in patients with SLVD [8,9].

PREVENTION OF SUDDEN CARDIAC DEATH

MR antagonists have also been shown to lower the risk of sudden cardiac death in patients with severe heart failure due to SLVD (risk ratio: 0.71 [0.54–0.95], p = 0.02) as well as in post-MI patients with SLVD (risk ratio: 0.79 [0.64–0.97], p = 0.03) [8,9]. Although death due to progressive heart failure is the most frequent cause of death in patients with severe heart failure, sudden cardiac death is more important in those with less severe heart failure and those post–myocardial infarction. A number of potential mechanisms may explain the effectiveness of MR antagonists in reducing sudden cardiac death, including a lower incidence of hypokalemic-induced ventricular arrhythmias, improved endothelial function, reduced oxidative stress, attenuation of platelet aggregation, decreased activation of matrix metalloproteinases, and improved ventricular remodeling [9]. Further, aldosterone blockade has also been reported to decrease sympathetic neuronal activation and improve heart-rate variability [27,49].

EFFECTS ON THE AUTONOMIC NERVOUS SYSTEM

MR antagonists have been shown to increase myocardial norepinephrine uptake and, therefore, reduce circulating norepinephrine levels [48]. This has been accompanied by a decrease in ventricular ectopic activity and ventricular arrhythmias. MR antagonists, administered systemically, have also been shown to reduce central sympathetic activity [49]. Recent experimental studies have suggested that TNF-α, which is elevated in heart failure, can cause an increase in PGE_2, which can cross the blood brain barrier and activate MRs in the paraventricular nucleus (PVN), resulting in an increase in sympathetic activity, salt craving, volume expansion, and a further release of TNF-α [49]. MR antagonists have also been shown to improve heart-rate variability, baroreceptor function, and QT dispersion [50]. Heart-rate variability and QT dispersion have been shown to be important predictors of sudden cardiac death. The explanation for the effectiveness of MR antagonists on heart-rate variability and baroreceptor function may potentially relate to the fact that they increase nitric oxide availability [51].

MYOCARDIAL FIBROSIS

Another mechanism important for both death due to progressive heart failure and sudden cardiac death is the effect of MR antagonists on collagen turnover. Progressive myocardial collagen formation is associated with an inhomogeneity in ventricular conduction, ventricular arrhythmias, and propensity to sudden cardiac death. Aldosterone blocks the uptake of norepinephrine into the myocardium and, therefore, increases circulating norepinephrine levels, whereas an MR antagonist increases myocardial uptake of norepinephrine, and decreases circulating norepinephrine levels [48,52]. A decrease in circulating norepinephrine levels, associated with an increase in heart-rate variability and baroreceptor function, could be of importance in the effectiveness of MR antagonists in reducing sudden cardiac death. Sudden cardiac death in some circumstances may also be related to thrombosis and to platelet embolization of the coronary arteries. MR antagonists have recently been shown to significantly decrease platelet P selectin and fibrinogen activity and, therefore, should decrease platelet activation [53]. MR antagonists have also been shown to alter fibrinolytic balance by decreasing PAI-1 levels [24]. An increase in PAI-1 and the ratio of PAI-1: tPA has been shown to be associated with an increase in ischemic events, and could be an important factor in sudden cardiac death.

EMERGING THEMES IN MR ANTAGONISM: IS IT THE LIGAND, THE RECEPTOR, OR BOTH?

Although the mechanisms previously outlined for the prevention of death due to progressive heart failure and sudden cardiac death are of importance, some further discussion as to why MR antagonists are effective is warranted. Aldosterone in conjunction with an increase in serum sodium intake, has been shown to have important pathophysiological effects on inflammation, subsequent myocardial and perivascular fibrosis, thrombosis, ventricular hypertrophy, and autonomic dysfunction. In support of these findings, aldosterone levels are predictive of cardiovascular mortality in patients with severe chronic heart failure [54]. Since ACE-inhibitors do not appear effective in suppressing angiotensin II or aldosterone formation over the long run in patients with heart failure or hypertension [55–58], it is not surprising that MR antagonists would be effective under these circumstances.

The predictive value of aldosterone levels in patients with mild-to-moderate heart failure or in hypertension is less certain because aldosterone levels do not predict events or hypertrophy. Nonetheless, MR antagonists have also been shown to be effective in correcting many of these pathophysiologic mechanisms. One possibility is that tissue levels of aldosterone may be elevated without a measurable increase in serum levels. MR antagonism could, therefore, exert a beneficial effect at the tissue level independent of any effect on serum levels. An alternate explanation that is particularly intriguing is the fact that inhibiting MR may block its activation by alternate ligands, such as cortisol. Under ordinary circumstances cortisol can bind to MR and activate it. However, owing to the presence of the enzyme 11 beta hydroxysteroid dehydrogenase (11βHSD-2), cortisol (corticosterone in rodents) is rapidly inactivated to cortisone (dehydrocorticosterone in rodents) (Fig. 5) [59]. The activity of this enzyme is such that cortisol is completely deactivated in the kidney. Another isoform of this enzyme 11bHSD 1, functions as a

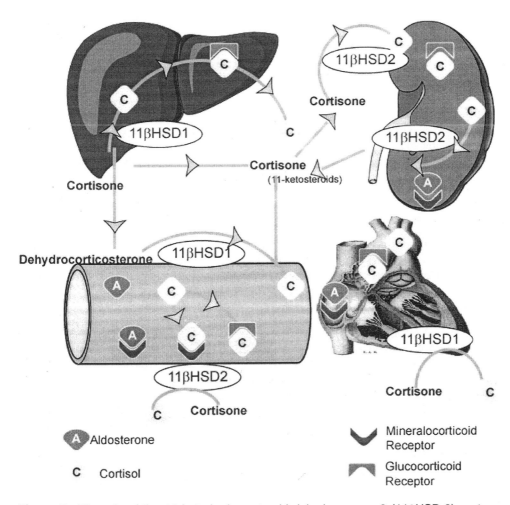

Figure 5 The role of the 11 beta hydroxysteroid dehydrogenase 2 (11βHSD-2) system in preserving mineralocorticoid receptor (MR) exclusivity to mineralocorticoids in humans. 11βHSD-1 plays an important role in regeneration of glucocorticoids in the liver as well as extra-hepatic tissues, such as the heart and vasculature.

reductase and is an important activator, and converts cortisone to cortisol [60]. Under conditions of 11bHSD deficiency, cortisol could almost exclusively occupy MR and activate it. The recent discovery of these enzymes in the vasculature and in the heart raises the possibility of glucocorticoid-mediated MR activation [61,62]. Further, these enzymes appear to be regulated by stressors such as inflammatory cytokines, hyperglycemia, and hypoxia [59,63,64]. For example, in the streptozotocin-induced diabetic rat model, aldosterone levels are reduced along with a concomitant decrease in renal 11HSD-2 activity [64]. These animals develop severe hypertension that can be corrected by spironolactone, which increases 11HSD-2 activity, thereby decreasing the availability of cortisol for occupying the mineralocorticoid receptor. Thus, it can be postulated that MR antagonists will be effective both in situations in which aldosterone levels are elevated, such as in severe chronic heart failure, but also in a variety of circumstances with increased oxidative stress, such as mild-moderate heart failure, essential hypertension, or atherosclerosis, in which circulating aldosterone levels may be within normal limits.

CONCLUSION

The demonstration of the effectiveness of MR antagonists in severe chronic heart failure in the RALES trial [14] and in postinfarction patients with left ventricular dysfunction in the EPHESUS trial, has expanded the horizon of utility of these agents. Although the mechanisms previously discussed are likely of pathophysiological importance, the further application of these principles to patients with mild heart failure secondary to SLVD, asymptomatic SLVD, and diastolic heart failure should await the application of well-designed prospective randomized studies with mortality and/or morbidity as endpoints.

REFERENCES

1. Packer M, Bristow MR, Cohn JN, Colucci WS, Fowler MB, Gilbert EM, Shusterman NH. The effect of carvedilol on morbidity and mortality in patients with chronic heart failure. U.S. Carvedilol Heart Failure Study Group. N Eng J Med. 1996; 334:1349–55.
2. Packer M, Coats AJ, Fowler MB, Katus HA, Krum H, Mohacsi P, Rouleau JL, Tendera M, Castaigne A, Roecker EB, Schultz MK, DeMets DL. Effect of carvedilol on survival in severe chronic heart failure. N Engl J Med. 2001; 344:1651–1658.
3. Rich S, McLaughlin VV. Endothelin receptor blockes in cardiovascular disease. Circulation 2003; 108:2184–90.
4. Bradham WS, Bozkurt B, Gunasinghe H, Mann D, Spinale FG. Tumor necrosis factor-alpha and myocardial remodeling in progression of heart failure: a current perspective. Cardiovasc Res 2002; 53:822–830.
5. Krum H. Tumor necrosis factor-alpha blockade as a therapeutic strategy in heart failure (RENEWAL and ATTACH): unsuccessful, to be specific. J Card Fail 2002; 8:365–368.
6. Cohn JN, Tognoni G. A randomized trial of the angiotensin-receptor blocker valsartan in chronic heart failure. N Engl J Med 2001; 345:1667–1675.
7. Packer M, Califf RM, Konstam MA, Krum H, McMurray JJ, Rouleau JL, Swedberg K. Comparison of omapatrilat and enalapril in patients with chronic heart failure: the omapatrilat versus enalapril randomized trial of utility in reducing events (OVERTURE). Circulation 2002; 106:920–926.
8. Pitt B, Zannad F, Remme W, Cody R, Castaigne A, Perez A, Palensky J, Wittes J. The effect of spironolactone on morbidity and mortality in patients with severe heart failure. N Engl J Med 1999; 341:709.

9. Pitt B, Remme W, Zannad F, Neaton J, Martinez F, Roniker B, Bittman R, Hurley S, Kleiman J, Gatlin M. Eplerenone, a selective aldosterone blocker, in patients with left ventricular dysfunction after myocardial infarction. N Engl J Med. 2003; 348:1309–1321.

10. Settel E. Further experience with spironolactone-hydrochlorothiazide (Aldactazide-A) in the long-term treatment of refractory cardiac edema. Am J Geriat Soc 1965:655–662.

11. Dahlstrom U, Karlsson E. Captopril and spironolactone therapy for refractory congestive heart failure. Am J Cardiol 1993; 71:29A–33A.

12. van Vliet AA, Donker AJ, Nauta JJ, Verheugt FW. Spironolactone in congestive heart failure refractory to high-dose loop diuretic and low-dose angiotensin-converting enzyme inhibitor. Am J Cardiol 1993; 71:21A–28A.

13. Bauersachs J, Heck M, Fraccarollo D, Hildemann SK, Ertl G, Wehling M, Christ M. Addition of spironolactone to angiotensin-converting enzyme inhibition in heart failure improves endothelial vasomotor dysfunction; role of vascular superoxide anion formation and endothelial nitric oxide synthase expression. J Am Coll Cardiol 2002; 39:351–358.

14. Pitt B, Zannad F, Remme WJ, Cody R, Castaigne A, Perez A, Palensky J, Wittes J. The effect of spironolactone on morbidity and mortality in patients with severe heart failure. Randomized Aldactone Evaluation Study Investigators. N Engl J Med 1999; 341:709–717.

15. Sharpe N, Murphy J, Smith H, Hannan S. Treatment of patients with symptomless left ventricular dysfunction after myocardial infarction. Lancet 1988; 1:255–259.

16. Cooper HA, Dries DL, Davis CE, Shen YL, Domanski MJ. Diuretics and risk of arrhythmic death in patients with left ventricular dysfunction. Circulation 1999; 100:1311–1315.

17. Funder JW. Aldosterone, salt and cardiac fibrosis. Clin Exp Hypertens 1997; 19:885–899.

18. Brilla CG, Pick R, Tan LB, Janicki JS, Weber KT. Remodeling of the rat right and left ventricles in experimental hypertension. Circ Res 1990; 67:1355–1364.

19. Kohler E, Bertschin S, Woodtli T, Resink T, Erne P. Does aldosterone-induced cardiac fibrosis involve direct effects on cardiac fibroblasts? J Vasc Res 1996; 33:315–326.

20. Robert V, Van Thiem N, Cheav SL, Mouas C, Swynghedauw B, Delcayre C. Increased cardiac types I and III collagen mRNAs in aldosterone-salt hypertension. Hypertension 1994; 24:30–36.

21. Sato A, Suzuki H, Murakami M, Nakazato Y, Iwaita Y, Saruta T. Glucocorticoid increases angiotensin II type 1 receptor and its gene expression. Hypertension 1994; 23:25–30.

22. Ullian ME, Walsh LG, Morinelli TA. Potentiation of angiotensin II action by corticosteroids in vascular tissue. Cardiovasc Res 1996; 32:266–273.

23. Brown NJ, Kim KS, Chen YQ, Blevins LS, Nadeau JH, Meranze SG, Vaughan DE. Synergistic effect of adrenal steroids and angiotensin II on plasminogen activator inhibitor-1 production. J Clin Endocrinol Metab 2000; 85:336–344.

24. Brown NJ, Nakamura S, Ma L, Nakamura I, Donnert E, Freeman M, Vaughan DE, Fogo AB. Aldosterone modulates plasminogen activator inhibitor-1 and glomerulosclerosis in vivo. Kidney Int 2000; 58:1219–1227.

25. Blasi ER, Frierdrich GE, De Ciechi PA, Coughenour MA, Amy RE, McMahon EG, Rocha R. Aldosterone/salt-induced myocardial injury: a vascular inflammatory disease. Am J Hyper 2001; 14:8A–9A.

25a. Weber KT. Aldosterone in congestive heart failure. NEJM 2001; 345:1689–97.

26. Cicoira M, Zanolla L, Rossi A, Golia G, Franceschini L, Brighetti G, Marino P, Zardini P. Long-term, dose-dependent effects of spironolactone on left ventricular function and exercise tolerance in patients with chronic heart failure. J Am Coll Cardiol 2002; 40:304–310.

27. Suzuki G, Morita H, Mishima T, Sharov VG, Todor A, Tanhehco EJ, Rudolph AE, McMahon EG, Goldstein S, Sabbah HN. Effects of long-term monotherapy with eplerenone, a novel aldosterone blocker, on progression of left ventricular dysfunction and remodeling in dogs with heart failure. Circulation 2002; 106:2967–2972.

28. Wang D, Liu YH, Yang XP, Rhaleb NE, Xy J, Carretero OA. Role of selective aldosterone blocker in mice with chronic heart failure following myocardial infarction. Hypertension 2002; 421:98–103.

29. Modena MG, Aveta P, Menozzi A, Rossi R. Aldosterone inhibition limits collagen synthesis and progressive left ventricular enlargement after anterior myocardial infarction. Am Heart J 2001; 141:41–46.

30. Zannad F, Alla F, Dousset B, Perez A, Pitt B. Limitation of excessive extracellular matrix turnover may contribute to survival benefit of spironolactone therapy in patients with congestive heart failure: insights from the randomized aldactone evaluation study (RALES). Circulation 2000; 102:2700–2706.

31. Weber KT, Brilla CG. Pathological hypertrophy and cardiac interstitium: fibrosis and renin-angiotensin-aldosterone system. Circulation 1991; 83:1849–1865.

32. Querejeta R, et al. Serum carboxy-terminal propeptide of procollagen type I is a marker of myocardial fibrosis in hypertensive heart disease. Circulation 2000; 101:1729–1735.

33. Rocha R, Martin-Berger CL, Yang P, et al. Selective aldosterone blockade prevents angiotensin II/salt-induced vascular inflammation in the rat heart. Endocrinology 2002; 143: 4828–4836.

34. Martinez DV, Rocha R, Matsumura M, Oestricher E, Ochoa-Maya M, Roubsanthisuk W, Williams GH, Adler GK. Cardiac damage prevention by eplerenone: comparison with low sodium diet or potassium loading. Hypertension 2002; 39:614–618.

35. Farquharson CA, Struthers AD. Increasing plasma potassium with amiloride shortens the QT interval and reduces ventricular extrasystoles but does not change endothelial function or heart rate variability in chronic heart failure. Heart 2002; 88:475–480.

36. Sato A, Funder JW, Saruta T. Involvement of aldosterone in left ventricular hypertrophy of patients with end-stage renal failure treated with hemodialysis. Am J Hypertens 1999; 12: 867–873.

37. Pitt B, Reichek N, Metscher B, Phillips R, Roniker B, Kleiman J, Burns Dobot EI. Efficacy and safety of eplerenone, enalapril, and eplerenone/enalapril combination therapy for essential hypertension and left ventricular hypertrophy: the 4E study. Am J Hypertension 2003; 15: 23A.

38. Rocha R, Chander PN, Zuckerman A, Stier CT. Role of aldosterone in renal vascular injury in stroke-prone hypertensive rats. Hypertension 1999; 33:232–237.

39. Rocha R, Chander PN, Khanna K, Zuckerman A, Stier CT. Mineralocorticoid blockade reduces vascular injury in stroke-prone hypertensive rats. Hypertension 1998; 31:451–458.

40. Virdis A, Neves MF, Amiri F, Viel E, Touyz RM, Schiffrin EL. Spironolactone improves angiotensin-induced vascular changes and oxidative stress. Hypertension 2002; 40:504–510.

41. Fiebeler A, Schmidt F, Muller DN, Park JK, Dechend R, Bieringer M, Shagdarsuren E, Breu V, Haller H, Luft FC. Mineralocorticoid receptor affects AP-1 and nuclear factor-{{kappa}}B activation in angiotensin II-induced cardiac injury. Hypertension 2001; 37:787–793.

42. Harada E, Yoshimura M, Yasue H, Nakagawa O, Nakagawa M, Harada M, Mizuno Y, Nakayama M, Shimasaki Y, Ito T, Nakamura S, Kuwahara K, Saito Y, Nakao K, Ogawa H. Aldosterone induces angiotensin-converting-enzyme gene expression in cultured neonatal rat cardiocytes. Circulation 2001; 104:137–139.

43. Wang J, Yu L, Solenberg PJ, Gelbert L, Geringer CD, Steinberg MI. Aldosterone stimulates angiotensin-converting enzyme expression and activity in rat neonatal cardiac myocytes. J Card Fail 2002; 8:167–174.

44. Drexler H, Hayoz D, Munzel T, Hornig B, Just H, Brunner HR, Zelis R. Endothelial function in chronic congestive heart failure. Am J Cardiol 1992; 69:1596–1601.

45. Katz SD. The role of endothelium-derived vasoactive substances in the pathophysiology of exercise intolerance in patients with congestive heart failure. Prog Cardiovasc Dis 1995; 38: 23–50.

46. Farquharson CA, Struthers AD. Spironolactone increases nitric oxide bioactivity, improves endothelial vasodilator dysfunction, and suppresses vascular angiotensin I/angiotensin II conversion in patients with chronic heart failure. Circulation 2000; 101:594–597.

47. Rajagopalan S, Duquaine D, King S, Pitt B, Patel P. Mineralocorticoid receptor antagonism in experimental atherosclerosis. Circulation 2002; 105:2212–2216.

48. Barr CS, Lang CC, Hanson J, Arnott M, Kennedy N, Struthers AD. Effects of adding spironolactone to an angiotensin-converting enzyme inhibitor in chronic congestive heart failure secondary to coronary artery disease. Am J Cardiol 1995; 76:1259–1265.

49. Zhang ZH, Francis J, Weiss RM, Felder RB. The renin-angiotensin-aldosterone system excites hypothalamic paraventricular nucleus neurons in heart failure. Am J Physiol-Heart Circ Physiol 2002; 283:H423–H433.

50. Yee KM, Pringle SD, Struthers AD. Circadian variation in the effects of aldosterone blockade on heart rate variability and QT dispersion in congestive heart failure. J Am Coll Cardiol 2001; 37:1800–1807.

51. Chowdhary S, Vaile JC, Fletcher J, Ross HF, Coote JH, Townend JN. Nitric oxide and cardiac autonomic control in humans. Hypertension 2000; 36:264–269.

52. Silvestre JS, Heymes C, Oubenaissa A, Robert V, Aupetit-Faisant B, Carayon A, Swynghe-dauw B, Delcayre C. Activation of cardiac aldosterone production in rat myocardial infarction: effect of angiotensin II receptor blockade and role in cardiac fibrosis. Circulation 1999; 99: 2694–2701.

53. Schafer A, Fraccarollo D, Hildemann SK, Christ M, Eigenthaler M, Kobsar A, Walter U, Bauersachs J. Inhibition of platelet activation in congestive heart failure by aldosterone receptor antagonism and ACE inhibition. Thromb Haemost 2003; 89:1024–1031.

54. Swedberg K, Eneroth P, Kjekshus J, et al. Hormones regulating cardiovascular function in patients with severe congestive heart failure and their relation to mortality. Circulation 1990; 82:1730–1736.

55. Staessen J, Lijnen P, Fagard R, Verschueren LJ, Amery A. Rise in plasma concentration of aldosterone during long-term angiotensin II suppression. J Endocrinol 1981; 91:457–465.

56. McKelvie RS, Yusuf S, Pericak D, Avezum A, Burns RJ, Probstfield J, Tsuyuki RT, White M, Rouleau J, Latini R, Maggioni A, Young J, Pogue J. Comparison of candesartan, enalapril, and their combination in congestive heart failure: randomized evaluation of strategies for left ventricular dysfunction (RESOLVD) pilot study. Circulation 1999; 100:1056–1064.

57. Struthers AD. Aldosterone escape during ACE inhibitor therapy in chronic heart failure. Eur Heart J 1995; 16:103–106.

58. Pitt B. ''Escape'' of aldosterone production in patients with left ventricular dysfunction treated with an angiotensin converting enzyme inhibitor: implications for therapy. Cardiovasc Drugs Ther 1995; 9:145–149.

59. Heiniger CD, Kostadinova RM, Rochat MK, Serra A, Ferrari P, Dick B, Frey BM, Frey FJ. Hypoxia causes down-regulation of 11 beta-hydroxysteroid dehydrogenase type 2 by induction of Egr-1. FASEB J 2003; 17:917–919.

60. Seckl JR, Walker BR. Minireview: 11beta-hydroxysteroid dehydrogenase type 1–a tissue-specific amplifier of glucocorticoid action. Endocrinology 2001; 142:1371–1376.

61. Brem AS, Bina RB, King T, Morris DJ. Bidirectional activity of 11 beta-hydroxysteroid dehydrogenase in vascular smooth muscle cells. Steroids 1995; 60:406–410.

62. Brem AS, Bina RB, King TC, Morris DJ. Localization of 2 11beta-OH steroid dehydrogenase isoforms in aortic endothelial cells. Hypertension 1998; 31:459–462.

63. Cai TQ, Wong B, Mundt SS, Thieringer R, Wright SD, Hermanowski-Vosatka A. Induction of 11beta-hydroxysteroid dehydrogenase type 1 but not -2 in human aortic smooth muscle cells by inflammatory stimuli. J Steroid Biochem Mol Biol 2001; 77:117–122.

64. Liu YJ, Nakagawa Y, Toya K, Wang Y, Saegusa H, Nakanishi T, Ohzeki T. Effects of spironolactone on systolic blood pressure in experimental diabetic rats. Kidney Int 2000; 57: 2064–2071.

16

New Pharmacologic Therapies in Heart Failure: Immunotherapy, Endothelin-1 Antagonists, Brain Natriuretic Peptides, and Neurohormonal Interventions

Cynthia K. Wallace and Kumudha Ramasubbu
*Baylor College of Medicine and The Methodist DeBakey Heart Center
Houston, Texas, USA*

Guillermo Torre-Amione
*The Methodist DeBakey Heart Center
Houston, Texas, USA*

SYNOPSIS

Approaches under clinical investigation to modify systemic mediators of heart failure progression include specific and broad-spectrum immunotherapies, agents targeting the activity of endothelin-1, the use of synthetic homologues of human B-type natriuretic peptide, vasopeptidase inhibitors, and vasopressin antagonists for both chronic and acute heart failure. Although experimental observations from the laboratory follow a logical process for development into clinical practice, it has become clear that the clinical utility of individual therapies requires meticulous clinical research that frequently encounters failure. Active clinical studies utilizing broad-spectrum antiinflammatory therapies, including immunomodulatory strategies, may provide the next generation of therapy in chronic heart failure. With regards to acute heart failure, we have seen clear documentation of hemodynamic benefits with the therapeutic use of recombinant type-B natriuretic peptide, and further investigation is ongoing with the nonspecific endothelin-1 antagonist tezosentan. Most importantly, the latest generation of clinical trials for heart failure has shown us that further development in this area will require the demonstration not only of hemodynamic, serologic, and symptomatic improvement, but also of disease-modifying effects on morbidity and mortality.

INTRODUCTION

The pathogenesis of heart failure has evolved from the relatively straightforward concept of heart failure as myocardial pump failure, to the understanding that the major determinant of heart failure progression is the persistent overactivation of various compensatory hormonal systems. Evidence has clearly demonstrated that intervention to modulate compensatory neuroendocrine systems through beta-adrenergic blockade and/or inhibition of the renin-angiotensin system can improve outcomes in chronic heart failure [1–4]. In contrast, clinical studies of ionotropes, such as dobutamine [5], vesnarinone [6], or milrinone [7], that directly address the mechanical pump failure by improving cardiac contractility have consistently been associated with increased mortality.

In addition to changes in the beta-adrenergic and renin-angiotensin pathways, it has now become clear that in the ''heart failure state'' there is activation of the inflammatory system that results in the production and release of proinflammatory cytokines, activation of the complement system, production of autoantibodies, and overexpression of class II MHC (major histocompatibility complex) molecules as well as adhesion molecules that may perpetuate the inflammatory state. The recognition of this new pathway of activation in heart failure has led to the investigation of new therapies aimed to block, modify, or prevent the systemic inflammatory state. In this chapter, we will discuss current approaches under investigation to modify systemic mediators of heart failure progression, including specific immunotherapy targeting cytokines, broad-spectrum immunotherapies–including immunoglobulin infusion, immunoadsorption and immunomodulatory therapy, therapies targeting the activity of endothelin 1 in both chronic and acute heart failure, the use of synthetic homologues of human B-type natriuretic peptide, vasopeptidase inhibitors, and vasopressin antagonists in chronic and acute heart failure.

IMMUNOTHERAPY IN HEART FAILURE

Ample evidence exists that heart failure is associated with the activation of the immune system resulting in elevated levels of proinflammatory cytokines. Cytokines play an essential role in the propagation and magnification of the immune response by recruiting cells to the area of inflammation, and stimulating cell proliferation and differentiation. In patients with heart failure, elevated levels of interleukin-1 (IL-1), interleukin-6 (IL-6) and tumor necrosis factor-α (TNF-α) are found [8–10]. Perhaps the best characterized inflammatory molecule in heart failure is TNF-α, and direct antagonism of this cytokine has been an area of intensive investigation.

Normal myocardium does not contain TNF-α but expresses both of its receptors, TNF-R1 and TNF-R2. In failing myocardium, however, there is increased expression of TNF-α and the receptors for TNF-α are downregulated [11]. Furthermore, circulating levels of TNF-α are also elevated in patients with heart failure, and the degree of elevation correlates with worsening of heart failure ([Fig. 1] [12]. These observations in humans, as well as the demonstration that in experimental animals TNF-α was capable of inducing reversible myocardial dysfunction [13] resulted in the evaluation of the role of this neurohormonal pathway as target of therapeutic intervention, and opened up a new area of investigation into inflammation as a contributor to heart failure.

Specific Cytokine Antagonism

Etanercept

Two large, randomized clinical trials in which patients with moderate-to-severe heart failure were treated with etanercept, a human recombinant TNF-α receptor that binds and inactivates circulating TNF-α molecules, were launched in the United States (Randomized Etanercept North American Strategy to Study Antagonism of Cytokines, RENAISSANCE)

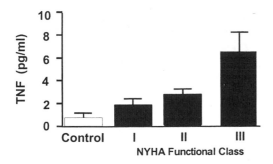

Figure 1 Level of tumor necrosis factor-α (TNF-α) in normal subjects and patients in New York Heart Association functional classes I–III. Patients' TNF-α levels were elevated in direct proportion to their functional class (p < 0.001 by analysis of variance). (From Ref. 12.)

and in Europe and Australia (Research into Etanercept Cytokine Antagonism in Ventricular Dysfunction, RECOVER). The RENAISSANCE trial randomized 925 patients with NYHA (New York Heart Association) class II, III, or IV heart failure and left ventricular ejection factor (LVEF) less than or equal to 30 to placebo or 25 mg etanercept 2 or 3 times per week (mean follow-up 12.7 months). The primary endpoint was a combined endpoint of all-cause mortality or hospitalization from CHF (chronic heart failure). No improvement was seen in either etanercept group, and in fact there was a nonsignificant trend toward an increase in the combined endpoint in the treated groups (Table 1) [14].

The RECOVER trial randomized 1123 patients with NYHA class II, III, or IV heart failure and LVEF 30 or less to placebo or 25 mg etanercept 1 or 2 times per week (mean follow-up 5.7 months). Again, the endpoint was a composite of all-cause mortality or hospitalization from CHF. No effect, positive or negative was seen in the treated groups as compared with placebo (Table 1). Both RENAISSANCE and RECOVER were terminated prematurely for lack of benefit [14].

Infliximab

Infliximab is a chimeric monoclonal antibody that binds and inactivates circulating TNF-α. The ATTACH trial (Anti-TNF-α Therapy Against CHF), a phase II study, enrolled 150

Table 1 Results of Trials of TNF-α Antagonism in Patients with NYHA Class II–IV CHF and LVEF 30 or Less

	Combined endpoint of all-cause mortality and CHF hospitalization relative risk (95% confidence interval)		
Etanercept	25 mg q Week	25 mg BIW	25 mg TIW
RENAISSANCE (n=925)		1.21 (0.92, 1.58)	1.23 (0.94, 1.61)
RECOVER (n=1123)	1.01 (0.72, 1.41)	0.87 (0.61, 1.24)	
Infliximab	5 mg/kg	10 mg/kg	
ATTACH (n=150)	0.80 (0.22, 2.99)	2.84 (1.01, 7.97)	

Source: From Ref. 14.

patients with NYHA class III–IV heart failure and randomized them to placebo or infliximab (5 mg/kg or 10 mg/kg IV infusion at 0, 2, and 6 weeks). The primary endpoint was improvement in clinical status at 14 weeks. The results revealed no effect on clinical status at 14 weeks in either infliximab dosing group, but the combined risk of death from any cause or hospitalization for heart failure through 28 weeks was increased in the patients randomized to 10 mg/kg infliximab (hazard ratio 2.84, 95% confidence interval 1.01 to 7.97; nominal P = 0.043), resulting in early termination of the trial (Fig. 2) [15].

Interestingly, circulating levels of TNF-α were reduced immediately after each infusion in both treatment groups, but remained elevated above baseline at all other time points throughout the study, although in vitro bioactivity assays indicated a reduction in biologically available TNF-α despite the apparent increase. C-reactive protein (CRP) and IL-6 levels decreased below baseline in both treatment groups and remained reduced through week 14. However, after week 14 the decrease reversed itself and by week 28, the levels of both approached baseline. Taken together, these results suggest a possible physiological compensation in response to TNF-α antagonism. Alternatively, there is the potential of late unbinding of TNF-α from the receptors, however the apparent decrease in biologically available TNF-α argues against this theory.

Table 1 shows a summary of the clinical trials of TNF-α antagonism. The absence of positive findings in large randomized clinical trials focused on a specific immune mediator in heart failure was obviously disappointing. However, the lack of clinical benefit may indicate a flaw in the approach of applying a highly specific intervention to a redundant immune system. TNF-α was a reasonable target for specific therapy, however, the failure of the clinical trials to establish benefit indicates that an approach that more diffusely targets the pro-inflammatory milieu may be more effective.

Broad-Spectrum Immunotherapy

Humoral immune activation in heart failure is evidenced by elevated serum levels of antibodies to myocardial proteins such as α-myosin (atrial myosin), and β-1 adrenoreceptors. [16–18], and the deposition of immunoglobulins in the myocardium of patients with cardiomyopathy [19]. The mechanisms through which autoantibodies may contribute to heart failure include not only antibody-mediated myocyte injury, but also, in the case of anti-β-1 adrenoreceptors, receptor agonism [20]. Therapies under investigation that seek to address this activation include: (a) intravenous gamma-globulin (IVIG), (b) immunoadsorption, and (c) immune modulation therapy.

Immunoglobulin Therapy

Immunoglobulin therapy (IVIG) modulates the immune system through several mechanisms. In autoimmune conditions, preparations of IVIG from pooled donors contain antiidiopathic antibodies that can bind to the F_{ab} fragment of the offending autoantibody and inactivate it [21]. Binding of the Fc fragment of the infused IVIG to endogenous macrophages may lead to saturation of these receptors with a resultant decrease in the number of macrophages available to respond to pathogenic antibody binding [22]. Treatment with IVIG has also been demonstrated to decrease pro-inflammatory mediators including IL_1, TNF-α, and $IL_{1\beta}$ [22–24]. In the setting of heart failure, IVIG may mitigate the contribution of autoimmune damage to disease progression. IVIG for the treatment of heart failure has been investigated in at least two randomized clinical trials.

In the Intervention in Myocarditis and Acute Cardiomyopathy (IMAC) trial, 62 patients who presented with recent onset cardiomyopathy (< 6 months) with a left ventricu-

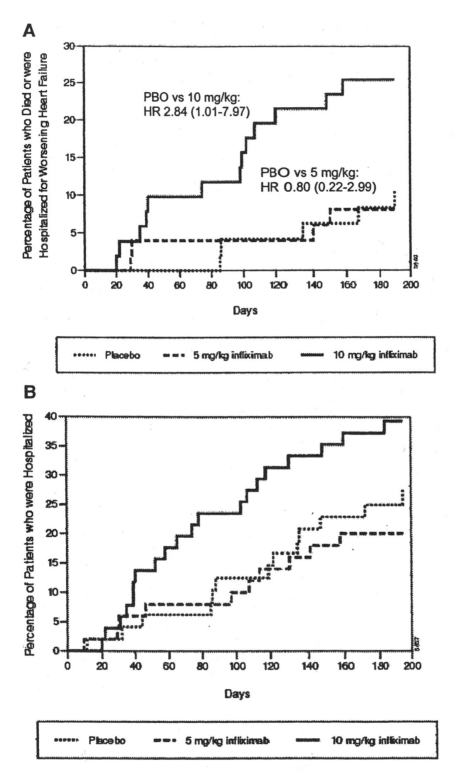

Figure 2 (**A**) Kaplan-Meier rates of death and hospitalization for heart failure. PBO indicates placebo; HR, hazard ratio. (**B**) Kaplan-Meier rates of hospitalization for any reason. (From Ref. 15.)

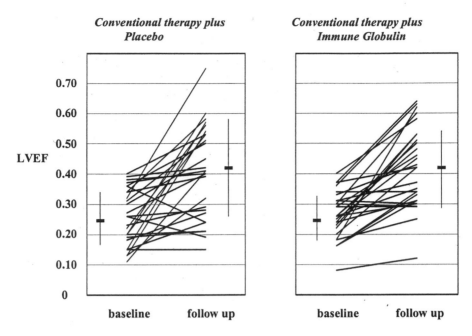

Figure 3 LVEF over time by treatment: LVEF by radionuclide scan at baseline and 12 months after randomization in patients randomized to placebo and IVIG. Overall, LVEF improved significantly over time (12-month LVEF significantly higher than baseline, $P <$ 0.001). However, no differences by treatment group were evident (P = NS for comparisons by treatment). (From Ref. 25.)

lar ejection fraction less than 40% and no evidence of coronary artery disease were random-ized to receive either 2 g/kg IVIG or placebo for two consecutive days in addition to conventional heart failure therapy. The primary end-point of the study was the change in left ventricular ejection fraction (LVEF) at 6 months. The mean LVEF in the placebo-treated patients increased from 23% at baseline to 42% at 6 months (Fig. 3). With this dramatic improvement in the placebo treated patients, there was no further effect observed in the IVIG treated patients (Table 2) [25]. However, a trial of IVIG in patients with chronic symptomatic CHF demonstrated quite different results. In this trial, 40 patients with chronic NYHA class II–IV CHF of either ischemic or nonischemic origin with an LVEF less than 40% were randomized to receive either IVIG induction therapy (1 daily infusion at 0.4 g/kg for 5 days) with subsequent monthly infusions (0.4 g/kg) for a total of 5 months, or an equivalent volume of placebo according to the same schedule. LVEF rose significantly from 26% to 31% in the treated patients, but did not increase significantly in the placebo group (28% to 29%) (Table 2). More interestingly, in this study it was found that there was an increase in at least three antiinflammatory peptides, IL-10 and the soluble receptors for IL-1 and TNF in the IVIG group [26].

Immunoadsorption

Immunoadsorption is an extracorporeal therapy that uses ligands or adsorbers to remove serum immunoglobulins and immune complexes. It has been hypothesized that idiopathic dilated cardiomyopathy is a direct result of autoantibody insult to the myocardium. In a small, prospective, case-control study of 34 patients listed for heart transplantation at the

Table 2 Results of Trials of Broad-Spectrum Immunotherapy Heart Failure

	Left ventricular ejection fraction				
IVIG	Treatment		Placebo		Patient Population
	Baseline	Increase at 6 mos	Baseline	Increase at 6 mos	
IMAC[25] (n=62)	0.25 ± 0.08	0.14 ± 0.12	0.25 ± 0.08	0.14 ± 0.14	New-onset cardiomyopathy, LVEF <40%
Gullestad, et al[26] (n=40)	0.26 ± 0.02	0.05 ± 0.03	0.28 ± 0.02	0.17 ± 0.02	Chronic CHF, LVEF < 40%
Immunoadsorption	Treatment		Placebo		
	Baseline	Increase at 1 year	Baseline	Increase at 1 year	
Staudt, et al.[28] (n=34)	0.22 ± 0.03	0.16 ± 0.08	0.24 ± 0.03	0.02 ± 0.06	Patients listed for HTX, elevated β-1 Ab
Staudt, et al.[29] (n=25)	0.21 ± 0.02	0.06 ± 0.01	0.18 ± 0.02	P = ns (value not reported)	DCM, elevated β-1 Ab, myocardial inflammation
Immune modulatory therapy	Combined endpoint of all-cause mortality and hospitalizations (No. of events)				
	Treatment		Placebo		
Torre-Amione, et al.[32] (n=75)	12		22		NYHA class III/IV

Source: From Refs. 25–29, 32.

German Heart Institute who had high titers of anti–beta-1 antibodies, immunoadsorption was performed over 5 consecutive days in 17 patients. In treated patients, LVEF improved from 22 % to 38% (Table 2), while both left ventricular end-systolic and end-diastolic volumes decreased. These changes were not observed in the control group. Three months after completing therapy there was no evidence of anti–beta 1 antibodies in the treated group [27], despite this group having had higher levels of these antibodies than the control group at baseline.

In a separate study, Staudt and colleagues randomized 25 patients with dilated cardiomyopathy, LVEF greater than 30% and evidence of β-1 receptor autoantibody to immunoadsorption followed by immunoglobulin (Ig) substitution vs. conventional therapy. The treatment group underwent monthly immunoadsorption followed by Ig substitution for 3 months. Consistent with earlier results, immunoadsorption and immunoglobulin substitution led to a significant decrease in β-1 receptor autoantibody levels, increase in LVEF (21.3% to 27.0%) (Table 2), and improvement in NYHA classification as compared with both baseline and controls. Treatment was also associated with a significant decrease in HLA class II antigen expression as compared with controls (Fig. 4)–an important finding since CD4+ T cell-mediated myocardial damage is dependent on peptide presentation by these antigens [28].

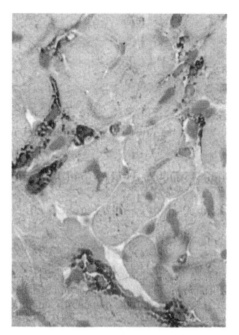
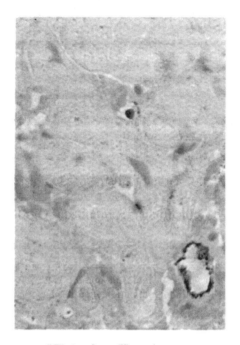

HLA-class II antigen
before IA/IgG therapy

HLA-class II antigen
post IA/IgG therapy

Figure 4   Changes in HLA class II antigen expression of same patient before and after 3-month therapy with IA and subsequent IgG substitution (magnification 3400). (From Ref. 28.)

A more recent investigation by the Staudt group sought to determine if a specific subclass of IgG, IgG-3, might play a more important role than others in the development of myocardial dysfunction. Two different immunoadsorption techniques were compared–Protein A immunoadsorption, which has a low affinity for IgG-3, and anti-IgG column, which has a high affinity for all classes. Eighteen DCM (dilated cardiomyopathy) patients were randomized to undergo immunoabsorption with one of the two techniques followed by IgG substitution at monthly intervals for 3 months. Although the total IgG adsorption was comparable in the two groups, IgG-3 was only effectively removed by the anti-IgG column technique. Consistent with the thought that IgG-3 might play an important role in cardiac dysfunction, CI (cardiac index), LVEF, and stroke volume index exhibited a significant increase in the anti-IgG group, while no significant improvements were noted in either the protein A or placebo group.

Column effluent (CE) was obtained from both treatment groups and its affect on rat cardiomyocytes was evaluated in vitro. The CE from the anti-IgG columns reduced Ca^{2+} transients and had a negative inotropic effect that was not observed when cells were treated with the protein A CE, lending further credence to the hypothesis that the IgG-3 class is integral to the development of cardiac dysfunction [29].

These are small studies, however, the magnitude of the changes observed merit further investigations. Unlike specific cytokine antagonism, immunoadsorption targets an early step in the inflammatory cascade, and may, therefore, succeed in modifying inflammatory contributors to heart failure by downregulating several proinflammatory pathways.

Immunomodulatory Therapy

Immune modulation therapy (IMT) involves the ex-vivo treatment of patients' blood with oxidative and thermal stressors (oxidizing agents, UV light and/or elevated temperatures), resulting in apoptosis of cells. These treated blood elements are then administered to the patient via intramuscular injection. Based on in-vitro evidence, the hypothesis is that the apoptotic cells may stimulate antiinflammatory cytokines and suppress proinflammatory cytokines (Fig. 5) [30]. In mouse models, this technique results in the increased expression of antiinflammatory cytokines in the circulation as well as beneficial effects on endothelial function [31].

In a recent trial, 75 patients with NYHA class III or IV heart failure, LVEF less than 40% and a 6-minute walk distance less than 300 meters were randomized to either IMT (38 patients) or placebo (37 patients). In the treatment group, IMT was given initially on two consecutive days. Two weeks later the patients began monthly injections for a total of eight treatments. The primary endpoint was change in 6-minute walk distance and NYHA class. Both the treatment and placebo groups showed an increase in the 6-minute

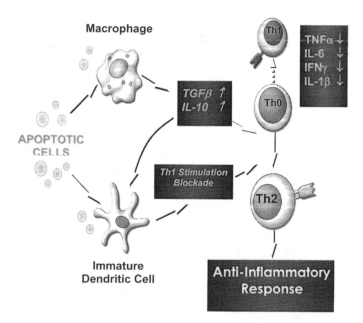

Figure 5 Modulation of T cell responses by apoptotic cells. Apoptotic cells or apoptotic bodies are engulfed by macrophages that following activation produce preferentially transforming growth factor- β and IL-10. The production of these cytokines creates preferential expansion of a T cell type, Th2 cell that by virtue of preferentially producing IL-10 perpetuates an antiinflammatory response. In addition to preferential expansion of Th2 cells, macrophage stimulation by apoptotic cells also decreases the proliferation of Th1 cells that promote inflammation. The resultant effect is to decrease the production of Interferon (IFN) γ, IL-1, TNFα and IL-6. The combined effect of preferentially stimulating Th2 and decreasing Th1 cell types is the reduction of proinflammatory cytokines (IL-1, IL-6, IFNγ and TNFα) and an increase in the production of anti-inflammatory cytokines (IL-10 and TGF-β)

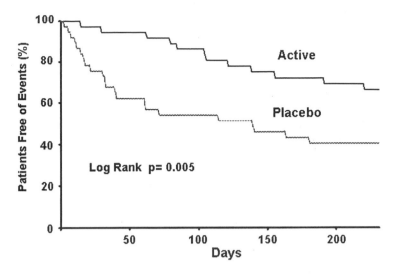

Figure 6   Survival free of events including all-cause mortality and hospitalizations due to worsening heart failure in patients treated with IMT (immune modulatory therapy; active) vs. those receiving placebo. (From Ref. 32.)

walk, but there was a nonsignificant trend toward increased improvement in NYHA class in the treated group as compared to placebo (15 vs. 9 patients improving by 1 or more class, p = 0.14). The IMT therapy significantly reduced both the risk of death (1 vs. 7, p = 0.022) and the risk of hospitalization (12 vs. 22, p = 0.005) (Fig. 6) [32]. A large randomized controlled trial, the Advanced Chronic Heart Failure Clinical Assessment of Immune Modulation Therapy (ACCLAIM) study, is now under way to further elucidate the effects of IMT on morbidity and mortality in this population.

Although several specific cytokine antagonists have not lived up to their early promise, the clinical benefits observed in novel trials of broad-spectrum antiinflammatory therapy are consistent with the hypothesis that ongoing inflammation contributes to the progression of heart failure. The reason for the failures of the TNF-α antagonists to show clinical benefit despite solid preclinical evidence for the hypothesis may be largely due to the redundancy of the immune system. Antagonism of a single cytokine, even if that cytokine is known to be elevated in heart failure quite possibly induces a compensatory response on the part of the immune system with as yet uncharacterized upregulations of other proinflammatory pathways. The promising results from early studies of broad-spectrum agents such as IVIG, immunoadsorption, and immune modulation therapy may be attributable to the fact that these therapies act at an earlier step in the proinflammatory cascade thereby inhibiting multiple pathways.

ENDOTHELIN-1 AS A THERAPEUTIC TARGET

It has been increasingly recognized that the vascular endothelium is an organ capable of synthesizing, secreting, and metabolizing multiple vasoactive substances. Endothelins are among the many such substances produced and metabolized by the vascular endothelium. Endothelins are now known as the most potent vasoconstrictive peptides with a prolonged effect. There are three isoforms of endothelin (ET-1, ET-2, and ET-3) [33] with the predominant form of endothelin produced by cardiac tissue and endothelial cells being ET-1. Plasma ET-1 concentrations are elevated in patients with chronic heart failure, correlate

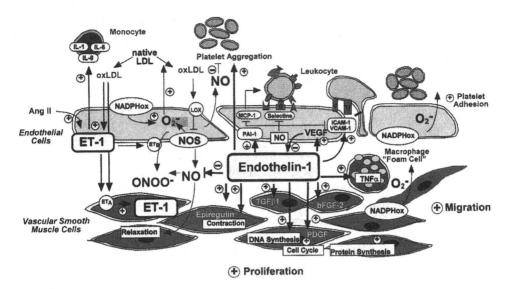

Figure 7 Vascular effects of ET-1. ET-1 is generated in endothelial and smooth muscle cells in response to oxidized LDL, angiotensin II (Ang II), etc. The stimulation of endothelial ET_B receptors increases the release of NO, whereas ET_A receptors mediate contraction and cell proliferation and migration. ET-1 stimulates interleukin (IL) and tumor necrosis factor-α (TNFα) expression in monocytes, leukocyte adherence, platelet aggregation, and adhesion molecule expression. ET-1 stimulates the production and action of growth factors, DNA and protein synthesis, and cell cycle progression. ONOO, indicates peroxynitrite; NOS, nitric oxide synthase; MCP-1, monocyte chemoattractant protein-1; ICAM-1, intracellular adhesion molecule-1; VCAM-1, vascular cell adhesion molecule-1; oxLDL, oxidized low density lipoprotein; O_2-, superoxide anion; LOX, lectin-like oxidized LDL receptor; TGF - 1, transforming growth factor-1; NADPHox, nicotinamide adenine dinucleotide phosphate oxidase; PAI-1, plasminogen activator inhibitor-1; VEGF, vascular endothelial growth factor; bFGF-2, basic fibroblast growth factor-2; PDGF, platelet-derived growth factor; +, stimulation; and -, inhibition. (From Ref. 43a.)

with both hemodynamic and symptom severity [34–37], and are strong independent predictors of death in these patients [38].

The two subtypes of endothelin receptors are endothelin-A and endothelin-B (ET_A, ET_B) [39]. ET_A is primarily localized to the vascular smooth muscle, cardiac myocytes, and fibroblasts [40]. Results from rat models indicate that ET_A may mediate vasoconstriction, inotropy, and mitogenesis (Fig. 7) [41]. ET_B is located on vascular endothelial cells and mediates vasodilation via an endothelial-derived relaxing factor (EDRF) dependent pathway that increases nitric oxide release [42,43] and prostacyclin production (Fig. 7) [44]. Furthermore, the ET_B plays a pivotal role in autocrine regulation by regulating ET-1 gene transcription [45] and the eventual pulmonary clearance and levels of ET-1 [46].

Endothelin-1 antagonists are of two classes, receptor-specific antagonists and dual receptor antagonists. Both types have been investigated in the setting of chronic congestive heart failure, and newer studies are investigating the use of dual receptor antagonists in the treatment of acute CHF exacerbations.

Et-1 Antagonists In Chronic Congestive Heart Failure

Several ET-1 antagonists have been investigated in the context of chronic CHF. Although these trials have frequently shown improvement in hemodynamic indicators of cardiac function, the results have been discouraging due to a neutral or negative impact on morbidity and mortality outcomes.

Darusentan

Darusentan, a selective ETA receptor blocker, was evaluated in an initial trial of a single oral dose (1, 10, 30, 100 or 300 mg) on cardiac index and other measures of hemodynamics in a group of 95 CHF patients. Following oral darusentan, a dose-dependent increase in CI and decrease mean arterial pressure, systemic vascular resistance, PCWP (pulmonary capillary wedge pressure) were observed. Improvements were also noted in other hemodynamic measurements during the immediate follow-up period [47].

The Heart Failure ET(A) Receptor Blockade Trial (HEAT) randomized 157 patients with CHF (present or recent NYHA class III of at least 3 months duration), pulmonary capillary wedge pressure greater than or equal to 12 mm Hg, and a cardiac index less than or equal to 2.6 L/min/m^2. to treatment with placebo or oral darusentan (30, 100, or 300 mg per day) for 3 weeks in addition to standard therapy to evaluate the effect of darusentan on cardiac index and pulmonary capillary wedge pressure. This study demonstrated an acute nonsignificant improvement in cardiac index of 1.3%, 7.9%, and 12.6% after 30, 100, and 300 mg of darusentan, respectively, with a significant improvement seen in all dosing groups at 3 weeks (Fig. 8A). Likewise, there was a significant decrease in systemic vascular resistance in the 300 mg group after 3 weeks of the darusentan treatment regimen (Fig. 8B). However, there was also a trend toward increased adverse events, particularly early exacerbations in heart failure that may limit the applicability of this therapy [48].

Importantly, darusentan was not associated with either an increase in heart rate or activation of other neurohormonal systems.

Bosentan

Bosentan is an ET-1 antagonist that acts on both ET_A and ET_B receptors [49]. In the Endothelin Antagonist Bosentan for Lowering Cardiac Events in Heart Failure (ENABLE) study, 1613 with class NYHA IIIb or IV heart failure patients were randomized to bosentan (125 mg twice daily) or placebo. The primary endpoint was a composite of all-cause mortality or hospitalization for heart failure. No significant difference was observed between bosentan and placebo (40% of patients on placebo, 39% receiving bosentan reached the endpoint). Additionally, as with the trials of darusentan, treatment with bosentan seemed to confer an early risk of worsening heart failure [50].

Thus, the chronic antagonism of ET-1, either via selective ET_A blockade or dual ET_A/ET_B antagonism does not appear to beneficially impact the chronic heart failure state.

Et-1 Antagonism in Acute Heart Failure Exacerbations

Tezosentan

Tezosentan is a highly potent dual ET receptor antagonist that inhibits ET-1 binding to both ET_A and ET_B receptors. It is water soluble, thus, allowing intravenous administration,

Figure 8 (**A**) Cardiac index, and (**B**) systemic vascular resistance at each time point during acute treatment and after 3 weeks of treatment with darusentan at different dosages compared with placebo. Values are mean ± SEM. Solid arrow indicates administration of standard medications at time point 0; dotted arrow, administration of study drug at 2 hours. (From Ref. 48.)

A)

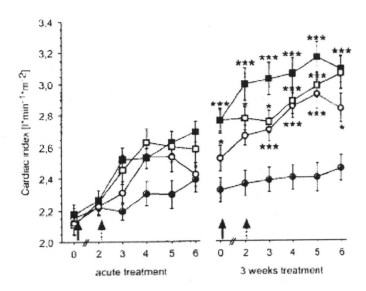

B)

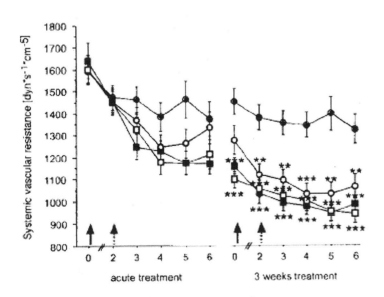

and has a short half-life (less than 10 minutes) that permits easy titration of its hemodynamic effects. Tezosentan was found to have a rapid onset of action in several animal models of heart failure, ischemic renal failure, and hypertension. It is excreted via bile with minimal metabolism [51].

The hemodynamic effects of tezosentan were initially investigated in patients with stable CHF. Sixty-one patients with NYHA class III–IV CHF and a LVEF less than 35% were randomized to either tezosentan (5,20,50, or 100 mg/hr) or placebo. The short-term intravenous use of tezosentan resulted in a statistically significant and dose-dependent increase in cardiac index and decrease in the pulmonary capillary wedge pressure, systemic vascular resistance (SVR), and mean arterial blood pressure (MAP). As seen in clinical trials of other ET-1 antagonists, these changes were not accompanied by an increase in heart rate suggesting that the increase in cardiac index was the result of the vasodilatory effects of tezosentan [52].

Tezosentan was further investigated to determine the safety of prolonged (48 hour) infusions in a randomized, active-controlled trial conducted on 14 patients with advanced heart failure. During tezosentan infusion, no episodes of hypotension requiring withdrawal of therapy occurred, and hemodynamic rebound was not observed after abrupt cessation of the infusion. Unlike some of the other investigational ET-1 antagonists, there were no reports of worsening heart failure in tezosentan-treated patients up to 28 days following the infusion [53].

These promising initial results were followed by the Randomized Intravenous Tezosentan study program (RITZ), which conducted several large-scale clinical trials of tezosentan, primarily in acute heart failure (summarized in Table 3). RITZ-1 and RITZ-2 were parallel studies conducted in patients with acute heart failure, with the critical difference that patients who were enrolled in RITZ-2 were those who, in the opinion of their physicians, required IV hemodynamic monitoring, while those in RITZ-1 did not. RITZ-1 enrolled 675 patients and evaluated the impact of 25 mg or 50 mg tezosentan therapy on dyspnea and time to worsening heart failure as compared with placebo. An evaluation of the RITZ-1 data showed no significant benefit, and the results of this study were never formally published [54].

RITZ-2 evaluated the use of tezosentan for acute decompensated heart failure with hemodynamic measurements assessed as the primary endpoints. In this trial, 292 patients

Table 3 A Summary of Large Randomized Clinical Studies of Tezosentan (RITZ: Randomized Intravenous TeZosentan Study Program)

Name of Trial (n)	Indication	Indication/end point	Outcome	Dose used
RITZ-1[54] (n=675)	Acute heart failure	Dyspnea at 6 hours	No significant benefit	50 mcg/kg/min
RITZ-2[55] (n=292)	Acute heart failure requiring IV hemodynamic monitoring	Cardiac index at 6 hours	Improved CI and PCWP	50 or 100 mcg/kg/min
RITZ-4[56] (n=193)	Acute heart failure (ischemic)	Composite index (death, worsening HF, new or recurrent MI)	No benefit, increased systemic hypotension	25mg/hr for 1 hr, then 50 mg/hr for 23 or 47 hours

Source: From Refs. 49–51.

admitted to the hospital for acute decompensated heart failure with CI less than or equal to 2.1 L/min/m^2 and PCWP 15 mm Hg or more were randomized to receive tezosentan (50mg/hr or 100 mg/hr) or placebo for 24 hours, then evaluated for hemodynamic and dyspnea changes. In both dosing groups, tezosentan resulted in significant improvements in CI and PCWP (Fig. 9). Although there was a dose-dependent increase in adverse events associated with tezosentan, there was a trend toward decreased worsening of heart failure in the treated groups at 24 hours [55]. The difference seen between the results of RITZ-1 and RITZ-2 may be due in part to the fact that the patients in RITZ-1 were less critically ill than the patients in RITZ-2, and, therefore, benefited less from the treatment.

RITZ-4 evaluated the use of IV tezosentan in the treatment of acute decompensated heart failure associated with acute coronary syndromes. One hundred ninety-three patients were randomized to tezosentan (25 mg/hr for 1 hr, then 50 mg/hr for 23 to 47 hr) or placebo, and followed for 72 hours to evaluate the occurrence of a composite end-point including death, worsening heart failure, worsening ischemia, and new or recurrent MI (myocardial infarction). At the end of the evaluation period, there was no significant difference in the composite endpoint between the treated group and the placebo group, but there was an increased risk of adverse events associated with tezosentan treatment. In the 48-hour follow-up period, more tezosentan-treated patients had cardiac failure (20.6% vs 12.6%), renal failure (7.2% vs. 2.1%), and hypotension (22.7% vs. 12.6%) compared with placebo-treated patients [56].

Both the selective and nonselective ET-1 antagonists have demonstrated a positive impact on clinical parameters of hemodynamics in patients with acute and chronic heart failure. However, these improvements have come at the cost of short-term worsening of heart failure in chronic patients, and increased risk of noncardiac adverse events in acute decompensated heart failure. With regards to their potential use in acute heart failure, it seems that the optimal dosing regimen and patient population has yet to be determined that can maximize the beneficial effects while maintaining an acceptable level of adverse events. Indeed, a dose-finding study has confirmed the hemodynamic efficacy of doses of tezosentan 10 times lower than those previously used in the RITZ program [57]. Based on this finding, a new trial called the Value of Endothelin Receptor Inhibition with Tezo-sentan in Acute Heart Failure (VERITAS) study is under way to evaluate low-dose tezosen-tan in acute heart failure with long-term morbidity and mortality as the primary endpoints.

HUMAN B-TYPE NATRIURETIC PEPTIDE

Human β-type natriuretic peptide, or brain natriuretic peptide (BNP) is elevated in acute heart failure, and correlates with severity of disease [58]. However, unlike other markers of heart failure, such as TNF-α and norepinephrine that are thought to exacerbate the heart failure state, the presence of BNP seems to serve a ameliorative role through its vasodila-tory and natriuretic effects. In acute heart failure, the stimulus for BNP release is myocytes stretch [59–61]. BNP binds preferentially to natriuretic peptide receptor A, leading to increased levels of cyclic guanine monophosphate. The end result of this activation is smooth muscle relaxation with consequent reductions in blood pressure and ventricular preload (Fig. 10). Following up on the beneficial effect of endogenous BNP production, clinical trials have focused on the impact of the administration of exogenous BNP on clinical indicators of heart failure.

Nesiritide

The first randomized placebo-controlled trial of nesiritide in heart failure was conducted in 103 subjects in NYHA class II–IV heart failure and LVEF less than or equal to 35%.

A)

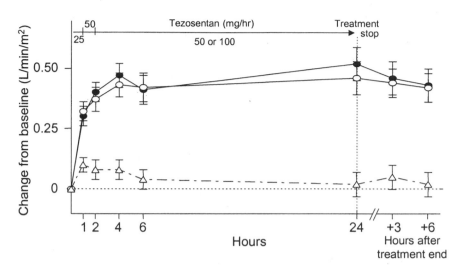

B)

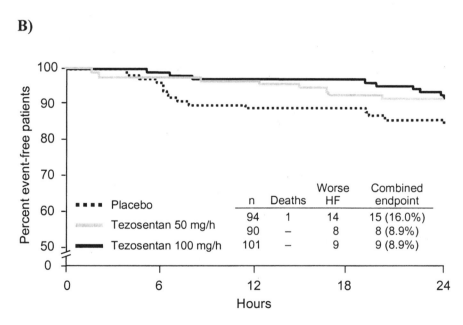

Figure 9 Results from RITZ-2. (**A**) Change in cardiac index from baseline through 30 hours, and (**B**)event-free (death and/or worsening heart failure) survival during 24 hours of treatment. (From Ref. 55.)

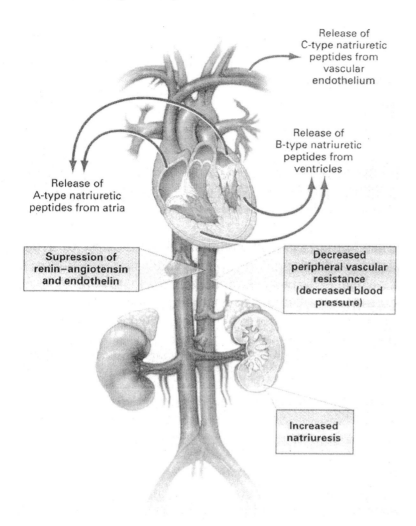

Release of
C-type natriuretic
peptides from
vascular
endothelium

Release of
B-type natriuretic
peptides from
ventricles

Release of
A-type natriuretic
peptides from atria

Supression of
renin–angiotensin
and endothelin

Decreased
peripheral vascular
resistance
(decreased blood
pressure)

Increased
natriuresis

Figure 10 The ABCs of Natriuretic Peptides. A-type natriuretic peptide is released by the atria, B-type natriuretic peptide primarily by the ventricles, and C-type natriuretic peptide by the vascular endothelium in response to increased filling pressure and volume of shear stress. The hormones have a short half-life and cause natriuresis and vasodilation, as well as suppression of renin-angiotensin and endothelin. (From Ref. 61a.)

Patients were randomized to receive one of three dosing regimens of nesiritide (0.015, 0.030, 0.06 mcg/kg/min) or placebo for 24 hours, and were assessed for changes in hemodynamic variables at 1,3, 6, 10 and 24 hours, as well as 2 and 4 hours after completion of the infusion. Nesiritide produced significant reductions in pulmonary wedge pressure (27% to 39% decrease by 6 hr), mean right atrial pressure and systemic vascular resistance, along with significant increases in cardiac index and stroke volume index, but had no significant effect on heart rate. Beneficial effects were evident at 1 hour and were sustained throughout the 24-hour infusion [62].

A second randomized, placebo-controlled trial was conducted in 127 patients hospitalized for symptomatic congestive heart failure with PCWP 18 mm Hg or higher and CI 2.7 L/min/m^2 or less to evaluate the effect of a 6-hour infusion of nesiritide at a rate of 0.015

or 0.030 μg/kg/min on PCWP, global clinical status, dyspnea, and fatigue. Hemodynamic variables were measured at baseline, and then every 1.5 hours through hour 6 of the infusion. Both dosing groups showed a significant improvement in hemodynamics and clinical status compared with placebo [63].

To further elucidate the effects of nesiritide therapy in acute decompensated heart failure, a large-scale, multicenter randomized trial of nesiritide was conducted comparing short-term (3 hr) nesiritide therapy to IV nitroglycerin and placebo, with another 24 hours of nesiritide therapy compared with IV nitroglycerin (Vasodilatation in the Management of Acute CHF, VMAC). The study population included 489 individuals with dyspnea at rest from decompensated CHF and evaluated the effect of treatment on change in PCWP among hemodynamically monitored patients and patient self-evaluation of dyspnea at 3 hours after initiation of study drug among all patients. At 3 hours, patients exhibited a significantly greater reduction in PCWP compared with either the nitroglycerin group or the placebo group, and a significant improvement in dyspnea compared with placebo (but not nitroglycerin). At 24 hours, PCWP decrease was greater in the nesiritide group than the nitroglycerin group, but patients' self-assessment of dyspnea were not significantly different [64]. The results of the VMAC study are summarized in Figure 11.

It remains to be seen whether nesiritide will provide a significant advantage over other therapies for the treatment of acute heart failure, either as a replacement for other vasodilators or an addition to current regimens. The clinical trials to-date have suggested that nesiritide has both safety advantages and disadvantages when compared with drugs in the current armamentarium. The PRECEDENT trial compared the arrhythmic effects of dobutamine with nesiritide in acute decompensated heart failure. Although both drugs were effective at improving the signs and symptoms of CHF, dobutamine significantly increased the risk of ventricular arrhythmias, whereas nesiritide had either a neutral or beneficial effect depending on the dose [65]. In addition, nesiritide did not increase heart rate despite the greater decrease in blood pressure as compared to dobutamine.

Concern has been raised regarding the renal impact of nesiritide due to increases in serum creatinine and cases of renal failure seen in some treated patients [66]. Since endogenous BNP is known to increase the glomerular filtration rate while decreasing blood pressure, the renal side effects seen in some trials may be a result of a prerenal state induced by BNP administration with concomitant diuretic use.

VASOPEPTIDASE INHIBITORS

Vasopeptidase inhibitors are a new group of agents under investigation for the treatment of hypertension and heart failure. They inhibit two enzymes, neutral endopeptidase (NEP) and angiotensin-converting enzyme (ACE), by virtue of the fact that these enzymes have a similar structure and catalytic site [67]. NEP is an endothelial cell surface zinc metallopeptidase predominantly found in the kidney that degrades the vasodilatory natriuretic peptides (A, B and C) [68]. ACE is well known to modulate the renin-angiotensin-aldosterone pathway by catalyzing the conversion of angiotensin I to the vasoconstrictor angiotensin II in the pulmonary vasculature. Both enzymes result in bradykinin degradation and have a net effect of increasing vasoconstriction and volume retention; therefore, inhibition of NEP and ACE results in increased vasodilation and improved diuresis [69]. Combined inhibition of NEP and ACE with vasopeptidase inhibitors has been shown to be effective and superior to ACE inhibition alone at improving cardiac geometry, hemodynamic measures, and survival in animal models of heart failure [69–71].

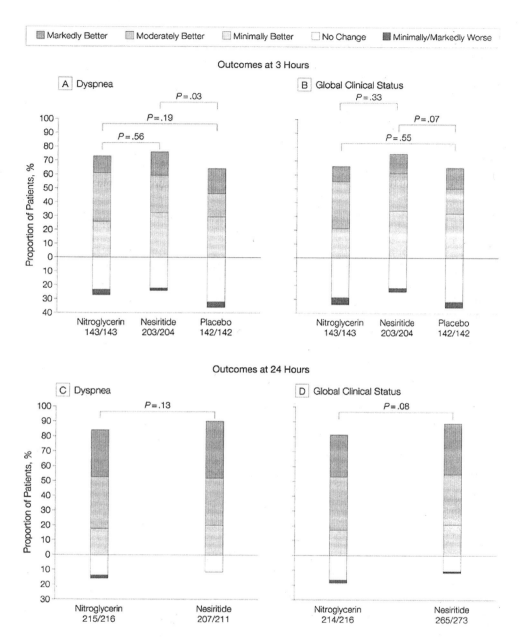

Figure 11 Outcomes at 3 and 24 hours for all treated patients by randomization group. (From Ref. 64.)

Omapatrilat

In an initial efficacy trial in humans, 48 patients with NYHA class II to III heart failure and LVEF greater than 40% were randomized to one of five dosing groups (2.5, 5, 10, 20, or 40 mg) of oral omapatrilat taken daily for 12 weeks. The 2.5 mg dosing group served as an active control group because this level of omapatrilat has been shown to produce ACE, but not NEP, inhibition. Forty patients were randomized to invasive hemodynamic monitoring, whereas the remaining eight participated in an exercise trial. All patients continued their regular cardiac medications (including ACE inhibitors) during the trial.

Patients in the 20 mg or 40 mg dosing groups showed a significant improvement in NYHA functional class at 12 weeks compared with the 2.5 mg active control group. These patients also exhibited improvements in functional status at 12 weeks as assessed by both the patient and the physician. All dosing groups exhibited a significant improvement in LVEF at 12 weeks compared with the control dose, with a greater improvement seen in the 20–40-mg group than the 5–10-mg group) (Table 4). Of the six hospitalizations for worsening heart failure during the study, all but one (5–10 mg) was in the 2.5 mg active control group. Omapratil was well-tolerated with the major adverse event being first-dose symptomatic hypotension (four patients in 20–40 mg), and intermittent hypotension (three patients in 20–40 mg, and 2 patients in 5–10 mg groups) [72].

The Immunosuppressive Therapy for the Prevention of Restenosis after Coronary Artery Stent Implantation (IMPRESS) trial randomized 573 patients with NYHA class II to IV heart failure and LVEF 40% or less to target doses of 40 mg oral omapatrilat or 20 mg oral lisinopril for 24 weeks. All patients were on stable doses of ACE inhibitors prior to beginning the study. The primary endpoint was improvement in maximum exercise treadmill test at week 12. The incidence of death, and comorbid events indicative of worsening heart failure were also assessed.

Maximum exercise treadmill test time improved slightly in both groups at 12 weeks with no significant difference observed between the two. Likewise, no significant difference was observed between the two groups in secondary endpoints; however, there was a consistent, nonsignificant reduction seen in the omapatrilat group in frequency of death, hospital admission, and supplemental diuretic use. The hazard ratio for the composite of death and admission for worsening heart failure was 0.52 (p = 0.052) favoring treatment with omapatrilat. Treatment with omapatrilat resulted in no increase in noncardiovascular adverse events, and a significant reduction in cardiovascular adverse events compared with lisinopril [73].

Further investigation of the acute and long-term hemodynamic effects of omapatrilat was conducted in 369 patients with symptomatic heart failure (NYHA class II–IV) randomized to receive 2.5, 5, or 10 mg oral omapatrilat (Panel I, n = 190) or 2.5, 20, or 40 mg of oral omapatrilat (Panel II, n = 179) for 12 weeks. Hemodynamic variables were assessed at baseline, 12 and 24 hours, and 12 weeks. Change in neurohormone levels including

Table 4 Omapatrilat Efficacy Trial Results

Outcome	Omapatrilat dose		
	2.5 mg (n = 15)	5–10 mg (n = 17)	20–40 mg (n = 13)
Patient assessment of functional status			
Greatly improved	0 (0%)	7 (41%)	5 (38%)
Moderately improved	5 (33%)	6 (35%)	5 (38%)
Clinician assessment of functional status			
Greatly improved	0 (0%)	2 (12%)	2 (15%)
Moderately improved	0 (0%)	7 (41%)	9 (69%)
LVEF	-3.4 ± 1.7	6.7 ± 1.6	7.4 ± 1.0

plasma ACE, ANP (atrial natriuretic peptide) , BNP, and renin among others were calculated at 3,12 and 24 hours after the first (day 1) and last (week 12) doses.

Acute hemodynamic improvement as indicated by 12 hour postdose change in PCWP was noted in the 10–40 mg groups on day 1, and the 20 mg and 40 mg groups at week 12 compared with the 2.5 mg active controls (Fig. 12). Plasma increases in ANP, BNP, and cGMP were noted in the 10, 20 and 40 mg dosing groups at 3 hours post–day 1 dose (all significant except change in BNP for 20 mg dose), with a return toward baseline levels at 12 hours postdose. At 12 weeks, no significant changes in these neurohormones were noted postdose, but there was a nonsignificant increase in ANP (+55 pmol/1; 95% CI −9,118) at 3 hours. No significant changes were noted at 12 weeks in potentially deleterious neurohormones, such as ET-1 and norepinephrine. Again, the most common adverse event observed was first-dose hypotension, which resulted in the withdrawal of four patients without serious consequences. One case of angioedema occurred in the 40 mg group after the first dose [74].

The Omapatrilat Versus Enalapril Randomized Trial of Utility in Reducing Events (OVERTURE) is the only randomized, controlled clinical trial of omapatrilat to date powered to evaluate morbidity and mortality outcomes. In this trial, 5770 patients with NYHA class II–IV heart failure or LVEF 30% or less were randomized to either enalapril (starting dose 2.5 mg, target dose 10 mg orally b.i.d., n = 2884) or omapatrilat (starting dose 10 mg, target dose 40 mg orally q.d., n = 2886). Patients were encouraged to receive all other appropriate therapy for heart failure, including ACE inhibitors and angiotensin

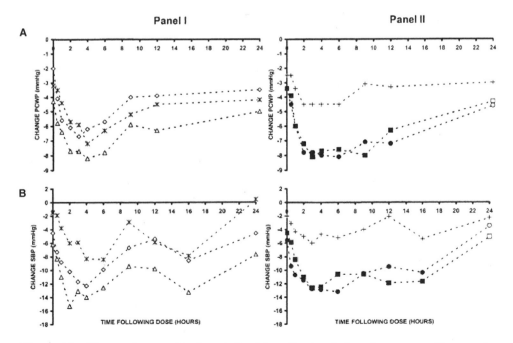

Figure 12 Change from pretreatment day 1 baseline levels in pulmonary capillary wedge pressure (PCWP) (**A**) and systolic blood pressure (SBP), (**B**) after the final dose of omapatrilat at 12 weeks. *Panel I:* open diamond, 2.5 mg; star, 5 mg; open triangle, 10 mg. *Panel II:* + = 2.5 mg; open square, 20 mg; open circle, 40 mg. Shaded symbols, indicate a significant difference (p = 0.05) in the 0-hr to 12-hr average change from predose day 1 for omapatrilat dose compared with the respective 2.5 mg group. (From Ref. 74.)

II receptor antagonists. The primary end-point was the combined risk of all-cause mortality or hospitalization for worsening heart failure, and the mean duration of follow-up was 14.5 months.

Of the 5770 patients, 970 died or were hospitalized requiring intravenous therapy for worsening heart failure during the study period in the enalapril group, and 914 in the omapatrilat group (hazard ratio 0.94, 95% CI 0.86, 1.03) (Fig. 13a). When all-cause mortality was evaluated alone, a similar hazard ratio was obtained (0.94, 95% CI 0.83, 1.07) (Fig. 13b). Although this met predefined criteria for noninferiority, there was no clear benefit seen with omapatrilat therapy. Adverse events were similar to those observed in other trial of omapatrilat with increases in hypotension and dizziness compared with enalapril, but decreases in heart failure exacerbation and renal impairment. Angioedema occurred in 24 patients (0.8%) in the omapatrilat arm as compared with 14 patients (0.5%) in the enalapril arm. Withdrawal rates due to adverse events were 17.9% in the omapatrilat group and 17.0% in the enalapril group [75].

The OVERTURE trial results were surprising as no benefit in dual inhibition of NEP and ACE could be seen in long-term morbidity and mortality outcomes, despite encouraging data from both preclinical and early clinical trials. In addition, in data submitted to the U.S. Food and Drug Administration for the new drug application for omapatrilat, 44 cases of angioedema among 6000 patients treated with omapatrilat were noted (0.7%) [76], which is consistent with the results of the OVERTURE trial. With no clear benefit established and legitimate concern regarding the incidence of angioedema, the utility of vasopeptidase inhibition in heart failure is currently in question.

VASOPRESSIN ANTAGONISTS

Arginine vasopressin (AVP) is a peptide hormone that is elevated in heart failure and associated with a poor prognosis [77,78]. AVP exerts its cardiac effects through two receptor subtypes: V_{1a} and V_2. V_{1a} is found on vascular smooth muscle cells and myocardiocytes. Activation of V_{1a} is initially inotropic but mediates a decrease in myocardial contractility with further increases in AVP, whereas V_{1a}-induced vasoconstriction occurs in a dose-dependent manner [79–81]. Stimulation of the V_{1a}-receptor further leads to increased myocardial protein synthesis resulting in myocardial hypertrophy [82,83]. V_2-receptors are found in the distal tubule of the kidney, and their activation results in water retention via upregulation of aquaporin channels [79,84]. Inhibition of AVP via V_{1a} and V_2 antagonism is an area of a current investigation in the treatment of heart failure.

Conivaptan

Conivaptan is a dual V_{1a}/V_2 receptor antagonist that has been investigated in the treatment of advanced heart failure. One hundred and forty-two patients with NYHA class III or IV heart failure were randomized to either a single IV dose of conivaptan (10, 20, or 40 mg) or placebo and evaluated over 12 hours for changes in hemodynamic parameters including CI, right atrial pressure (RAP) and PCWP. Both PCWP and RAP were significantly reduced in the 20 mg and 40 mg treatment groups compared with placebo at 3 to 6 hours, but CI was not improved. Urine output in the 20 mg and 40 mg groups was significantly higher over the 12-hour follow-up than that of the placebo group. Conivaptan was associated with fewer side-effects during the follow-up period than placebo [85].

A

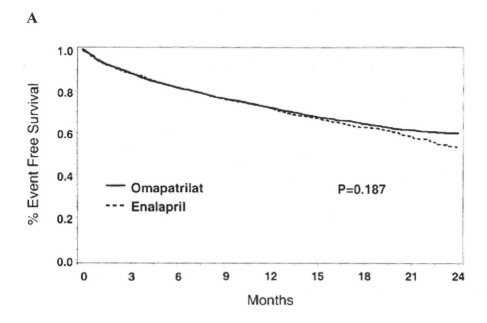

B

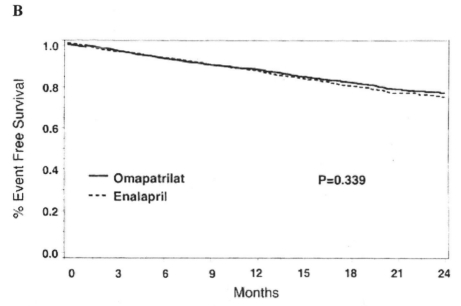

Figure 13 (**A**) Kaplan-Meier analysis of time to death or hospitalization for heart failure requiring intravenous treatment in the omapatrilat and enalapril groups. (**B**) Kaplan-Meier analysis of time to death in the omapatrilat or enalapril groups. (From Ref. 75.)

Tolvaptan

Chronic administration of tolvaptan, a nonpeptide V_2 receptor antagonist, was studied in 254 patients with a diagnosis of CHF irrespective of LVEF and NYHA functional class. Patients were randomized to receive oral tolvaptan (30, 45 or 60 mg) or placebo daily for

25 days and maintained on stable doses of furosemide. The primary efficacy variable was change in body weight from baseline to study day 14.

All treatment groups had an initial weight loss compared with baseline at study day 1 that was significantly greater than that of the placebo arm. This weight loss was maintained throughout the treatment period, but no further benefit of treatment was seen after day 1. Urine sodium excretion over the first 24-hour period was significantly greater in all dosing tolvaptan groups compared with placebo, but serum sodium stayed within normal ranges throughout the study for most individuals in both the active treatment and placebo groups. Only dry-mouth, thirst, and polyuria were reported more frequently with tolvaptan than placebo, leading to drug discontinuation in two patients in the 60 mg group [86].

Antagonism of AVP through the V_{1a} and V_2 has theoretical appeal given the physiological consequences of excess AVP. Initial clinical trials have established that these drugs are relatively safe, and that treatment is associated with improvements in some hemodynamic and clinical parameters associated with heart failure. However, no study has yet evaluated the impact of either single or dual receptor antagonism on long-term morbidity and mortality.

CONCLUSIONS

The clinical studies presented in this chapter represent novel areas of research that highlight the complexity of developing new therapies from the bench to the bedside. Although experimental observations from the laboratory follow a logical process for development into clinical practice, it has become clear that the clinical utility of individual therapies require meticulous clinical research and frequently encounters failures. The clinical trials of TNF-α antagonism and neuropeptidase inhibitors are good examples of treatment models that failed the test of large-scale clinical utility despite encouraging preclinical and early clinical data.

Perhaps in the current armamentarium for chronic heart failure further antagonism of various pathways is not possible due to the inability to demonstrate clinical benefit beyond currently established therapies. It remains to be seen whether the benefits shown in early trials of vasopressin antagonists can result in improved quality of life and/or survival in heart failure patients.

Active clinical studies utilizing broad-spectrum antiinflammatory therapies, including immunomodulatory strategies, may provide the next generation of therapy in chronic heart failure. With regards to acute heart failure, we have seen clear documentation of hemodynamic benefits with the therapeutic utilization of recombinant type-B natriuretic peptide, and further investigation is ongoing with the nonspecific endothelin-1 antagonist tezosentan. Ongoing clinical research will better define the appropriate use of these and other drugs in acute heart failure. Most importantly, the experience of the latest generation of clinical trials of new therapies for heart failure has shown us that further development in this area will require the demonstration not only of hemodynamic, serologic, and symptomatic improvement, but also of disease-modifying effects on morbidity and mortality.

REFERENCES

1. MERIT-HF Investigators Effect of metoprolol CR/XL in chronic heart failure: metoprolol CR/XL Randomized Intervention Trial in Congestive Heart Failure (MERIT-HF). Lancet 1999 Jun 12; 353(9169):2001–2007.

2. Packer M, Poole-Wilson PA, Armstrong PW, Cleland JG, Horowitz JD, Massie BM, Ryden L, Thygesen K, Uretsky BF. Comparative effects of low and high doses of the angiotensin-converting enzyme inhibitor, lisinopril, on morbidity and mortality in chronic heart failure. ATLAS Study Group. Circulation 1999 Dec 7; 100(23):2312–2318.

3. The CONSENSUS Trial Study Group. Effects of enalapril on mortality in severe congestive heart failure: results of the Cooperative North Scandinavian Enalapril Survival Study. N Engl J Med 1987; 316:1429–1435.

4. The SOLVD Investigators. Effect of enalapril on survival in patients with reduced left ventricular ejection fractions and congestive heart failure. N Engl J Med 1991; 325:292–302.

5. Thackray S, Easthaugh J, Freemantle N, Cleland JG. The effectiveness and relative effectiveness of intravenous inotropic drugs acting through the adrenergic pathway in patients with heart failure-a meta-regression analysis. Eur J Heart Fail 2002; 4:515–529.

6. Cohn JN, Goldstein SO, Greenberg BH, Lorell BH, Bourge RC, Jaski BE, Gottlieb SO, McGrew F, DeMets DL, White BG. A dose-dependent increase in mortality with vesnarinone among patients with severe heart failure. Vesnarinone Trial Investigators. N Engl J Med 1998; 339:1810–1816.

7. Packer M, Carver JR, Rodeheffer RJ, Ivanhoe RJ, DiBianco R, Zeldis SM, Hendrix GH, Bommer WJ, Elkayam U, Kukin ML, et al. Effect of oral milrinone on mortality in severe chronic heart failure. The PROMISE Study Research Group. N Engl J Med 1991; 325: 1468–1475.

8. Francis SE, Holden H, Holt CM, Duff GW. Interleukin-1 in myocardium and coronary arteries of patients with dilated cardiomyopathy. J Mol Cell Cardiol 1998; 30:215–223.

9. Munger MA, Johnson B, Amber IJ, Callahan KS, Gilbert EM. Circulating concentrations of proinflammatory cytokines in mild or moderate heart failure secondary to ischemic or idiopathic dilated cardiomyopathy. Am J Cardiol 1996; 77:723–727.

10. Levine B, Kalman J, Mayer L, Fillit HM, Packer M. Elevated circulating levels of tumor necrosis factor in severe chronic heart failure. N Engl J Med 1990; 223:236–241.

11. Torre-Amione G, Kapadia S, Lee J, Bies RD, Lebovitz R, Mann DL. Expression and functional significance of tumor necrosis factor receptors in human myocardium. Circulation 1995; 92:1487–1493.

12. Torre-Amione G, Kapadia S, Benedict C, Oral H, Young JB, Mann DL. Proinflammatory cytokine levels in patients with depressed left ventricular ejection fraction: a report from the Studies of Left Ventricular Dysfunction (SOLVD). J Am Coll Cardiol 1996; 27:1201–1206.

13. Bozkurt B, Kribbs SB, Clubb FJ, Michael LH, Didenko VV, Hornsby PJ, Seta Y, Oral H, Spinale FG, Mann DL. Pathophysiologically relevant concentrations of tumor necrosis factor-alpha promote progressive left ventricular dysfunction and remodeling in rats. Circulation 1998; 97:1382–1391.

14. Anker SD, Coats AJ. How to RECOVER from RENAISSANCE? The significance of the results of RECOVER, RENAISSANCE, RENEWAL and ATTACH. Int J Cardiol 2002 Dec; 86(2–3):123–30.

15. Chung ES, Packer M, Lo KH, Fasanmade AA, Willerson JT. Anti-TNF Therapy Against Congestive Heart Failure Investigators. Randomized, double-blind, placebo-controlled, pilot trial of infliximab, a chimeric monoclonal antibody to tumor necrosis factor-alpha, in patients with moderate-to-severe heart failure: results of the anti-TNF Therapy Against Congestive Heart Failure (ATTACH) trial. Circulation 2003 Jul 1; 107(25):3133–3140.

16. Caforio AL, Goldman JH, Baig MK, Haven AJ, Dalla Libera L, Keeling PJ, McKenna WJ. Cardiac autoantibodies in dilated cardiomyopathy become undetectable with disease progression. Heart 1997; 77:62–67.

17. Caforio AL, Goldman JH, Haven AJ, Baig KM, McKenna WJ. Evidence for autoimmunity to myosin and other heart-specific autoantigens in patients with dilated cardiomyopathy and their relatives. Int J Cardiol 1996; 54:157–163.

18. Magnusson Y, Hjalmarson A, Hoebeke J. Beta 1-adrenoceptor autoimmunity in cardiomyopathy. Int J Cardiol 1996 May; 54(2):137–141.

19. Hatle L, Melbye OJ. Immunoglobulins and complement in chronic myocardial disease. A myocardial biopsy study. Acta Med Scand 1976; 200(5):385–389.

20. Wallukat G, Muller J, Podlowski S, Nissen E, Morwinski R, Hetzer R. Agonist-like beta-adrenoceptor antibodies in heart failure. Am J Cardiol 1999 Jun 17; 83(12A):75H–79H.

21. Dietrich G, Kaveri SV, Kazatchkine MD. Modulation of autoimmunity by intravenous immune globulin through interaction with the function of the immune/idiotypic network. Clin Immunol Immunopathol 1992 Jan; 62(1 Pt 2):S73–S81.

21. Dalakas MC. Mechanisms of action of IVIg and therapeutic considerations in the treatment of acute and chronic demyelinating neuropathies. Neurology 2002 Dec 24; 59(12 Suppl 6): S13–21.

22. Sharief MK, Ingram DA, Swash M, Thompson EJ. I.V. immunoglobulin reduces circulating proinflammatory cytokines in Guillain-Barre syndrome. Neurology 1999 Jun 10; 2(9): 1833–1838.

24. Aukrust P, Muller F, Svenson M, Nordoy I, Bendtzen K, Froland SS. Administration of intravenous immunoglobulin (IVIG) in vivo–down-regulatory effects on the IL-1 system. Clin Exp Immunol 1999 Jan; 115(1):136–143.

25. McNamara DM, Holubkov R, Starling RC, Dec GW, Loh E, Torre-Amione G, Gass A, Janosko K, Tokarczyk T, Kessler P, Mann DL, Feldman AM. Controlled trial of intravenous immune globulin in recent-onset dilated cardiomyopathy. Circulation 2001; 103:2254–2259.

26. Gullestad L, Aass H, Fjeld JG, Wikeby L, Andreassen AK, Ihlen H, Simonsen S, Kjekshus J, Nitter-Hauge S, Ueland T, Lien E, Froland SS, Aukrust P. Immunomodulating therapy with intravenous immunoglobulin in patients with chronic heart failure. Circulation 2001; 103:220–225.

27. Muller J, Wallukat G, Dandel M, Bieda H, Brandes K, Spiegelsberger S, Nissen E, Kunze R, Hetzer R. Immunoglobulin adsorption in patients with idiopathic dilated cardiomyopathy. Circulation 2000; 101:385–391.

28. Staudt A, Schaper F, Stangl V, Plagemann A, Bohm M, Merkel K, Wallukat G, Wernecke KD, Stangl K, Baumann G, Felix SB. Immunohistological changes in dilated cardiomyopathy induced by immunoadsorption therapy and subsequent immunoglobulin substitution. Circulation 2001 Jun 5; 103(22):2681–2686.

29. Staudt A, Bohm M, Knebel F, Grosse Y, Bischoff C, Hummel A, Dahm JB, Borges A, Jochmann N, Wernecke KD, Wallukat G, Baumann G, Felix SB. Potential role of autoantibodies belonging to the immunoglobulin G-3 subclass in cardiac dysfunction among patients with dilated cardiomyopathy. Circulation 2002 Nov 5; 106(19):2448–2453.

30. Fadok VA, Bratton DL, Konowal A, Freed PW, Westcott JY, Henson PM. Macrophages that have ingested apoptotic cells in vitro inhibit proinflammatory cytokine production through autocrine/paracrine mechanisms involving TGF-beta, PGE2, and PAF. J Clin Invest 1998; 101:890–898.

31. Shivji GM, Suzuki H, Mandel AS, Bolton AE, Sauder DN. The effect of VAS972 on allergic contact hypersensitivity. J Cutan Med Surg 2000; 4:132–137.

32. Torre-Amione GT, Young J, Sestier F. A novel immune modulation therapy reduces the risk of death and hospitalization in patients with advanced congestive heart failure: results of a randomized, controlled, multi-center Phase II trial. Submitted.

33. Inoue A, Yanagisawa M, Kimura S, Kasuya Y, Miyauchi T, Goto K, Masaki T. The human endothelin family: distinct isopeptides predicted by three separate genes. Proc Natl Acad Sci U S A 1989; 86:2863–2867.

34. Cody RJ, Haas GJ, Binkley PF, Capers Q, Kelley R. Plasma endothelin correlates with the extent of pulmonary hypertension in patients with chronic congestive heart failure. Circulation 1992 Feb; 85(2):504–509.

35. Kiowski W, Sutsch G, Hunziker P, Muller P, Kim J, Oechslin E, Schmitt R, Jones R, Bertel O. Evidence for endothelin-1-mediated vasoconstriction in severe chronic heart failure. Lancet 1995 Sep 16; 346(8977):732–736.

36. Pacher R, Bergler-Klein J, Globits S, Teufelsbauer H, Schuller M, Krauter A, Ogris E, Rodler S, Wutte M, Hartter E. Plasma big endothelin-1 concentrations in congestive heart failure patients with or without systemic hypertension. Am J Cardiol 1993 Jun 1; 71(15):1293–1299.

37. Wei CM, Lerman A, Rodeheffer RJ, McGregor CG, Brandt RR, Wright S, Heublein DM, Kao PC, Edwards WD, Burnett JC. Endothelin in human congestive heart failure. Circulation 1994 Apr; 89(4):1580–1586.

38. Pacher R, Stanek B, Hulsmann M, Koller-Strametz J, Berger R, Schuller M, Hartter E, Ogris E, Frey B, Heinz G, Maurer G. Prognostic impact of big endothelin-1 plasma concentrations compared with invasive hemodynamic evaluation in severe heart failure. J Am Coll Cardiol 1996 Mar 1; 27(3):633–641.

39. Sakurai T, Yanagisawa M, Masaki T. Molecular characterization of endothelin receptors. Trends Pharmacol Sci 1992; 13:103–108.

40. Hosoda K, Nakao K, Tamura N, Arai H, Ogawa Y, Suga S, Nakanishi S, Imura H. Organization, structure, chromosomal assignment, and expression of the gene encoding the human endothelin-A receptor. J Biol Chem 1992; 267:18797–18804.

41. Mulder P, Richard V, Derumeaux G, Hogie M, Henry JP, Lallemand F, Compagnon P, Mace B, Comoy E, Letac B, Thuillez C. Role of endogenous endothelin in chronic heart failure: effect of long-term treatment with an endothelin antagonist on survival, hemodynamics, and cardiac remodeling. Circulation 1997; 96:1976–1982.

42. Maemura K, Kurihara H, Morita T, Oh-hashi Y, Yazaki Y. Production of endothelin-1 in vascular endothelial cells is regulated by factors associated with vascular injury. Gerontology 1992; 38(suppl 1):29–35.

43. Haynes WG, Webb DJ. Contribution of endogenous generation of endothelin-1 to basal vascular tone. Lancet 1994(344):852–854.

43a. Luscher TF, Barton M. Endothelins and endothelin receptor antagonists: therapeutic considerations for a novel class of cardiovascular drugs. Circulation 2000 Nov 7; 102(19):2434–2440.

44. Haynes WG, Webb DJ. Endothelium-dependent modulation of responses to endothelin-1 in human veins. Clin Sci (Colch) 1993(84):427–433.

45. Iwasaki S, Homma T, Matsuda Y, Kon V. Endothelin receptor subtype B mediates autoinduction of endothelin-1 in rat mesangial cells. J Biol Chem 1995; 270:6997–7003.

46. Sakai S, Miyauchi T, Sakurai T, Yamaguchi I, Kobayashi M, Goto K, Sugishita Y. Pulmonary hypertension caused by congestive heart failure is ameliorated by long-term application of an endothelin receptor antagonist: increased expression of endothelin-1 messenger ribonucleic acid and endothelin-1-like immunoreactivity in the lung in congestive heart failure in rats. J Am Coll Cardiol 1996; 28:1580–1588.

47. Spieker LE, Mitrovic V, Noll G, Pacher R, Schulze MR, Muntwyler J, Schalcher C, Kiowski W, Luscher TF. Acute hemodynamic and neurohumoral effects of selective ET(A) receptor blockade in patients with congestive heart failure. ET 003 Investigators. J Am Coll Cardiol 2000 Jun; 35(7):1745–1752.

48. Luscher TF, Enseleit F, Pacher R, Mitrovic V, Schulze MR, Willenbrock R, Dietz R, Rousson V, Hurlimann D, Philipp S, Notter T, Noll G. Ruschitzka F; Heart Failure ET(A) Receptor Blockade Trial. Hemodynamic and neurohumoral effects of selective endothelin A (ET(A)) receptor blockade in chronic heart failure: the Heart Failure ET(A) Receptor Blockade Trial (HEAT). Circulation 2002 Nov 19; 106(21):2666–2672.

49. Clozel M, Breu V, Gray GA, Kalina B, Löffler BM, Burri K, Cassal JM, Hirth G, Muller M, Neidhart W, Ramuz H. Pharmacological characterization of bosentan, a new potent orally active nonpeptide endothelin receptor antagonist. J Pharmacol Exp Ther 1994; 270:228–235.

50. Kalra PR, Moon JC, Coats AJ. Do results of the ENABLE (Endothelin Antagonist Bosentan for Lowering Cardiac Events in Heart Failure) study spell the end for non-selective endothelin antagonism in heart failure?. Int J Cardiol 2002 Oct; 85(2–3):195–197.

51. Clozel M, Ramuz H, Clozel JP, Breu V, Hess P, Loffler BM, Coassolo P, Roux S. Pharmacology of tezosentan, a new endothelin receptor antagonist designed for parenteral use. J Pharmacol Exp Ther 1999; 290:840–846.

52. Torre-Amione G, Young JB, Durand J-B, Bozhurt B, Mann DL, Kobrin F, Pratt CM. Hemodynamic effects of tezosentan, an intravenous dual endothelin receptor antagonist, in patients with Class III to IV congestive heart failure 2001; 103:973–980.

53. Torre-Amione G, Durand JB, Nagueh S, Vooletich MT, Kobrin I, Pratt C. A pilot safety trial of prolonged (48 h) infusion of the dual endothelin-receptor antagonist tezosentan in patients with advanced heart failure. Chest 2001 Aug; 120(2):460–466.

54. Teerlink JR, Massie BM, Cleland JG, Tzivoni D. for the RITZ- 1 Investigators. A double-blind, parallel-group, multicenter, placebo-controlled study to investigate the efficacy and

safety of tezosentan in reducing the symptoms in patients with acute decompensated heart failure (RITZ-1) (abstr). Circulation 2001; 104(II):526.

55. Torre-Amione G, Young JB, Colucci WS, Lewis BS, Pratt C, Cotter G, Stangl K, Elkayam U, Teerlink JR, Frey A, Rainisio M, Kobrin I. Hemodynamic and clinical effects of tezosentan, an intravenous dual endothelin receptor antagonist, in patients hospitalized for acute decompensated heart failure. J Am Coll Cardiol 2003 Jul 2; 42(1):140–147.

56. O'Connor CM, Gattis WA, Adams KF, Hasselblad V, Chandler B, Frey A, Kobrin I, Rainisio M, Shah MR, Teerlink J, Gheorghiade M. Randomized Intravenous TeZosentan Study-4 Investigators. Tezosentan in patients with acute heart failure and acute coronary syndromes: results of the Randomized Intravenous TeZosentan Study (RITZ-4). J Am Coll Cardiol 2003 May 7; 41(9):1452–1457.

57. Cotter G, Kaluski E, Pacher R, Stangl K, Perchenet L, Kobrin I, Rainisio M, Frey A, Neuhart E, Dingemanse J, Torre-Amione G. Low doses of tezosentan are hemodynamically active and decrease type-B natriuretic peptide levels in patients with acute heart failure. (submitted).

58. McCullough PA, Omland T, Maisel AS. B-type natriuretic peptides: a diagnostic breakthrough for clinicians. Rev Cardiovasc Med 2003 Spring; 4(2):72–80.

59. Edwards BS, Zimmerman RS, Schwab TR, Heublein DM, Burnett JC. Atrial stretch, not pressure, is the principal determinant controlling the acute release of atrial natriuretic factor. Circ Res 1988; 62:191–195.

60. Bruneau BG, Piazza LA, de Bold AJ. BNP gene expression is specifically modulated by stretch and ET-1 in a new model of isolated rat atria. Am J Physiol 1997; 273:H2678–H2686.

61. Wiese S, Breyer T, Dragu A, et al. Gene expression of brain natriuretic peptide in isolated atrial and ventricular human myocardium: influence of angiotensin II and diastolic fiber length. Circulation 2000; 102:3074–3079.

61a. Baughman A. B-type natriuetic peptide—a window to the heart. N Engl J Med 2002 July 18; 347(3):158–159.

62. Mills RM, LeJemtel TH, Horton DP, Liang C, Lang R, Silver MA, Lui C, Chatterjee K. Sustained hemodynamic effects of an infusion of nesiritide (human B-type natriuretic peptide) in heart failure: a randomized, double-blind, placebo-controlled clinical trial. Natrecor Study Group. J Am Coll Cardiol 1999 Jul; 34(1):155–162.

63. Colucci WS, Elkayam U, Horton DP, Abraham WT, Bourge RC, Johnson AD, Wagoner LE, Givertz MM, Liang CS, Neibaur M, Haught WH, LeJemtel TH. Intravenous nesiritide, a natriuretic peptide, in the treatment of decompensated congestive heart failure. Nesiritide Study Group. N Engl J Med 2000 Jul 27; 343(4):246–253.

64. Publication Committee for the VMAC Investigators (Vasodilatation in the Management of Acute CHF). Intravenous nesiritide vs nitroglycerin for treatment of decompensated congestive heart failure: a randomized controlled trial. JAMA 2002 Mar 27; 287(12):1531–1540.

65. Burger AJ, Horton DP, LeJemtel T, Ghali JK, Torre G, Dennish G, Koren M, Dinerman J, Silver M, Cheng ML, Elkayam U. Prospective randomized evaluation of cardiac ectopy with dobutamine or natrecor therapy. Effect of nesiritide (B-type natriuretic peptide) and dobutamine on ventricular arrhythmias in the treatment of patients with acutely decompensated congestive heart failure: the PRECEDENT study. Am Heart J 2002 Dec; 144(6): 1102–1108.

66. Grines CL. Safety and effectiveness of dofetilide for conversion of atrial fibrillation and nesiritide for acute decompensation of heart failure: a report from the cardiovascular and renal advisory panel of the Food and Drug Administration. Circulation 2000 May 30; 101(21): E200–1.

67. Trindade PT, Rouleau JL. Vasopeptidase inhibitors: potential role in the treatment of heart failure. Heart Fail Monit 2001; 2(1):2–7.

68. Turner AJ, Isaac RE, Coates D. The neprilysin (NEP) family of zinc metalloendopeptidases: genomics and function. Bioessays 2001 Mar; 23(3):261–269.

69. Trippodo NC, Fox M, Monticello TM, Panchal BC, Asaad MM. Vasopeptidase inhibition with omapatrilat improves cardiac geometry and survival in cardiomyopathic hamsters more than does ACE inhibition with captopril. J Cardiovasc Pharmacol 1999 Dec; 34(6):782–790.

70. Burrell LM, Farina NK, Balding LC, Johnston CI. Beneficial renal and cardiac effects of vasopeptidase inhibition with S21402 in heart failure. Hypertension 2000 Dec; 36(6): 1105–1111.

71. Farina NK, Johnston CI, Burrell LM. Reversal of cardiac hypertrophy and fibrosis by S21402, a dual inhibitor of neutral endopeptidase and angiotensin converting enzyme in SHRs. J Hypertens 2000 Jun; 18(6):749–755.

72. McClean DR, Ikram H, Garlick AH, Richards AM, Nicholls MG, Crozier IG. The clinical, cardiac, renal, arterial and neurohormonal effects of omapatrilat, a vasopeptidase inhibitor, in patients with chronic heart failure. J Am Coll Cardiol 2000; 36:479–486.

73. Rouleau JL, Pfeffer MA, Stewart DJ, Isaac D, Sestier F, Kerut EK, Porter CB, Proulx G, Qian C, Block AJ. Comparison of vasopeptidase inhibitor, omapatrilat, and lisinopril on exercise tolerance and morbidity in patients with heart failure: IMPRESS randomized trial. Lancet 2000 Aug 19; 356(9230):615–620.

74. McClean DR, Ikram H, Mehta S, et al. Omapatrilat Hemodynamic Study Group. Vasopeptidase inhibition with omapatrilat in chronic heart failure: acute and long-term hemodynamic and neurohumoral effects. J Am Coll Cardiol 2002 Jun 19; 39(12):2034–2041.

75. Packer M, Califf RM, Konstam MA, et al. Comparison of omapatrilat and enalapril in patients with chronic heart failure: the Omapatrilat Versus Enalapril Randomized Trial of Utility in Reducing Events (OVERTURE). Circulation 2002 Aug 20; 106(8):920–926.

76. Messerli FH, Nussberger J. Vasopeptidase inhibition and angio-edema. Lancet 2000; 356: 608–609.

77. Goldsmith SR, Francis GS, Cowley AW, et al. Increased plasma arginine vasopressin levels in patients with congestive heart failure. J Am Coll Cardiol 1983; 1:1385–1390.

78. Francis GS, Benedict C, Johnstone DE, et al. Comparison of neuroendocrine activation in patients with left ventricular dysfunction with and without congestive heart failure: a substudy of the Studies of Left Ventricular Dysfunction. Circulation 1990; 82:1724–1729.

79. Walker BR, Childs ME. Adams EM. Direct cardiac effects of vasopressin: role of V1- and V2-vasopressinergic receptors. Am J Physiol 1988 Aug; 255(2 Pt 2):H261–H265.

80. Kaygisiz Z, Kabadere TE, Dernek S, Erden SH. The effects of vasopressin in isolated rat hearts. Indian J Physiol Pharmacol 2001 Jan; 45(1):54–62.

81. Briner VA, Tsai P, Choong HL, Schrier RW. Comparative effects of arginine vasopressin and oxytocin in cell culture systems. Am J Physiol 1992 Aug; 263(2 Pt 2):F222–F227.

82. Nakamura Y, Haneda T, Osaki J, Miyata S, Kikuchi K. Hypertrophic growth of cultured neonatal rat heart cells mediated by vasopressin V(1A) receptor. Eur J Pharmacol 2000 Mar 10; 391(1–2):39–48.

83. Fukuzawa J, Haneda T, Kikuchi K. Arginine vasopressin increases the rate of protein synthesis in isolated perfused adult rat heart via the V1 receptor. Mol Cell Biochem 1999 May; 195(1–2):93–98.

84. Xu DL, Martin PY, Ohara M, St John J, Pattison T, Meng X, Morris K, Kim JK, Schrier RW. Upregulation of aquaporin-2 water channel expression in chronic heart failure rat. J Clin Invest 1997 Apr 1; 99(7):1500–1505.

85. Udelson JE, Smith WB, Hendrix GH, Painchaud CA, Ghazzi M, Thomas I, Ghali JK, Selaru P, Chanoine F, Pressler ML, Konstam MA. Acute hemodynamic effects of conivaptan, a dual V(1A) and V(2) vasopressin receptor antagonist, in patients with advanced heart failure. Circulation 2001 Nov 13; 104(20):2417–2423.

86. Gheorghiade M, Niazi I, Ouyang J, Czerwiec F, Kambayashi J, Zampino M, Orlandi C. Tolvaptan Investigators. Vasopressin V2-receptor blockade with tolvaptan in patients with chronic heart failure: results from a double-blind, randomized trial. Circulation 2003 Jun 3; 107(21):2690–2696. Epub 2003 May 12.

17

Treatment of Diastolic Heart Failure

William H. Gaasch
Department of Cardiovascular Medicine, Lahey Clinic
Burlington, Massachusetts, and the University of Massachusetts Medical School,
Worcester, Massachusetts, USA

Theo E. Meyer
Department of Medicine, the University of Massachusetts Memorial Health Center
and the University of Massachusetts Medical School,
Worcester, Massachusetts, USA

Heart failure is a clinical syndrome that is manifest by dyspnea, fatigue, and edema. The syndrome is caused by cardiac dysfunction and activation of neurohormonal mechanisms that promote fluid retention. The signs and symptoms of congestive heart failure (CHF) have long been known to occur in the presence of a normal left ventricular (LV) ejection fraction and this led to the use of terms such as "backward failure"–indicating a failure of the heart to accept venous return at normal filling pressures. It is now recognized that CHF in the presence of a normal ejection fraction is primarily caused by abnormalities in the diastolic properties of the ventricle and consequently, the term "diastolic heart failure" has replaced backward failure [1–7].

TERMINOLOGY

Diastolic dysfunction refers to abnormal LV diastolic distensibility, filling, or relaxation–regardless of whether the ejection fraction is normal or abnormal and whether the patient is symptomatic or asymptomatic. In this chapter, the term "asymptomatic diastolic dysfunction" is used to refer to an asymptomatic patient with a normal LV ejection fraction, and echo-Doppler evidence of an abnormal pattern of LV filling [5]. This has also been referred to as "preclinical heart disease" [8]; it is often a reflection of early hypertensive heart disease. If a patient with asymptomatic diastolic dysfunction exhibits effort intolerance and dyspnea, especially if there is evidence of venous congestion and edema, the terms "diastolic heart failure" (i.e., "symptomatic diastolic dysfunction") is used. This terminology parallels that used in asymptomatic and symptomatic patients with systolic dysfunction and it facilitates the use of a clinical, pathophysiological, diagnostic, and therapeutic framework that includes virtually all patients with LV dysfunction–whether or not they have cardiac symptoms [5].

363

PATHOPHYSIOLOGY

The diastolic properties of the left ventricle are determined by the volume of the chamber, the thickness and passive stiffness of the ventricular wall, and the active process of myocardial relaxation. An increase in myocardial mass and/or alterations in the extra myocardial collagen network may cause or contribute to an increase in passive elastic stiffness of the ventricle. Disorders of the active process of myocardial relaxation, acting alone or in concert with abnormal passive properties of the ventricle, can also stiffen the ventricle. LV compliance or distensibility is reduced and the dynamics of filling are altered. Under these circumstances, relatively small increments in venous return can produce substantial increases in LV end-diastolic pressure as well as left atrial and pulmonary venous pressures. The most common causes of diastolic dysfunction are LV hypertrophy and myocardial ischemia [1,2] (Table 1).

The basic mechanisms that underlie diastolic dysfunction may be intrinsic to the cardiomyocyte (e.g., abnormal calcium homeostatis) or extracellular matrix (e.g., alterations in collagen). In addition, neurohormonal and cardiac endothelial activity modulate ventricular stiffness and relaxation. Knowledge of these mechanisms offers potential therapeutic targets [2].

Abnormalities of systolic function are often present in patients with predominant diastolic heart failure, and a normal ejection fraction at rest does not necessarily mean that myocardial contractile function is truly normal. Likewise, abnormalities of diastolic function are generally present in patients with systolic heart failure. In this chapter, the

Table 1 Causes of Diastolic Dysfunctional

Myocardial disease
  Impaired relaxation
    Myocardial ischemia
    Myocyte hypertrophy
    Cardiomyopathy
    Aging
    Hypothyroidism
  Increase passive stiffness
    Diffuse fibrosis
    Postmyocardial infarction scarring and fibrosis
    Myocyte hypertrophy
    Infiltrative processes (e.g., amyloidosis, hemochromatosis)
Endocardial disease
    Fibroelastosis
Pericardial disease
    Constriction
    Tamponade
Abnormal coronary circulation
    Capillary compression
    Venous engorgement
Other disease
    Volume overload of the right ventricle
    Extrinsic compression by tumor

Source: Ref. 8a

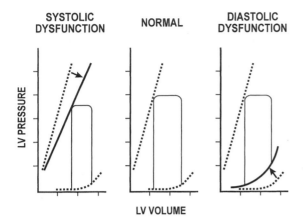

Figure 1 Diagram of left ventricular pressure-volume loops in systolic dysfunction and diastolic dysfunction. In systolic dysfunction, contractility is depressed and the end-systolic pressure-volume line is displaced downward and to the right; there is diminished capacity to eject blood into a high-pressure aorta. In diastolic dysfunction, chamber stiffness is increased and the diastolic pressure-volume relation is displaced up and to the left; there is diminished capacity to fill at low diastolic pressures. The left ventricular ejection fraction is low in systolic dysfunction and normal in diastolic dysfunction.

emphasis is on management of diastolic heart failure in which the dominant abnormality is in diastole.

In predominant diastolic heart failure, the left ventricle exhibits a limited ability to fill and LV diastolic pressures are abnormally elevated over the encountered normal physiological range of LV rest and/or exercise pressure-volume conditions. The ventricle is typically not enlarged and the ejection fraction at rest is normal or near normal. By contrast, in systolic failure the dominant abnormality is a defect in contractile function and the ventricle exhibits a limited ability to eject; the ventricle is generally enlarged and the ejection fraction is depressed. The differences and similarities between systolic and diastolic heart failure are compared and contrasted in Figure 1 and Table 2. Despite certain pathophysiological differences, patients with diastolic heart failure and those with systolic heart failure exhibit a similar reduction in exercise capacity and impairment in the quality of life [6]. Thus, morbidity is similar in systolic and diastolic heart failure, but long-term survival is generally better in patients with diastolic heart failure (Chapter 9).

DIAGNOSTIC CRITERIA

The clinical diagnosis of diastolic heart failure requires reliable evidence of CHF in a patient with a normal LV ejection fraction at rest. At the bedside, it is virtually impossible to differentiate patients with diastolic heart failure from patients with systolic heart failure (Table 3); echocardiographic (or other modality) confirmation of a normal ejection fraction at rest is mandatory for the diagnosis of diastolic heart failure. Plasma levels of brain natriuretic peptide (BNP) may be used to confirm the diagnosis of congestive heart failure, either systolic or diastolic [9]. Serum BNP levels have been shown to correlate with echocardiographically derived measures of diastolic dysfunction (e.g., impaired relaxation, "pseudonormalization," and restriction) [9] (Fig. 2). However, further study will be re-

Table 2 Differences and Similarities Between Systolic and Diastolic Heart Failure

	Systolic Heart Failure	Diastolic Heart Failure
Signs and Symptoms of HF	Present	Present
BNP	↑↑	↑
Exercise Testing		
Duration	↓	↓
Systolic BP	↑	↑↑
Pulse pressure	↑	↑↑
VO$_2$	↓↓	↓
LV Remodeling		
End-diastolic volume	↑↑	N
End-systolic volume	↑↑	N–↓
Myocardial mass	↑ (eccentric LVH)	↑ (concentric LVH)
Relative wall thickness	↓	↑↑
Cardiomyocyte	↑ length	↑ diameter
EC matrix (collagen)	↓	↑↑
LV Systolic Function		
Ejection fraction	↓↓	N–↑
Stroke volume	N–↓	N–↓
Myocardial contractility	↓↓	↓
LV Diastolic Function		
Chamber stiffness	N–↓	↑↑
Myocardial stiffness	N–↑	↑
Relaxation time-constant	↑–↑↑	↑–↑↑
Filling dynamics	Abnormal	Abnormal
End-diastolic pressure	↑↑	↑↑
Preload reserve	Exhausted	Limited
Morbidity (hosp/recurrent HF)	↑↑	↑↑
Survival	↓↓	↓

BNP, brain natriuretic peptide; BP, blood pressure; V0$_2$, peak oxygen consumption; EC, extracellular; LV, left ventricular.

quired before BNP levels can be recommended as a noninvasive method of differentiating systolic from diastolic heart failure.

At present, there is no consensus whether measurements of diastolic function are necessary in order to establish a diagnosis of diastolic heart failure. Some cardiologists propose cardiac catheterization or echocardiographic ''···evidence of abnormal LV relaxation, filling, diastolic distensibility or diastolic stiffness···'' [7] . Others rely only upon cardiac catheterization to document the presence of diastolic dysfunction before making a diagnosis of diastolic heart failure [3]. Still others propose that if valvular heart disease is excluded, virtually all patients with CHF and a normal LV ejection fraction exhibit diastolic dysfunction and that echocardiographic or other measurements of diastolic function are merely confirmatory [4]. In such instances, consideration must be given to other causes of heart failure with a normal ejection fraction (e.g., aortic or mitral valve disease, cor pulmonale, extremes of volume overload, etc.) [1].

In this chapter, *asymptomatic diastolic dysfunction* is defined as the presence of abnormal indices of diastolic function in patients with a normal ejection fraction and no cardiac symptoms. *Diastolic heart failure* is defined as the presence of signs and symptoms of CHF (often acute pulmonary edema) in the presence of a normal ejection fraction.

Table 3 Prevalence of Signs and Symptoms in Systolic and Diastolic Heart Failure

	Diastolic HF (LVEF > 50%)	Systolic HF (LVEF < 50%)
Symptoms		
Dyspnea on exertion	85%	96%
Paroxysmal nocturnal dyspnea	55%	50%
Orthopnea	60%	73%
Physical Examination		
Jugular venous distension	35%	46%
Rales	72%	70%
Displaced apical impulse	50%	60%
S3	45%	65%
S4	45%	66%
Hepatomegaly	15%	16%
Edema	30%	40%
Chest film		
Cardiomegaly	90%	96%
Pulmonary venous hypertension	75%	80%

Source: From Ref. 2.

Patients who remain symptomatic despite apparently successful treatment and resolution of congestion are referred to as having *chronic diastolic heart failure*.

MANAGEMENT

The recommendations presented in this chapter are based primarily on the results of small clinical studies, anecdotal experience, and an understanding of the pathophysiology of

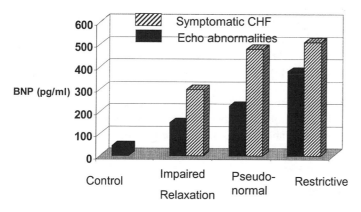

Figure 2 Progressive elevation in circulating brain natriuretic peptide levels is observed among patients with asymptomatic echocardiographic abnormalities. Each abnormal group was different from normal controls (p < 0.001). Higher levels are seen for patients who had symptomatic diastolic heart failure. The extent of diastolic dysfunction is based upon transmitral Doppler-flow parameters, which included impaired relaxation, pseudonormalization, and restrictive filling abnormalities. (From Ref. 9.)

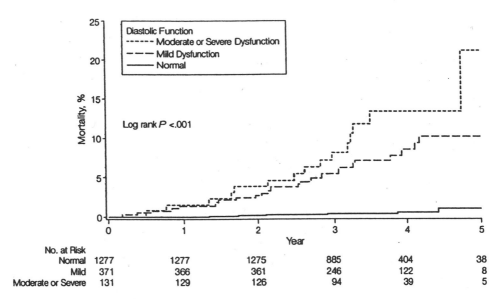

Figure 3 Kaplan-Meier mortality curves for subjects following in an community population study from Olmstead county who demonstrated normal diastolic function vs. those who had echocardiographic evidence for mild, moderate, or severe diastolic dysfunction. (From Ref. 8.)

diastole (Table 4). There is currently only one large placebo-controlled clinical trial that supports blockade of the renin-angiotensin-aldosterone system in patients with chronic diastolic heart failure [10] (see following text and Chapter 14).

Asymptomatic Diastolic Dysfunction

The prevalence of asymptomatic diastolic dysfunction is not known, but there is reason to believe that the condition is not rare–especially in patients with hypertension. The finding of diastolic dysfunction in an asymptomatic patient is a risk factor for the future development of CHF, and the early identification of such patients provides a window of opportunity to prevent progression of what appears to be "preclinical heart disease" [8,11] (Fig. 3). At present, there are no long-term data supporting effective pharmacological therapy directed primarily at the myocardial mechanisms resulting in diastolic dysfunction per se. Rather, the goal of chronic pharmacological therapy should be aggressive management of the preventable causes of diastolic dysfunction (e.g., hypertension) and similarly aggressive management of the modifiable factors that precipitate or exacubate diastolic heart failure [1].

Acute Diastolic Heart Failure

The initial management of acute diastolic heart failure and pulmonary edema consists of measures that relieve pulmonary congestion while maintaining oxygenation, arterial pressure, and perfusion of vital organs. With few exceptions the initial treatment of patients with diastolic heart failure is similar to that used in those with systolic heart failure. On presentation to the Emergency Department, the diagnosis of heart failure should be confirmed and associated or complicating problems should be considered and appropriately

Table 4 Management of Diastolic Heart Failure

INITIAL MANAGEMENT
Treat the Presenting Syndrome
    Pulmonary edema/congestive state
    Systemic arterial hypertension
    Acute myocardial ischemia
    Atrial fibrillation/flutter/sinus tachycardia
Clarify the Diagnosis
    History and physical examination
    Echocardiography
    Cardiac catheterization/angiography (when clinically
       necessary)
    Biopsy (rarely needed but can be useful in
       differentiating myocardial from pericardial disease)
LONG-TERM MANAGEMENT
Consider Mechanisms
    Promote regression of left ventricular hypertrophy
    Prevention/promotion of regression of interstitial
       fibrosis
    Modify cellular/extracellular mechanisms
Correct the pathophysiology
    Sodium restriction and diuretics
    Blockade of the renin-angiotensin aldosterone system
    Maintenance of atrial contraction and atrioventricular
       synchrony
    Prevention of excessive tachycardia
    Treatment of systemic hypertension
    Prevention of myocardial ischemia

excluded (e.g., pneumonia, myocardial infarction, pulmonary embolism, dissection of the aorta). At the same time, treatment should be initiated.

Treatments

    Oxygen. In most patients arterial hypoxemia can be reversed by oxygen administration with nasal prongs or a Venturi mask. If this is not effective, continuous positive airway pressure should be used. Endotracheal intubation may be required if arterial oxygenation cannot be maintained or if there is progressive hypercapnia.

    Morphine. This agent (administered intravenously in a dose of 3–5 mg. over several minutes) diminishes distress and the work of breathing. Morphine achieves its beneficial hemodynamic effects by acting as a vasodilator and, thereby, pooling blood in the splanchnic circulation. Special caution is necessary if the pulmonary edema is associated with hypotension, stroke, or independent pulmonary disease–especially in patients with hypercapnia.

    Preload Reduction. A decrease in left atrial and pulmonary venous pressure is obviously desirable in patients with acute pulmonary edema. In patients with LV systolic dysfunction and acute exacerbation of chronic heart failure (most of whom have an expanded central blood volume), a substantial reduction in pulmonary venous pressure can be achieved without a significant decline in arterial pressure. However, patients with diastolic heart failure may develop a substantial and sudden decrease in arterial pressure

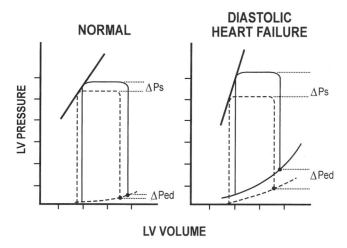

Figure 4   Effect of a reduction in central blood volume on LV pressure-volume loops in a normal heart (*left panel*) and in diastolic heart failure (*right panel*). The solid lines represent the baseline state and the broken lines represent the effects of preload reduction. In the normal heart a small reduction in LV end-diastolic volume results in a small decrease in end-diastolic pressure and a modest decrease in systolic pressure. By contrast, in diastolic heart failure, a similar decrease in LV end-diastolic volume results in a substantial decrease in diastolic pressure and a large decrease in systolic pressure. The result may be marked systemic hypotension. (From Ref. 8.)

when attempts are made to reduce preload acutely. This occurs as a consequence of: (a) the steep ventricular diastolic pressure-volume relation (and a preload or strain dependent change in compliance), and (b) a right ventricular and pericardial effect with a shift to a lower pressure-volume curve (i.e., a strain independent change) [12]. Thus, a small reduction in diastolic volume can result in relatively large reductions in LV diastolic pressure and arterial pressure (Fig. 4). Therefore, if there is reason to believe that diastolic heart failure is present, more conservative doses of diuretics, nitrates, or nesiritide should be considered than used in patients with systolic heart failure.

Diuretics are effective and commonly used in the initial treatment. Furosemide is administered intravenously at an initial dose of 40–80 mg; subsequent doses depend on the response to the initial dose. Intravenous nitroglycerine may also be used to reduce preload. The initial infusion rate is 10 micrograms/min and the rate may be increased to 300 micrograms/min to achieve the desired effect. Nitroglycerin has the advantage of being antiischemic and does not result in electrolyte abnormalities. Indeed, when treatments with nitrates, furosemide, and morphine are compared, optimal clinical outcomes are observed with nitrates [13]. One advantage of nitroglycerin is its rapid reversibility in the event that hypotension ensues. Rotating tourniquets also provide a rapidly reversible reduction in central venous pressures but are seldom necessary in the current era. Nesiritide produces a dose-dependent decrease in pulmonary capillary wedge pressure and systemic vascular resistance, and an increase in cardiac output; it is administered as a continuous intravenous infusion (dose: 0.015–0.06 mg/kg/min) after a bolus (0.25–1.0 mg/kg/min). Although useful in decompensated systolic heart failure, there is very little experience with this agent in diastolic heart failure and no controlled trials have examined it safety or efficacy.

Afterload Reduction.   Many, but not all, patients with acute pulmonary edema and diastolic heart failure are hypertensive [14]. While nitroglycerin or nesiritide are both effective in reducing blood pressure and relieving pulmonary edema, sodium nitroprusside is the vasodilator of choice when a *substantial* reduction in pressure is required. It is administered by intravenous infusion at an initial dose of 10–25 mg/min; the dose is adjusted to obtain the desired hemodynamic effects. Sodium nitroprusside is used only in situations requiring short-term therapy; early arrangements should be made to substitute other intravenous or oral antihypertensive agents.

Long-Term Management

Any long-term therapeutic pharmacologic program must be based on a careful consideration of the putative cause or causes of diastolic dysfunction in the individual patient and the potential individualized response to and benefit of treatment. For example, verapamil may be effective in symptomatic patients who have hypertrophic cardiomyopathy [15], but is contraindicated in patients who have cardiac amyloidosis [16]. Coronary artery disease, hypertensive heart disease, chronic constrictive pericarditis, and aortic stenosis provide relatively specific surgical and/or pharmacologic therapeutic targets, but the most commonly encountered clinical entity, namely diastolic heart failure in the elderly, often affords less specific targets in a more challenging and fragile population [17]. In general, emphasis is placed on control of arterial hypertension and intravascular volume, prevention of myocardial ischemia, management of the congestive state, and maintenance of normal sinus rhythm. (Table 3)

Given the paucity of clinical trials in diastolic heart failure to date, there are few ''evidence-based'' recommendations regarding chronic pharmacologic therapy, including the selection, optimal dosing, and duration of therapy for nearly all pharmacologic agents. The chronic pharmacologic treatment of diastolic heart failure is under investigation in several large randomized clinical studies; the design of these trials are summarized elsewhere [1]. One large trial of an angiotensin-receptor blocking agent has been completed to date and provides data that supports the use of these agents in diastolic heart failure [10]. In the Candesartan in Heart Failure: Assessment of Reduction in Mortality and Morbidity (CHARM)–Preserved Trial, the effects of the angiotensin-receptor type 1 blocker, candesartan, was studied in 3023 patients with clinical evidence of heart failure and an ejection fraction greater than 40% [10]. After 6 months, two-thirds of the patients were taking the target dose of 32 mg of candesartan once daily. After 3 years of treatment, no reduction in cardiovascular mortality was observed; however, candesartan treatment resulted in a significant reduction in hospitalizations for heart failure (Chapter 14). These results, especially when viewed in the context of the overall CHARM program [18], support the use of chronic, high-dose candesartan to reduce morbidity, especially hospitalization, in patients with diastolic heart failure. At present, it is unclear if this benefit extends to other angiotensin-receptor type 1 blocking agents. There have been no large scale clinical trials of angiotensin converting enzyme inhibitors, beta-blockers, diuretics, nitrates, calcium channel blockers, digoxin or aldosterone antagonists completed to date in patients with diastolic heart failure.

Specific Therapeutic Targets

Venous Congestion. The renin-angiotensin-aldosterone system is activated in patients who have chronic diastolic heart failure [6], but the mechanisms that evoke its activation remain unclear in patients who have LV diastolic dysfunction. In some, myocardial ischemia, uncontrolled hypertension, and excessive dietary sodium may promote to the development of congestion, while in others, low systemic vascular resistance or low arterial pressure may contribute to salt and water retention [19]. Despite a limited understanding of the pathogenesis of salt and water retention in patients with diastolic dysfunction, diuretics remain the mainstay of therapy for venous congestion.

After treatment of the presenting syndrome, salt restriction is necessary and long-term administration of a diuretic is usually required. By reducing the central blood volume and lowering ventricular diastolic pressures, these agents alleviate congestive symptoms. The potential for diuretics to reduce cardiac output, especially in patients with small LV chambers and preserved ejection fraction at rest, must be considered and overdosing should be avoided. With the exception of their antihypertensive effects (and possibly by promoting subendocardial blood flow by lowering the LV diastolic pressure), diuretics do not alter the primary disease processes that lead to diastolic dysfunction.

Thiazide diuretics may suffice for management of mild heart failure, but the adverse effects of glucose intolerance, hypokalemia, hyperuricemia and hyponatremia (the latter especially in fragile elderly patients) can be undesirable. Loop diuretics, such as furosemide, are more potent than the thiazide diuretics, especially when the glomerular filtration rate is reduced. The combination of furosemide and a thiazide diuretic can be especially useful when edema is refractory to either agent alone. For patients who develop hypokalemia, the potassium-sparing diuretic spironolactone may be added. Spironolactone also has the potential to retard the fibrosis that contributes to abnormal chamber stiffness, although there is no compelling evidence to date that this effect is realized in any clinically significant way. As stated, the effects of spironolactone on survival in diastolic heart failure have not been prospectively studied to date.

The reduction in blood volume by diuretics triggers an increase in sympathetic tone and intensification of renin-angiotensin activation, which can lead to further vasoconstriction and worsening of the congestive state. Some vasodilators, particularly nitrates and pure arteriolar vasodilators, evoke a similar response. ACE inhibitors, angiotensin-receptor blockers, and beta-adrenergic blockers blunt this neurohormonal activation and decrease the salt and water retention that complicates heart failure treatment. In addition, these agents may also have salutary effects on the active and passive properties of the left ventricle. If hypotension does not limit their use, ACE inhibitors can, at the very least, provide useful adjunctive therapy in patients with diastolic dysfunction, particularly those with evidence of a chronic congestive state. Since neurohormonal activation occurs in patients with diastolic heart failure, albeit at a lesser degree of intensity than in patients with systolic heart failure, some experts have anecdotally recommended empiric application of the consensus guidelines for stepwise pharmacologic therapy of systolic heart failure in patients with diastolic heart failure. Although unproven to date, the application of such stepwise neurohormonal antagonism may forestall remodeling and other aspects of disease progression in patients with diastolic heart failure.

Atrial Arrhythmias.   Atrial fibrillation in patients with LV diastolic dysfunction is usually accompanied by a substantial increase in ventricular diastolic and atrial filling pressures that may lead to pulmonary edema and hypotension. Overt decompensation occurs partly because of inadequate time for complete ventricular relaxation and partly because of the loss of organized atrial systole and its substantial contribution to ventricular filling. An attempt to restore and maintain sinus rhythm is mandatory. Direct current cardioversion may be required on an emergency basis. In less urgent situations, electrical or chemical cardioversion can be performed after rate control with beta-blockers, calcium channel blockers, or digitalis. Sinus rhythm is rarely restored when atrial fibrillation complicates diastolic heart failure due to cardiac amyloidosis. Even if sinus rhythm is restored, patients with advanced cardiac amyloidosis may exhibit impaired atrial systolic contraction.

Rate control. Excessive tachycardia is poorly tolerated in diastolic heart failure. Atrial tachyarrhythmias and even sinus tachycardia have a negative impact on diastolic function for several reasons. A rapid heart rate causes an increase in myocardial oxygen demand and decrease in coronary perfusion time that can promote ischemic diastolic dysfunction even in the absence of coronary artery disease. In addition, tachycardia does not allow sufficient time for ventricular relaxation and, as a result, there is incomplete relaxation between beats, which causes an increase in diastolic pressure relative to volume. Tachycardia also reduces the diastolic filling time, which may limit ventricular filling. Accordingly, most clinicians use beta-blockers or calcium channel blockers to prevent excessive tachycardia and produce a relative bradycardia in patients who have diastolic dysfunction. It should be recognized, however, that excessive or inappropriate bradycardia can result in a fall in cardiac output despite some potential for improved filling pressures. Such considerations underscore the need for individualizing therapeutic interventions that affect heart rate.

The optimal target heart rate at rest and during exercise in diastolic heart failure is not known, but it is likely that hearts evidencing diastolic heart failure would function most efficiently at relatively slow rates. A relative bradycardia has several potentially beneficial effects that are largely related to the salutary effects on myocardial energetics and the prolonged diastolic interval that allows complete relaxation between beats. Furthermore, hypertrophied and failing hearts exhibit a flat or even negative force-frequency relationship, and in contrast to normal hearts, function may improve as the rate is slowed [20,21]. Attempts to control heart rates must be individualized, but an initial goal should be a resting rate of approximately 65 to 70 bpm with a blunted exercise-induced increase in heart rate. Most beta-blockers and some calcium channel blockers exert a substantial negative chronotropic effect, but the use of such agents can be limited by hypotension or other side effects. These agents actually exert *negative* lusitropic effects; their putative benefit in diastolic heart failure is principally through control of heart rate and blood pressure (see previous text).

Myocardial Ischemia. Extensive clinical and experimental literature documents the deleterious effect of intermittent or chronic myocardial ischemia on diastolic function of the left ventricle. A transient increase in LV stiffness and diastolic pressure develops during myocardial ischemia caused by coronary spasm, exercise, rapid atrial pacing, angioplasty balloon inflation, and spontaneous angina [22]. Ischemia can be treated with nitrates, beta-blockers, and calcium channel blockers, percutaneous coronary intervention, or coronary artery bypass surgery. When the signs and symptoms of ischemic diastolic dysfunction are prominent, coronary revascularization should be considered when favorable coronary artery anatomy is delineated on coronary angiography [23]. Nonetheless, signs and symptoms of heart failure may persist despite successful revascularization due to chronic residual abnormalities of myocardial function.

Hypertension and Hypertrophy. Several factors contribute to the diastolic dysfunction seen in hypertensive heart disease, especially hypertensive hypertrophic cardiomyopathy of the elderly [17,24]. First, the abnormal loading conditions imposed by arterial hypertension reduce LV relaxation and filling rates. Second, concentrically hypertrophied hearts exhibit increased passive stiffness (caused by a low LV volume–mass ratio and fibrosis of the myocardium) and impaired relaxation that is independent of hemodynamic loads. Third, limited coronary vascular reserve can be responsible for myocardial ischemia, even in the absence of epicardial coronary disease. Each of these factors should be considered in the treatment of patients with hypertensive heart disease and diastolic dysfunction. Abnormalities of diastolic function can be detected in asymptomatic hypertensive patients with or without measurable ventricular hypertrophy [25]. Adequate control of the arterial pressure in these patients with preclinical heart disease should favorably alter loading conditions in the short term, while promoting regression of hypertrophy.

Although the short-term treatment of elevated systemic arterial pressure tends to augment diastolic function, the effect of load reduction is difficult to demonstrate during long-term therapy; indeed, there is considerable variation in the effects of different antihypertensive agents on myocardial relaxation. For example, despite an equivalent reduction in arterial pressure, nifedipine augments LV filling rate and other relaxation indices, but propranolol does not [26]. Some studies of patients who have hypertensive heart disease indicate that diastolic dysfunction improves as LV hypertrophy regresses [27,28]. Other studies have confirmed improved diastolic function, prolonged exercise duration, and better heart failure scores in verapamil-treated patients who have hypertensive heart disease and clinically significant LV diastolic dysfunction, but these clinical benefits were not closely related to changes in blood pressure or heart rate [29]. Differences in the effects of treatment on diastolic function probably depend on the amount of hypertrophy regression, the alterations in LV loading conditions, the direct myocardial effect of the antihypertensive agent, and possibly changes in coronary flow reserve.

Progressive interstitial fibrosis accompanies the hypertrophic response to arterial hypertension; fibrosis can also be prominent in the hypertrophy seen with aortic stenosis and hypertrophic cardiomyopathy. This abnormal accumulation of fibrillar collagen is a result of enhanced collagen synthesis by cardiac fibroblasts that is partially related to the activity of the renin-angiotensin-aldosterone system. The important functional consequences of progressive interstitial and perivascular fibrosis include increased myocardial stiffness and impaired coronary flow reserve. In experimental studies, ACE inhibitors or spironolactone appears to protect against this exaggerated fibrous tissue response [30]. In hypertensive patients, ACE-inhibitor therapy has been shown to result in regression of myocardial fibrosis and improvement in diastolic function; these improvements were not closely related to changes in left ventricular mass [31]. Thus, the imperative to aggressively treat arterial hypertension includes prevention of the deleterious effects of elevated levels of angiotensin II and aldosterone. ACE inhibitors and angiotensin-receptor blockers are widely used and effective antihypertensive agents that can produce regression of LV hypertrophy and a salutary effect on cardiac fibrosis.

Hypertrophic Cardiomyopathy and Relaxation.   Although hypertrophic cardiomyopathy (HCM) is a unique entity, diastolic dysfunction is a most important component of its pathophysiology; thus, it may provide additional insight into the more general problem of diastolic dysfunction. The diastolic dysfunction of HCM is caused by increased passive stiffness of the ventricle, (due to a low LV volume–mass ratio, fibrosis, and fiber disarray) and abnormal myocardial relaxation (due to abnormal calcium metabolism, altered loading conditions and nonuniformity) [32].

As a result of depressed calcium sequestration by the sarcoplasmic reticulum and perhaps an increase in membrane calcium channels, myocardial calcium overload contributes to a slow or delayed myocardial relaxation (a slow and prolonged dissociation of actin-myosin), which leads to increased diastolic tension [33]. Such prolonged relaxation can persist throughout the entire diastolic interval, especially in the presence of tachycardia. Assuming that the alterations in passive stiffness are relatively fixed and irreversible (which may not be true), medical therapy has generally been directed toward the relaxation abnormalities and control of myocardial loads.

The calcium channel blockers (verapamil, diltiazem, and nifedipine) can improve many of the abnormal indices of relaxation and provide symptomatic relief [33]. Verapamil, the most widely used calcium channel blocker in hypertrophic cardiomyopathy, has a beneficial effect on angina and dyspnea; it also improves exercise capacity [15].

Therapy is initiated at a low dosage (120–240mg per day) and gradually increased to 360–480mg per day; the optimal dose is determined by the symptomatic response of the patient. Unfortunately, the vasodilating effects of calcium channel blockers can lead unpredictably to intensification of an outflow obstruction or hypotension even in the absence of obstruction.

Although beta-blockers do not directly augment ventricular relaxation rate, they are commonly used in patients who have hypertrophic cardiomyopathy. Angina, dyspnea, and presyncopal symptoms tend to improve during treatment. Angina seems to respond more favorably than dyspnea. Thus, treatment with metoprolol may be initiated at 25 to 50 mg twice a day; the dose is then gradually increased to 100 to 200 mg depending on the clinical response. Some patients require higher doses to achieve a beneficial effect on exercise capacity and symptoms.

Exercise Intolerance. Patients who have a history of diastolic heart failure (as well as those who have diastolic dysfunction and little or no congestion) exhibit exercise intolerance that has two major causes. First, elevated LV diastolic, left atrial, and pulmonary venous filling pressures cause a reduction in lung compliance that increases the work of breathing and evokes the symptom of dyspnea. Increased LV diastolic pressures during exercise may also limit subendocardial blood flow during periods of increased myocardial oxygen demand, further worsening diastolic function. Second, an inadequate cardiac output during exercise contributes to fatigue of the skeletal muscles and the accessory muscles of respiration. However, neither of these pathophysiological mechanisms provides a complete explanation for substantial exercise intolerance observed in many of these patients with heart failure [34]. Given the limited understanding of the precise factors responsible for dyspnea and fatigue, it has been difficult to develop a standardized treatment plan for patients with chronic diastolic heart failure. Certainly, hypertension, myocardial ischemia, and clinically apparent congestion must be treated, but caution must be exercised to avoid even mild volume depletion that can contribute to a reduced cardiac output.

A most important (and largely ignored) treatment should be directed against the physical deconditioning that is prominent in many patients with diastolic heart failure. Cardiac rehabilitation programs can be very helpful in improving symptoms and functional capacity but have not been shown to favorably alter prognosis [35].

Although calcium channel blockers and beta-blockers improve symptoms in some patients with LV diastolic dysfunction, the benefit on exercise capacity is not always paralleled by improved measures of LV diastolic function. For example, in symptomatic patients who have hypertrophic cardiomyopathy, a placebo-controlled, double-blind comparison of the effects of verapamil and propranolol on exercise tolerance indicated that both agents produced an increase in exercise duration; however, relaxation rate increased with verapamil and decreased with propranolol treatment [36]. The observation that verapamil effects persisted in the long-term [15], and can be effective in relieving symptoms in patients who have other causes of diastolic dysfunction [29] has made this agent a treatment of choice for exercise intolerance. Beta-blockers remain an acceptable alternative. Despite their direct depressant effects on myocardial relaxation, these agents can sometimes improve exercise tolerance.

ACE inhibitors or angiotensin II-receptor blocking agents also have the potential to improve exercise tolerance in patients who have diastolic dysfunction. Treatment with losartan has been shown to produce an increase in exercise capacity and to improve quality of life in patients who have hypertensive cardiovascular disease and documented diastolic dysfunction [37]. These responses are similar to those reported for patients treated with verapamil [29]. The salutary effects of losartan and verapamil are, at least in part, related to their antihypertensive effect.

Positive Inotropic Drugs

Positive inotropic agents are generally not used in the long-term treatment of patients with diastolic heart failure because the ejection fraction is preserved and there is little potential for an acute or chronic beneficial effect. Such agents also carry substantial risk, especially in the typical elderly patient with acutely decompensated diastolic heart failure. Anecdotally, positive inotropic agents may have a short-term beneficial effect in a very small number of acutely or severely ill patients, particularly those with advanced restrictive cardiomyopathies, perhaps by primarily redistributing a limited cardiac output to hypoperfused vital circulatory beds rather than increasing total cardiac output. However, virtually all positive inotropic agents have the potential to worsen the pathophysiological processes that cause more typical diastolic dysfunction in patients without advanced restrictive cardiomyopathies. For example, digitalis, by inhibiting the sodium-potassium adenosine triphosphatase pump, augments intracellular calcium through a sodium-calcium exchange mechanism and enhances the contractile state. By doing so, digitalis produces an increase in systolic energy demands while adding to a diastolic calcium overload. These effects may not be clinically apparent in many circumstances, but during hemodynamic stress or ischemia, digitalis may promote or contribute to diastolic dysfunction [38]. Data from the DIG (Digitalis Investigators Group) study, however, suggest that digitalis might have a modest beneficial effect, despite a normal LVEF on some clinical outcome measures, such as heart failure hospitalizations [39]. However, this trial also reported a corresponding increase in endpoints related to myocardial ischemia and ventricular arrhythmias during digoxin administration. Recognizing conflicting opinions on this issue, most clinicians do not use digitalis in patients with diastolic heart failure.

Beta-adrenergic agonists, by increasing intracellular cyclic adenosine monophosphate, enhance calcium sequestration by the sarcoplasmic reticulum and promote a more rapid and complete myocardial relaxation between beats [40]. Beta-agonists can also increase venous capacitance, which leads to a reduction in ventricular filling pressures. Phosphodiesterase inhibitors can produce similar salutary effects on myocardial relaxation and venous capacitance [41]. Unfortunately, all cyclic adenosine monophosphate-dependent agents promote calcium influx into the cell and augment myocardial energy demands. Thus, milrinone, enoximone, and similar agents should be used only in the short-term management of acute, severely decompensated diastolic heart failure. As is the case with the use of any positive inotropic agent in patients with heart disease, the therapeutic risk-benefit ratio must be considered in detail, and such agents must be used with appropriate caution and acknowledgement of their risk. As stated, the patients most likely to benefit are those rare patients with advanced or end-stage restrictive cardiomyopathies. In the absence of advanced restrictive cardiomyopathy, the typical patient with hypertensive or age-dependent diastolic heart failure is unlikely to benefit either acutely or chronically from inotropic therapy compared with more conventional therapies. The routine use of positive inotropic agents in patients with acute or chronic diastolic heart failure is not recommended.

SUMMARY

The management of diastolic heart failure has two major objectives. The first is to reverse the consequences of diastolic dysfunction (e.g., venous congestion and exercise intolerance). The second is to eliminate or reduce the factors responsible for diastolic dysfunction (e.g., ischemia, hypertrophy, and fibrosis). Thus, the long-term management of patients with diastolic heart failure includes salt restriction, a diuretic, and inhibition of the renin-angiotensin-aldosterone system. In selected patients, beta-adrenergic blocking agents, calcium channel blocking agents and antiischemic therapies can be beneficial. Randomized clinical trials are needed to assess the efficacy and optimal dosage of pharmacological therapy in diastolic heart failure.

REFERENCES

1. Gaasch WH, Zile MR. Left ventricular diastolic dysfunction and diastolic heart failure. Ann Rev Med 2004; 55:08.1–08.22.
2. Zile MR, Brutsaert DL. New concepts in diastolic dysfunction and heart failure: Part II: causal mechanisms and treatment. Circulation 2002; 105:1503–1508.
3. Vasan RS, Levy D. Defining diastolic heart failure: a call for standardized diagnostic criteria. Circulation 2000; 101:2118–2121.
4. Zile MR, Gaasch WH, Carroll JD, Feldman MD, Aurigemma GP, Schaer GL, Ghali JK, Liebson PR. Heart failure with a normal ejection fraction: is measurement of diastolic function necessary to make the diagnosis of diastolic heart failure? Circulation 2001; 104:779–782.
5. Gaasch WH. Diagnosis and treatment of heart failure based on left ventricular systolic or diastolic dysfunction. JAMA 1994; 271:1276-1280.
6. Kitzman DW, Little WC, Brubaker PH, Hundley WG, Marburger CT, Brosnihan B, Morgan TM, Stewart KP. Pathophysiological characterization of isolated diastolic heart failure in comparison to systolic heart failure. JAMA 2002; 288:2144–2150.
7. Paulus WJ. and the European Study Group on Diastolic Heart Failure. How to diagnose diastolic heart failure. Eur Heart J 1998; 19:990–1003.
8. Redfield MM, Jacobsen SJ, Burnett JC, Mahoney DW, Bailey KR, Rodeheffer RJ. Burden of systolic and diastolic ventricular dysfunction in the community. JAMA 2003; 289:194–202.
8a. Angeja BG, Grossman W. Evaluation and management of diastolic heart failure. Circulation 2003; 107:659–63.
9. Lubien E, DeMaria A, Krishnaswamy P, Clopton P, Koon J, Kazanegra R, Gardetto N, Wanner E, Maisel AS. Utility of B-natriuretic peptide in detecting diastolic dysfunction: comparison with Doppler velocity recordings. Circulation 2002; 105(5):595–601.
10. Yusuf S, Pfeffer MA, Swedberg K, Granger CB, Held P, McMurray JJV, Michelson EL, Olofsson B, Ostergren J. Effects of candesartan in patients with chronic heart failure and preserved left ventricular ejection fraction: the CHARM-Preserved Trial. Lancet 2003; 362: 777–781.
11. Aurigemma GP, Gottdiener JS, Shemanski L, Gardin J, Kitzman D. Predictive valve of systolic and diastolic function for incident congestive heart failure in the elderly: the cardiovascular health study. Am J Coll Cardiol 2001; 37:1042–1048.
12. Smith ER, Smiseth OA, Kingma I, Manyari D, Belenkie I, Tyberg JV. Mechanism of action of nitrates: role of changes in venous capacitance and in the left ventricular diastolic pressure-volume relation. Am J Med 1984; 76(6A):14–21.
13. Hoffmann JR, Reynolds S. Comparison of nitroglycerine, morphine, and furosemide in treatment of presumed pre-hospital pulmonary edema. Chest 1987; 92(4):586–593.
14. Gandhi SK, Powers JC, Nomeier AM, Fowle K, Kitzman DW, Rankin KM, Little WC. The pathogenesis of acute pulmonary edema associated with hypertension. N Engl J Med 2001; 344:17–22.
15. Bonow RO, Dilsizian V, Rosing DR, Maron BJ, Bacharach SL, Green MV. Verapamil-induced improvement in left ventricular filling and increased exercise tolerance in patients with hypertrophic cardiomyopathy: short and long term results. Circulation 1985; 72:853–864.
16. Pollak A, Falk RH. Left ventricular systolic dysfunction precipitated by verapamil in cardiac amyloidosis. Chest 1993; 104:618–622.
17. Topol EJ, Traill TA, Fortuin NJ. Hypertensive hypertrophic cardiomyopathy of the elderly. N Engl J Med 1985; 312:277–283.

18. Pfeffer MA, Swedberg K, Granger CB, Held P, McMurray JJV, Michelson EL, Olofsson B, Ostergren J, Yusuf S. Effects of candesartan on mortality and morbidity in patients with chronic heart failure: the CHARM-Overall Program. Lancet 2003; 362:759–766.

19. Anand IS, Chandrashekhar Y, Ferrari R, Sarma R, Guleria R, Jindal SK, Wahi PL, Poole-Wilson PA, Harris P. Pathogenesis of congestive state in chronic obstructive pulmonary disease: studies of body water and sodium, renal function, hemodynamics and plasma hormones during edema and after recovery. Circulation 1992; 86:12–21.

20. Liu CP, Ting CT, Lawrence W, Maughan WL, Chang MS, Kass DA. Diminished contractile response to increased heart rate in intact human left ventricular hypertrophy: systolic versus diastolic determinants. Circulation 1993; 88:1893–1906.

21. Mulieri LA, Hasenfuss G, Leavitt B, Allen PD, Alpert NR. Altered myocardial force–frequency relation in human heart failure. Circulation 1992; 85:1743–1750.

22. Paulus WJ, Bronzwaer JGF, de Bruyne B, Grossman W. Different effects of 'supply' and 'demand' ischemia on left ventricular diastolic function in humans. In: Gaasch WH, LeWinter MM, Eds. Left Ventricular Diastolic Dysfunction and Heart Failure. Philadelphia: Lea and Febiger, 1994:286–305.

23. Kunis R, Greenberg H, Yeoh CG, Garfein OB, Pepe AJ, Pinkemall BH, Sherrid MV, Dwyer EM. Coronary revascularization for recurrent pulmonary edema in elderly patients with ischemic heart disease and preserved ventricular function. N Engl J Med 1985; 313:1207–1210.

24. Hoit BD, Walsh RA. Diastolic function in hypertensive heart disease. In: Gaasch WH, LeWinter MM, Eds. Left Ventricular Diastolic Dysfunction and Heart Failure. 1994. Philadelphia: Lea and Febiger:354–372.

25. Inouye I, Massie B, Loge D, Topic N, Silverstein D, Simpson P, Tubau J. Abnormal left ventricular filling: an early finding in mild to moderate systemic hypertension. Am J Cardiol 1984; 53:120–126.

26. Zusman RM. Nifedipine but not propranolol improves left ventricular systolic and diastolic function in patients with hypertension. Am J Cardiol 1989; 64:51F–61F.

27. Smith VE, White WB, Meeran MK, Karimeddini MK. Improved left ventricular filling accompanies reduced left ventricular mass during therapy of essential hypertension. J Am Coll Cardiol 1986; 8:1449–1454.

28. Schulman SP, Weiss JL, Becker LC, Gottlieb SO, Woodruff KM, Weisfeldt ML, Gerstenblith G. The effects of antihypertensive therapy on left ventricular mass in elderly patients. N Engl J Med 1990; 322:1350–1356.

29. Setaro JF, Zaret BL, Schulman DS, Black HR, Soufer R. Usefulness of verapamil for congestive heart failure associated with abnormal left ventricular diastolic filling and normal left ventricular systolic performance. Am J Cardiol 1990; 66:981–986.

30. Weber KT, Brilla CG. Pathological hypertrophy and cardiac interstitium: fibrosis and renin–angiotensin–aldosterone system. Circulation 1991; 83:1849–1865.

31. Brilla CG, Reinhard RC, Rupp H. Lisinopril mediated regression of myocardial fibrosis in patients with hypertensive heart disease. Circulation 2000; 102:1388–1393.

32. Wigle ED, Sasson Z, Henderson MA, Ruddy TD, Fulop J, Rakowski H, Williams WG. Hypertrophic cardiomyopathy: the importance of the site and the extent of hypertrophy. Prog Cardiovasc Dis 1985; 28:1–83.

33. Udelson JE, Bonow RO. Left ventricular diastolic function and calcium channel blockers in hypertrophic cardiomyopathy. In: Gaasch WH, LeWinter MM, Eds. Left Ventricular Diastolic Dysfunction and Heart Failure. 1994. Philadelphia: Lea and Febiger:465–489.

34. Chikamori T, Counihan PJ, Doi YL, Takata J, Stewart JT, Frenneaux MP, McKenna WJ. Mechanisms of exercise limitation in hypertrophic cardiomyopathy. J Am Coll Cardiol 1992; 19:507–512.

35. Kitzman DW, Brubaker PH, Anderson RA, Morgan T, Miller HS, Stewart KP, Ettinger SW, Hundley WG. Exercise training improves aerobic capacity in elderly patients with diastolic heart failure: a randomized, controlled trial. Circulation 1999; 100:I-296.

36. Rosing DR, Kent KM, Maron BJ, Epstein SE. Verapamil therapy: a new approach to the pharmacologic treatment of hypertrophic cardiomyopathy. II. effects on exercise capacity and symptomatic status. Circulation 1979; 60:1208–1213.

37. Warner JG, Metzger DC, Kitzman DW, Wesley DJ, Little WC. Losartan improves exercise tolerance in patients with diastolic dysfunction and a hypertensive response to exercise. J Am Coll Cardiol 1999; 33:1567–1572.

38. Lorell BH, Isoyama S, Grice WN, Weinberg EO, Apstein CS. Effects of ouabain and isoproterenol on left ventricular diastolic function during low-flow ischemia in isolated, blood-perfused rabbit hearts. Circ Res 1988; 63:457–467.

39. Massie BM, Abdalla I. Heart failure in patients with preserved left ventricular systolic function: do digitalis glycosides have a role?. Prog Cardiovasc Dis 1998; 40:357–369.

40. Lang RM, Carroll JD, Nakamura S, Itoh H, Rajfer SI. Role of adrenoceptors and dopamine receptors in modulating left ventricular diastolic function. Circ Res 1988; 63:126–134.

41. Monrad ES, McKay R, Baim DS, Colucci WS, Fifer MA, Heller GV, Royal HD. Improvement in indexes of diastolic performance in patients with congestive heart failure treated with milrinone. Circulation 1984; 70:1030–1037.

18

Cardiac Resynchronization Therapy

William T. Abraham
The Davis Heart and Lung Research Institute, The Ohio State University
Columbus, Ohio, USA

INTRODUCTION

Electrophysiological disturbances are common in the setting of chronic left ventricular dysfunction with or without heart failure. Approximately one-third of patients with systolic heart failure have a QRS duration greater than 120 millisecond, which is most commonly manifested as left bundle branch block [1,2]. Such electrical disturbances result in left ventricular (i.e., *intra*ventricular) dyssynchrony with paradoxical septal wall motion, which further impairs the pumping ability of an already struggling heart [3–6]. In particular, left ventricular dyssynchrony causes suboptimal ventricular filling, prolonged duration of mitral regurgitation, and a reduction in left ventricular pressure development (dP/dt). *Inter*ventricular dyssynchrony also occurs in the setting of bundle branch block, adversely affecting the timing of left and right ventricular ejection. Ventricular dyssynchrony, defined electrocardiographically by a prolonged QRS duration, has been associated with increased mortality in heart failure patients [7–10].

Despite equivocal results from early attempts to use right-sided, dual chamber pacing to treat advanced systolic heart failure [11–16], atrial-synchronized biventricular pacing has proved useful in the management of certain patients with chronic systolic heart failure and ventricular dyssynchrony. This form of pacing therapy is now referred to as cardiac resynchronization therapy. The development of cardiac resynchronization therapy for the treatment of heart failure has progressed rapidly over the past several years. Early studies provided proof of concept, supporting the benefit of biventricular pacing in heart failure, via mechanistic, short-term, and longer-term observational studies [5,6,17–25]. Cazeau and colleagues [17] performed the first application of atrial-synchronized biventricular pacing by using four chamber pacing in a 54-year-old man with NYHA (New York Heart Association) class IV heart failure and significant conduction disturbances (QRS duration of 200 milliseconds, PR interval of 200 milliseconds, and an interatrial conduction interval of 90 milliseconds). After placing standard transvenous pacing leads in the right atrium and right ventricle, the left atrium was paced by a lead placed in the coronary sinus, while the left ventricle was paced by an epicardial lead located on the left ventricular free wall. After 6 weeks of pacing, the patient experienced a marked improvement in his clinical status with a weight loss of 17 kg and a disappearance of peripheral edema. His functional class improved to NYHA class II.

Such favorable anecdotal experiences lead to small studies evaluating the acute hemodynamic effects of biventricular pacing. Positive results were achieved in studies by Foster and colleagues [18] and Saxon and associates [5], who evaluated the effects of temporary epicardial, atrial-synchronized biventricular pacing in postoperative cardiac surgery patients with reduced left ventricular function. Overall, patients demonstrated acute improvements in cardiac hemodynamic performance. The consequences of the acute and longer-term effects of biventricular pacing in heart failure were evaluated soon after and were equally encouraging, with patients showing consistent, often sustained, improvement in exercise tolerance, NYHA functional class, and cardiac output [19–25].

The first randomized controlled trials designed to evaluate the effects of cardiac resynchronization therapy on quality of life, functional status, and exercise capacity were begun in 1998–1999 [26–35]. These trials affirmed that cardiac resynchronization therapy was safe and clinically effective in heart failure patients. In addition, cardiac resynchronization therapy was shown to improve left ventricular size and function. Finally, randomized controlled trials to assess the effects of cardiac resynchronization therapy on morbidity and mortality were initiated, starting in 2000 [36–38]. The first of these trials reported demonstrated improved morbidity as well as reduced mortality for patients with moderate-to-severe heart failure [37]. This study showed that the addition of defibrillation therapies in conjunction with cardiac resynchronization further improved patient outcomes.

The mechanisms of action and proven clinical benefits of cardiac resynchronization therapy are reviewed in this chapter. In addition, recommendations for patient selection based on the results of randomized controlled trials are made, to encourage the evidence-based application of cardiac resynchronization in heart failure patients.

MECHANISMS OF ACTION

Early studies of biventricular pacing provided important insight into the mechanisms of action of cardiac resynchronization therapy through electrocardiographic and echocardiographic data. The hemodynamic improvement seen with cardiac resynchronization therapy is related to its ability to increase left ventricular filling time, decrease septal dyskinesis, and reduce mitral regurgitation or the deleterious effects of ventricular dyssynchrony in the failing heart. Over time, these effects of resynchronization therapy result in improvements in ventricular geometry and function, compatible with reverse remodeling of the heart. Other mechanisms, as yet undetermined, may contribute to the clinical benefits of cardiac resynchronization therapy.

Increased Left Ventricular Filling Time

In the presence of a long AV (atrioventricular) delay and/or an interventricular conduction delay (IVCD), left ventricular activation is delayed, but atrial activation is not. Hence, both early passive left ventricular filling and the atrial ''kick'' may occur simultaneously, resulting in deceased total transmitral blood flow and diminished preloading of the left ventricle [39]. These events are often seen as a fusion of the E and A waves on Doppler echocardiogram of transmitral blood flow. With atrial-synchronized biventricular pacing, both ventricles are activated simultaneously; thus, the left ventricle is able to complete contraction and begin relaxation earlier, which increases filling time. The effect of cardiac resynchronization can be seen by the return of normal E and A wave separation on Doppler echocardiogram of transmitral blood flow.

Decreased Septal Dyskinesis

Although left ventricular activation and contraction are delayed in the presence of an IVCD, septal activation and contraction are not. This timing mismatch results in septal dyskinesis or paradoxical septal wall motion, as the septum moves away from the left ventricular free wall during systole. This paradoxical septal wall motion impairs mitral valve function, thereby increasing mitral regurgitation and reducing the septum's contribution to left ventricular stroke volume [40]. With cardiac resynchronization therapy, the ventricles are activated simultaneously, thus improving ventricular contraction pattern by allowing left ventricular ejection to occur prior to relaxation of the septum, resulting in decreased mitral regurgitation and increased left ventricular stroke volume [27].

Reduced Mitral Regurgitation

In the presence of a long PR interval and/or an IVCD, mitral valve closure may not be complete, since atrial contraction is not followed by a properly timed ventricular systole. If the time lag is long enough, a ventricular-atrial pressure gradient may develop and cause diastolic mitral regurgitation [41]. By resynchronizing AV activation and contraction, normal mitral valve timing is restored and regurgitation is potentially reduced or eliminated. In addition, the improvement in left ventricular contraction pattern also serves to minimize regurgitant flow across the mitral valve, as previously noted. Serial evaluations in large numbers of heart failure patients with ventricular dyssynchrony have confirmed a marked reduction in mitral regurgitant flow following initiation of cardiac resynchronization therapy [31].

Left Ventricular Reverse Remodeling

Numerous small mechanistic studies and the results of randomized controlled trials suggest a beneficial effect of cardiac resynchronization therapy on ventricular remodeling. Left ventricular end-systolic and end-diastolic dimensions have been shown to decrease and ejection fraction to increase modestly during chronic resynchronization therapy. Yu and colleagues [42] evaluated 25 NYHA class III or IV heart failure patients with baseline ejection fractions less than 40% and QRS durations greater than 140 milliseconds treated with biventricular pacing therapy. Subjects were assessed serially during 3 months of pacing and after pacing had been withheld for 4 weeks. During cardiac resynchronization therapy, there was a progressive improvement in ventricular structure and function. At 3 months, significant improvements were noted in ejection fraction, dP/dt, myocardial performance index, and mitral regurgitation. Left ventricular end-diastolic and end-systolic volumes were significantly reduced from 205 ± 68 to 168 ± 67 ml and from 162 ± 54 to 122 ± 42 ml, respectively. However, withholding pacing resulted in a progressive but not immediate loss of effect (i.e., pathophysiological adverse remodeling again ensued resulting in increased ventricular volumes and a reduction in ejection fraction).

Such observations have since been made in studies of hundreds of heart failure patients. In the Multicenter InSync Randomized Clinical Evaluation (MIRACLE), serial Doppler echocardiograms were obtained at baseline, 3, and 6 months in 323 optimally treated NYHA class III and IV heart failure patients [31]. Cardiac resynchronization therapy for 6 months was associated with reduced end-diastolic and end-systolic volumes (both $p < 0.001$), reduced left ventricular mass ($p < 0.01$), increased ejection fraction

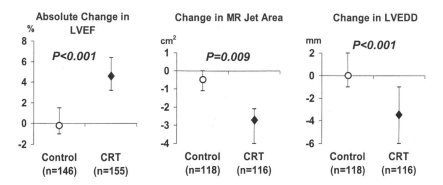

Figure 1 Effects of cardiac resynchronization therapy on measures of left ventricular structure and function. From *left to right*, paired median change from baseline at 6 months is shown for left ventricular ejection fraction (LVEF), mitral regurgitant (MR) jet area, and left ventricular end-diastolic dimension (LVEDD) determined echocardiographically. Baseline values for LVEF, MR jet area, and LVEDD were 22 ± 6%, 7.2 ± 4.9 cm², and 69 ± 10 mm, respectively, in the control group (*open circles*) and 22 ± 6%, 7.6 ± 6.4 cm², and 70 ± 10 mm, respectively, in the resynchronization group (*solid diamonds*). (From Ref. 31; adapted.)

($p < 0.001$), reduced mitral regurgitant blood flow ($p < 0.001$), and improved myocardial performance index ($p < 0.001$) as compared with control (Fig. 1).

MAJOR CLINICAL TRIALS OF CARDIAC RESYNCHRONIZATION THERAPY

A number of observational as well as randomized, controlled trials have recently been completed and others are currently under way to evaluate the safety, efficacy, and long-term effects of cardiac resynchronization therapy in the heart-failure population. The weight of evidence supporting the beneficial effects of cardiac resynchronization therapy for the treatment of heart failure is now quite substantial. To date, more than 4000 patients have been evaluated in randomized single- or double-blinded controlled trials, and several hundred more patients have been assessed in uncontrolled or observational studies. Table 1 reviews the inclusion criteria and current status of completed and of some ongoing randomized controlled trials of cardiac resynchronization in heart failure. These studies include the Pacing Therapies in Congestive Heart Failure (PATH-CHF) trial [26–28], the Multisite Stimulation in Cardiomyopathy (MUSTIC) studies [29,34], the MIRACLE trial [31], MIRACLE ICD [35], the VENTAK CHF/CONTAK CD Trials [32], the Cardiac Resynchronization in Heart Failure (CARE HF) trial [38], and the Comparison of Medical Therapy, Pacing and Defibrillation in Heart Failure (COMPANION) trials [36,37].

PATH-CHF

The PATH-CHF study [26–28] was a single-blind, randomized, controlled crossover trial designed to evaluate the effects of biventricular pacing on acute hemodynamic function and to assess any chronic clinical benefit in NYHA class III or IV heart failure patients with idiopathic or ischemic dilated cardiomyopathy. Primary endpoints were the effect of pacing on oxygen consumption at peak exercise and at anaerobic threshold during

Table 1 Major Randomized Controlled Trials of Cardiac Resynchronization Therapy

Study (N Random)	NYHA	QRS	SINUS	ICD?	Status
MIRACLE (524[a])	III, IV	$\geq$130	NORMAL	NO	PUBLISHED
MUSTIC SR (58)	III	>150	NORMAL	NO	PUBLISHED
MUSTIC AF (43)	III	>200[d]	AF	NO	PUBLISHED
PATH CHF (42)	III, IV	$\geq$120	NORMAL	NO	PUBLISHED
CONTAK CD (581[b])	III–IV	$\geq$120	NORMAL	YES	PUBLISHED
MIRACLE ICD (362[c])	III–IV	$\geq$130	NORMAL	YES	PUBLISHED
PATH CHF II (89)	III, IV	$\geq$120	NORMAL	NO	PRESENTED
COMPANION (1520)	III, IV	$\geq$120	NORMAL	NO	PUBLISHED
PACMAN (328)	III	$\geq$150	NORMAL	NO	ENROLLED
MIRACLE ICD II (186)	II	$\geq$130	NORMAL	YES	PRESENTED
VECTOR (420)	II–IV	$\geq$140	NORMAL	NO	ENROLLING
CARE HF (800)	III, IV	$\geq$120[e]	NORMAL	NO	ENROLLED

LVEF 35% or less for all trials.
[a] Includes 71 patients enrolled in 3-month pilot study.
[b] Includes 248 patients enrolled in 3-month crossover phase.
[c] Excludes class II patients.
[d] RV paced QRS.
[e] Echo-based criteria for QRS less than 150 milliseconds.

cardiopulmonary exercise testing and 6-minute hall walk. Secondary endpoints included changes in NYHA class, quality of life (assessed by the Minnesota Living with Heart Failure questionnaire), and hospitalization frequency. Changes in echocardiographic parameters, LVEF, cardiac output, and filling pattern, were also assessed.

The PATH-CHF study consisted of four phases: (a) preoperative patient evaluation phase, (b) an intraoperative acute testing phase using a proprietary computer and software to guide the selection of an optimal AV delay and pacing site for the chronic pacing phase, (c) a randomized crossover protocol using two different pacing modes, each 4 weeks in duration with a 4-week control phase in between, and (d) a chronic pacing phase.

The study began in the summer of 1995 and enrolled 42 patients. An interim analysis assessing the differences in benefit between pacing and no pacing was performed in the spring of 1998, and the results were encouraging, with a trend toward improvement in all primary and secondary endpoints during pacing [28]. However, the results are weakened by the small number of patients studied, the study's single-blind design, and the observation that functional endpoints did not return to baseline during the "pacing off" control or wash-out period.

MUSTIC

Begun in March 1998, the MUSTIC trial was designed to evaluate the safety and clinical efficacy of cardiac resynchronization in patients with severe heart failure of either an idiopathic, or ischemic origin [29,34]. MUSTIC was really two studies. The first study involved 58 randomized patients with NYHA class III heart failure, normal sinus rhythm, and QRS duration of at least 150 milliseconds. All patients were implanted with a device, and after a run-in period, patients were randomized in a single-blind fashion to receive either active pacing or no pacing. After 12 weeks, patients were crossed-over and remained in the alternate study assignment for 12 weeks. After completing this second 12-week period, the device was programmed to the patient's preferred mode of therapy.

The second MUSTIC study involved few patients (only 37 completers) with atrial fibrillation and slow ventricular rates (either spontaneously or from radiofrequency ablation). A VVIR biventricular pacemaker and leads for each ventricle were implanted, and the same randomization procedure described above was applied. However, biventricular VVIR pacing vs. single-site right ventricular VVIR pacing, instead of no pacing, were compared in this group.

The primary endpoints for MUSTIC were exercise tolerance (assessed by measurement of peak VO_2 or the 6-minute hall walk test) and quality of life (assessed using the Minnesota Living with Heart Failure questionnaire). Secondary endpoints included rehospitalizations and/or drug therapy modifications for worsening heart failure. Results from the normal sinus rhythm arm of MUSTIC showed that during the active pacing phase, the mean distance walked in 6 minutes was 23% greater than during the inactive pacing phase (P < 0.001) [29]. Significant improvement was also seen in quality of life and NYHA class. Fewer hospitalizations occurred during active resynchronization therapy as well. Similar effects have been reported in the atrial fibrillation arm of MUSTIC [34], although the magnitude of benefit appeared to be somewhat less than that seen in patients in normal sinus rhythm.

MIRACLE

The early, positive results from observational studies and from single-blinded controlled trials led to the development of the MIRACLE trial [30]. As the first prospective, randomized, double-blind, parallel-controlled clinical trial, MIRACLE was designed to validate the results from previous cardiac resynchronization studies and to further evaluate the therapeutic efficacy and identify mechanisms of potential benefit of cardiac resynchronization therapy. Primary endpoints were NYHA class, quality of life score (using the Minnesota Living with Heart Failure questionnaire), and 6-minute hall walk distance. Secondary endpoints included assessments of a composite clinical response, cardiopulmonary exercise performance, neurohormone and cytokine levels, QRS duration, cardiac structure and function, and a variety of measures of worsening heart failure and combined morbidity and mortality.

The MIRACLE trial began in October 1998 and was completed late in 2000. Four hundred fifty-three patients with moderate-to-severe symptoms of heart failure associated with a left ventricular ejection fraction 35% or less and a QRS duration of 130 ms or more were randomized (double-blind) to either cardiac resynchronization (n = 228) or to a control group (n = 225) for 6 months, while conventional therapy for heart failure was maintained [31]. Compared with the control group, patients randomized to cardiac resynchronization demonstrated a significant improvement in quality of life score (−18.0 vs. −9.0 points, p = 0.001), 6-minute walk distance (+39 vs. +10 meters, p = 0.005), NYHA functional class ranking (−1.0 vs. 0.0 class, p < 0.001), treadmill exercise time (+81 vs. +19 sec, p = 0.001), peak VO_2 (+1.1 vs. 0.1 ml/kg/min, p < 0.01), and left ventricular ejection fraction (+4.6% vs. −0.2%, p < 0.001). Cardiac resynchronization therapy patients demonstrated a highly significant improvement in the composite clinical heart failure response endpoint, as compared with control subjects, suggesting an overall improvement in heart failure clinical status. Further, fewer patients in the cardiac resynchronization group required hospitalization (8% vs. 15%) or intravenous medications (7% and 15%) for the treatment of worsening heart failure (both p < 0.05) when compared with the control group (Fig. 2). This 50% reduction in hospitalization for the cardiac resynchronization group was accompanied by a significant reduction in length of stay, resulting in a 77% decrease in total days hospitalized over 6 months compared with the

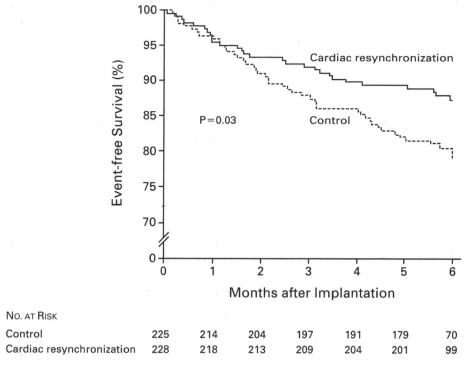

No. at Risk

Control	225	214	204	197	191	179	70
Cardiac resynchronization	228	218	213	209	204	201	99

Figure 2 Effect of cardiac resynchronization on the composite endpoint of death or hospitalization for heart failure. Kaplan-Meier estimates of the time to death or hospitalization for worsening heart failure among patients randomized to the control group and those randomized to cardiac resynchronization. The risk of an event was 40% lower in the resynchronization group (95% confidence level, 4% to 63%; p = 0.03). (From Ref. 31.)

control group. Implantation of the device was successful in 92% of patients. The results of this trial led to the U.S. Food and Drug Administration (FDA) approval of the InSync system in August 2001.

MIRACLE ICD

MIRACLE ICD was a prospective, multicenter, randomized, double-blind, parallel-controlled clinical trial intended to assess the safety and clinical efficacy of a combined implantable cardioverter-defibrillator (ICD) and cardiac resynchronization system in patients with dilated cardiomyopathy (LVEF ≤ 35%, LVEDD ≥ 55 mm), NYHA class III or IV heart failure (a cohort of class II patients was also enrolled), IVCD (QRS ≥ 130 millisecond), and an indication for an ICD. The MIRACLE ICD study was designed to be nearly identical to the MIRACLE trial. Primary and secondary efficacy measures were essentially the same as those evaluated in the MIRACLE trial, but measures of cardioverter-defibrillator function (including the efficacy of antitachycardia therapy with biventricular pacing) were also included.

Of 369 patients receiving devices and randomized, 182 were controls (cardioverter defibrillator activated, cardiac resynchronization *off*) and 187 were in the resynchronization group (cardioverter defibrillator activated, cardiac resynchronization *on*) [35]. At 6 months, patients assigned to cardiac resynchronization had a greater improvement in median quality

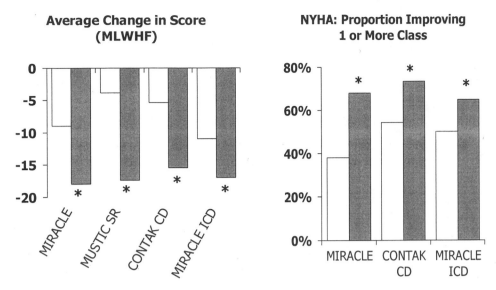

Figure 3 Effects of cardiac resynchronization therapy on quality of life and functional status. *Left panel* demonstrates the effect of resynchronization therapy on quality of life determined by the Minnesota Living with Heart Failure Questionnaire (MLWHF) whereas the *right panel* depicts the proportion of patients with an improvement in NYHA functional class ranking of at least one class. Data are taken from four independent randomized controlled trials of resynchronization therapy, as indicated on the figure. Improvements seen in patients actively treated with cardiac resynchronization (*shaded bars*) significantly exceed those observed in the control groups (*white bars*), with all p-values less than 0.05 as depicted by the *. The consistency of effect is visible across the four studies.

of life score (-17.5 vs. -11.0, p $=$ 0.02) and functional class (-1 vs. 0, p $=$ 0.007) than controls, but were no different than controls in the change in distance walked in 6 minutes (55 m vs. 53 m, p $=$ 0.36). Peak oxygen consumption increased by 1.1 ml/kg/min in the cardiac resynchronization group, vs. 0.1 ml/kg/min in controls (p $=$ 0.04), while treadmill exercise duration increased by 56 sec in the resynchronization group and decreased by 11 sec in controls (p $=$ 0.0006). The magnitude of improvement was comparable to that seen in the MIRACLE trial (Figs. 3 and 4), suggesting that heart failure patients with an ICD indication benefit as much from cardiac resynchronization therapy as those patients without an indication for an ICD.

Of note in the MIRACLE ICD trial, the efficacy of biventricular antitachycardia pacing was significantly greater than that seen in right ventricular antitachycardia pacing. This observation suggests another potential benefit of an ICD combined with a resynchronization device in such patients. Finally, no proarrhythmia was observed and arrhythmia termination capabilities were not impaired by the addition of resynchronization therapy. This device was approved for use in NYHA class III and IV systolic heart failure patients with ventricular dyssynchrony and an ICD indication in June 2002.

CONTAK CD

The CONTAK CD trial enrolled 581 symptomatic heart failure patients with ventricular dyssynchrony and malignant ventricular tachyarrhythmias, who were all candidates for

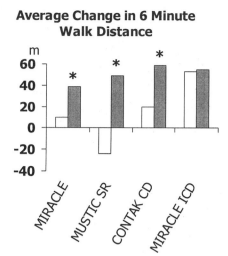
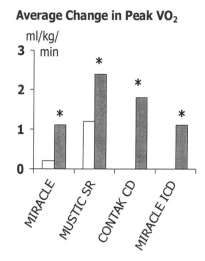

Figure 4 Effects of cardiac resynchronization therapy on exercise capacity. The effects of resynchronization therapy on the 6-minute hall walk distance and on peak oxygen consumption (VO_2) are shown on the *right* and *left* panels, respectively. Data are taken from four independent randomized controlled trials of resynchronization therapy, as indicated on the figure. Improvements seen in patients actively treated with cardiac resynchronization (*shaded bars*) significantly exceed those observed in the control groups (*white bars*), with all p-values less than 0.05 as depicted by the *. As in Fig. 3, the consistency of effect is visible across the four studies with the exception of the 6-minute hall walk finding observed in MIRACLE ICD.

an implantable cardioverter-defibrillator. Following unsuccessful implant attempts and withdrawals, 490 patients were available for analysis [32]. The study did not meet its primary endpoint of a reduction in disease progression, defined by a composite endpoint of morbidity (heart failure hospitalization), mortality, and ventricular arrhythmia requiring defibrillator therapies, although the trends were in a direction favoring cardiac improved outcome with resynchronization therapy. However, the CONTAK CD trial did demonstrate statistically significant improvements in peak oxygen uptake and quality of life in the resynchronization group compared with control subjects, although quality of life was improved only in NYHA class III and IV patients without right bundle branch block. Left ventricular dimensions were also reduced, and left ventricular ejection fractions increased, as seen in other trials of cardiac resynchronization therapy. Importantly, the improvement seen in peak VO_2 with cardiac resynchronization was again comparable to that observed in the MIRACLE trial. Improvements in NYHA functional class were not observed in this study. The CONTAK CD device was approved for use in NYHA class III and IV systolic heart failure patients with ventricular dyssynchrony and an ICD indication in May 2002.

COMPANION

Begun in early 2000, COMPANION was a multicenter, prospective, randomized, controlled clinical trial designed to compare drug therapy alone to drug therapy in combination with cardiac resynchronization in patients with dilated cardiomyopathy, an IVCD, NYHA class III or IV heart failure, and no indication for a device [36,37]. COMPANION randomized 1520 patients into one of three treatment groups in a 1:2:2 allocation: Group 1 (308 patients) received optimal medical care only, Group II (617 patients) received optimal medical care and the Guidant CONTAK TR (biventricular pulse generator), and Group III (595 patients) received optimal medical care and the CONTAK CD (combined heart failure/bradycardia/tachycardia device). The primary endpoint of the COMPANION trial was a composite of all-cause mortality and all-cause hospitalization (measured as time to first event) beginning from time of randomization. Secondary endpoints included all-cause mortality and a variety of measures of cardiovascular morbidity. When compared with optimal medical therapy alone, the combined endpoint of mortality or heart failure hospitalization was reduced by 35% for patients receiving cardiac resynchronization therapy and 40% for patients receiving cardiac resynchronization plus defibrillator therapy (both $p <$ 0.001). For the mortality endpoint alone, cardiac resynchronization therapy patients had a 24% risk reduction ($p = 0.060$) and cardiac resynchronization therapy plus defibrillator implanted patients experienced a risk reduction of 36% ($p < 0.003$), when compared with optimal medical therapy. COMPANION confirmed the results of earlier cardiac resynchronization therapy trials in improving symptoms, exercise tolerance, and quality of life for heart failure patients with ventricular dyssynchrony. In addition, COMPANION showed for the first time the impact of cardiac resynchronization plus defibrillator therapy in reducing all-cause mortality.

CARE-HF

Another randomized controlled morbidity and mortality trial is CARE-HF. This study compares optimal medical therapy alone to optimal medical therapy plus cardiac resynchronization in 800 patients with NYHA class III or IV systolic heart failure and ventricular dyssynchrony determined by either electrocardiographic (QRS duration > 150 milliseconds) or echocardiographic (QRS duration ≥ 120 and < 150 milliseconds plus echocardiographic evidence of dyssynchrony) criteria [38]. CARE-HF is now fully enrolled with results expected in late 2004.

LIMITATIONS OF CARDIAC RESYNCHRONIZATION THERAPY

The success rate for placement of a transvenous cardiac resynchronization system has ranged from about 88% to 92% in clinical trials. This means that 8% to 12% of patients undergoing an implant procedure will not attain a functioning system using this approach. Patients with failed implants must then settle for either another attempt at transvenous placement of the left ventricular lead or epicardial placement of the lead, or they must resign themselves to the absence of cardiac resynchronization therapy. Implant-related complications are similar to those seen with standard pacemaker and defibrillator technologies, with the additional risk of dissection or perforation of the coronary sinus during placement of the left ventricular lead. Although rare, this event may lead to substantial morbidity and even mortality in heart failure patients. Finally although many patients benefit from resynchronization therapy, about one-quarter to one-third of patients have no demonstrable benefit as measured in clinical trials. In such responders, the risk-benefit ratio for cardiac resynchronization is likely unfavorable. Unfortunately, there exist no reliable prospective predictors of responsiveness to resynchronization therapy at the present time.

CANDIDATES FOR CARDIAC RESYNCHRONIZATION THERAPY

The criteria for selecting patients for cardiac resynchronization therapy are primarily determined by the inclusion/exclusion criteria of the major randomized controlled trials, especially MIRACLE, MIRACLE ICD, CONTAK CD and COMPANION. In general, patients with chronic, moderate or severe (NYHA class III–IV) heart failure despite optimal standard medical therapy, a left ventricular ejection fraction less than 35%, left ventricular end diastolic diameter greater than 55 to 60 mm, QRS duration greater than 120 to 130 milliseconds, and with or without an indication for an ICD, benefit the most from cardiac resynchronization therapy. Future randomized clinical trials should help to further define exactly which patients will be the best candidates for cardiac resynchronization therapy and thus potentially extend the promise of this therapy to patients with milder degrees of heart failure and/or ventricular dyssynchrony.

SUMMARY

Cardiac resynchronization therapy is a newer therapeutic modality for patients with ventricular dyssynchrony and moderate-to-severe heart failure. Experience has shown it to be safe and effective, with patients demonstrating significant improvement in both clinical symptoms, measures of functional status and exercise capacity, and echocardiographic parameters. Ongoing and future clinical trials should help to further define the ideal patient with systolic heart failure for cardiac resynchronization.

REFERENCES

1. Farwell D, Patel NR, Hall A, et al. How many people with heart failure are appropriate for biventricular resynchronization? Eur Heart J 2000; 21:1246–1250.
2. Aaronson KD, Schwartz JS, Chen TM, et al. Development and prospective validation of a clinical index to predict survival in ambulatory patients referred for cardiac transplant evaluation. Circulation 1997; 95:2660–2667.
3. Xiao HB, Brecker SJ, Gibson DG. Effects of abnormal activation on the time course of the left ventricular pressure pulse in dilated cardiomyopathy. Br Heart J 1992; 68:403–407.
4. Littmann L, Symanski JD. Hemodynamic implications of left bundle branch block. J Electrocardiol 2000; 33(Suppl):115–121.
5. Saxon LA, Kerwin WF, Cahalan MK, et al. Acute effects of intraoperative multisite ventricular pacing on left ventricular function and activation/contraction sequence in patients with depressed ventricular function. J Cardiovasc Electrophysiol 1998; 9:13–21.
6. Kerwin WF, Botvinick EH, O'Connell JW, et al. Ventricular contraction abnormalities in dilated cardiomyopathy: effect of biventricular pacing to correct interventricular dyssynchrony. J Am Coll Cardiol 2000; 35:1221–1227.
7. Xaio HB, Roy C, Fujimoto S, et al. Natural history of abnormal conduction and its relation to prognosis in patients with dilated cardiomyopathy. Int J Cardiol 1996; 53:163–170.
8. Unverferth DV, Magorien RD, Moeschberger ML, et al. Factors influencing the one-year mortality of dilated cardiomyopathy. Am J Cardiol 1984; 54:147–152.
9. Shamim W, Francis DP, Yousufuddin M, et al. Intraventricular conduction delay: a prognostic marker in chronic heart failure. Int J Cardiol 1999; 70:171–178.
10. Brophy JM, Deslauriers G, Rouleau JL. Long-term prognosis of patients presenting to the emergency room with decompensated congestive heart failure. Can J Cardiol 1994; 10:543–547.
11. Hochleitner M, Hortnagl H, Ng CK, et al. Usefulness of physiologic dual-chamber pacing in drug-resistant idiopathic dilated cardiomyopathy. Am J Cardiol 1990; 66:198–202.

12. Hochleitner M, Hortnagl H, Ng C, Hortnagl H, Gschnitzer F, Zechman W. Long-term efficacy of physiologic dual-chamber pacing in the treatment of end-stage idiopathic dilated cardiomyopathy. Am J Cardiol 1992; 70:1320–1325.

13. Brecker SJ, Xiao HB, Sparrow J, et al. Effects of dual-chamber pacing with short atrioventricular delay in dilated cardiomyopathy. Lancet 1992; 340:1308–1312.

14. Innes D, Leitch JW, Fletcher PJ. VDD pacing at short atrioventricular intervals does not improve cardiac output in patients with dilated heart failure. PACE 1994; 17:959–965.

15. Linde C, Gadler F, Edner M, et al. Results of atrioventricular synchronous pacing with optimized delay in patients with severe congestive heart failure. Am J Cardiol 1995; 75:919–923.

16. Gold MR, Feliciano Z, Gottlieb SS, Fisher ML. Dual-chamber pacing with a short atrioventricular delay in congestive heart failure: a randomized study. J Am Coll Cardiol 1995; 26:967–973.

17. Cazeau S, Ritter P, Bakdach S, et al. Four chamber pacing in dilated cardiomyopathy. PACE 1994; 17:1974–1979.

18. Foster AH, Gold MR, McLaughlin JS. Acute hemodynamic effects of atrio-biventricular pacing in humans. Ann Thorac Surg 1995; 59:294–300.

19. Bakker P, Meijburg H, de Vries J, et al. Biventricular pacing in end-stage heart failure improves functional capacity and left ventricular function. J Interv Card Electrophysiol 2000; 4:395–404.

20. Cazeau S, Ritter P, Lazarus A, et al. Multisite pacing for end-stage heart failure: early experience. Pacing Clin Electrophysiol 1996; 19:1748–1757.

21. Blanc JJ, Etienne Y, Gilard M, et al. Evaluation of different ventricular pacing sites in patients with severe heart failure: results of an acute hemodynamic study. Circulation 1997; 96: 3273–3277.

22. Leclercq C, Cazeau S, Le Breton H, et al. Acute hemodynamic effects of biventricular DDD pacing in patients with end-stage heart failure. J Am Coll Cardiol 1998; 32:1825–1831.

23. Kass DA, Chen CH, Curry C, et al. Improved left ventricular mechanics from acute VDD pacing in patients with dilated cardiomyopathy and ventricular conduction delay. Circulation 1999; 99:1567–1573.

24. Gras D, Mabo P, Tang T, et al. Multisite pacing as a supplemental treatment of congestive heart failure: preliminary results of the Medtronic Inc. InSync Study. Pacing Clin Electrophysiol 1998; 21:2249–2255.

25. Gras D, Leclercq C, Tang A, Bucknall C, Oude Luttikhuis H, Kirstein-Pedersen A. Cardiac resynchronization therapy in advanced heart failure: the multicenter InSync clinical study. Eur J Heart Fail 2002; 4:311–320.

26. Auricchio A, Stellbrink C, Sack S, et al. The Pacing Therapies for Congestive Heart Failure (PATH-CHF) Study: rationale, design, and endpoints of a prospective randomized multicenter study. Am J Cardiol 1999; 83:130D–135D.

27. Auricchio A, Stellbrink C, Block M, et al. for the Pacing Therapies for Congestive Heart Failure Study Group. Effect of pacing chamber and atrioventricular delay on acute systolic function of paced patients with congestive heart failure. Circulation 1999; 99:2993–3001.

28. Auricchio A, Klein H, Spinelli J. Pacing for heart failure: selection of patients, techniques, and benefits. Eu J Heart Fail 1999; 1:275–279.

29. Cazeau S, Leclercq C, Lavergne T, et al. for the Multisite Stimulation in Cardiomyopathies (MUSTIC) Study Investigators. Effects of multisite biventricular pacing in patients with heart failure and intraventricular conduction delay. N Engl J Med 2001; 344:873–880.

30. Abraham WT. on behalf of the Multicenter InSync Randomized Clinical Evaluation (MIRACLE) Investigators and Coordinators. Rationale and design of a randomized clinical trial to assess the safety and efficacy of cardiac resynchronization therapy in patients with advanced heart failure: the Multicenter InSync Randomized Clinical Evaluation (MIRACLE). J Card Fail 2000; 6:369–380.

31. Abraham WT, Fisher WG, Smith AL, et al. for the Multicenter InSync Randomized Clinical Evaluation (MIRACLE) Investigators and Coordinators. Double-blind, randomized controlled trial of cardiac resynchronization in chronic heart failure. N Engl J Med 2002; 346:1845–1853.

32. Higgins SL, Hummel JD, Niazi IK, et al. Cardiac resynchronization therapy for the treatment of heart failure in patients with intraventricular conduction delay and malignant ventricular tachyarrhythmias. J Am Coll Cardiol 2003; 42:1454–1459.

33. Linde C, Leclercq C, Rex S, et al. on behalf of the Multisite Stimulation in Cardiomyopathies (MUSTIC) Study Group. Long-term benefits of biventricular pacing in congestive heart failure: results from the Multisite Stimulation in Cardiomyopathy (MUSTIC) Study. J Am Coll Cardiol 2002; 40:111–118.

34. Leclercq C, Walker S, Linde C, et al. Comparative effects of permanent biventricular and right-univentricular pacing in heart failure patients with chronic atrial fibrillation. Eur Heart J 2002; 23:1780–1787.

35. Young JB, Abraham WT, Smith AL, et al. Safety and efficacy of combined cardiac resynchronization therapy and implantable cardioversion defibrillation in patients with advanced chronic heart failure. The Multicenter InSync ICD Randomized Clinical Evaluation (MIRACLE ICD) trial. JAMA 2003; 289:2685–2694.

36. Bristow MR, Feldman AM, Saxon LA. for the COMPANION Steering Committee and COMPANION Clinical Investigators. Heart failure management using implantable devices for ventricular resynchronization: Comparison of Medical Therapy, Pacing, and Defibrillation in Chronic Heart Failure (COMPANION) trial. J Card Fail 2000; 6:276–285.

37. Bristow MR, Saxon LA, Boehmer J, Kreuger S, Kuss DA, De Marco T, Carson P, DiCarlol L, De Mets D, White RG, DeVries DW, Feldman AM for the COMPANION Investigators. Effect of cardiac resynchronization therapy with or without an implantable defibrillator in advanced heart failure: N Engl J Med 2004; 350:2140–2150.

38. Cleland JGF, Daubert JC, Erdmann E, et al. on behalf of The CARE-HF study Steering Committee and Investigators. The CARE-HF study (Cardiac Resynchronisation in Heart Failure study): rationale, design and end-points. Eur J Heart Fail 2001; 3:481–489.

39. Nishimura RA, Hayes DL, Holmes DR, et al. Mechanism of hemodynamic improvement by dual-chamber pacing for severe left ventricular dysfunction: an acute Doppler and catheterization hemodynamic study. J Am Coll Cardiol 1995; 25:281–288.

40. Grines CL, Bashore TM, Boudoulas H, et al. Functional abnormalities in isolated left bundle branch block. The effect of interventricular asynchrony. Circulation 1989; 79:845–853.

41. Panidis IP, Ross J, Munley B, et al. Diastolic mitral regurgitation in patients with atrioventricular conduction abnormalities: a common finding by Doppler echocardiography. J Am Coll Cardiol 1986; 7:768–774.

42. Yu CM, Chau E, Sanderson JE, et al. Tissue doppler echocardiographic evidence of reverse remodeling and improved synchronicity by simultaneously delaying regional contraction after biventricular pacing therapy in heart failure. Circulation 2002; 105:438–445.

19

Management of Atrial and Ventricular Arrhythmias in Heart Failure

Usha Tedrow and William G. Stevenson
Cardiovascular Division, Brigham and Women's Hospital
Boston, Massachusetts, USA

SYNOPSIS

Atrial and ventricular cardiac arrhythmias, nearly ubiquitous in the heart failure patient population, often accompany and contribute to clinical decompensations. Atrial fibrillation and flutter are the most common supraventricular arrhythmias, and are managed with a combination of rate control, anticoagulation, antiarrhythmic drugs, and ablation where appropriate. Nonsustained ventricular arrhythmias are common, but sudden cardiac death risk varies depending on etiology of heart failure and other clinical features. In addition to implantable cardiac defibrillators to prophylax against arrhythmic sudden death, antiarrhythmic drugs and occasionally catheter ablation are required. In summary, arrhythmia management in the heart failure population is complex, requiring careful integration of varied strategies including medication and procedures. Equally important are device therapies, such as implantable defibrillators for prophylaxis of sudden death, and adjunctive left ventricular pacing for cardiac resynchronization therapy. Because of the potential risks and benefits of these therapeutic modalities peculiar to the heart failure population, it is essential that management is integrated between patient, heart failure specialist, and electrophysiologist.

In the heart failure patient population, cardiac arrhythmias frequently contribute to worsened symptoms, periodic decompensations, and increased mortality in the form of sudden death. Arrhythmia recognition and management is an important aspect of caring for these patients. Chronic heart failure predisposes to both supraventricular and ventricular arrhythmias. The etiologic diversity of patients with heart failure has an impact on the incidence of arrhythmias and on diagnostic and therapeutic strategies. Arrhythmia prevention and management plans, taking into account the potential benefits and risks of implantable defibrillators, left ventricular pacing for cardiac resynchronization therapy, antiarrhythmic drugs and ablation, often require careful integration with heart failure management.

ANTIARRHYTHMIC DRUGS

Antiarrhythmic drugs must be used cautiously with careful assessment of risk and benefit in patients with heart failure. The potential for drug toxicity is increased by diminished hepatic or renal excretion and drug interactions are common. In addition, depressed ventricular function is associated with a greater risk of drug induced proarrhythmia, such as drug-induced polymorphic VT (e.g., torsades de pointes). Many drugs have negative inotropic effects that can aggravate heart failure.

Antiarrhythmic Effects of Beta-Adrenergic Blockers

Beta-adrenergic blockers are a first-line therapy for many arrhythmias. These agents have antiarrhythmic effects and demonstrated efficacy for improving mortality and reducing sudden death in heart failure. [1–3] Beta-adrenergic blockers can help control the ventricular response to atrial fibrillation and diminish symptoms of palpitations from supraventricular arrhythmias and premature ventricular contractions. [4] Many ventricular arrhythmias are aggravated by sympathetic stimulation. Beta-adrenergic blockers are also effective in reducing many ventricular arrhythmias. In addition, sympathetic stimulation can blunt or reverse the electrophysiological effects of amiodarone and other antiarrhythmic drugs. A combination of a beta-adrenergic blocker with another antiarrhythmic drug can be useful. Aggravation of bradyarrhythmias is the major arrhythmia-related adverse effect.

Class I Sodium Channel Blocking Antiarrhythmic Drugs

The class I antiarrhythmic drugs are largely reserved for control of frequent symptomatic arrhythmias in patients who have an implantable defibrillator when amiodarone, dofetilide, or sotalol are less attractive options. Class I sodium channel blocking drugs (mexiletine, tocainide, procainamide, quinidine, disopyramide, flecainide, and propafenone) have negative inotropic effects (with the possible exception of quinidine) [5,6]. Blockade of sodium channels diminishes intracellular sodium and, thereby, may decrease intracellular calcium by its effect on the sodium calcium exchanger (the opposite effect of digitalis). Quinidine may lack negative inotropic effects because vasodilation and QT interval prolongation, which allow additional time for calcium to enter during the plateau phase of the action potential, may offset the negative inotropic effects of the sodium channel blockade. In addition to a long-term risk of drug-induced systemic lupus erythematosus, procainamide is metabolized to N-acetylprocainamide (NAPA), which is a Class III antiarrhythmic drug that has QT prolonging effects of its own and accumulates in patients with renal insufficiency.

Class I antiarrhythmic drugs also have a potential for proarrhythmia that is likely aggravated by the electrophysiological changes of heart failure and hypertrophy [7,8]. These adverse effects of Class I antiarrhythmic drugs likely explain the increases in mortality observed when these agents were administered to patients with prior myocardial infarction, to patients with heart failure and atrial fibrillation, and to patients who had been resuscitated from a cardiac arrest [2,7,9].

Amiodarone

Amiodarone is the major option for antiarrhythmic drug therapy in patients with heart failure, largely because it is a relatively safe from a cardiac standpoint [10–12]. Amiodarone blocks cardiac sodium, potassium, and calcium currents and has sympatholytic effects. It has activity against both ventricular and supraventricular arrhythmias. Individual trials have found either benefit, or no effect on mortality [10,11]. A meta-analysis of randomized trials in patients with heart failure concluded that amiodarone reduced mortality by 17% and reduced sudden death by 23% [13]. Although benefit is controversial, a major adverse impact on mortality is unlikely. Noncardiac toxicities are the major limitation (see following text).

Subgroup analysis suggests that amiodarone may be more likely to be beneficial for patients with nonischemic cardiomyopathy, those who have a relatively elevated resting heart rate ($\geq$ 90/min), and for those who are being concomitantly treated with beta blockade [10,11]. Ventricular proarrhythmia is unusual. Amiodarone has been initiated in the outpatient setting without an increase in mortality [10,11,13]. Bradyarrhythmias due to potent effects on the sinus and AV (atrioventricular) nodes are the major cardiac risk, occurring in 1% to 7 % of patients in randomized trials, and in up to a third of patients in some case series [13,14].

In patients with compensated heart failure, amiodarone is well tolerated from a hemodynamic standpoint when administered at a loading dose of 600 to 800 mg daily for 1 to 2 weeks [10–12,14,15]. In patients with advanced heart failure, administration of the loading dose and, in particular, large oral doses (e.g., > 1200 mg daily) can exacerbate heart failure [16].

Noncardiac toxicities are a major problem. In randomized trials 41% of patients discontinue therapy by 2 years due to real or perceived side effects. The true incidence of side effects is lower, as indicated by the observation that placebo was discontinued in 27% of patients in these trials [13]. However, it is often difficult to distinguish an amiodarone-induced side effect from symptoms of heart failure. Amiodarone induced pulmonary toxicity occurs in approximately 1% of patients per year of therapy [17]. Chronic therapy at doses exceeding 300 mg per day increases the risk. A chest radiograph should be obtained annually. Annual pulmonary function tests are recommended by some physicians, particularly for those patients taking a daily dose in excess of 300 mg. A decrease in diffusing capacity can indicate development of pulmonary toxicity [18]. When pulmonary toxicity is suspected, a right heart catheterization to assess the possibility of pulmonary vascular congestion, and a high resolution chest computed tomography scan to assess interstitial fibrosis can be helpful in distinguishing pulmonary toxicity from heart failure [18,19].

Thyroid abnormalities occur in up to 18% of patients [20]. Hypothyroidism is easily managed with thyroid replacement therapy and does not generally warrant discontinuation of amiodarone. Hyperthyroidism is a much more difficult problem, and can be refractory to management with antithyroid medications. Because the gland is saturated with iodine from the amiodarone, thyroid ablation with radioactive iodine is not possible. Discontinuation of the drug and medical therapy for hyperthyroidism in consultation with an endocrinologist is often required. Routine thyroid stimulating hormone (TSH) assay every 6 months, as well as assessment of hepatic transaminases at those times for potential liver toxicity, are reasonable.

Additionally, long-term use of amiodarone is associated with corneal and cutaneous deposits, which are usually mainly cosmetic difficulties for the patient. In contrast, optic neuritis and peripheral neuropathy are also associated with use of amiodarone, and warrant discontinuation of the drug to prevent further neurologic deterioration.

Amiodarone increases the energy required for defibrillation and can render an implantable cardiac defibrillator (ICD) ineffective in some patients. It can also impair arrhythmia detection by slowing the rate of ventricular tachycardia. These concerns warrant careful testing of ICD function and defibrillation after amiodarone therapy is initiated in patients with ICDs.

Dofetilide

Dofetilide is a Class III antiarrhythmic drug that is approved for therapy of atrial fibrillation. It blocks the repolarizing potassium current I_{Kr}, increasing action potential duration and the QT interval. Its major toxicity is proarrhythmia from torsades de pointes, which occurs in more than 3% of patients [21]. It is primarily renally excreted with a plasma half-life of 9.5 hours. It requires initiation in-hospital with continuous electrocardiographic monitoring for a minimum of 72 hours to detect the development of QT prolongation and torsades de pointes. It should not be administered to patients with significant renal insufficiency (calculated creatinine clearance < 20 ml/min). Taking these precautions and avoiding drug administration to patients with prolonged QT intervals, dofetilide can be administered safely to patients with heart failure. The Danish Investigations of Arrhythmia and Mortality on Dofetilide Study (DIAMOND) showed that, in patients with class III of IV heart failure, during a median follow-up of 18 months, there was no difference in mortality between dofetilide-treated and placebo groups [21]. Dofetilide-treated patients were less likely to be rehospitalized for exacerbation of heart failure (30% compared with 38%), possibly due to a reduction in atrial fibrillation.

Sotalol

Sotalol is a mixture of two stereoisomers. The d isomer has Class III effects similar to dofetilide, from block of the potassium current I_{Kr}. The l isomer is a potent nonselective beta-adrenergic blocker. Sotalol has not been specifically evaluated in heart failure patients. In survivors of myocardial infarction who have depressed ventricular function, chronic therapy with the d isomer of sotalol increases mortality [22]. Sotalol causes torsades de pointes with a similar incidence to that of dofetilide and can aggravate bradyarrhythmias and heart failure through its beta-blocking effects. Therapy should be initiated in-hospital during continuous electrocardiographic monitoring. It also has a renal route of excretion and should be avoided in patients with renal insufficiency. Its antiarrhythmic efficacy for atrial fibrillation is less than that of amiodarone [23].

Azimilide

Azimilide is a new type III antiarrhythmic drug which blocks potassium channels I_{Ks} and I_{Kr}. In the Azimilide Post-infarct Survival Evaluation (ALIVE) trial, presented in preliminary form, 3717 patients, 15 to 21 days after myocardial infarction, with ejection fractions less than 35% were randomized to placebo or azimilide [24,25]. There was no difference in all-cause mortality at 1 year, and fewer patients in the drug group developed atrial fibrillation. The incidence of torsades de pointes was very low: 0.3% in the drug group vs. 0.1% of the placebo group. There was, however, a 1% incidence of neutropenia, within 48 days of initiation of azimilide; all patients had spontaneous recovery of cell lines after stopping the drug.

SUPRAVENTRICULAR TACHYCARDIAS

Atrial fibrillation and atrial flutter are the most common supraventricular arrhythmias encountered. Rarely, an incessant supraventricular tachycardia (SVT) from ectopic atrial tachycardia or atrioventricular reentry from an accessory pathway causes a tachycardia-induced cardiomyopathy [26]. Such SVTs typically have a rate greater than 120 beats per minute and despite depressed systolic function, marked ventricular dilation is often absent. Control of the arrhythmia can be followed by return of ventricular function to normal over weeks to several months. A persistently rapid response to atrial fibrillation can also cause a clinical picture of tachycardia-induced cardiomyopathy.

Atrial Fibrillation

The prevalence of atrial fibrillation increases with the severity of heart failure. Atrial fibrillation is found in 6% of patients with mild heart failure and more than 40% of patients with advanced heart failure (Fig. 1) [8,21,27–31]. The potential adverse effects of atrial fibrillation include loss of A-V synchrony, rapid or slow ventricular rate responses that are no longer under optimal physiological control, variable time for cardiac filling due to oscillations of R-R intervals and risk of thromboembolism [4,8,32–34]. In some, but not all, studies atrial fibrillation has been associated with increased mortality and more frequent hospitalizations [8,27,28,31,35].

Patients with atrial fibrillation and heart failure are at increased risk of stroke; anticoagulation with warfarin is warranted [36–38]. Adequate control of heart rate is important. Whether attempting to restore and maintain sinus rhythm (rhythm control) is better than simply controlling the ventricular rate and maintaining anticoagulation is not known [4,39], but has been investigated in the Atrial Fibrillation Follow-up Investigation of Rhythm Management (AFFIRM) trial. Although most of the patients in AFFIRM had normal ejection fractions, 26% had low ejection fractions, and 939 (23%) had a history of congestive heart failure. Overall, there was a trend toward increased mortality for the strategy of administering antiarrhythmic drugs to attempt to maintain sinus rhythm (rhythm control group). However, the prespecified subgroup analysis of the patients with a history of heart failure shows a neutral effect on mortality, with an absolute odds ratio for mortality slightly in favor of the rhythm control strategy [40].

In the congestive heart failure survival trial of antiarrhythmic therapy (CHF-STAT) trial, patients who converted from atrial fibrillation to sinus rhythm during therapy with amiodarone had better survival compared with those who did not convert [21,29]. Similarly, patients treated with dofetilide who achieved sinus rhythm had fewer hospitalizations for heart failure exacerbations [21]. It remains unclear whether atrial fibrillation has adverse effects that increase mortality, or is simply a marker of more severe heart failure.

For heart failure patients with a first episode of atrial fibrillation and those with symptomatic paroxysms of atrial fibrillation, antiarrhythmic drug therapy to attempt to maintain sinus rhythm is reasonable. Amiodarone, dofetilide, and sotalol are the major antiarrhythmic drug options. Amiodarone is most likely to be effective [14,41]. In a ran-

% Patients with Atrial Fibrillation

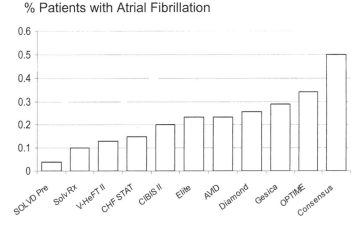

Figure 1   The incidence of atrial fibrillation in recent heart failure and arrhythmia trials is shown. (From Ref. 151.)

domized trial of patients with atrial fibrillation without heart failure, maintenance of sinus rhythm for 1 year was achieved in 69% of patients treated with amiodarone compared with 39% of those treated with sotalol or the Class I antiarrhythmic drug propafenone [23]. In the DIAMOND trial, 12% of patients who had atrial fibrillation on entry to the study converted to sinus rhythm by 1 month when treated with dofetilide; only 1% of atrial fibrillation patients in the placebo group converted to sinus rhythm. Dofetilide also reduced the risk of recurrent atrial fibrillation once sinus rhythm had been restored (hazard ratio 0.35) [21]. Amiodarone and dofetilide have not been directly compared.

When sinus rhythm cannot be maintained, adequate rate control during atrial fibrillation is of paramount importance [12,26,32,38,42,43]. A poorly controlled ventricular rate can exacerbate heart failure and contribute to further deterioration in ventricular function. A resting heart rate below 80 to 90 beats/min and remaining below 100 beats/min with comfortable ambulation is a reasonable goal. Beta-adrenergic blockers and digoxin are the first line options for rate control [38]. Digoxin is less effective when sympathetic tone is elevated, but useful because it lacks adverse hemodynamic effects. The calcium channel blockers diltiazem and verapamil slow heart rate but should be avoided in patients with advanced heart failure due to their negative inotropic effects and potential for increasing mortality in patients with heart failure due to coronary artery disease [44]. Amiodarone is an effective drug for rate control but other agents are preferable due to its toxicities.

When adequate rate control cannot be achieved with pharmacologic means, catheter ablation of the AV junction with implantation of a permanent pacemaker should be considered. AV junction ablation achieves rate control and regularizes the heart rhythm. The atria continue to fibrillate, necessitating anticoagulation. Although the atrial contribution to ventricular filling is not restored, exertional symptoms and palpitations improve and recurrent hospitalizations may be reduced [43,45–51]. Although symptoms improve, objective demonstration of improvement in exercise time or oxygen uptake are not usually observed [32,46]. In some patients left ventricular ejection fraction improves, which may be a consequence of the decrease in rate, or better ability to measure ejection fraction once the heart rate is regularized [52].

Two problems are of concern with this procedure. Occasional patients experience deterioration in heart failure after this procedure [53,54]. A change in ventricular activation sequence produced by right ventricular pacing might be responsible, as discussed in Chapter 18. Patients at greatest risk for hemodynamic deterioration have severely depressed ventricular function and functional mitral regurgitation. Whether biventricular pacing (left ventricular and right ventricular pacing, discussed in Chapter 18) would reduce this risk is not known. Secondly, sudden death due to torsades de pointes has occurred after ablation, potentially the result of the sudden reduction in heart rate. Pacing at 90 beats per minute for the initial 1 to 3 months after ablation appears to reduce this risk [55].

If a heart failure patient with atrial fibrillation is being considered for cardiac surgery to correct a valvular lesion or to revascularize, left atrial appendage removal or ligation has been suggested, in the hope of reducing the risk thrombus formation and embolism. This is the subject of the Left Atrial Appendage Occlusion Study (LAAOS), a randomized trial currently in the recruitment phase [56]. In addition, the possibility of a surgical MAZE operation can be considered to reduce the burden of arrhythmia. More recently, catheter ablation for pulmonary vein isolation has been useful in selected patients with atrial fibrillation [57], but is likely to have limited efficacy in patients with heart failure and associated atrial dilation.

Atrial Flutter

As for atrial fibrillation, rate control and anticoagulation are important [38,58–60]. Although some studies suggest less risk of left atrial thrombus formation in patients with

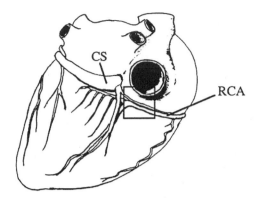

Figure 2 (A) Shown is a posterior (diaphragmatic) view of heart with arterial and venous anatomy and its relationship to right atrial inferior isthmus (highlighted with rectangle). RCA indicates right coronary artery; CS, coronary sinus.

atrial flutter than that observed in patients with atrial fibrillation, others suggest a similar risk in these two groups [58–62]. Chronic anticoagulation with warfarin is prudent. Recurrent atrial flutter responds poorly to pharmacologic therapy and rate control is often more difficult to achieve than for atrial fibrillation [63]. Antiarrhythmic drugs that slow the rate of atrial flutter without blocking AV nodal conduction, such as Class I antiarrhythmic drugs, can lead to life-threatening 1:1 AV conduction.

The most common form of atrial flutter is due to circulation of a single reentry wave front around the tricuspid annulus. Radiofrequency catheter ablation is an excellent option for patients with this type of atrial flutter and is more effective than antiarrhythmic drug therapy [64,65]. Ablation of the isthmus between the tricuspid valve annulus and inferior vena cava abolishes atrial flutter in more than 95% of patients (Fig. 2) [66]. Procedural risk is minimal. Less commonly an apparent atrial flutter is due to reentry involving an area of scar in the right or left atrium. Ablation of these types of flutter is more difficult, with somewhat lower efficacy. Ablation of flutter in the left atrium is associated with a risk of arterial embolism from left atrial catheter manipulation.

Despite effective ablation of atrial flutter, atrial fibrillation recurs in 20% to 30% of patients within the following 2 years. Emergence of atrial fibrillation likely increases

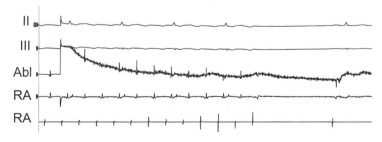

Figure 2 (B) Shown is termination of atrial flutter to normal sinus rhythm with completion of a line of radiofrequency lesions from the tricuspid annulus to the inferior vena cava. The upper two tracings are surface ECG leads II and III, followed by the intracardiac ablation catheter showing artifact from ongoing ablation. The lower two tracings are intracardiac atrial electrograms initially showing rapid regular activity that suddenly stops when the flutter terminates.

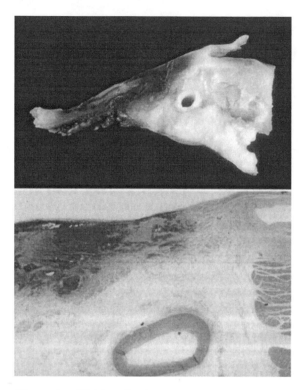

Figure 2 (C) *Top view* is a longitudinal section of posterior aspect of right AV groove with atrium, ventricle, tricuspid valve, and right coronary artery in AV groove fat pad. Dark lesions are areas of coagulation necrosis corresponding to sites at which RF current was applied. Maximal depth of lesion is 2 mm. Distance from endocardial surface at ablation site to edge of coronary artery is 4 mm. *Bottom view* is a low-power microscopic section (hematoxylin and eosin, magnification ×33) of RF ablation site at right AV groove. There is a clear-cut coagulation necrosis of myocardium with surrounding loose granulation tissue and fat necrosis. (Parts A and C of this figure from Ref. 66.)

with poor left ventricular function. Those with atrial flutter and prior atrial fibrillation appear to have a recurrence rate of atrial fibrillation in excess of 70% over 20 months [65]. When atrial flutter develops during chronic drug therapy for atrial fibrillation, ablation of flutter may allow maintenance of sinus rhythm, but continued drug therapy for prevention of atrial fibrillation is still likely to be required [67].

VENTRICULAR ARRHYTHMIAS AND SUDDEN CARDIAC DEATH

Sudden cardiac death accounts for 20% to 50% of the mortality in patients with heart failure. Ventricular arrhythmias are a major etiology, and implantable defibrillators (ICDs) are warranted for many high-risk patients. Other mechanisms of sudden death also occur [68–71]. Bradyarrhythmias caused 41% of in-hospital unexpected cardiac arrests in one series [71]. Conduction disease associated with heart failure, myocardial ischemia, antiarrhythmic and beta-adrenergic blocking drugs, and hyperkalemia are important potential etiologies. Bradyarrhythmias and pulseless electrical rhythm may be a more common presentation of cardiac arrest in nonischemic cardiomyopathies (NICM) as compared with ischemic cardiomyopathies (ICM). Similarly, compared with stable outpatients, patients

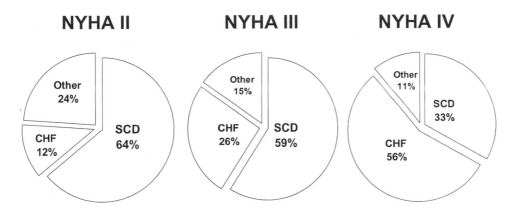

Figure 3 Shown is mode of death grouped by heart failure class. Categories are sudden cardiac death (SCD), death due to congestive heart failure (CHF), and other causes, over the 21-month follow-up period in the Metoprolol Randomized Intervention Trial in Congestive Heart Failure (MERIT-HF) trial. (From Ref. 74.)

hospitalized with advanced heart failure may have a higher incidence of electromechanical dissociation as a cause of sudden death [68,72]. Unexpected and unrecognized acute myocardial infarction, pulmonary embolism, stroke, and ruptured aortic aneurysms also cause some of these deaths.

In chronic dilated heart failure, the incidence of sudden death increases with the severity of heart failure [30,73–81]. In patients with minimal-to-modest symptoms of heart failure, the annual risk of sudden death ranges from 2% to 6% per year. Those with more advanced symptoms, New York Heart Association functional class III to IV, have risk of 5% to 12% per year. As the severity of heart failure increases, deaths due to pump failure increase to a greater extent than sudden deaths (Fig. 3) [74]. Thus, the *proportion* of sudden deaths decreases from 50% to 80% in mild-to-moderate heart failure, to only 5% to 30% for severe heart failure. The risk of sudden death is approximately similar for a given severity of ventricular dysfunction regardless of whether heart failure is due to ICM as compared with NICM [69,82,83].

ICDs provide effective therapy for most episodes of ventricular tachycardia or fibrillation and are warranted for many high risk patients. The superiority of ICDs to therapy with amiodarone has been convincingly demonstrated for patients who have been resuscitated from a cardiac arrest [9,15,84–86]. In the Antiarrhythmics Versus Implantable Defibrillator (AVID) trial total mortality at 3 years was reduced from 36% to 25%; an 11% absolute reduction in mortality and a 31% relative reduction in mortality compared with antiarrhythmic drug therapy (amiodarone in more than 95% of patients). Two smaller trials also show similar trends [9,84,85]. The arrhythmia history, etiology of heart failure, severity of ventricular dysfunction, and, in advanced heart failure, the candidacy for cardiac transplantation or destination left ventricular assist device therapy are important considerations in selecting patients for ICDs. Whether the patient may benefit from LV pacing for cardiac resynchronization is also an important consideration (Chapter 18).

Monomorphic Ventricular Tachycardia

Patients with ICM typically have large areas of infarction (Fig. 4a). Surviving myocyte bundles present within the infarction create channels for conduction set up reentry circuits

A

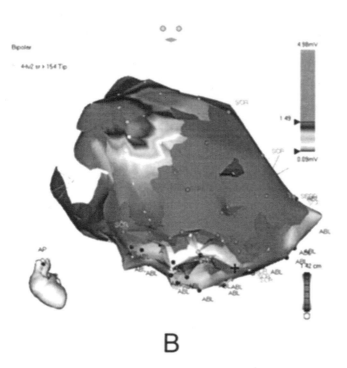

B

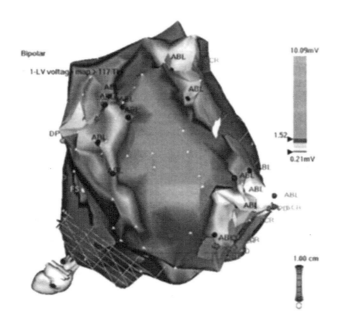

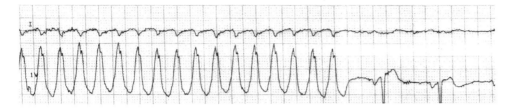

Figure 5 Shown is an episode of spontaneously terminating monomorphic ventricular tachycardia in a patient with ischemic cardiomyopathy.

[87,88]. The ventricular tachycardia (VT) that results is typically monomorphic, with each QRS complex resembling the preceding and following QRS complex (Fig. 5). Because the arrhythmia substrate is relatively fixed and stable, VT is usually inducible with programmed stimulation, allowing electrophysiological testing to be used to detect these reentry circuits, thereby identifying patients at risk of spontaneous episodes. Although, in general, absence of inducible VT at electrophysiological testing indicates a reasonably low risk of sudden arrhythmic death after myocardial infarction, in patients with poor ventricular function, absence of inducible VT does not necessarily convey a low sudden death risk [89,90].

In patients with idiopathic NICM, large areas of scar or infarction are usually absent (Fig. 4b) and programmed stimulation rarely induces sustained monomorphic VT if it has not occurred spontaneously [91,92]. A negative electrophysiology study has little prognostic value [93–97]. Interestingly, of the uncommon NICM patients who develop sustained monomorphic VT, most have evidence of large areas of ventricular scar associated with a reentry circuit [98]. The scar may be a consequence of replacement fibrosis from the myopathic process itself or due to infarcts from embolism of left ventricular or atrial thrombus to a coronary artery. Scars causing VT in the absence of coronary artery disease should prompt consideration of sarcoidosis, Chagas' disease, and arrhythmogenic right ventricular dysplasia [99–106].

Approximately 20% to 40% of NICM patients with monomorphic VT have reentry through the bundle branches causing their VT [98,107]. This tachycardia is also inducible by programmed stimulation, and is amenable to cure by catheter ablation of the right bundle branch.

Chronic Therapy for Sustained Monomorphic VT

Following restoration of sinus rhythm, potential precipitating and aggravating factors should be sought and corrected. However, it should be recognized that sustained monomor-

◄─────────────────────────────────

Figure 4 A and B. Left ventricular electroanatomic maps from two patients with VT due to ischemic (**A**) and nonischemic (**B**) cardiomyopathy are shown. Maps were created during LV mapping by moving a catheter from point to point on the ventricle. Points on the map are color coded for electrogram amplitude in millivolts (mV). Dark areas represent normal myocardium. Low voltage pale (yellow, green and red regions pale (<1.5 mV) are abnormal scars or infarcts and areas of gray represent unexcitable scar. Notably the ischemic cardiomyopathy has a large area of low voltage anteroapical scar, whereas the nonischemic cardiomyopathy has patchy low voltage disease.

phic VT is associated with an underlying structural abnormality in the vast majority of cases, and that the risk of recurrence during long-term follow-up likely exceeds 20% regardless of antiarrhythmic drug therapy, or correction of myocardial ischemia, or other potential aggravating factors. When monomorphic VT occurs with elevated serum cardiac enzymes indicating infarction, the risk of recurrent VT remains high despite treatment for ischemia [108]. The major role of electrophysiological testing is to confirm the diagnosis when supraventricular tachycardia with aberrancy is a consideration, and guiding ablation therapy, if needed.

If ventricular tachycardia is incessant, it should be suppressed with antiarrhythmic drug therapy or catheter ablation [109]. The possibility of idiopathic VT causing tachycardia-induced cardiomyopathy should be considered. Implantation of an ICD is recommended for the majority of patients with sustained VT as previously discussed. The device can often terminate the arrhythmia by painless, antitachycardia pacing. If VT recurs causing symptomatic ICD therapies, antiarrhythmic drugs, or catheter ablation can be considered at that time.

Sustained Polymorphic Ventricular Tachycardia

Polymorphic VT has a continually changing QRS complex. It is often caused by potentially reversible conditions. Acute myocardial ischemia or infarction is a common etiology and warrants evaluation. Torsades de pointes associated with QT interval prolongation is the other major form of polymorphic VT. Less commonly, polymorphic VT is associated with cardiomyopathy or prior infarction without clear precipitating triggers.

Torsades de Pointes

Polymorphic ventricular tachycardia associated with QT interval prolongation is referred to as torsades de pointes [110]. Any cause of QT interval prolongation can cause torsades de pointes [111–114]. Hypokalemia, bradycardia, drugs–such as sotalol, dofetilide, ibutilide, quinidine, n-acetylprocainamide, haloperidol, and erythromycin– are relatively common causes. A more extensive list is available at the www.QTdrugs.org Web site maintained by Georgetown University. Electrophysiological changes that accompany ventricular hypertrophy in chronic heart failure may increase susceptibility to torsades de pointes.

Torsades de pointes is often ''bradycardia-dependent'' or ''pause dependent,'' with a characteristic initiating sequence (Fig. 6). A sudden increase in R–R interval as may occur following a premature beat, creates a pause. The QT interval of the beat terminating the pause is prolonged. The first beat of the tachycardia interrupts the T-wave of that beat. Interventions that increase heart rate and shorten refractoriness are protective. Emergent

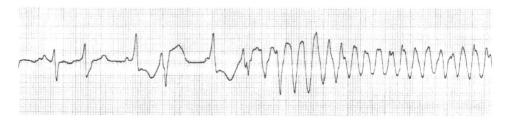

Figure 6   Shown is an episode of torsades de pointes initiated by a long-short RR interval.

treatment is intravenous administration of 1 to 2 gm of magnesium sulfate. If episodes continue, therapy directed at accelerating the heart rate with intravenous administration of isoproterenol and/or transvenous pacing is warranted.

Patients who have had torsades de pointes should avoid all drugs that prolong the QT interval. Although amiodarone prolongs the QT interval, it rarely causes torsades de pointes, possibly because it also blocks ionic currents that also cause the arrhythmia. Patients with heart failure are particularly susceptible to torsades de pointes and therapy with amiodarone is not protective [115,116]. Treatment with an ICD is reasonable. ICDs also provide pacing to prevent bradycardia and suppress pauses following premature beats that may help prevent polymorphic VT [117].

Syncope

There are a variety of causes of syncope and determining the etiology is often challenging. Among 491 consecutive patients with advanced heart failure, Middlekauff and co-workers found that 12% had a history of syncope [118]. In 45% of patients, syncope was attributed to a cardiac arrhythmia. Orthostatic hypotension or a noncardiac cause was identified in 25%, and no clear cause was identified in 30% of patients. The rate of sudden death during the following year was 45%. The sudden death risk was similar for patients with identifiable cardiac causes and presumptively identified noncardiac causes of syncope, suggesting that even when an apparently benign explanation is found, patients with heart failure and syncope remain at high risk for sudden death.

In patients with NICM and syncope, a negative electrophysiological study does not indicate a low risk. Knight and co-workers implanted ICDs in 14 patients with nonischemic cardiomyopathy, unexplained syncope, and a negative electrophysiology study. During an average follow-up of 2 years, half of the patients received therapy from the ICD for ventricular tachycardia or ventricular fibrillation [119]. Of 639 consecutive patients with nonischemic cardiomyopathy referred for heart transplantation reported by Fonarow and co-workers, 147 (23%) had a history of syncope [120]. Twenty-five of these patients received an ICD; 40% received an appropriate shock for VT, and none died suddenly during a mean follow-up of 22 months. Of the 122 patients who had a history of syncope but did not receive an ICD, 15% died suddenly during follow-up. Actuarial survival at 2 years was 84.9% with an ICD therapy and 66.9% with conventional therapy.

Based on the these data, implantation of an ICD is a reasonable consideration for most patients with heart failure and unexplained syncope [119–121].

PRIMARY PREVENTION OF SUDDEN DEATH IN HEART FAILURE

Identifying patients at risk for a cardiac arrest prior to its occurrence (primary prevention) is the focus of much research. For a marker of risk to be useful clinically requires demonstration that: (a) the marker identifies a high-risk group, and (b) specific therapy directed at the high-risk group improves survival. Several noninvasive markers of potential electrical instability, such as ambient ventricular ectopy including nonsustained VT, signal-averaged ECG, heart rate variability, QT dispersion and T wave alternans, have a physiological basis for predicting arrhythmia risk. However, in most cases, the prevalence of abnormal markers increases in parallel to the severity of heart failure and, disappointingly, has not been found to be specific for arrhythmia risk [122].

Nonsustained VT and Ventricular Ectopic Activity

Ventricular ectopic activity and nonsustained VT of 3 or more consecutive beats are common in heart failure patients; 34% to 79% of patients have one or more runs of nonsustained VT on 24-hour ambulatory recordings [82,123,124]. These are typically short; only 30% of patients have runs more than 5 beats in duration [82]. Fast, long runs of nonsustained VT and polymorphic VT should prompt a careful search for possible myocardial ischemia and possible causes of torsades de pointes.

Frequent ventricular ectopy and nonsustained VT are markers for increased mortality and sudden death, but appear to reflect the severity of underlying heart failure and ventricular dysfunction, rather than a specific arrhythmia risk [82,123,124]. Furthermore, suppression of nonsustained VT, such as by amiodarone, does not necessarily improve survival. Occasionally ventricular ectopic activity is due to an aggravating factor that requires treatment, or is a marker for hemodynamic deterioration. Hyperkalemia or hypokalemia, hypoxemia, apneic periods during sleep, and myocardial ischemia are potential causes that deserve evaluation when a marked change in the frequency of ectopic activity occurs [125–128]. Asymptomatic arrhythmias should, in general, not receive specific antiarrhythmic therapy unless there is concern that very frequent arrhythmias are having a negative impact on ventricular function.

Coronary Artery Disease with Depressed Left Ventricular Function

The multicenter automatic defibrillator implantation trial investigators (MADIT) II trial demonstrated that ICDs improve survival (from 80.2% to 85.8% at 2 years) in patients with coronary artery disease and a left ventricular ejection fraction less than 0.30 who had not had an infarct or revascularization procedure within 30 days (Table 1). It is important to recognize that although the average LVEF was 23% in the 1232 randomized patients, patients with class IV symptoms in the preceding 3 months were excluded, and approximately 70% of patients were in functional class I or II. The 9% 1-year mortality in the control group is consistent with mild-to-moderate heart failure, limiting the applicability of this trial to patients with more advanced disease [129].

Coronary Artery Disease with Depressed LV Function and Nonsustained VT

The multicenter unsustained tachycardia trial (MUSTT) provided strong evidence that ICDs improve survival in a select group of patients with prior myocardial infarction, left ventricular ejection fraction less than 0.4 and nonsustained VT [89,130] who also have inducible VT at electrophysiology testing (Table 1). Of 2202 patients who qualified for electrophysiological study, 35% had inducible VT; 704 of these patients were randomized either to a control group who did not receive antiarrhythmic therapy or to a treatment group who received antiarrhythmic drug therapy guided by electrophysiological testing, or an ICD. The 5-year rate of sudden death or resuscitation from cardiac arrest was 32% for the patients who did not receive antiarrhythmic therapy compared with 25% for those assigned to antiarrhythmic therapy (relative risk, 0.73; 95 percent confidence interval, 0.53 to 0.99). The benefit of treatment was due to ICDs, which were implanted in 46% of patients in the treatment group. Patients with an ICD had a 5-year rate of sudden death or cardiac arrest of 9% compared with 37% for patients treated with antiarrhythmic drugs. Although symptomatic heart failure was not required for trial entry, the mean left ventricular ejection fraction was 0.30, class II or III symptoms were present in 63% of patients,

Table 1 ICD Primary Prevention Trials

	MADIT I	CABG-Patch	MUSTT	MADIT II
Target population	Post–myocardial infarction	Post-coronary artery bypass grafting	Nonsustained VT	Post–myocardial infarction
Treatment	ICD vs. best-available drug therapy	ICD vs. control	ICD vs. EPS-guided drug therapy or no therapy	ICD vs. best available therapy
Patients enrolled	196	900	704	1232
Arrhythmia qualifier	Spontaneous NSVT + inducible, nonsuppressible VT/VF	None (abnormal signal averaged ECG)	Spontaneous NSVT + inducible VT/VF	None
LVEF (%) qualifier	≤ 35	< 36	None	30
CHF qualifier	None	None	None	None
NYHA II (%)	67 vs. 63[a]	71 vs. 74[a]	41 36 38[b]	35
NYHA III (%)	See above	See above	26 20 25[b]	25
NYHA IV (%)	Excluded	Excluded	Excluded	5
Mean LVEF (%)	26	27	30	23
ACE inhibitors (%)	50	50	75	70
Beta-blockers (%)	29% ICD vs. 16% drug group	24% ICD vs. 17% control	51% ICD vs. 29% non-ICD	70% in both groups
Outcome	*Survival advantage in ICD group*	*No difference in survival*	*Survival advantage in ICD group*	*Survival advantage in ICD group*
Total mortality rate	16% ICD vs. 34% drug at 1 year (hazard ratio 0.46)	27% ICD vs. 24% control at 4 years	24% ICD vs. 48% no treatment vs. 55% drug treatment at 5 years	14.2% ICD vs. 19.8% control at 20 months
Comments	Drug therapy: 80% amiodarone, 11% Class IA, 9% no antiarrhythmic drug at discharge.	1. ICDs implanted surgically and intraoperatively. 2. Post–CABG ejection fractions unknown	Most patients randomized to drug therapy were taking Class IA agents.	1. Survival curves diverge at 9 months rather than soon after implant. 2. Survival advantage mitigated by worsened heart failure in ICD arm. 3. Concentrated benefit among those with prolonged QRS duration.

[a] Conventional therapy vs. ICD therapy, Class II and III combined
[b] EP study guided drug therapy with ICD, EP study guided drug therapy without ICD, No antiarrhythmic therapy, respectively.

and 72 % to 75% were treated with ACE inhibitors. That ICDs improve survival in this group is also consistent with a smaller primary prevention trial (MADIT I) of 196 patients with prior infarction, left ventricular ejection fraction less than 35% and inducible VT at electrophysiological study that was not suppressed by administration of intravenous procainamide (Table 1) [90].

Whether recent surgical revascularization should influence selection of patients for an ICD is not clear. The Coronary Artery Bypass Graft (CABG) Patch Trial enrolled patients undergoing coronary artery bypass surgery who had a left ventricular ejection fraction less than 36% and an abnormal signal-averaged electrocardiogram (Table 1) [131]. Patients were randomized to receive an ICD (an epicardial lead system) at the time or surgery or to no ICD. During follow-up there was no difference in mortality even though ICD shocks were frequent. One possible explanation is that coronary artery revascularization reduces sudden death risk[89].

Based on the available evidence, an ICD should be considered for patients with heart failure due to coronary artery disease and LV ejection fraction less than 0.3, or less than 0.4 with inducible VT, provided that the severity of heart failure and other comorbidities do not preclude an ICD.

Nonischemic Dilated Cardiomyopathy

For patients with NICM who have not had a sustained ventricular arrhythmia or syncope, electrophysiological testing for risk stratification is not useful [91–97]. Furthermore, an ICD has yet to be shown to be beneficial. The Cardiac Arrhythmia Trial (CAT) enrolled 104 patients with angiographically documented dilated cardiomyopathy diagnosed within 9 months, left ventricular ejection fraction 30% or less, and New York Heart Association class II or III heart failure. Patients were randomized to amiodarone or ICD. The overall mortality in this trial was much lower than expected, and there was no significant difference between the two populations, even after 7 years of follow-up.

A meta-analysis suggests that amiodarone may improve mortality in patients with heart failure and those with NICM may be more likely to benefit [10,124,132], [11]. The amiodarone vs. ICD randomized trial (AMIOVIRT) enrolled 103 patients with nonischemic dilated cardiomyopathy, nonsustained VT, and left ventricular ejection fraction less than 0.35 to therapy with amiodarone or an ICD [133]. There was no difference in survival between the two groups.

In the older Gruppo de Estudo de la Sobreveda en la Insufficiencia Cardiaca en Argentina (GESICA) trial, which randomized 516 patients to amiodarone vs. placebo, the majority of whom did not have known coronary artery disease, the benefit of amiodarone was confined to those patients who had a relatively rapid resting heart rate (> 90 beats/ min) after optimization of heart failure therapies, suggesting that slowing of heart rate may have conferred benefit [10,12]. Since these trials were conducted, beta-blocker use has become a routine therapy. Whether the addition of amiodarone to beta-blockers is beneficial, as appears to be the case in patients with prior myocardial infarction, is not known [134].

Other trials will hopefully clarify arrhythmia management in this group. The Sudden Cardiac Death in Heart Failure trial (SCD HeFT) has randomized approximately 2500 patients with NYHA class II and III heart failure and ejection fraction less than 35% to placebo, ICD, and amiodarone arms and is in the follow-up phase. The Defibrillators in Nonischemic Cardiomyopathy Treatment Evaluation (DEFINITE) trial is randomizing patients with ejection fraction less than 35%, nonsustained VT or frequent ventricular ectopy to ICD or standard medical therapy.

For the present, we consider chronic therapy with amiodarone for patients with symptomatic palpitations from nonsustained VT and for patients with nonischemic cardiomyopathy who have relatively rapid resting heart rates, particularly if they are not able to tolerate beta-adrenergic blocking agents. Administration of amiodarone is also considered for patients who have a very high density of ventricular ectopy, such as incessant ventricular bigeminy, based on the unproven assumption that suppression of ectopic activity may improve hemodynamic performance in some of these patients [135].

Heart Failure Severity and ICDs

The severity of heart failure is an important consideration in assessing whether an ICD is warranted (Table 2) [136]. Successful termination of VT or ventricular fibrillation meaningfully extends survival when the patient has well compensated heart failure and returns to the prearrhythmia functional state. As previously noted, trials showing benefit of ICDs have generally selected patients with relatively preserved functional capacity and the control group mortality in these trials is consistent with that of a mild-to-moderate heart failure

Table 2   Use of Implantable Defibrillators in Patients with Heart Failure[a]

Class I
• Cardiac arrest due to ventricular fibrillation (VF) or ventricular tachycardia (VT) not due to transient or reversible cause
• Spontaneous sustained VT in association with structural heart disease
• Syncope of undetermined origin with clinically relevant sustained VT or VF induced at electrophysiological study
• Nonsustained VT with coronary artery disease, prior myocardial infarction and inducible, nonsupressible VT

Class IIa
• Left ventricular ejection fraction less than or equal to 30%, at least 1 month following myocardial infarction and 3 months after surgical revascularization[b]

Class IIb
• Cardiac arrest presumed to be due to VF when electrophysiologic testing is precluded by other medical conditions
• Severe symptoms, such as syncope, in patients awaiting cardiac transplantation
• Nonsustained VT with sustained VT at electrophysiologic study in patients with ischemic heart disease
• Recurrent syncope of undetermined etiology in the presence of ventricular dysfunction

Class III-Contraindicated
• Incessant VT or VF (ICD may be indicated after arrhythmia control)
• VT or VF due to a transient or reversible condition
• Projected life expectancy less than 6 months
• Significant psychiatric illness that may be aggravated by device implantation or that may preclude device follow up
• NYHA class IV heart failure in patients who are not candidates for cardiac transplantation

Note: Class I recommendations are those for which there is general agreement that the treatment is effective. Class II recommendations represent areas of some debate, with class IIa recommendations areas of greater consensus in favor of treatment, and class IIb areas where treatment is less favorably regarded. Class III conditions are felt to be contraindications to use of the treatment.
[a] based on current guidelines from Ref. 136
[b] Present Centers for Medicare and Medicaid Services (CMS) guidelines specify QRS duration greater than 120 milliseconds.

severity. Extension of survival is limited when deteriorating heart failure or associated complications leads to death from pump failure soon after an episode of VT. Patients with severely decompensated heart failure are less likely to benefit from an ICD and are at increased risk for harm from the implantation and testing procedure.

The risk benefit balance of ICDs is difficult to assess for patients with advanced heart failure. In a post hoc analysis of subgroups in the AVID trial there was a survival benefit demonstrable for patients with ejection fractions between 0.20 and 0.34, but patients with worse left ventricular function (ejection fraction < 0.20) did not have a statistically significant improvement in survival. In a post hoc analysis of the Canadian Implantable Defibrillator Study (CIDS), the study population was divided into quartiles of risk based on age, ejection fraction, and functional class. ICD therapy was associated with a 50% reduction in death in the highest risk quartile, but conferred no benefit in the three lower risk quartiles [85]. In the MADIT I study, benefit appeared to be largely confined to patients with ejection fractions less than the median value of 26% [137].

Thus, the benefit of ICD therapy as reflected by an extension of survival appears to follow a bell-shaped curve. Patients with mild heart failure generally have a lower risk of arrhythmia events and as a population receive less benefit during initial follow-up. With increasing severity of heart failure the incidence of arrhythmic events (VT and ventricular fibrillation) increase such that the benefit of the ICD increases, until, mortality from pump failure increases to the extent that effective arrhythmia termination minimally extends survival [138]. In some cases, heart failure symptoms become intolerable and patients seek to have the tachyarrhythmia therapies of the device turned off to avoid painful shocks as death approaches. Extrapolating data from trials to an individual patient is often difficult.

In general, patients with compensated heart failure are candidates for ICD implantation when they have an indication for an ICD. Some patients with decompensated heart failure should not receive an ICD, even though the risk of ventricular arrhythmias is high. For some of these patients, amiodarone may be a better option. However, some patients with transient class IV symptoms survive for years after resuscitation from a cardiac arrhythmia [139].

The possibility for cardiac transplantation and left ventricular assist devices as home destination therapy also impacts on the potential benefit of an ICD. Most patients who are accepted onto elective transplantation waiting lists are sufficiently compensated to wait at home for a donor heart to become available. Sudden death is a significant risk for these patients. Of 434 patients accepted onto the elective transplantation list between 1984 and 1997 at one center, 25% received a donor heart, 26% of patients died, and 72% of these deaths were sudden [77]. Even for patients who have very poor functional capacity, a dramatic extension of survival occurs when successful defibrillation allows a patient to receive a transplant. Protection from sudden arrhythmic death with an ICD allows some patients with advanced heart failure to await cardiac transplantation at home, avoiding or delaying in-patient waiting until hemodynamic deterioration necessitates inotropic support. Implantation of an ICD is reasonable in these patients even though progressive hemodynamic deterioration is anticipated [77,140,141].

Bradycardia Pacing with ICDs

All ICDs incorporate pacing for bradycardia. Dual chamber (atrioventricular) pacing, activity responsiveness, and mode switching for atrial arrhythmias are available. Approximately 50% of patients who require ICD therapy have indications for or subsequently evolve the need for permanent pacing for bradyarrhythmia. Use of the ICD for bradycardia pacing is preferable to placement of a separate pacemaker, thereby avoiding adverse interactions between the devices and minimizing the number of leads implanted. If sinus rhythm rather than atrial fibrillation is present, maintenance of AV synchrony is generally preferred. This is achieved with a dual chamber defibrillator that requires placement of an atrial lead as well as the ventricular lead [142].

Although dual chamber (right atrial and right ventricular) pacing is generally preferred to ventricular pacing alone for patients with bradycardia, the consequences of AV pacing warrant careful consideration due to the potential for adverse hemodynamic effects of right ventricular apical pacing (RVAP). As discussed in Chapter 18, RVAP produces QRS prolongation similar to left bundle branch block, and is associated with worse ventricular performance than ventricular activation over the normal His-Purkinje system which produces a shorter QRS duration [143–145]. The Dual Chamber Pacing or Ventricular Backup Pacing in patients with an Implantable Defibrillator (DAVID) trial randomized 506 ICD patients with ejection fractions less than 40% to dual chamber pacing at a base rate of 70 beats per minute vs. ventricular backup pacing at a rate of 40 beats per minute [146]. It was expected that dual chamber pacing would allow better medical management of heart failure and lower incidence of atrial fibrillation. However, the trial was stopped early in November 2002 for increased hospitalizations for heart failure in the group receiving dual chamber pacing. The adverse effect was attributed to a 60% rate of RVAP in the dual chamber pacing group vs. a 1% rate of RVAP in patients with ventricular backup pacing. It is, therefore, desirable to avoid RVAP when there is normal ventricular activation (i.e., narrow QRS duration). In some patients, back-up ventricular pacing below the intrinsic heart rate, which results in supraventricular conduction and rare ventricular pacing, might be preferable to chronic RVAP in the dual chamber mode. The implementation of left ventricular pacing leads (discussed in Chapter 18) may obviate this concern, but further investigation is required.

ICD Implantation Considerations

The ICD implantation procedure usually includes initiation of ventricular fibrillation and testing of defibrillation from the ICD to make certain that the lead configuration and energy available will effectively defibrillate. Induced ventricular fibrillation is associated with mild, transient ventricular dysfunction, which is well tolerated in the majority of patients. [147] In patients with advanced heart failure defibrillation threshold testing occasionally precipitates a hemodynamic deterioration [141]. In one series three of 59 patients (5%) who were being evaluated for cardiac transplantation developed electromechanical dissociation after successful defibrillation. In decompensated patients ICD implantation should be deferred until medical therapy has been optimized and heart failure improved. In general, the mortality from defibrillation implantation is less than 1%, but this has not been specifically assessed in heart failure populations.

Continuing Care

Patients with ICDs should be followed in a specialized clinic. Routine device interrogations assessing sensing and pacing function, remaining battery life, and arrhythmias detected by the ICD is generally performed every 3 to 4 months.

Up to 40% of patients receive inappropriate therapies from the ICD at some point during follow-up. Heart rate is the major criterion for arrhythmia detection. A rate exceeding the programmed detection threshold will trigger therapy with either antitachycardia pacing (ATP) or high voltage shocks. Thus, sinus tachycardia or a rapid supraventricular tachycardia can lead to painful shocks. Inappropriate therapy, as for rapid atrial fibrillation or flutter can often be recognized and managed with reprogramming of the ICD. Occasionally inappropriate therapy is due to oversensing of diaphragmatic activity or T-waves. Electrical noise indicating a lead fracture or loose connection of the lead in the pulse generator header can also cause inappropriate shocks.

Following the first symptomatic therapy from the ICD after implantation, patient assessment with interrogation of the device is usually warranted to confirm appropriate function of the ICD (Fig. 7a) and assess the possibility that therapy was inappropriate, triggered by a supraventricular arrhythmia. If the patient receives more than one shock in a short period of time or has symptoms of arrhythmia or a change in symptoms that persists following an ICD shock, urgent evaluation is required. Failure of ICD therapy to terminate the arrhythmia, persistence of a ventricular tachycardia at a rate that is slower than the programmed detection criteria, or persistence of a supraventricular arrhythmia, such as atrial fibrillation, are possible causes. Repeated episodes of ventricular tachycardia or ventricular fibrillation are a marker for greater mortality, and are often associated with hemodynamic deterioration and warrant urgent assessment [148–150]. Myocardial ischemia, electrolyte disturbances and intercurrent illness are important potential causes of arrhythmia exacerbations that should be considered. Patients who have infrequent episodes of ventricular tachycardia usually do not require immediate evaluation when symptoms indicate that another episode of tachycardia has been terminated by the ICD, provided that the episode is similar to previous episodes.

Occasionally it is necessary to temporarily disable an ICD to prevent incessant shocks or antitachycardia pacing such as may be triggered by an "electrical storm" of recurrent ventricular tachycardia or atrial fibrillation with a rapid ventricular response (Fig. 7b) in a patient in the intensive care unit [150]. Application of a magnet over the

A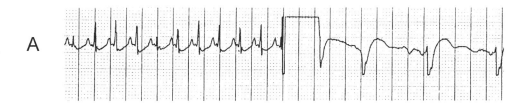

B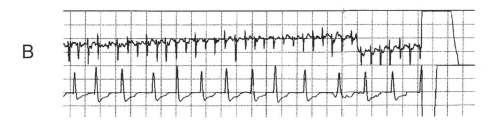

Figure 7 A and B. Shown are two examples of implantable defibrillator shock delivery. In the upper (**A**) tracing, a ventricular electrogram (EGM) and is shown. Rapid ventricular tachycardia is terminated by a shock from the device. In the lower (**B**) tracing, simultaneous atrial and ventricular EGMs are shown. The atrial EGM shows very rapid irregular signals consisted with atrial fibrillation, and the irregular response on the ventricular channel is also consistent with atrial fibrillation. In this case, an inappropriate shock occurred due to atrial fibrillation with rapid ventricular response.

ICD pulse generator suspends arrhythmia detection as long as the magnet is in place, allowing time for implementation of other therapy. While the magnet is in place the patient must be closely monitored and external cardioversion used as appropriate to treat arrhythmias.

Antiarrhythmic Drug Interactions with ICDs

Many patients with ICDs require antiarrhythmic drug therapy to control supraventricular arrhythmias (most commonly atrial fibrillation and flutter) or reduce episodes of ventricular tachycardia (Table 3). In the presence of an ICD, the potential for fatal drug-induced proarrhythmia is low. The ICD will terminate torsades de pointes and provide pacing for bradyarrhythmias. Antiarrhythmic drugs can impede effective ICD termination of arrhythmias and should be used cautiously.

Some antiarrhythmic drugs increase the energy required for defibrillation. At the time of ICD implantation, defibrillation testing is performed by inducing ventricular fibrillation and observing that an ICD shock will terminate fibrillation. Most ICDs are capable of providing a 28 to 35 Joule shock. A 10 Joule safety margin is recommended and confirmed by demonstrating that ventricular fibrillation is terminated by a shock 10 Joules below the maximum energy available from the ICD. Amiodarone therapy typically increases the energy required for defibrillation. If the defibrillation threshold is close to the maximal energy of the ICD, antiarrhythmic drug therapy may increase it such that maximal energy shocks from the ICD are no longer effective. Class III antiarrhythmic drugs that block potassium channels–sotalol and dofetilide–may decrease the defibrillation threshold. In general, repeat defibrillation testing is warranted when chronic therapy with an antiarrhythmic drug is administered, with the possible exceptions of beta-blockers, sotalol, and dofetilide.

Table 3 Preferred Antiarrhythmic Drugs for Atrial Fibrillation in Heart Failure

Drug	Typical dose	Contraindication	Side effects
1. Amiodarone	• Load 600–800 mg/day for 2 weeks, • then 400 mg/day for 2 weeks, • then continue at 200 mg/day	• Resting bradycardia or heart block without backup pacing • baseline significant hepatic or pulmonary disease	Bradycardia, negative ionotropy, pulmonary, thyroid, hepatic, neurologic toxicities
2. Dofetilide	• 250–500 mg twice a day • Dose reduction for renal insufficiency and for increase in QTc by 15% or QT >500 ms with initial dose	• QTc greater than 440 msec • CrCl <20 mL/min	Proarrhythmia (Torsades de pointes)
3. Sotalol	• 80–160 mg twice a day • Dose reduction for renal insufficiency and for increase in QTc by 15% or QT >520 ms with initial dose	• QTc greater than 440 milliseconds • Resting bradycardia or heart block without backup pacing • CrCl <40 mL/min	Bradycardia, negative ionotropy

Psychological Support

The presence of an ICD "safety-net" is greatly reassuring for most patients. Those who have experienced repeated, painful ICD shocks, however, often live in fear of an arrhythmia recurrence [150–158]. Some patients needlessly restrict activities and suffer significant depression and anxiety. Patient support groups and counseling are often beneficial. Some patients require therapy with anxiolytics and antidepressant medications.

Conclusion

ICDs provide effective and reliable treatment of sustained ventricular tachycardia and fibrillation and can be expected to decrease the risk of arrhythmic death in patients with heart failure. Whether this benefit translates to an overall improvement in survival depends on the severity of pump dysfunction. Appropriate patient selection for ICDs is an important aspect of arrhythmia management. Future devices will incorporate features that hope to reduce atrial arrhythmias, improve ventricular function, and monitor hemodynamics, as well as prevent sudden arrhythmic death.

REFERENCES

1. Exner DV, et al. Beta-adrenergic blocking agent use and mortality in patients with asymptomatic and symptomatic left ventricular systolic dysfunction: a post hoc analysis of the Studies of Left Ventricular Dysfunction. J Am Coll Cardiol 1999; 33(4):916–923.
2. Kennedy HL, et al. Beta-blocker therapy in the Cardiac Arrhythmia Suppression Trial. CAST Investigators. Am J Cardiol 1994; 74(7):674–680.
3. Exner DV, et al. Beta-blocker use and survival in patients with ventricular fibrillation or symptomatic ventricular tachycardia: the Antiarrhythmics Versus Implantable Defibrillators (AVID) trial. J Am Coll Cardiol 1999; 34(2):325–333.
4. Khand AU, et al. Systematic review of the management of atrial fibrillation in patients with heart failure. Eur Heart J 2000; 21(8):614–632.
5. Ravid S, et al. Congestive heart failure induced by six of the newer antiarrhythmic drugs. J Am Coll Cardiol 1989; 14(5):1326–1330.
6. Stevenson WG. Mechanisms and management of arrhythmias in heart failure. Curr Opin Cardiol 1995; 10(3):274–281.
7. Flaker GC, et al. Antiarrhythmic drug therapy and cardiac mortality in atrial fibrillation. The Stroke Prevention in Atrial Fibrillation Investigators. J Am Coll Cardiol 1992; 20(3): 527–532.
8. Stevenson WG, et al. Improving survival for patients with atrial fibrillation and advanced heart failure. (erratum appears in J Am Coll Cardiol 1997 Dec; 30(7):1902.). J Am Coll Cardiol 1996; 28(6):1458–1463.
9. Kuck KH, et al. Randomized comparison of antiarrhythmic drug therapy with implantable defibrillators in patients resuscitated from cardiac arrest: the Cardiac Arrest Study Hamburg (CASH). Circulation 2000; 102(7):748–754.
10. Nul DR, et al. Heart rate is a marker of amiodarone mortality reduction in severe heart failure. The GESICA-GEMA Investigators. Grupo de Estudio de la Sobrevida en la Insuficiencia Cardiaca en Argentina-Grupo de Estudios Multicentricos en Argentina. J Am Coll Cardiol 1997; 29(6):1199–1205.
11. Singh SN, et al. Amiodarone in patients with congestive heart failure and asymptomatic ventricular arrhythmia. Survival Trial of Antiarrhythmic Therapy in Congestive Heart Failure.(comment). N Engl J Med 1995; 333(2):77–82.
12. Massie BM, et al. Importance of assessing changes in ventricular response to atrial fibrillation during evaluation of new heart failure therapies: experience from trials of flosequinan. Am Heart J 1996; 132(1 Pt 1):130–136.

13. anonymous. Effect of prophylactic amiodarone on mortality after acute myocardial infarction and in congestive heart failure: meta-analysis of individual data from 6500 patients in randomized trials. Amiodarone Trials Meta-Analysis Investigators. Lancet 1997; 350(9089): 1417–1424.

14. Weinfeld MS, et al. Early outcome of initiating amiodarone for atrial fibrillation in advanced heart failure. J Heart Lung Transplantation 2000; 19(7):638–643.

15. anonymous. A comparison of antiarrhythmic-drug therapy with implantable defibrillators in patients resuscitated from near-fatal ventricular arrhythmias. The Antiarrhythmics versus Implantable Defibrillators (AVID) Investigators. N Engl J Med 1997; 337(22):1576–1583.

16. Gottlieb SS, et al. High dose oral amiodarone loading exerts important hemodynamic actions in patients with congestive heart failure. J Am Coll Cardiol 1994; 23(3):560–564.

17. Dusman RE, et al. Clinical features of amiodarone-induced pulmonary toxicity. Circulation 1990; 82(1):51–59.

18. Singh SN, et al. Pulmonary effect of amiodarone in patients with heart failure. The Congestive Heart Failure-Survival Trial of Antiarrhythmic Therapy (CHF-STAT) Investigators (Veterans Affairs Cooperative Study No. 320). J Am Coll Cardiol 1997; 30(2):514–517.

19. Siniakowicz RM, et al. Diagnosis of amiodarone pulmonary toxicity with high-resolution computerized tomographic scan. J Cardiovasc Electrophysiol 2001; 12(4):431–436.

20. Loh KC. Amiodarone-induced thyroid disorders: a clinical review.(comment). Postgraduate Medical Journal 2000; 76(893):133–40.

21. Torp-Pedersen C, et al. Dofetilide in patients with congestive heart failure and left ventricular dysfunction. Danish Investigations of Arrhythmia and Mortality on Dofetilide Study Group. N Engl J Med 1999; 341(12):857–865.

22. Pratt CM, et al. Mortality in the Survival With ORal D-sotalol (SWORD) trial: why did patients die? Am J Cardiol 1998; 81(7):869–876.

23. Roy D, et al. Amiodarone to prevent recurrence of atrial fibrillation. Canadian Trial of Atrial Fibrillation Investigators. N Engl J Med 2000; 342(13):913–920.

24. Pratt CM, Singh SN, Al-Khalidi HR, Brum JM, Holroyde MJ, Marcello SR, Schwartz PJ, Camm AJ ALIVE Investigators. The efficacy of azimilide in the treatment of atrial fibrillation in the presence of left ventricular systolic dysfunction: results from the Azimilide Postinfarct Survival Evaluation (ALIVE) trial. Journal of the American College of Cardiology. 43(7):1211–1216, 2004.

25. Camm AJ, Karam R, Pratt CM. The azimilide post-infarct survival evaluation (ALIVE) trial. Am J Cardiol 1998; 81(6A):35D–39D.

26. Shinbane JS, et al. Tachycardia-induced cardiomyopathy: a review of animal models and clinical studies. J Am Coll Cardiol 1997; 29(4):709–715.

27. Mahoney P, et al. Prognostic significance of atrial fibrillation in patients at a tertiary medical center referred for heart transplantation because of severe heart failure. Am J Cardiol 1999; 83(11):1544–1547.

28. Dries DL, et al. Atrial fibrillation is associated with an increased risk for mortality and heart failure progression in patients with asymptomatic and symptomatic left ventricular systolic dysfunction: a retrospective analysis of the SOLVD trials. Studies of Left Ventricular Dysfunction. J Am Coll Cardiol 1998; 32(3):695–703.

29. Deedwania PC, et al. Spontaneous conversion and maintenance of sinus rhythm by amiodarone in patients with heart failure and atrial fibrillation: observations from the Veterans Affairs congestive heart failure survival trial of antiarrhythmic therapy (CHF-STAT). The Department of Veterans Affairs CHF-STAT Investigators. Circulation 1998; 98(23): 2574–2579.

30. anonymous. Effects of enalapril on mortality in severe congestive heart failure. Results of the Cooperative North Scandinavian Enalapril Survival Study (CONSENSUS). The CONSENSUS Trial Study Group. N Engl J Med 1987; 316(23):1429–1435.

31. Crijns HJ, et al. Prognostic value of the presence and development of atrial fibrillation in patients with advanced chronic heart failure. Eur Heart J 2000; 21(15):1238–1245.

32. Kay GN, et al. The Ablate and Pace Trial: a prospective study of catheter ablation of the AV conduction system and permanent pacemaker implantation for treatment of atrial fibrillation. APT Investigators. J Intervent Cardiac Electrophysiol 1998; 2(2):121–135.

33. Pardaens K, et al. Atrial fibrillation is associated with a lower exercise capacity in male chronic heart failure patients. Heart 1997; 78(6):564–568.

34. Verma A, et al. Effects of rhythm regularization and rate control in improving left ventricular function in atrial fibrillation patients undergoing atrioventricular nodal ablation. Can J Cardiol 2001; 17(4):437–445.

35. Carson PE, et al. The influence of atrial fibrillation on prognosis in mild to moderate heart failure. The V-HeFT Studies. The V-HeFT VA Cooperative Studies Group. Circulation 1993; 87(6 Suppl):VI102–VI110.

36. Dries DL, et al. Effect of antithrombotic therapy on risk of sudden coronary death in patients with congestive heart failure. Am J Cardiol 1997; 79(7):909–913.

37. anonymous. Predictors of thromboembolism in atrial fibrillation: I. clinical features of patients at risk. The Stroke Prevention in Atrial Fibrillation Investigators. (comment). Ann of Intern Med 1992; 116(1):1–5.

38. Fuster V, et al. ACC/AHA/ESC guidelines for the management of patients with atrial fibrillation: executive summary. A Report of the American College of Cardiology/American Heart Association Task Force on Practice Guidelines and the European Society of Cardiology Committee for Practice Guidelines and Policy Conferences (Committee to Develop Guidelines for the Management of Patients With Atrial Fibrillation): developed in Collaboration With the North American Society of Pacing and Electrophysiology. J Am Coll Cardiol 2001; 38(4):1231–1266.

39. Tuinenburg AE, et al. Lack of prevention of heart failure by serial electrical cardioversion in patients with persistent atrial fibrillation. Heart (British Cardiac Society) 1999; 82(4): 486–493.

40. Wyse DG, et al. A comparison of rate control and rhythm control in patients with atrial fibrillation. (comment). N Engl J Med 2002; 347(23):1825–1833.

41. Roy D, et al. Amiodarone to prevent recurrence of atrial fibrillation. Canadian Trial of Atrial Fibrillation Investigators. N Engl J Med 2000; 342(13):913–920.

42. Grogan M, et al. Left ventricular dysfunction due to atrial fibrillation in patients initially believed to have idiopathic dilated cardiomyopathy. Am J Cardiol 1992; 69(19):1570–1573.

43. Ueng KC, et al. Acute and long-term effects of atrioventricular junction ablation and VVIR pacemaker in symptomatic patients with chronic lone atrial fibrillation and normal ventricular response. (comment). J Cardiovas Electrophysiol 2001; 12(3):303–309.

44. Heywood JT. Calcium channel blockers for heart rate control in atrial fibrillation complicated by congestive heart failure. Can J Cardiol 1995; 11(9):823–826.

45. Brown CS, et al. Clinical improvement after atrioventricular nodal ablation for atrial fibrillation does not correlate with improved ejection fraction. Am J Cardiol 1997; 80(8): 1090–1091.

46. Brignole M, et al. Assessment of atrioventricular junction ablation and VVIR pacemaker versus pharmacological treatment in patients with heart failure and chronic atrial fibrillation: a randomized. controlled study. (comment). Circulation 1998; 98(10):953–960.

47. Proclemer A, et al. Radiofrequency ablation of atrioventricular junction and pacemaker implantation versus modulation of atrioventricular conduction in drug refractory atrial fibrillation. Am J Cardiol 1999; 83(10):1437–1442.

48. Fitzpatrick AP, et al. Quality of life and outcomes after radiofrequency His-bundle catheter ablation and permanent pacemaker implantation: impact of treatment in paroxysmal and established atrial fibrillation. Am Heart J 1996; 131(3):499–507.

49. Manolis AG, et al. Ventricular performance and quality of life in patients who underwent radiofrequency AV junction ablation and permanent pacemaker implantation due to medically refractory atrial tachyarrhythmias. J Intervent Cardiac Electrophysiol 1998; 2(1):71–76.

50. Levy T, et al. Importance of rate control or rate regulation for improving exercise capacity and quality of life in patients with permanent atrial fibrillation and normal left ventricular function: a randomized controlled study. Heart (British Cardiac Society) 2001; 85(2): 171–178.

51. Falk RH. Atrial fibrillation. (comment) (erratum appears in. N Engl J Med 2001 Jun 14; 344(24):1876.

51. N Engl J Med. 2001; 344(14):1067–1078.

52. Edner M, et al. Prospective study of left ventricular function after radiofrequency ablation of atrioventricular junction in patients with atrial fibrillation. Br Heart J 1995; 74(3):261–267.

53. Twidale N, et al. Mitral regurgitation after atrioventricular node catheter ablation for atrial fibrillation and heart failure: acute hemodynamic features. Am Heart J 1999; 138(6 Pt 1): 1166–1175.

54. Vanderheyden M, et al. Hemodynamic deterioration following radiofrequency ablation of the atrioventricular conduction system. Pacing Clin Electrophysiol 1997; 20(10 Pt 1): 2422–2428.

55. Geelen P, et al. Ventricular fibrillation and sudden death after radiofrequency catheter ablation of the atrioventricular junction. Pacing Clin Electrophysiol 1997; 20(2 Pt 1):343–348.

56. Crystal E, et al. Left Atrial Appendage Occlusion Study (LAAOS): a randomized clinical trial of left atrial appendage occlusion during routine coronary artery bypass graft surgery for long-term stroke prevention. Am Heart J 2003; 145(1):174–178.

57. Haissaguerre M, et al. Spontaneous initiation of atrial fibrillation by ectopic beats originating in the pulmonary veins. N Engl J Med 1998; 339(10):659–666.

58. Corrado G, et al. Thromboembolic risk in atrial flutter. The FLASIEC (FLutter Atriale Societa Italiana di Ecografia Cardiovascolare) multicentre study. Eur Heart J 2001; 22(12): 1042–1051.

59. Lanzarotti CJ, Olshansky B. Thromboembolism in chronic atrial flutter: is the risk underestimated? J Am Coll Cardiol 1997; 30(6):1506–1511.

60. Schmidt H, et al. Prevalence of left atrial chamber and appendage thrombi in patients with atrial flutter and its clinical significance. J Am Coll Cardiol 2001; 38(3):778–784.

61. Seidl K, et al. Risk of thromboembolic events in patients with atrial flutter. Am J Cardiol 1998; 82(5):580–583.

62. Wood KA, et al. Risk of thromboembolism in chronic atrial flutter. Am J Cardiol 1997; 79(8):1043–1047.

63. Crijns HJ, et al. Long-term outcome of electrical cardioversion in patients with chronic atrial flutter. Heart 1997; 77(1):56–61.

64. Natale A, et al. Prospective randomized comparison of antiarrhythmic therapy versus first-line radiofrequency ablation in patients with atrial flutter. J Am Coll Cardiol 2000; 35(7): 1898–1904.

65. Paydak H, et al. Atrial fibrillation after radiofrequency ablation of type I atrial flutter: time to onset, determinants, and clinical course. Circulation 1998; 98(4):315–322.

66. Delacretaz E, et al. Radiofrequency ablation of atrial flutter. Circulation 1999; 99(14): E1–E2.

67. Huang DT, et al. Hybrid pharmacologic and ablative therapy: a novel and effective approach for the management of atrial fibrillation. J Cardiovasc Electrophysiol 1998; 9(5):462–469.

68. Pratt CM, et al. Exploration of the precision of classifying sudden cardiac death. Implications for the interpretation of clinical trials. Circulation 1996; 93(3):519–524.

69. Uretsky BF, et al. Acute coronary findings at autopsy in heart failure patients with sudden death: results from the assessment of treatment with lisinopril and survival (ATLAS) trial. Circulation 2000; 102(6):611–616.

70. Stevenson WG, Sweeney MO. Arrhythmias and sudden death in heart failure. Jpn Circ J 1997; 61(9):727–740.

71. Faggiano P, et al. Mechanisms and immediate outcome of in-hospital cardiac arrest in patients with advanced heart failure secondary to ischemic or idiopathic dilated cardiomyopathy. American Journal of Cardiology 2001; 87(5):655–7.

72. Grubman EM, et al. Cardiac death and stored electrograms in patients with third-generation implantable cardioverter-defibrillators. J Am Coll Cardiol 1998; 32(4):1056–1062.

73. anonymous. Effect of enalapril on survival in patients with reduced left ventricular ejection fractions and congestive heart failure. The SOLVD Investigators. N Engl J Med 1991; 325(5):293–302.

74. anonymous. Effect of metoprolol CR/XL in chronic heart failure: Metoprolol CR/XL Randomized Intervention Trial in Congestive Heart Failure (MERIT-HF). Lancet 1999; 353(9169):2001–2007.

75. Cohn JN, et al. Ejection fraction, peak exercise oxygen consumption, cardiothoracic ratio, ventricular arrhythmias, and plasma norepinephrine as determinants of prognosis in heart failure. The V-HeFT VA Cooperative Studies Group. Circulation 1993; 87(6 Suppl): VI5–V16.

76. anonymous. The Cardiac Insufficiency Bisoprolol Study II (CIBIS-II): a randomized trial. Lancet 1999; 353(9146):9–13.

77. Nagele H, Rodiger W. Sudden death and tailored medical therapy in elective candidates for heart transplantation. J Heart Lung Transplant 1999; 18(9):869–876.

78. Uretsky BF, Sheahan RG. Primary prevention of sudden cardiac death in heart failure: will the solution be shocking? J Am Coll Cardiol 1997; 30(7):1589–1597.

79. Cohn JN, et al. A dose-dependent increase in mortality with vesnarinone among patients with severe heart failure. Vesnarinone Trial Investigators. N Engl J Med 1998; 339(25): 1810–1816.

80. Pitt B, et al. Effect of losartan compared with captopril on mortality in patients with symptomatic heart failure: randomised trial—the Losartan Heart Failure Survival Study ELITE II. Lancet 2000; 355(9215):1582–1587.

81. Pitt B, et al. The effect of spironolactone on morbidity and mortality in patients with severe heart failure. Randomized Aldactone Evaluation Study Investigators. N Engl J Med 1999; 341(10):709–717.

82. Teerlink JR, et al. Ambulatory ventricular arrhythmias in patients with heart failure do not specifically predict an increased risk of sudden death. PROMISE (Prospective Randomized Milrinone Survival Evaluation) Investigators. Circulation 2000; 101(1):40–46.

83. Stevenson WG, et al. Sudden death prevention in patients with advanced ventricular dysfunction. Circulation 1993; 88(6):2953–2961.

84. Connolly SJ, et al. Canadian implantable defibrillator study (CIDS): a randomized trial of the implantable cardioverter defibrillator against amiodarone. Circulation 2000; 101(11): 1297–1302.

85. Sheldon R, et al. Identification of patients most likely to benefit from implantable cardioverter-defibrillator therapy: the Canadian Implantable Defibrillator Study. Circulation 2000; 101(14):1660–1664.

86. Connolly SJ, et al. Meta-analysis of the implantable cardioverter defibrillator secondary prevention trials. AVID, CASH and CIDS studies. Antiarrhythmics vs Implantable Defibrillator study. Cardiac Arrest Study Hamburg. Canadian Implantable Defibrillator Study. Eur Heart J 2000; 21(24):2071–2078.

87. de Bakker JM, et al. Slow conduction in the infarcted human heart. 'Zigzag' course of activation. Circulation 1993; 88(3):915–926.

88. Stevenson WG, et al. Exploring postinfarction reentrant ventricular tachycardia with entrainment mapping. J Am Coll Cardiol 1997; 29(6):1180–1189.

89. Buxton AE, et al. A randomized study of the prevention of sudden death in patients with coronary artery disease. Multicenter Unsustained Tachycardia Trial Investigators (erratum appears in. N Engl J Med 2000 Apr 27; 342(17):1300. N Engl J Med 1999; 341(25): 1882–1890.

90. Moss AJ, et al. Improved survival with an implanted defibrillator in patients with coronary disease at high risk for ventricular arrhythmia. Multicenter Automatic Defibrillator Implantation Trial Investigators. N Engl J Med 1996; 335(26):1933–1940.

91. Stevenson WG, et al. Inducible ventricular arrhythmias and sudden death during vasodilator therapy of severe heart failure. Am Heart J 1988; 116(6 Pt 1):1447–1454.

92. Turitto G, et al. Risk stratification for arrhythmic events in patients with nonischemic dilated cardiomyopathy and nonsustained ventricular tachycardia: role of programmed ventricular stimulation and the signal-averaged electrocardiogram. J Am Coll Cardiol 1994; 24(6): 1523–1528.

93. Hammill SC, et al. Influence of ventricular function and presence or absence of coronary artery disease on results of electrophysiologic testing for asymptomatic nonsustained ventricular tachycardia. Am J Cardiol 1990; 65(11):722–728.

94. Lindsay BD, et al. Prospective detection of vulnerability to sustained ventricular tachycardia in patients awaiting cardiac transplantation. Am J Cardiol 1992; 69(6):619–624.

95. Das SK, et al. Prognostic usefulness of programmed ventricular stimulation in idiopathic dilated cardiomyopathy without symptomatic ventricular arrhythmias. Am J Cardiol 1986; 58(10):998–1000.

96. Meinertz T, et al. Determinants of prognosis in idiopathic dilated cardiomyopathy as determined by programmed electrical stimulation. Am J Cardiol 1985; 56(4):337–341.

97. Poll DS, et al. Usefulness of programmed stimulation in idiopathic dilated cardiomyopathy. Am J Cardiol 1986; 58(10):992–997.

98. Delacretaz E, et al. Mapping and radiofrequency catheter ablation of the three types of sustained monomorphic ventricular tachycardia in nonischemic heart disease. J Cardiovasc Electrophysiol 2000; 11(1):11–17.

99. Ellison KE, et al. Entrainment mapping and radiofrequency catheter ablation of ventricular tachycardia in right ventricular dysplasia. J Am Coll Cardiol 1998; 32(3):724–728.

100. Pinski SL. The right ventricular tachycardias. J Electrocardiol 2000(33 Suppl):103–114.

101. Corrado D, et al. Spectrum of clinicopathologic manifestations of arrhythmogenic right ventricular cardiomyopathy/dysplasia: a multicenter study. J Am Coll Cardiol 1997; 30(6): 1512–1520.

102. anonymous. Case records of the Massachusetts General Hospital. Weekly clinicopathological exercises. Case 20-2000. A 61-year-old man with a wide-complex tachycardia. N Engl J Med 2000; 342(26):1979–1987.

103. Marcus FI, Fontaine G. Arrhythmogenic right ventricular dysplasia/cardiomyopathy: a review. Pacing Clin Electrophysiol 1995; 18(6):1298–1314.

104. Fontaine G, et al. Arrhythmogenic right ventricular dysplasia. Ann Rev Med 1999(50): 17–35.

105. Inoue S, et al. Myocarditis and arrhythmia: a clinico-pathological study of conduction system based on serial section in 65 cases. Jpn Circ J 1989; 53(1):49–57.

106. Delacretaz E, et al. Ablation of ventricular tachycardia with a saline-cooled radiofrequency catheter: anatomic and histologic characteristics of the lesions in humans. J Cardiovasc Electrophysiol 1999; 10(6):860–865.

107. de Bakker JM, et al. Fractionated electrograms in dilated cardiomyopathy: origin and relation to abnormal conduction. J Am Coll Cardiol 1996; 27(5):1071–1078.

108. Woelfel A, Wohns DH, Foster JR. Implications of sustained monomorphic ventricular tachycardia associated with myocardial injury. Ann Intern Med 1990; 112(2):141–143.

109. Soejima K, et al. Catheter ablation in patients with multiple and unstable ventricular tachycardias after myocardial infarction: short ablation lines guided by reentry circuit isthmuses and sinus rhythm mapping. Circulation 2001; 104(6):664–669.

110. Passman R, Kadish A. Polymorphic ventricular tachycardia, long Q-T syndrome, and torsades de pointes. Med Clin North Am 2001; 85(2):321–341.

111. MacNeil M. The side effect profile of Class III antiarrhythmic drugs focus on DL Sotalol. Am J Cardiol 1997; 80:90G–98G.

112. Kowey PR, VanderLugt JT, Luderer JR. Safety and risk/benefit analysis of ibutilide for acute conversion of atrial fibrillation/flutter. Am J Cardiol 1996; 78(8A):46–52.

113. Mazur A, et al. Pause-dependent polymorphic ventricular tachycardia during long-term treatment with dofetilide: a placebo-controlled, implantable cardioverter-defibrillator-based evaluation. J Am Coll Cardiol 2001; 37(4):1100–1105.

114. Maor N, Weiss D, Lorber A. Torsade de pointes complicating atrioventricular block: report of two cases. Int J Cardiol 1987; 14(2):235–238.

115. Tomaselli GF, Rose J. Molecular aspects of arrhythmias associated with cardiomyopathies. Curr Opin Cardiol 2000; 15(3):202–208.

116. Middlekauff HR, et al. Amiodarone and torsades de pointes in patients with advanced heart failure. Am J Cardiol 1995; 76(7):499–502.

117. Viskin S. Cardiac pacing in the long QT syndrome: review of available data and practical recommendations. J Cardiovasc Electrophysiol 2000; 11(5):593–600.

118. Middlekauff HR, et al. Syncope in advanced heart failure: high risk of sudden death regardless of origin of syncope. J Am Coll Cardiol 1993; 21(1):110–116.

119. Knight BP, et al. Outcome of patients with nonischemic dilated cardiomyopathy and unexplained syncope treated with an implantable defibrillator. J Am Coll Cardiol 1999; 33(7): 1964–1970.

120. Fonarow GC, et al. Improved survival in patients with nonischemic advanced heart failure and syncope treated with an implantable cardioverter-defibrillator. Am J Cardiol 2000; 85(8): 981–985.

121. Fruhwald FM, et al. Syncope in dilated cardiomyopathy is a predictor of sudden cardiac death. Cardiology 1996; 87(3):177–180.

122. Moss AJ. MADIT-II and implications for noninvasive electrophysiologic testing. Ann Noninvasive Electrocardiol 2002; 7(3):179–180.

123. Singh SN, et al. Prevalence and significance of nonsustained ventricular tachycardia in patients with premature ventricular contractions and heart failure treated with vasodilator therapy. Department of Veterans Affairs CHF STAT Investigators. J Am Coll Cardiol 1998; 32(4):942–947.

124. Doval HC, et al. Nonsustained ventricular tachycardia in severe heart failure. Independent marker of increased mortality due to sudden death. GESICA-GEMA Investigators. Circulation 1996; 94(12):3198–3203.

125. Davies SW, et al. Overnight studies in severe chronic left heart failure: arrhythmias and oxygen desaturation. Br Heart J 1991; 65(2):77–83.

126. Javaheri S. Effects of continuous positive airway pressure on sleep apnea and ventricular irritability in patients with heart failure. Circulation 2000; 101(4):392–397.

127. Javaheri S, Corbett WS. Association of low PaCO2 with central sleep apnea and ventricular arrhythmias in ambulatory patients with stable heart failure. Ann Intern Med 1998; 128(3): 204–207.

128. Javaheri S, et al. Sleep apnea in 81 ambulatory male patients with stable heart failure. Types and their prevalences, consequences, and presentations. Circulation 1998; 97(21): 2154–2159.

129. Moss AJ, et al. Prophylactic implantation of a defibrillator in patients with myocardial infarction and reduced ejection fraction. N Engl J Med 2002; 346(12):877–883.

130. Buxton AE, et al. Electrophysiologic testing to identify patients with coronary artery disease who are at risk for sudden death. Multicenter Unsustained Tachycardia Trial Investigators. N Engl J Med 2000; 342(26):1937–1945.

131. Bigger JT, et al. Mechanisms of death in the CABG Patch trial: a randomized trial of implantable cardiac defibrillator prophylaxis in patients at high risk of death after coronary artery bypass graft surgery. Circulation 1999; 99(11):1416–1421.

132. Doval HC, et al. Randomised trial of low-dose amiodarone in severe congestive heart failure. Grupo de Estudio de la Sobrevida en la Insuficiencia Cardiaca en Argentina (GESICA). Lancet 1994; 344(8921):493–498.

133. Strickberger SA, et al. Amiodarone versus implantable cardioverter-defibrillator:randomized trial in patients with nonischemic dilated cardiomyopathy and asymptomatic nonsustained ventricular tachycardia—AMIOVIRT. J Am Coll Cardiol 2003; 41(10):1707–1712.

134. Connolly SJ. Meta-analysis of antiarrhythmic drug trials. Am J Cardiol 1999; 84(9A): 90R–93R.

135. Barold HS, et al. Concealed mechanical bradycardia: an indication for permanent pacemaker implantation. Pacing Clin Electrophysiol 1998; 21(10):2007–2008.

136. Gregoratos G, et al. ACC/AHA/NASPE 2002 guideline update for implantation of cardiac pacemakers and antiarrhythmia devices: summary article: a report of the American College of Cardiology/American Heart Association Task Force on Practice Guidelines (ACC/AHA/ NASPE Committee to Update the 1998 Pacemaker Guidelines). Circulation 2002; 106(16): 2145–2161.

137. Moss AJ. Implantable cardioverter defibrillator therapy: the sickest patients benefit the most. Circulation 2000; 101(14):1638–1640.

138. Bocker D, et al. Potential benefit from implantable cardioverter-defibrillator therapy in patients with and without heart failure. Circulation 1998; 98(16):1636–1643.

139. Mecca A, et al. Implantable cardioverter defibrillator therapy for patients with life- threatening ventricular arrhythmias and severe heart failure. Am J Cardiol 2000; 86(8):875–877.

140. Saxon LA, et al. Implantable defibrillators for high-risk patients with heart failure who are awaiting cardiac transplantation. Am Heart J 1995; 130(3 Pt 1):501–506.

141. Sweeney MO, et al. Influence of the implantable cardioverter/defibrillator on sudden death and total mortality in patients evaluated for cardiac transplantation. Circulation 1995; 92(11): 3273–3281.

142. Best PJ, Hayes DL, Stanton MS. The potential usage of dual chamber pacing in patients with implantable cardioverter defibrillators. Pacing Clin Electrophysiol 1999; 22(1 Pt 1): 79–85.

143. Grines CL, et al. Functional abnormalities in isolated left bundle branch block. The effect of interventricular asynchrony. Circulation 1989; 79(4):845–853.

144. Nielsen JC, et al. Regional myocardial blood flow in patients with sick sinus syndrome randomized to long-term single chamber atrial or dual chamber pacing—effect of pacing mode and rate. J Am Coll Cardiol 2000; 35(6):1453–1461.

145. Tse HF, Lau CP. Long-term effect of right ventricular pacing on myocardial perfusion and function. J Am Coll Cardiol 1997; 29(4):744–779.

146. Wilkoff BL, et al. Dual-chamber pacing or ventricular backup pacing in patients with an implantable defibrillator: the Dual Chamber and VVI Implantable Defibrillator (DAVID) Trial. JAMA 2002; 288(24):3115–3123.

147. Spotnitz HM. Does ventricular fibrillation cause myocardial stunning during defibrillator implantation? J Card Surg 1993; 8(2 Suppl):249–256.

148. Pires LA, et al. Sudden death in implantable cardioverter-defibrillator recipients: clinical context, arrhythmic events and device responses. J Am Coll Cardiol 1999; 33(1):24–32.

149. Villacastin J, et al. Incidence and clinical significance of multiple consecutive, appropriate, high-energy discharges in patients with implanted cardioverter-defibrillators. Circulation 1996; 93(4):753–762.

150. Exner DV, et al. Electrical storm presages nonsudden death: the Antiarrhythmics Versus Implantable Defibrillators (AVID) Trial. Circulation 2001; 103(16):2066–2071.

150a. Stevenson WG, Epstein LM, Maisel WH, Sweeney MO, Stevenson LW. Clinical approaches to tachyarrhythmias. In: Camm AJ, Ed. Clinical Approach to Tachyarrhythmias. Vol. 15. Futura Publishing. Inc., 2002.

151. Thomas SA, Friedmann E, Kelley FJ. Living with an implantable cardioverter-defibrillator: a review of the current literature related to psychosocial factors. AACN Clin Iss 2001; 12(1): 156–163.

152. Sears SF, et al. Assessing the psychosocial impact of the ICD: a national survey of implantable cardioverter defibrillator health care providers. (comment). Pacing Clin Electrophysiol 2000; 23(6):939–945.

153. Dunbar SB, et al. Association of mood disturbance and arrhythmia events in patients after cardioverter defibrillator implantation. Depres Anxiety 1999; 9(4):163–168.

154. Heller SS, et al. Psychosocial outcome after ICD implantation: a current perspective. Pacing Clin Electrophysiol 1998; 21(6):1207–1215.

155. Fricchione GL, Vlay LC, Vlay SC. Cardiac psychiatry and the management of malignant ventricular arrhythmias with the internal cardioverter-defibrillator. Am Heart J 1994; 128(5): 1050–1059.

20
Heart Failure in Special Populations

Clyde W. Yancy
Heart Failure/Transplantation, University of Texas Southwestern Medical Center
Dallas, Texas, USA

SYNOPSIS

Despite considerable elucidation of the heart failure syndrome, two important special clinical situations arise that require additional perspectives: ''special populations'' of patients affected with heart failure; and important clinical comorbidities that may accompany heart failure. The prototypical special populations are women, the elderly, and minorities. Each of these groups is frequently underrepresented in clinical trials but is seemingly overrepresented in clinical practice. Available data, largely derived from post-hoc subgroup analyses of the major clinical initiatives in heart failure, have yielded several prevailing themes pertinent to all three groups: the compelling influence of hypertension on the genesis of heart failure; questions regarding efficacy of current medical treatment regimens; and the concern that morbidity and possibly mortality due to heart failure may be more problematic. Despite these concerns, there are no substantial data to suggest that treatment algorithms should vary as a function of gender, age, or race. Whereas most clinical trials in heart failure exclude the patient with significant renal, pulmonary, or thyroid diseases, the prevalence of these comorbidities in heart failure is not insignificant and the contribution to excess morbidity and mortality in heart failure can be substantial.

INTRODUCTION

Heart failure is no longer a diagnosis of futility with a poor quality of life and dismal outcome. Rather, significant strides in elucidation of the pathophysiology of left ventricular dysfunction have led to the emergence of therapeutic options that have yielded marked improvements in the quality and quantity of life for persons affected with heart failure. The use of angiotensin converting enzyme inhibitors [1], beta-blockers [2], aldosterone antagonists [3], and angiotensin-receptor antagonists for the ACE-I-intolerant patient [4] now represent standards of care and should be regarded as quality benchmarks in any ambulatory heart failure disease management program. With appropriate introduction of comprehensive neurohormonal antagonism, the risk of death due to heart failure in all but the most severely ill patient can be reduced by 50% and the corresponding decrease in the risk for hospitalization is of nearly the same magnitude.

The target of therapy for heart failure is shifting from a focus based solely on increased longevity to one that aims to improve the quality of life and to reduce the consumption of health care resources. This is a laudable evolution in the treatment of one of the most common medical maladies, but a disturbing question emerges. Do these treatment successes and the favorable momentum now established include *all* patients with heart failure? Such a question appears perfunctory at first contemplation, but the demographics of major clinical trials have been overwhelmingly male, late middle-age, and white. As well, the majority of clinical trials in heart failure exclude by definition patients who have other important systemic illnesses. *Thus, the majority of patients with heart failure are excluded from participation in clinical trials.* Nevertheless, favorable results of clinical trials have been extrapolated to the general population with the presumption that the results are applicable in a more general population. Renewed analyses have begun to address the applicability of the findings from important clinical trials in the broader population and to establish nuances in the natural history of heart failure in subgroups of interest and perhaps differences in the response to medical therapy.

This chapter will address two important groups; those patients in special populations affected with heart failure, especially women, the elderly, and African Americans; and those patients with common comorbidities, including renal disease, pulmonary disease, and thyroid disease.

Prior to embarking upon a discussion of the important subgroups in heart failure, it is important to acknowledge limitations of the currently available datasets. Virtually all of the available information on treatment emanates from post-hoc analyses of clinical trial data that did not have as an a priori objective a statistically valid population of any of these important subgroups. Data regarding important comorbidities are even less reliable as these patients were often excluded from clinical trial participation. Despite these obvious limitations, consistent themes have emerged that define the patient groups in question, enlighten their unique natural history, and address their response to medical therapy for heart failure.

SPECIAL POPULATIONS AT RISK

Women

Women are significantly affected by heart failure [5] (Fig. 1). The highest incidence of heart failure is observed in older women and in African American women. In addition, in younger women (age <50 years), the high prevalence of obesity and diabetes may predispose to heart failure. Hypertension is a known risk factor for heart failure in as many as 90% of all cases of the disease [5,6]. This is especially true in women. Both men and especially women who demonstrate obesity have been shown to have corresponding linear increases in sympathetic nervous system activation [7]. This pattern is present in both African-American and Caucasian women. The correlation is even more striking in women with significant visceral fat deposits. Obesity, which is present in at least 35% of the U.S. population [8], predisposes to sympathetic activation in women, which in turn predisposes to hypertension. Given the correlation of hypertension as an antecedent illness in the eventual development of heart failure [6], it is plausible that the obesity epidemic is partially responsible for the occurrence of heart failure in women. The obesity epidemic likewise contributes to the alarming rates of type II diabetes seen in women, and the striking prevalence of the metabolic syndrome, thus, establishes an important substrate for aggressive cardiovascular disease in women.

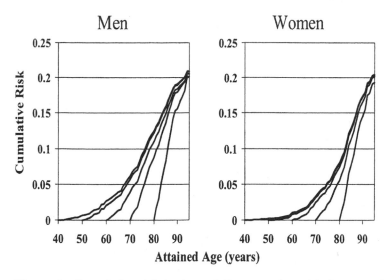

Figure 1 Cumulative risk for heart failure at selected index ages for men and women. Lifetime risk of heart failure for a given index age is cumulative risk through age 94 years. (From Ref. 5a.)

As a consequence, the natural history of heart failure in women is typified by hypertension, diabetes, obesity and African American race. The incidence of documented epicardial coronary artery disease is lower as is the concomitant presence of tobacco abuse [9].

Women with heart failure may fare slightly better than men. In the original Framingham Study, women with heart failure had a 5-year survival of 50% compared with only 33% for men [5]. A more recent analysis, Resource Utilization Among Congestive Heart Failure Study [REACH] [10], confirmed yet again a better prognosis for women than for men. REACH was a 10-year epidemiological survey of heart failure (n = 29,686) using ICD-9 codes as a probe with incidence, prevalence, and mortality identified. The incidence of heart failure in the Framingham study was 4.7 cases/1000 for women and 7.2/1000 for men. In REACH, the incidence for women was 5.3 and for men, 5.5/1000. The prevalence of heart failure in the Framingham study was 7.7/1000 in women and 7.4/1000 in men. In REACH, the prevalence was 10.5/1000 in women and 10.9/1000 in men. The overall median survival seen in REACH for women was 4.5 years vs. 3.7 years for men. (Fig. 2) [10]. The corresponding median survivals seen in the Framingham study were 3.2 and 1.7 years for women and men, respectively. For women in REACH who were less than 65 years of age, the median survival was 6 years. Thus, women with heart failure have a lower incidence of the disease, similar prevalence, and a decided survival advantage compared with men. The REACH survey included nearly 45% African Americans compared with virtually zero in the Framingham Study. Given the excess incidence of heart failure in African Americans, i.e., 50% to 75% greater incidence [11], the findings from REACH may have been largely impacted by the very different demographic features.

The survival advantage seen in women with heart failure is not clear and within recent clinical trials, is not manifest. If there is a difference in mortality, it may be influenced by a higher incidence of heart failure with preserved systolic function, which is known to have a somewhat better prognosis than heart failure with systolic dysfunction. These data should not be interpreted to represent heart failure as a benign disease in women. The diagnosis of heart failure in women is associated with a greater 5-year risk of death than

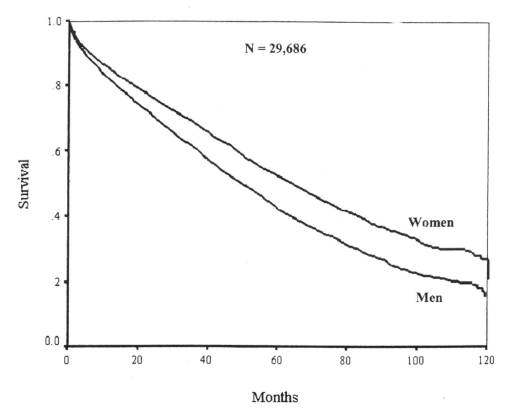

Figure 2 Age-adjusted and race-adjusted mortality for men and women with heart failure in an integrated health care system, 1989 to 1999; p < 0.0001. (From Ref. 10.)

an acute myocardial infarction, breast cancer, and colon cancer; and a similar rate of death as ovarian cancer. Only female lung cancer patients fare worse than heart failure patients [12].

The pathophysiological explanations for these gender differences in heart failure have not been fully explored and are largely theoretical. Several observations vis-à-vis ventricular pathology are pertinent. In response to hypertension, women do express a less malignant pattern of left ventricular hypertrophy than men. Women appear to be quite sensitive to the effects of chemotherapeutic agents, especially anthracyclines and the HER-2-neu oncogene antibody (herceptin). These differences may be gender specific or may be seen in women simply due to breast cancer therapy. One also notes the pathology associated with peripartum cardiomyopathy and the slightly higher incidence of primary pulmonary hypertension. If a pathophysiological basis for ventricular/vascular disease is present, a culprit etiology would reside in the cardiovascular influences of estrogen. Estrogen stimulates genes responsible for prostacyclin, endothelin-1, E-selectin, vascular endothelial growth factor and matrix metalloproteinase-2. Estrogen also stimulates genes regulating fibrinogen, tPA and PAI-1, platelet derived growth factor, transforming growth factor beta 1 and protein S [9]. Thus, an environment is created that predisposes to vascular smooth muscle growth, fibrosis, and thrombosis. Much work needs to be done to fully understand the nuances of estrogen effect on the cardiovascular system.

The treatment of heart failure in women has not been studied in a prospective, controlled manner nor are any such trials contemplated. Moreover, the representation of

Table 1 Participation of Women in Major Clinical Trials of Heart Failure

Trial	Number of Women	% Women
V-HeFT I	0	0
CONSENSUS I	75	30
SOLVD-Treatment	504	19.5
U.S. Carvedilol Heart Failure Trials	256	23.5
COPERNICUS	465	25
DIG	1520	22.5

women in major heart failure trials has been quite variable, ranging from 0% to 30%. (Table 1)

Data from 30 randomized trials of ACE inhibitors in heart failure due to left ventricular systolic dysfunction *failed to demonstrate a mortality benefit* of ACE inhibitors in women [13]. (Fig. 3) There are no data from the direct vasodilator experience in women, i.e., V-HeFT I and II trials. A review of the Digitalis Investigators Group (DIG trial) determined that not only did women fail to derive a benefit from digoxin therapy for heart failure, but that a risk existed when the digoxin level was high normal but still well within the recommended therapeutic range [14]. The absence of benefit on outcome for ACE - inhibitors, vasodilators, and digoxin in women may reflect selection bias in these early trials.

The experience with beta-adrenergic receptor antagonists is more encouraging, but questions of efficacy have also been raised. (Fig. 4) A review of key beta-blocker trials reveals that the representation of women in these trials was not controlled and in only one study was a randomization target specified. The Beta-Blocker Evaluation of Survival Trial, [BEST], prespecified a randomization target for women and incentivized investigators to recruit women. The target was at least 20% of enrolled patients and this threshold was achieved. In BEST, 593 women were enrolled. Unfortunately, the overall trial results failed to meet the primary endpoint of a reduction in all-cause mortality [15]. This was especially evident in women and within the African American cohorts in the trial. Prior to surmising that these findings cast doubt on the efficacy of beta-blockers in women with heart failure, it must be acknowledged that bucindolol has a very different pharmacologic profile from other beta-blockers used in heart failure (Chapter 13). It exerts a much more profound reduction in plasma norepinephrine levels and has been demonstrated to have at least partial intrinsic sympathomimetic activity [16]. Both of these characteristics have been separately shown to contribute to excess mortality in heart failure.

The BEST trial demonstrated that women with heart failure are overrepresented by African Americans—30% of the women in BEST were African American. Women were more likely to have a nonischemic etiology for their left ventricular dysfunction. The degree of neurohormonal activation was less in women than men, measured as plasma norepinephrine levels. The presence of atrial fibrillation imparted a two-fold increase in the risk of death for women in the BEST trial [17].

The Metoprolol Extended Release Randomized Intervention Trial in Heart Failure [MERIT-HF] study included nearly 900 women (29% of the overall cohort). A benefit on all-cause mortality was not seen within this group but the combined endpoint of all-cause mortality and all cause hospitalization was achieved with a 21% reduction in events. The reduction in all-cause hospitalizations was 29% and for hospitalizations due to heart failure, there was a 42% reduction in hospitalizations. Within the MERIT-HF experience,

MALE

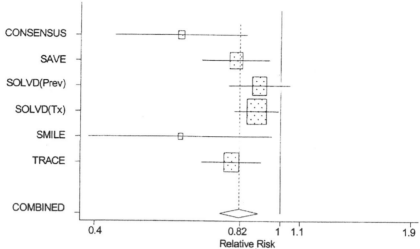

FEMALE

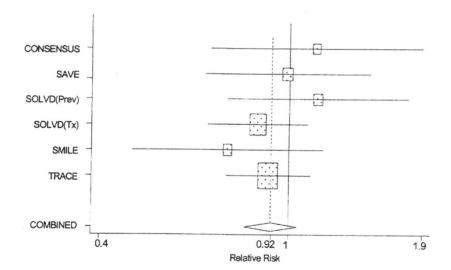

Figure 3 Effect of angiotensin-converting enzyme inhibitors on mortality in patient with heart failure. For each study, *the size of the box* is proportional to the sample size, and the lines denote the 95% confidence interval. For the combined results, the *ends of the diamond shape* denote the 95% confidence interval. Trial abbreviations are contained in the text. Prev, prevention trial; Tx, treatment trial. (From Ref 13a.)

183 women were identified as having severe heart failure. The influence of beta-blocker therapy on that group yielded a 57% decrease in all-cause hospitalization and 72% reduction in heart failure hospitalization [18].

The favorable benefit of beta-blocker therapy in women was further supported by results from the carvedilol trials. In the U.S. Carvedilol Heart Failure Trials Program, the relative risk reduction for mortality was 0.32 (p = 0.028) in women and 0.43 (p = 0.007) in men. Mortality was not a prespecified endpoint in these trials [19]. The Carvedilol

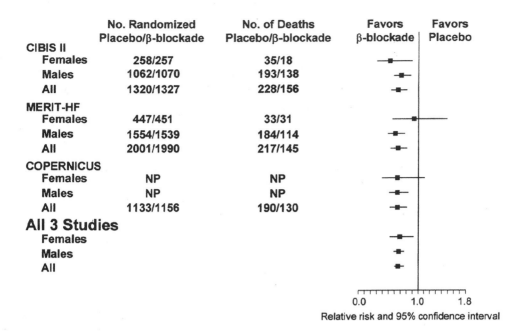

	No. Randomized Placebo/β-blockade	No. of Deaths Placebo/β-blockade	Favors β-blockade	Favors Placebo
CIBIS II				
Females	258/257	35/18		
Males	1062/1070	193/138		
All	1320/1327	228/156		
MERIT-HF				
Females	447/451	33/31		
Males	1554/1539	184/114		
All	2001/1990	217/145		
COPERNICUS				
Females	NP	NP		
Males	NP	NP		
All	1133/1156	190/130		
All 3 Studies				
Females				
Males				
All				

0.0   1.0   1.8
Relative risk and 95% confidence interval

Figure 4   Point estimates for hazard ratios and 95% confidence intervals for total mortality by gender and overall in the CIBIS II, MERIT-HF and COPERNICUS trial. Trial abbreviations are contained in the text. (From Ref. 18.) NP; not published

Prospective Randomized Cumulative Survival study (COPERNICUS) trial evaluated the efficacy of carvedilol when added to an ACE inhibitor in the management of severe heart failure. The overall trial results were overwhelmingly positive and demonstrated a 35% survival advantage attributable to carvedilol. Among the 465 women randomized (25% of the overall population), a similar relative risk reduction in mortality was seen when compared to men. The confidence intervals were broad and crossed the line of identity; however, for the combined endpoint of death plus hospitalization for any reason or death plus hospitalization for heart failure, the relative risk reduction was not only identical to men but did, in fact, reach statistical significance [20,21].

The aggregate experience using beta-blocker therapy in women clearly demonstrates efficacy of this drug class and there should be no hesitancy to utilize neurohormonal antagonism with beta-blockers plus ACE inhibitors as primary therapy of heart failure in women with a goal of reducing both morbidity and mortality.

Elderly

The burden of heart failure and its public health implications are perhaps greatest in the elderly population. The prevalence of heart failure in persons beyond the age of 65 years exceeds 5% and for those beyond the age of 80 years, the prevalence is at least 10% of the population. Among patients hospitalized with heart failure, 80% are older than 65 years [22]. In the Acute Decompensated Heart Failure Registry [ADHERE], the *median age* of 27,000 patients admitted for heart failure to 250 U.S. hospitals was 75 years. The in-hospital mortality rate for all participants was 4% but was substantially higher in the cohort greater than 75 years of age [23]. The mortality rate attributable to heart failure hospitalization is highest in the elderly and approximates the average mortality rate of acute myocardial infarction. The expense attributable to in-patient care for hospitalization represents nearly 50% of the annual $30 billion expenditure on heart failure, and the majority of this hospitalization expense is observed in the elderly population admitted with heart failure–*oftentimes with preventable precipitating causes for the admission.* The ability of any treatment strategy to impact these costs has considerable public health implications.

Comprehensive disease-management programs that encourage compliance with optimal medical treatment strategies, promote flexible diuretic regimens, and provide nursing based education are particularly helpful in the elderly population. Emerging data from these programs are clearly demonstrating a decrease in hospitalization usage and an improvement in mortality [24].

As a disease entity, heart failure in the elderly is a peculiar process. There are several explanations for the high prevalence of heart failure in the elderly. More patients now survive acute myocardial infarction and are spared premature death due to sudden cardiac events. Thus, more patients are surviving with impaired ventricular function and undergo ventricular remodeling, the natural history of which leads to symptomatic heart failure. Another plausible explanation for the high prevalence of heart failure in the elderly is hypertension [25]. Nearly *90%* of all individuals above the age of 80 years have hypertension, which places this population at high risk for the development of heart failure [26]. (Fig. 1) Yet another potential explanation for the prevalence of heart failure in the elderly is the natural senescence of the myocardium. The loss of functioning myocytes is approximately 5% per year in patients beyond the age of 65 years, which, along with the corresponding increase in extracellular matrix, contributes to changes in left ventricular compliance. Consequently, ventricular phenotypic changes exist that predispose to ''heart failure with preserved systolic function.'' Clinical data support this physiological construct. Consistently, 50% of heart failure admissions in the elderly occur in the setting of preserved systolic function [23]. Evidence-based algorithms for the treatment of diastolic heart failure are currently lacking (Chapter 17).

Management of heart failure in the elderly should be aimed at its prevention. As noted, hypertension imparts a considerable risk in the development of heart failure, at least two-fold above the general population. This risk is even higher in the setting of hypertension with a prior myocardial infarction and/or diabetes [27]. Encouraging data from the hypertension literature demonstrate the ability to significantly limit the progression from hypertension to heart failure in the elderly.

The Systolic Hypertension in the Elderly Project [SHEP] was a placebo-controlled, randomized trial of thiazide diuretics with or without beta-blockers in patients older than 60 years with systolic hypertension. The entry systolic blood pressure was 160 to 219 mm Hg. The treated group experienced an annual reduction in the onset of heart failure of at least 50%. The magnitude of this benefit was even greater in the elderly patient with systolic hypertension and a past history of a myocardial infarction. The number of hypertensive patients needed to treat to save one life with thiazide diuretic plus beta-blocker was 48; in the setting of a prior myocardial infarction, that number was reduced to only 15 [27]. (Fig. 5) The Swedish Trial of Older Persons [STOP] with systolic hypertension supported these findings by demonstrating that the use of thiazide diuretics plus beta-blockers reduced annual mortality by 43% [28].

More recent data from the Second Australian National Blood Pressure Study Group demonstrated that for patients aged 65 to 84 years with hypertension (defined as systolic greater than 160 mmHg and/or diastolic pressure greater than 90 mm Hg) the use of an ACE inhibitor led to a 17% decrease in the rate of a cardiovascular event or death in men

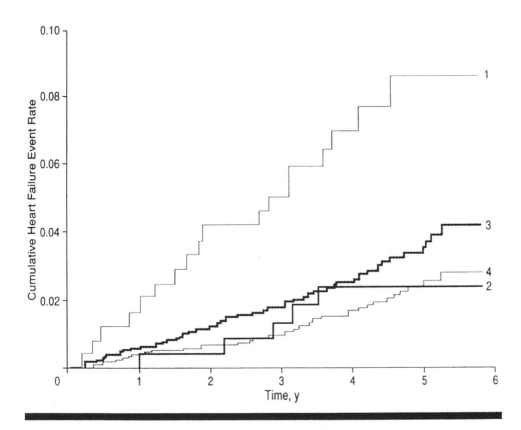

Figure 5 Occurrence of fatal and hospitalized nonfatal heart failure in the active therapy and placebo groups of the Systolic Hypertension in the Elderly Program [SHEP] among participants who had a history or electrocardiographic evidence of myocardial infarction (MI) at baseline and among those who did not have a history or electrocardiographic evidence of MI at baseline. *Line 1* indicates the placebo group (patients with a history of MI at baseline); *line 2*, active therapy group (patients with history of MI at baseline); *line 3*, placebo group (patients with no history of MI at baseline); and *line 4*, active therapy group (patients with no history of MI at baseline). (From Ref. 27.)

(*but not in women*) compared with the use of a thiazide alone [29]. There was no difference in outcomes within women. The HOPE trial enrolled patients 55 years of age or older with known risk factors for atherosclerosis to ramipril, vitamin E or placebo. The use of ramipril in this at-risk group was associated with a 17% decrease in the incidence of heart failure [30]. These trial data suggest that effective therapy of hypertension may decrease the incidence of heart failure and improve cardiovascular outcomes. Consequently, the argument for the implementation of *preventive* strategies for heart failure is quite compelling.

Once the disease is established, data regarding treatment becomes of paramount importance. Therapeutic options to manage heart failure are not only effective in the elderly, but are perhaps *most effective* due to the very high event rate in this population. Depending on the age threshold defining ''elderly,'' the majority of heart failure trials were actually conducted in elderly cohorts and, thus, the findings are ideally suitable to the usual patient population. A review of the MERIT-HF, U.S. Carvedilol Heart Failure

Trials Program and COPERNICUS trials demonstrates in a most convincing way that patients older than 65 years in these trials responded to medical therapy of heart failure using the combination of an ACE inhibitor and beta-blocker. The magnitude of benefit in each trial for those patients younger than 65 and older than 65 years of age was identical [19,20,31]. Observations in patients older than 75 years support, yet again, the benefit of medical therapy in heart failure [32].

Available data would suggest that heart failure in the elderly is a major public health problem and deserves more attention. The event rate is quite high and the expenditure of resources is considerable. The very high penetration of symptomatic heart failure with preserved systolic function further complicates disease management in this group. Prevention is the best strategy and effective evidence based management of hypertension appears to be the most appropriate strategy. This is especially evident in the group with systolic hypertension of the elderly. When the elderly patient has symptomatic heart failure due to systolic dysfunction, it must be emphasized that there are no data to substantiate the appropriateness of a more conservative strategy. Unfortunately, elderly patients when exposed to appropriate therapies for heart failure are often *underdosed*, thus, limiting the efficacy of these agents. Long-term disease management in the elderly should also address end-of-life decision-making and the application of expensive device and surgical treatment alternatives in the setting of advance heart failure and limited longevity.

Ethnic Minorities

The most salient discussion of ''special populations'' in the realm of heart failure focuses on ethnic minority groups. Conclusions from these limited data sets must be qualified. The best data points available are for African Americans with heart failure as no other ethnic minority has been studied to any significant degree. Heart failure occurs in the African American population with a higher incidence, perhaps as much as 50% higher than in other racial groups. The overall incidence of heart failure in the population is 2% [~5 million patients] but within the African American cohort, the incidence is 3% [33]. The SOLVD [Studies of Left Ventricular Dysfunction] Prevention trial confirmed that African Americans develop heart failure at a statistically higher incidence rate than non–African Americans [34]. There are also several differences in the presentation of this disease in African Americans. Symptoms are generally associated with a more advanced stage of left ventricular dysfunction. The clinical classification is likewise more advanced—thus, the African American patient with heart failure presents with a much more malignant disease process. Disease etiology also differs from the general population. The SOLVD Registry first identified a striking dissimilarity in the etiology of left ventricular dysfunction in African Americans compared to non–African Americans [35]. Whereas hypertension as a lone etiology of left ventricular dysfunction was present in only 4% of the non–African American cohort, more than 30% of the African American cohort had hypertension as the probable cause of left ventricular dysfunction. Data reported from major clinical trials in heart failure support this variance in disease etiology. The documented presence of either a prior myocardial infarction or known ischemic heart disease is present in nearly 70% of cases of heart failure in non–African Americans, but only 40% for African Americans [33]. (Fig. 6). By inference, the proportion of nonischemic disease associated with left ventricular dysfunction and heart failure is much higher in African American patients. The distribution of nonischemic etiologies may include hypertensive heart disease, dilated cardiomyopathies, alcohol and obesity related cardiomyopathies and postinflammatory cardiomyopathies. Although difficult to precisely quantify,

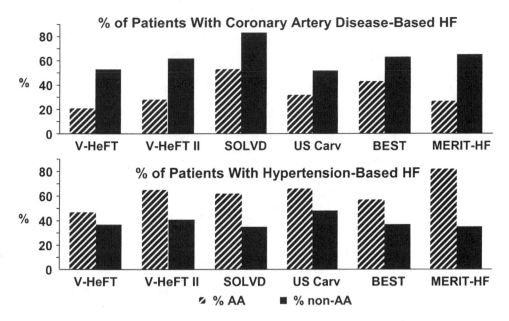

Figure 6 Etiology of heart failure among African-American men and women who participated in major heart failure clinical trial. Trial abbreviations are contained in the text.

the incidence of hypertension varies from 30% to nearly 60% depending on the database
analyzed [33].

Outcomes seen within the African American group with heart failure are perhaps
most troublesome. Both morbidity *and mortality* outcomes appear to be higher in this
population. Heart failure hospitalization rates in African Americans are higher than for
non–African Americans. Whether this variance is related to more advanced disease or
differences in access to standard medical care is unclear. Within the SOLVD treatment
trial, African Americans had a higher rate of hospitalization despite being cared for by
the same investigator/infrastructure as the overall study.

Mortality issues are quite debatable. The SOLVD experience suggested that an increased mortality risk does exist within the African American patient with heart failure.
The relative risk of race as a contributor to mortality was 1.75-fold increased for African
American men and 2.4-fold increased for African American women. Despite controlling
for quantifiable measures of socioeconomic status (i.e., financial stress and educational
level), differences in outcomes still persisted [36]. These data strongly suggest that important physiological differences do exist. However, these issues have been challenged since
the data were not risk-adjusted. A subsequent reanalysis matched African American patients with non–African American patients for the same degree of left ventricular dysfunction, clinical classification, and trial participation, i.e., Prevention or Treatment trial. The
characteristics of this overall matched population weighed heavily toward a lower risk
population. In this lower-risk matched cohort, there were no differences in mortality noted.
Hospitalizations did, however, vary as a function of race. After initiation with ACE inhibitor therapy, the rate of hospitalization was unaffected in African American patients while
being reduced by 44% in non–African American patients. Although this observation might
suggest poorer outcomes in heart failure as a function of race, the impact of the prescribed
dose of ACE inhibition on blood pressure reduction was much less—6/3 mmHg in the

non–African American group and 0/0 mm Hg in the African American group. Thus, the observed difference in the rate of hospitalization might have been attributable to drug effect and be dose dependent [37].

Unique Pathophysiological Considerations of Heart Failure in African Americans

The foregoing data suggest that a credible argument can be made that heart failure in African Americans is a different disease process. If the influence of the socioeconomic milieu is insufficient to account for observed differences, then certain pathophysiological differences must be implicated. Hypertension is a more malignant vascular process in African Americans [33,38,39]. It is associated with a three-fold incidence of left ventricular hypertrophy, a nearly 10-fold incidence of end-stage renal disease, and a higher rate of stroke, hemorrhagic stroke, and fatality due to stroke [38].

Plausible pathophysiological explanations do exist, but proven mechanisms are still lacking. The emerging field of population biology with specific identification of single nucleotide polymorphisms (SNPs) that affect protein expression provides candidate genetic mechanisms that may add insight regarding the pathophysiology of hypertensive heart disease. Candidate single nucleotide polymorphisms include but are not limited to genes for; ACE [40]; aldosterone synthase [40]; eNOS (nitric oxide synthase) [40]; alpha 1, beta 1 and beta 2 adrenergic receptors [41,42]; natriuretic peptide receptors and G proteins [43]. (Table 2)

Taken in aggregate, one or more of these polymorphisms may contribute to accelerated fibrosis, impaired vasodilation, blunted renin-angiotensin-aldosterone system function, blunted sympathetic nervous system function, and impaired nitric oxide homeostasis.

An especially attractive hypothesis implicates accelerated fibrosis. Transforming growth factor beta-1, (TGF-beta-1), is a cytokine that is stimulated by angiotensin II production, promotes collagen turnover, stimulates mRNA for endothelin, and is associated with both left ventricular hypertrophy and glomerular hypertrophy. Within a hypertensive cohort of African Americans, TGF-beta-1 levels are remarkably elevated even when compared with similarly hypertensive non–African Americans. A described polymorphism at codon 10 for TGF-beta 1 is present in African Americans that leads to a 40% increase in TGF-beta-1 levels that subsequently leads to an increase in endothelin-1 levels [44]. A similarly attractive hypothesis can be constructed that incorporate variations in the expression of adrenergic receptors. Within a small cohort of African Americans with respiratory

Table 2 Plausible Genetic Polymorphisms Responsible for Left Ventricular Dysfunction in African Americans

Genetic Polymorphism	Clinical Implications
Beta 1 adrenergic receptor; Gly-389	Subsensitive beta-1- receptor; decreased affinity for agonist and less cAMP generation (41)
Beta 1 adrenergic receptor; ARG-389/alpha 2C Del322–325 receptor	Presence of both polymorphisms is associated with increased risk for heart failure in blacks; RR 10.11 when both are present (42)
eNOS	Subsensitive Nitric Oxide system (40)
Aldosterone Synthase	? Excessive fibrosis (40)
TGF-Beta 1	40% higher TGF Beta 1 levels;? Higher endothelin levels;? More fibrosis (44)
G Protein 825-T Allele	Marker of low renin HTN, LVH and stroke (43)

illnesses, there is a described polymorphism of the β_1 adrenergic receptor that exists at position 389 and involves a glycine substitution for arginine. When exposed to isoproterenol, this SNP results in a blunted production of cyclic AMP (adenosine monophosphate) and would be a plausible explanation for a subsensitive sympathetic nervous system [41,42]. (Fig. 7) Within the Vasodilator Heart Failure Trials (V-HeFT), African Americans had lower norepinephrine levels despite similar measures of left ventricular dysfunction, thus supporting the concept that the sympathetic nervous system may be subsensitive in this population [45]. However, data from a population of patients with heart failure analyzed for the apparent loss-of-gain Gly-389 SNP yielded a remarkable observation. The combination of the *arginine-389* substituted β_1 adrenergic receptor *plus* a separate SNP of the α-receptor, that increases the presynaptic release of norepinephrine, was associated with a striking incidence of heart failure *only in African Americans* [42]. (Fig. 8) Clearly this field of investigation requires more data but observations regarding poorer outcomes in African Americans with heart failure may ultimately be explained less so by the arbitrary descriptor of race and more so by the distribution of at-risk genetic markers.

Response to Medical Therapy for Heart Failure in African Americans

Vasodilator Therapy. The Vasodilator Heart Failure Trials (V-HeFT I and II) tested the benefit of isosorbide dinitrate and hydralazine given in combination vs. placebo in patients with NYHA class II -III ambulatory heart failure due to systolic dysfunction [46,47]. V-HeFT I is considered a landmark trial because it first demonstrated that the natural history of heart failure could be altered with medical therapy, specifically vasodilator therapy [46]. V-HeFT II later compared vasodilator therapy and ACE inhibitor therapy and demonstrated superiority of ACE inhibitor therapy [47]. When those trials were reevaluated as a function of race, no statistically significant benefit was evident in non–African Americans [45]. The entirety of the positive response seen in V-HeFT-I was observed in African Americans. Within V-HeFT II, the non–African American group demonstrated a

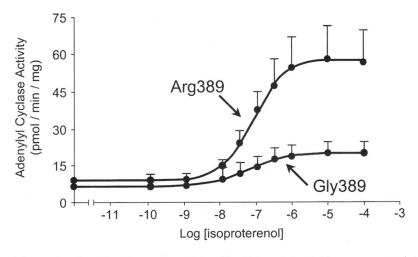

Figure 7 Functional coupling of the Gly-389 and Arg-389 receptors to adenylyl cyclase. Results illustrate absolute adenylyl cyclase activity based on studies with clonal lines expressing each receptor. The Arg-389 receptor demonstrates small increases in basal activity and marked increases in agonist-stimulated activity compared with the Gly-389 receptor. (From Ref. 41.)

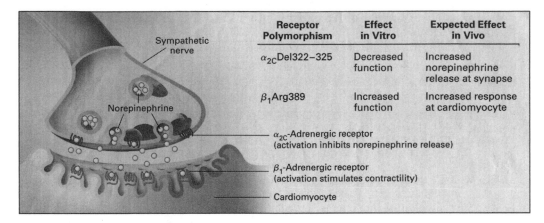

Receptor Polymorphism	Effect in Vitro	Expected Effect in Vivo
α_{2C}Del322–325	Decreased function	Increased norepinephrine release at synapse
β_1Arg389	Increased function	Increased response at cardiomyocyte

α_{2C}-Adrenergic receptor
(activation inhibits norepinephrine release)

β_1-Adrenergic receptor
(activation stimulates contractility)

Cardiomyocyte

Figure 8 Basis of the hypothesis that the α_{2C}Del322–325 and β_1Arg389 receptors act synergistically as risk factors for heart failure. The α_{2C}-adrenergic receptor (along with the α_{2A}-adrenergic receptor) inhibits norepinephrine release at cardiac presynaptic nerve endings through negative feedback. The presence of the dysfunctional α_{2C}Del322–325 receptor would be expected to result in enhance norepinephrine release. The β_1-adrenergic receptor is the receptor for norepinephrine on the cardiomyocyte, and the presence of the hyperfunctional β_1Arg389 receptor would be expected to increase contractile response at the myocyte. The combination of increased norepinephrine release and increased responsiveness of the receptor may increase the risk of over heart failure. (From Ref. 42.)

benefit of ACE-inhibitor therapy over vasodilator therapy. However, there was no statistically significant difference between vasodilator therapy and ACE-inhibitor therapy in the African-American cohort [45]. These data do not mean that ACE inhibitors did not work in the African-American group but rather that the vasodilator regimen worked particularly well. The prevailing hypothesis is that the combination of isosorbide dinitrate and hydralazine functions as a potent nitric oxide donor/antioxidant, which may be uniquely beneficial in the African-American population. This potential benefit of vasodilator therapy in African Americans is being tested prospectively in a randomized, placebo-controlled clinical trial, African American Heart Failure Trial (A-HeFT) [48]. A proprietary combination of isosorbide dinitrate and hydralazine, BiDil, is being given in addition to standard therapy for heart failure that includes ACE inhibitors and beta-blockers.

ACE-Inhibitor Therapy. Prevailing theories from the hypertension literature have consistently suggested that African Americans do not respond as favorably to ACE inhibitors. Supporting data are underwhelming and mechanistic information on variances in the renin angiotensin aldosterone system are likewise absent. The SOLVD trial provides the best data on the use of ACE inhibitors in African Americans with heart failure [35,36]. Despite early reports of differences in mortality, there has not been any conclusive evidence within the SOLVD experience that African Americans have a dissimilar response to ACE inhibitors when mortality is the end-point [37]. Any apparent mortality differences are likely related to a differential incidence of disease and not a failure to respond to medical therapy. Data from the V-HeFT II trial corroborate that finding by demonstrating that the annual mortality rate in both African Americans and non–African Americans was similar in the groups on ACE-inhibitor therapy, ~13% annual mortality rate [45]. Hospitalization rates were dissimilar in SOLVD for reasons as previously stated [37]. Whether this hospitalization risk can be reduced with higher dose ACE inhibition has not been tested. (Fig. 9)

Angiotensin- receptor antagonists (ARBs) have emerged as appropriate therapy in ACE inhibitor intolerant patients and as adjunctive therapy for some patients already receiving an ACE inhibitor [49]. However, no published data are available to either support or refute their benefit in African Americans with heart failure. In the absence of prospectively acquired data, ARB therapy should be prescribed when clinically indicated irrespective of race.

Beta Blocker Therapy. The greatest recent advance in medical therapy for heart failure has been the addition of beta-blocker therapy to ACE inhibitors as preferred management for heart failure. Beta-blockers have been convincingly shown to prolong survival, diminish hospitalizations, and improve symptoms in large-scale clinical trials. As with ACE inhibitors, questions have been raised regarding the efficacy of beta-blockers in African Americans.

The possibility of diminished efficacy was strongly suggested in the Beta-Blocker Evaluation of Survival Trial [BEST]. Within the African-American group (n = 623), bucindolol failed to demonstrate a survival advantage. Although a 17% survival benefit was seen in non–African American patients, a 17% *decrement* in survival was observed in the African-American group [15]. (Fig. 10) However, the disparate outcomes seen in both African Americans and women in the BEST trial may be explained more by significant differences in the drug than in specific racial or gender differences [16].

The experience with carvedilol has been quite different and strongly supports the addition of beta-blockers to ACE inhibitors in the management of heart failure in African Americans. The U.S. Heart Failure Trials Program randomized 1094 patients to one of four concurrent trials according to disease severity [19]. Twenty per cent of the patients were African American. Analysis of outcomes by race demonstrated a benefit attributable

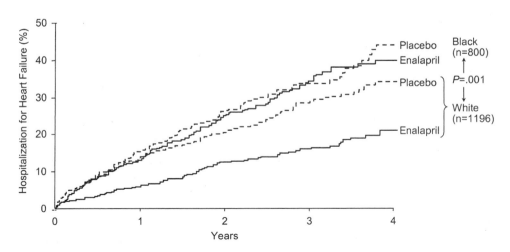

Figure 9 Rates of hospitalization for heart failure among black patients and matched white patients randomly assigned to enalapril or placebo treatment in the Studies of Left Ventricular Dysfunction (SOLVD) trial. The rate of hospitalizations for heart failure among black patients assigned to enalapril was significantly higher than that observed among matched white patients assigned to enalapril treatment (p < 0.001 by Fisher's exact test). (From Ref. 37.)

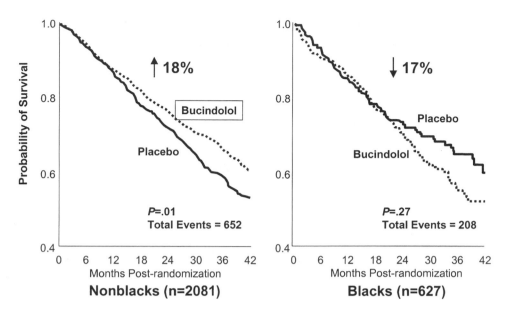

Figure 10 Survival by treatment group for black and non-black patients who received bucindolol or placebo therapy during the Beta-blocker Evaluation of Survival Trial. Bucindolol treatment was associated with improved survival among non-black participants but a trend toward worse survival among black participants in the trial. (From Ref. 15.)

to carvedilol plus ACE inhibitors of the same magnitude as that seen in non–African Americans. Disease progression, identified as death, hospitalization due to heart failure or intensification of medical therapy, was reduced by 54% in the African-American cohort and by 51% in the non–African American group [50]. (Fig. 11)

To substantiate that these findings were not spurious, hemodynamic efficacy and the effect on ventricular function data were evaluated. The improvement in left ventricular ejection fraction was identical for both groups, ~10 EF units. The impact on blood pressure (~1.5 mmHg), and the effect on heart rate (~ −13 bpm) were identical for both groups [50]. Further support for the benefit of carvedilol can be found in the COPERNICUS study [20]. In this mortality trial of advanced heart failure, the African-American cohort was proportionately smaller than that enrolled in the U.S. Heart Failure Trials Program (6% vs. 20%) but fared equally well compared to the non–African-American group. These two trials taken show a striking similarity of outcomes in African Americans with heart failure in all clinical classes when therapy consists of ACE inhibitors and carvedilol.

In the MERIT-HF trial, only 5% of the study population was African American. The sample size and correspondingly the number of events were too small to reach statistical significance but the direction of benefit was consistent with efficacy of beta-blocker therapy [31].

Data from controlled clinical trials using other agents (i.e., omapatrilat, aldosterone antagonists, nesiritide) have either been devoid of sufficient African Americans to justify analysis or the results have been unavailable.

The ongoing A-HeFT trial represents the first effort to accumulate data in a prospective manner that will not only identify drug effect, if any, of isosorbide dinitrate and hydralazine but also it should illuminate the natural history of heart failure within this very important ''subpopulation'' [48]. It is imperative that more physiological and mecha-

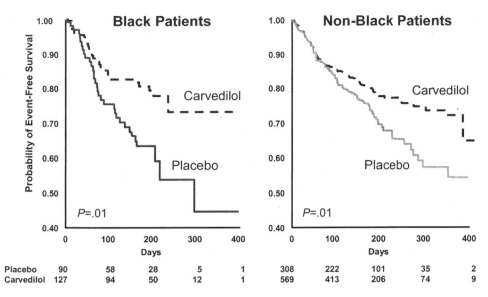

Figure 11 Kaplan-Meier analysis of cumulative rates of survival without hospitalization among black patients (*left panel*) and among non-black patients (*right panel*). Within the cohort of black patients, those randomly assigned to receive carvedilol had a 48% lower risk of death from any cause or hospitalization for any reason than those assigned to receive placebo (p = 0.01); among the non-black cohort, the risk reduction was 30% (p = 0.01). There was no significant difference in the magnitude of the drug's effect between the two racial cohorts (p = 0.33). (From Ref. [50].)

nistic data be obtained in this group—especially within the realm of genetic predispositions for disease. This may prove difficult as race as a physiological factor for disease is compromised and confounded by the heterogeneity of the African Americans.

IMPORTANT COMORBIDITIES

Renal Disease

Renal disease, either chronic renal insufficiency (CRI) or end-stage renal disease (ESRD), is strongly associated with both heart disease and heart failure. Available data demonstrate that even mild degrees of renal insufficiency impart a worse prognosis and may influence medical therapy for heart failure [51,52]. (Fig. 12) The concomitant presence of CRI, defined as a serum creatinine greater than 1.4mg/dL in women and 1.5 mg/dL in men, has been shown to be associated with an increased relative risk (RR = 1.43) of death due to heart failure [51]. Within hospitalized patients, as many as 70% will develop evidence of worsening renal function during treatment. An increase of only 0.1mg/dL predicts a worse outcome with a high sensitivity but low specificity [53]. The sensitivity and specificity are strengthened for in-hospital mortality and length of stay more than 10 days when the rise in serum creatinine approximates 0.3mg/dL (81% and 62%, respectively). The specificity increases to nearly 90% when the rise in serum creatinine is above 1.5mg/dL. Twenty percent of hospitalized patients will develop an increase in serum creatinine of 0.5mg/dL, thus, a sizeable number of heart failure admissions are at risk for poor outcomes based on concomitant renal diseases [53].

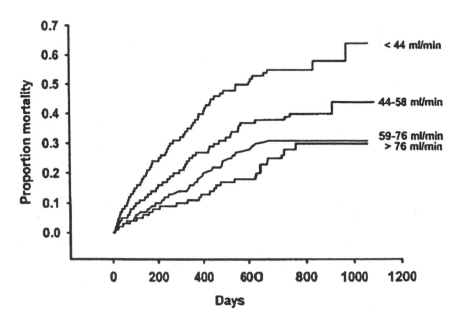

Figure 12 Relationship between baseline calculated glomerular filtration rate (CFRc) and survival among 1196 patient with chronic heart failure. GFRc was estimated using the Cockroft Gault equation and corrected for gender. (From Ref 52a.)

In most clinical trials, patients with significant renal insufficiency were excluded; thus, data on the benefits of ACE inhibitors, angiotensin-receptor antagonists, beta-blockers and especially aldosterone antagonists are not available for heart failure associated with advanced renal insufficiency. However, data are available for the influence of ACE inhibitors in the setting of mild renal dysfunction [54,55]. The use of ACE inhibitors is associated with a rise in serum creatinine that is generally ascribed to a reduction in intraglomerular pressures. Angiotensin II selectively vasoconstricts the efferent renal arteriole in the setting of heart failure. Removal of the influence of angiotensin II leads to a decrease in intraglomerular pressure and a rise in serum creatinine that is further exacerbated by the use of diuretics. Thus, serum creatinine values may rise as much as 200% in heart failure patients treated with ACE inhibitors [55,56]. This would seem to lead to a worrisome limitation of the use of these agents in heart failure complicated by moderate renal insufficiency. However, clinical trial data are much more encouraging. In the Evaluation of Losartan in the Elderly (ELITE) study, either captopril or losartan was administered to patients with a creatinine value up to 3.5 mg/dL. Only 2% of patients required discontinuation of therapy because of worsening of renal function [55,57]. Smaller trials in elderly patients have demonstrated that for heart failure patients with a creatinine greater than 2.5mg/dL, the mortality reduction with ACE inhibitors was 66% compared with a 42% reduction in those patients with a serum creatinine less than 2.5mg/dL [58]. Similarly, heart failure outcomes that occurred in the post-MI setting and associated with a creatinine of greater than 3 mg/dL were still benefited by the use of ACE inhibitors [59].

Chronic renal insufficiency does increase the risk of hyperkalemia by nearly fivefold, but the concomitant use of diuretics reduces that risk substantially. ESRD, results in a unique pathophysiological cardiovascular construct that accelerates adverse outcomes and is uniquely associated with cardiovascular disease. The interrelatedness of cardiac and renal disease emanates from similar etiological considerations, especially hypertension, diabetes, and atherosclerosis. Once severe renal disease has become established, the result-ant anemia, fibrosis, and cardiomyopathy of overload become operative.

Anemia represents an independent predictor of adverse outcomes in heart failure (Chapter 10). The Canadian cohort study of chronic renal disease demonstrated that for every 0.5g/dL of hemoglobin decrease, the odds ratio for LVH was 1.32 or a 32% increase. Each 10gm/dL decrease was associated with an odds ratio of LV dilation of 1.46 or 46% [60]. It is not yet clear that correction of the anemia will result in improved outcomes, but progressive LV dilatation may be prevented and quality of life appears to be improved at a target hematocrit of 33% to 36% as reported in the national Kidney Foundation Dialysis Outcomes Quality Initiative. Ongoing clinical trials in heart failure are specifically addressing the impact of anemia and its correction.

The mechanisms of ventricular remodeling appear to be related to chronically in-creased cardiac output and heart rate with concomitant neurohormonal activation. In the setting of dialysis, 80% of patients will either have left ventricular hypertrophy or systolic dysfunction [54]. Thirty-seven per cent will have had a previous episode of heart failure and the rate of development of heart failure approximates 10%/year [54]. Hypertension is an important contributor to LV dysfunction in dialysis patients. For each 10 mmHg increment in blood pressure, there is a 48% higher risk of developing LVH [54]. A target BP of 140/90 is recommended for the dialysis patient and 130/80 mm Hg for the nondialysis dependent patient with chronic renal insufficiency [54].

In addition to the careful initiation of ACE inhibitors as therapy for heart failure, other proven strategies should be considered. Angiotensin-receptor antagonists appear to have a similar risk profile as ACE inhibitors and should be considered. A known history of hyperkalemia, renal artery stenosis, or glomerular filtration rates significantly less than 30 ml/min represents major contraindications to therapy with ACE inhibitors or angioten-sin-receptor antagonists. There is no reason to withhold beta-blocker therapy for heart failure in either CRI or ESRD unless a usual contraindication to beta-blocker therapy exists [60a]. Loop diuretics can be quite effective in CRI, albeit at higher doses but aldosterone antagonists should be avoided. For the diuretic nonresponder, acute ultrafiltra-tion may be an effective means to rapidly reduce blood volume. Digoxin can be safely given but dosing will likely need to be on alternate days and levels should be followed carefully. For the patient being dialyzed, care should be taken to avoid low potassium dialysate, as this will predispose to arrhythmias. Long-acting nitrates and hydralazine would be a reasonable alternative treatment choice but the true impact of these agents on mortality is at best modest and more effective therapies should be considered as initial therapy.

Pulmonary Disease

The concomitant presence of pulmonary disease represents an important comorbidity in heart failure. Pulmonary disease impacts both the diagnosis and therapy of heart failure. The presenting complaint of dyspnea is just as likely for obstructive or reactive airway disease as it is for heart failure. The emerging utility of B-type natriuretic peptide as a marker of left ventricular stress/stretch helps to reconcile the origin of dyspnea as either cardiac or pulmonary [61].

Pulmonary function is often abnormal in the setting of heart failure, perhaps as many as 60% of patients with heart failure will have abnormal pulmonary function studies. In the acute setting of decompensated heart failure, obstructive pulmonary defects can be seen but these clear rapidly with effective therapy of heart failure. Chronic obstructive defects are uncommon in heart failure alone [62,63].

Pulmonary function testing typically reveals a restrictive defect and reduced transfer of carbon monoxide (DLCO). This restrictive defect is typically multifactorial in etiology. Respiratory muscles work less efficiently, lung volumes are smaller due to cardiomegaly, lung compliance is altered due to chronic pulmonary edema, chronic pleural effusions may be present, and alveolar fluid may be present [62]. Patients with heart failure who have heart failure and an FEV_1 less than 60% fare less well with a more advanced NYHA classification and poorer gas exchange on cardiopulmonary stress testing [64]. Even following heart transplantation, pulmonary function tests may not normalize and the DLCO may remain impaired.

The limitation of beta-blocker use in concomitant pulmonary disease refers only to reactive airway disease. Obstructive pulmonary disease does not appear to be affected by the administration of these agents. No good benchmarks are available, but significant reversibility of the FEV_1 with bronchodilators of at least 15% appears to be a contraindication to beta-blocker therapy. Status asthmaticus has been described and can be life threatening.

Thyroid Disease

The concomitant presence of thyroid disease and/or disorders in heart failure is quite important. Thyroid hormone has a substantial impact on cardiac function. The changes are both hemodynamic and structural [65]. Cardiac myocytes take up T3, not T4. T3 receptor proteins regulate the cellular effects of T3. These receptor proteins are bound to the promoter region of T3 responsive genes. The alpha myosin heavy chain gene, sarcoplasmic reticulum Ca^{2+} adenosine triphosphate, and voltage-gated potassium channels genes are all upregulated by thyroid hormone while beta myosin heavy chain, and phospholamban are downregulated by thyroid hormone. Excess thyroid hormone results in an increase in the positively influenced genes and their subsequent protein expression and deficient thyroid hormone leads to an increase in the negatively regulated genes and their protein expression [66]. Even subclinical hypothyroidism has demonstrable systolic and diastolic dysfunction present along with increased systemic vascular resistance [65].

Hyperthyroidism occurs much less frequently in association with heart failure. It typically leads to high-output heart failure seemingly through a direct toxic effect on the myocardium, both chronotropic and inotropic and can likewise lead to a dilated cardiomyopathy. Correction of the hyperthyroid state leads to resolution of the cardiac findings.

Clinical issues regarding thyroid disease in heart failure are frequently amplified in the setting of amiodarone use. Amiodarone affects the conversion of triiodothyronine to tetraiodothyronine and can cause the full gamut of thyroid disorders. The more common situation is amiodarone-induced hypothyroidism due to the decrease in available T4. Thyroid hormone supplementation is frequently all that is required to correct this syndrome. Acute thyroiditis as well as an autoimmune thyroiditis can occur during amiodarone therapy resulting in clinical hyperthyroidism. Reduction and/or cessation of amiodarone therapy is often required and, occasionally, thyroidectomy may be indicated if the indication for amiodarone is indeed life threatening [67].

The clinical condition of 'the low triiodothyronine state'' or the ''low T3 syndrome'' should be recognized in heart failure patients [68]. A survey of thyroid function testing in heart failure patients reveals that fewer than 10% will have true hypothyroidism, i.e., an increased TSH. But 30% or more will have a low T3 and normal T4 and TSH levels. This low T3 state correlates with the severity of heart failure and may be prognostically important [68]. Whether or not these patients would benefit from T3 replacement is not yet known. Small studies have suggested an improvement in exercise tolerance [69] and cardiac output, but the risk of increased myocardial oxygen consumption, especially in the setting of ischemic heart disease remains a concern. Because of the significant influence of thyroid hormone on cardiac structure and function, the assessment of thyroid function should be an obligatory component of any evaluation for heart failure.

REFERENCES

1. The SOLVD Investigators. Effect of enalapril on survival in patients with reduced left ventricular ejection fractions and congestive heart failure. N Engl J Med 1991; 325:293–302.
2. Packer M, Coats AAJ, Fowler MB, et al. Effect of carvedilol on survival in severe chronic heart failure. N Engl J Med 2001; 344:1651–1658.
3. Pitt B, Zannad F, Remme WJ. Randomized aldactone evaluation study. N Engl J Med 1999; 341:709–717.
4. Cohn JN, Tognoni G, et al. A randomized trial of the angiotensin receptor blocker valsartan in chronic heart failure. N Engl J Med 2001; 345:1667–1675.
5. Kannel WB, Belanger AJ. Epidemiology of heart failure. Am Heart J 1991; 121:951–957.
5a. Lloyd-Jones DM, Larson MG, Leip EP, Berser A, D'Agostino RB, Kannel WB, Murabito JM, Vasan RS, Benjamin EJ, Levy D; Framington Heart Study Circulation 2002; 106:3068–72.
6. Levy D, Larson MG, Vasan RS. The progression from hypertension to congestive heart failure. JAMA 1996; 275:1557–1562.
7. Victor RG, Mark AL. The sympathetic nervous system in human hypertension. In: Laragh JH, BB, Eds. Pathophysiology, Diagnosis and Management. New York: Raven Press, 1995: 863–878.
8. Gillum RF, Mussolino ME, Madans JH. Body fat distribution and hypertension incidence in women and men. The NHANES I epidemiologic follow-up study. Int J Obesity 1998; 22: 127–134.
9. Wenger NK. Women, heart failure, and heart failure therapies. Circulation 2002; 105: 1526–1528.
10. McCullough PA, Philbin EF, Spertus JA, Kaatz S, Sandberg KR, Weaver WD. Confirmation of a heart failure epidemic: findings from the resource utilization among congestive heart failure (REACH) study. J Am Coll Cardiol 2002; 39:60–69.
11. Kannel WB, Ho K, Thom T. Changing epidemiological features of cardiac failure. Br Heart J 1994; 72(Supplement S):3–9.
12. Stewart S. Prognosis of patients with heart failure compared with common types of cancer. Heart Fail Monitor 2003; 3:87–94.
13. Garg R, Yusef S. for the Collaborative Group on ACE Inhibitor Trials. Overview of the randomized trials of angiotensin-converting enzyme inhibitors on mortality and morbidity in patients with heart failure. JAMA 1995; 273:1450–1456.
13a. Shekelle PG, Rich MW, Morton SC, Atkinson SW, Tu W, Maglione M, Rhodes S, Barrett M, Fongrow GC, Greenberg B, Heidenreich PA, Knabel T, Konstum MA, Steimle A, Stevenson LW. Efficacy of angiotensin-converting enzyme inhibitors and beta-blockers in the management of left ventricular systolic dysfunction according to race, gender and diabetic status. A meta-analysis of major clinical trials. J Am Coll Cardiol 2003; 41:1529–38.
14. Rathore SS, Wang Y, Krumholz HM. Sex-based differences in the effect of digoxin for the treatment of heart failure. N Engl J Med 2002; 347:1403–1411.
15. The Beta Blocker Evaluation of Survival Trial Investigators. A trial of the beta blocker bucindolol in patients with advanced chronic heart failure. N Engl J Med 2001; 344: 1659–1667.
16. Andreka P, Aiyar N, Olson LC, Wei JQ, Turner MS, Webster KA, Ohlstein EH, Bishopric NH. Bucindolol displays intrinsic sympathomimetic activity in human myocardium. Circulation 2002; 105:2429–2434.

17. Ghali JK, Jalal K, Krause-Steinrauf HJ, Adams KF, Khan SS, Rosenberg YD, Yancy CW, Young JB, Goldman S, Peberdy MA, Lindenfeld JA. Gender differences in advanced heart failure: insights from the BEST study. J Am Coll Cardiol 2003 Dec 17; 42(12):2128–34.

18. Ghali JK, Pina IL, Gottleib SS, Deedwania PC, Wikstrand JC. The MERIT-HF Study Group. Metoprolol CR/XL in female patients with heart failure: analysis of the experience in metoprolol extended-release randomized intervention trial in heart failure (MERIT-HF). Circulation 2002; 105:1585–1591.

19. Packer M, Bristow MR, Cohn JN, et al. The effect of carvedilol on morbidity and mortality in patients with chronic heart failure. N Engl J Med 1996; 334:1349–1355.

20. Packer M, Coats AJS, Fowler MB, et al. Effect of carvedilol on survival in severe chronic heart failure. N Engl J Med 2001; 344:1651–1658.

21. Packer M, Fowler MB, Roecker EB, et al. Effect of carvedilol on the morbidity of patients with severe chronic heart failure: results of the Carvedilol Prospective Randomized Cumulative Survival (COPERNICUS) Study. Circulation 2002; 106:2194–2199.

22. Hunt SA, et al. ACC/AHA guidelines for the evaluation and management of chronic heart failure in the adult: executive summary: a report of the American College of Cardiology/ American Heart Association Task Force on Practice Guidelines (Committee to Revise the 1995 Guidelines for the Evaluation and Management of Heart Failure.). J Am Coll Cardiol 2001; 38:2101–2113.

23. Fonarow GC. The acute decompensated heart failure national registry (ADHERE); opportunities to improve care of patients hospitalized with acute decompensated heart failure. Reviews in Cardiovasc Med 2003; 4(suppl 7):S21–S30.

24. Stewart S, Horowitz JD. Home-based intervention in congestive heart failure; long term implications on readmission and survival. Circulation 2002; 205:2861–2866.

25. ALLHAT Officers and Coordinators for the ALLHAT Collaborative Research Group. Major outcomes in high-risk hypertensive patients randomized to angiotensin-converting enzyme inhibitor or calcium channel blocker vs. diuretic. The Antihypertensive and Lipid Lowering Treatment to Prevent Heart Attack Trial (ALLHAT). JAMA 2002; 288:2981–2997.

26. Vasan RS, Beiser A, Seshadri S, et al. Residual lifetime risk for developing hypertension in middle-aged women and men: The Framingham Heart Study. JAMA 2002; 287:1003–1010.

27. Kostis JB, Davis BR, Cutler J, et al. for the SHEP Cooperative Research Group. Prevention of heart failure by antihypertensive drug treatment in older persons with isolated systolic hypertension. JAMA 1997; 278:212–216.

28. Dahlof B, Lindholm LH, Hansson L, et al. Morbidity and mortality in the Swedish trial in Old Persons with Hypertension. (STOP-Hypertension). Lancet 1991; 338:1281–1285.

29. Wing LMH, Reid CM, Ryan P, Beilin LJ, Brown MA, et al. A comparison of outcomes with angiotensin converting enzyme inhibitors and diuretics for hypertension in the elderly. N Engl J Med 2003; 348:583–592.

30. The Heart Outcomes Prevention Evaluation Study Investigators. Effects of an angiotensin-converting-enzyme inhibitor, ramipril, on cardiovascular events in high-risk patients. N Engl J Med 2000; 342:145–153.

31. MERIT-HF Study Group. Effect of metoprolol CR/XL in chronic heart failure: Metoprolol CR/XL Randomised Intervention Trial in Congestive Heart Failure (MERIT-HF). Lancet 1999; 353:2001–2007.

32. Cioffi G, Stefenelli C. Tolerability and clinical effects of carvedilol in patients over 70 years of age with chronic heart failure due to left ventricular dysfunction. Italian Heart J 2001; 2: 1319–1329.

33. Yancy CW. Heart failure in African Americans: a cardiovascular enigma. J Card Fail 2000; 6:183–186.

34. Dries DL, Strong MH, Cooper RS, Drazner M. Efficacy of angiotensin-converting enzyme inhibition in reducing progression from asymptomatic left ventricular dysfunction to symptomatic heart failure in black and white patients. J Am Coll Cardiol 2002; 40:311–317.

35. Bourassa MG, Gurne O, Bangdiwala SI, et al. Natural history and patterns of current practice in heart failure. The Studies of Left Ventricular Dysfunction (SOLVD) Investigators. J Am Coll Cardiol 1993; 22:14A–19A.

36. Dries DL, Exner DV, Gersh BJ, Cooper HA, Carson PE, Domanski MJ. Racial differences in the outcome of left ventricular dysfunction (published erratum appears in N Engl J Med 1999; 3414:298). N Engl J Med 1999; 340:609–616.

37. Exner DV, Dries DL, Domanski MJ, Cohn JN. Lesser response to angiotensin-converting-enzyme inhibitor therapy in black as compared with white patients with left ventricular dysfunction. N Engl J Med 2001; 344:1351–1357.

38. Saunders E. Hypertension in minorities: blacks. Am J Hypertens 1995; 8:115s–119s.

39. Flack JM, Ferdinand KC, Nasser SA. Epidemiology of hypertension and cardiovascular disease in African Americans. J Clin Hypertens (Greenwich) 2003; 5:5–11.

40. McNamara DM, Holub Rov R, Janosko K, Halmer A, Wang JJ, MacGown GA, Murali S, Rosenblum WD, London B, Feldman AM. Pharmacogenetic interactions between β-blocker therapy and the angiotensin converting enzyme deletion polymorphism in patients with congestive heart failure. Circulation 2001; 103:1644–48.

41. Mason DA, Moore JD, Green SA, Liggett SB. A gain of function polymorphism in a G-protein coupling domain of the human beta-1 adrenergic receptor. J Biologic Chem 1999; 274:12670–12674.

42. Small KM, Wagoner LE, Levin AM, Kardia SLR, Liggett SB. Synergistic polymorphisms of beta 1 and alpha 2C adrenergic receptors and the risk of congestive heart failure. N Engl J Med 2002; 347(15):1135–1142.

43. Siffert W. Molecular genetics of G proteins and atherosclerotic risk. Basic Res Cardiol 2001; 96:606–611.

44. Suthanthiran M, Li B, Song JO, et al. Transforming growth factor-beta1 hyperexpression in African-American hypertensives: a novel mediator of hypertension and/or target organ damage. Proc Natl Acad Sci USA 2000; 97:3479–3484.

45. Carson P, Ziesche S, Johnson G, Cohn JN. Racial differences in response to therapy for heart failure: analysis of the Vasodilator-Heart Failure Trials. J Cardiac Fail 1999; 5:178–187.

46. Cohn JN, Archibald DG, Ziesche S, Franciosa JA, Harston WE, Tristani FE, Dunkman WB, Jacobs W, Francis GS, Flohr KH, Goldman S, Cobb FR, Shah PM, Saunders R, Fletcher RD, Loeb HS, Hughes VC, Baker B. Effect of vasodilator therapy on mortality in chronic congestive heart failure: Results of the Veterans Administration Cooperative Study. N Engl J Med 1986; 314:1547–1552.

47. Cohn JN, Johnson G, Ziesche S, Cobb F, Francis GS, Tristani FE, Smith R, Dunkman WB, Loeb H, Wong M, Bhat G, Goldman S, Fletcher RD, Doherty J, Hughes CV, Carson P, Cintron G, Shabetai R, Haakenson C. A comparison of enalapril with hydralazine-isosorbide dinitrate in the treatment of chronic congestive heart failure. N Engl J Med 1991; 325: 303–310.

48. Franciosa JA, Taylor AL, Cohn JN, Yancy CW, Ziesche S, Olukotun A, Ofili E, Fredinand K, Loscalzo J, Worcel W. for the A-HeFT Investigators. African American Heart Failure Trial (A-HeFT): rationale, design, and methodology. J Cardiac Fail 2002; 8:128–135.

49. McMurray J, Ostergren J, Swedberg K, Granger CB, Held P, Michelson EL, Olofsson B, Yusef S, Pfeffer MA. for the CHARM Investigators. Effects of candesartan in patients with chronic heart failure and reduced left ventricular systolic function taking angiotensin-converting enzyme inhibitors; the CHARM-Added trial. Lancet. 2003; 362:767–71.

50. Yancy CW, Fowler MB, Colucci WS, et al. Race and the response to adrenergic blockade with carvedilol in patients with heart failure. N Engl J Med 2001; 344:1358–1365.

51. McClellan WM, Flanders WD, Langston RD, Jurkovitz C, Presley R. Anemia and renal insufficiency are independent risk factors for death among patients with congestive heart failure admitted to community hospitals; a population-based study. J Am Soc Nephrol 2002; 13:1928–1936.

52. Culleton BF, Larson MG, Wilson PWF, et al. Cardiovascular disease and mortality in a community based cohort with mild renal insufficiency. Kidney Int 1999; 56:2214–2219.

52a. Hillege HL, Girbes ARJ, de Kam RJ, Boomsma F, de Zeeuw D, Charlesworth A, Hampton JR, Van Veldhuisen DJ. Renal function in neurohormonal activation, and survival in patients with chronic heart failure. Circulation 2000; 102:203–10.

53. Gottlieb SS, Abraham W, Butler J, Forman DE, Loh E, Massie BM, O'Connor CM, Rich MW, Stevenson LW, Young J, Krumholz HM. The prognostic importance of different definitions of worsening renal function in congestive heart failure. J Cardiac Fail 2002; 8:136–41.

54. Murphy S. Management of heart failure and coronary artery disease in patients with chronic kidney disease. Semin Dialysis 2003; 16(2):165–172.

55. Ahmed A. Use of angiotensin-converting enzyme inhibitors in patients with heart failure and renal insufficiency: how concerned should we be by the rise in serum creatinine? J Am Geriatr Soc 2002; 50:1297–1300.

56. Bakris Gl, Weir MR. Angiotensin-converting enzyme inhibitor-associated elevations in serum creatinine: is this cause for concern? Arch Intern Med 2000; 160:685–693.

57. Pitt B, Segal R, Martinez FA, et al. Randomised trial of losartan versus captopril in patients over 65 with heart failure (Evaluation of Losartan in the Elderly Study, ELITE). Lancet 1997; 349:747–752.

58. Ahmed A, Kiefe CI, Allman RM, et al. Survival benefits of angiotensin-converting enzyme inhibitors in older heart failure patients with perceived contraindications. J Am Geriatr Soc 2002; 50:1659–1666.

59. Frances CD, Noguchi H, Massie BM, et al. Are we inhibited? Renal insufficiency should not preclude the use of ACE inhibitors for patients with myocardial infarction and depressed left ventricular function. Arch Intern Med 2000; 160:2645–2650.

60. Levin A, Thompson CR, Ethier J, Carlisle EJF, Tobe S, et al. Left ventricular mass index increase in early renal disease: impact of decline in hemoglobin. Am J Kidney Dis 1999; 34: 125–134.

60a. Cice G, Ferrara L, D'Andrea A, D'Isa S, Di Beneditto A, Cittadini A, Russo PE, Golino P, Calabro R. Carvedolol increases 2 year survival in dialysis patients with dilated cardiomyopathy. A prospective placebo-controlled trial. J Am Coll Cardiol 2003; 41:1438–44.

61. McCullough PA, Hollander JE, Nowak RM, Storrow AB, Duc P, et al. Uncovering heart failure in patients with a history of pulmonary disease; rationale for the early use of B-type natriuretic peptide in the emergency department. Acad Emerg Med 2003; 10:198–204.

62. Kotlyar E, Keogh AM, Macdonald PS, Arnold RH, McCaffrey DJ, et al. Tolerability of carvedilol in patients with heart failure and concomitant chronic obstructive pulmonary disease or asthma. J Heart Lung Transplantation 2002; 21:1290–1295.

63. Chua TP, Coats AJS. The lungs in chronic heart failure. Eur Heart J 1995; 16:882–887.

64. Lawless C, Malinowska K, Mullen G, Mendez J, Pisani B. Can beta blockers be safely titrated in patients with abnormal pulmonary function tests? J Heart Lung Transplantation 2000; 19: 73.

65. Klein I, Ojamaa K. Mechanisms of disease: thyroid hormone and the cardiovascular system. N Engl J Med 2001; 344:501–509.

66. Danzi S, Klein I. Thyroid hormone-regulated cardiac gene expression and cardiovascular disease. Thyroid 2002; 12:467–472.

67. Bogazzi F, Bartelena L, Gasperi M, Braverman LE, Martino E. The various effects of amiodarone on thyroid function. Thyroid 2001; 11:511–519.

68. Ascheim DD, Hryniewicz K. Thyroid hormone metabolism in patients with congestive heart failure: the low triiodothyronine state. Thyroid 2002; 12:511–515.

69. Hamilton MA, Stevenson LW, Fonarow GC, Steimle A, Goldhaber JI, et al. Safety and hemodynamic effects of intravenous triiodothyronine in advanced congestive heart failure. Am J Cardiol 1998; 81:443–447.

21

Practice Guidelines for Heart Failure Management

Thomas H. Lee
Harvard Medical School
Boston, Massachusetts, USA

SYNOPSIS

Underutilization of pharmacologic and diagnostic interventions that have been shown to improve patient outcomes remains evident for chronic heart failure (HF) management. Practice guidelines define therapeutic interventions that are viewed as most important, whereas care plans help ensure that these interventions are delivered to all appropriate patients. The extensive, peer-reviewed ACC/AHA (American College of Cardiology/ American Heart Association) heart failure guidelines are reviewed in detail. Critical pathways for hospitalized heart failure patients can also improve overall quality of care and often shorten hospital length of stay. Disease-management programs for ambulatory heart failure treatment have been shown to improve quality of life and decrease hospitalizations for recurrent heart failure in virtually all controlled and observational studies. Strategies to improve quality of care should include continuous quality improvement (CQI) measures to ensure prompt adoption of published guidelines in the clinical care of heart failure patients.

The growing interest in practice guidelines for heart failure has been encouraged by three trends that have accompanied improvement in the effectiveness of therapies detailed throughout this book. First, research has provided increasing sophistication in the measurement of quality of care of heart failure. Second, heart failure is one of the few syndromes in which better care not only improves patient outcomes, but also reduces costs. Third, the rise of consumerism has intensified interest in quality of care, particularly for chronic conditions affecting the aging baby boomer generation and their parents.

As increasing amounts of data on the quality of care become available, and often are made public, underutilization of interventions known to improve patient outcomes has become apparent. The Joint Commission on Accreditation of Healthcare Organizations (JCAHO) is collecting and disseminating publicly data on the quality of care for patients with heart failure on a hospital-specific basis. Pilot data from a large sample of hospitals show that about 14% of patients with heart failure and left ventricular dysfunction did not receive ACE inhibitors at discharge, despite the absence of contraindications. This initiative has also found that 61% of hospitalized smokers with heart failure did not receive counseling on smoking cessation; 21% of patients did not receive an evaluation of left

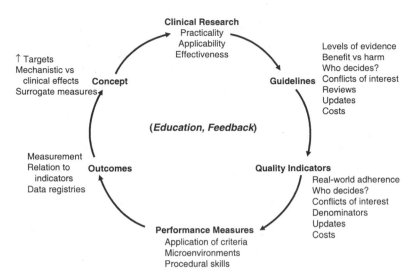

Figure 1 Model for the integration of quality into the therapeutic development cycle. (From Ref. 1.)

ventricular function; and 72% did not receive adequate discharge instructions (http://www.jcaho.org/pms/core + measures/hf_overview.htm; accessed on August 15, 2003).

The result of this convergence of trends and the availability of such data have led to a fundamental change in attitudes of clinicians toward practice guidelines for heart failure, and widespread adoption of tactics for their implementation, such as disease management programs. This acceptance has not come easily, as physicians often view practice guidelines as a threat to professional autonomy. Nevertheless, the fear that "cookbook medicine" might erode quality of care has been tempered by convincing evidence that care for patients with heart failure is characterized by frequent gaps in quality. Instead, the development of guidelines and quality measures, the implementation of interventions aimed at improving quality, and the measurement of their impact are now recognized as critical contributors to medical progress (Fig. 1) [1].

This chapter will, therefore, be divided into four sections. The first will provide a general discussion of practice guidelines and quality of care, with a focus on how they are relevant to congestive heart failure. The second will summarize the key recommendations of the leading set of practice guidelines for heart failure. The third will describe tactics for implementation of these guidelines, with a particular focus on team management. The final section will summarize recommendations for measurement of quality of care in heart failure for the purpose of improvement.

PRACTICE GUIDELINES AND QUALITY OF CARE

A variety of terms related to practice guidelines and quality of care are often used interchangeably, but their distinctions are useful and reflect perspectives of quality of care that vary among the key parties in health care [2]. A simple framework for quality that reflects these varying perspectives describes three basic types of errors–*under*-use, *over*-use, and *mis*-use. Underuse is the failure to provide a medical intervention when it is likely to produce a favorable outcome for a patient, such as failing to use an ACE inhibitor for a patient with known left ventricular dysfunction. Overuse occurs when the benefits of an intervention do not justify the potential harm or costs, such as use of a brand-named drug when an equally effective lower-cost generic is available. Misuse occurs when a preventable complication eliminates the benefit from a health care intervention. An example is initiation of a beta-blocker in a patient with decompensated heart failure leading to admission to hospital.

Physicians have traditionally been most interested in ''underuse''–that is, the *reliability* with which patients receive interventions that evidence indicates will improve patient outcomes. Accordingly, ''practice guidelines'' (Table 1) define which interventions are most important [3], and ''care plans'' help ensure that these interventions are delivered to all patients, unless the patient has contraindications. These care plans are often in the form of checklists that describe all the interventions that should be considered for a patient with heart failure on the inpatient or outpatient basis. Such plans can reduce the chances of gaps in quality for patients with heart failure, including those subsets that are less likely to receive optimal care routinely, such as women, minorities, or the elderly [4].

''Critical pathways'' are usually used for hospitalized patients, and are in a sense an adaptation of care plans. Like care plans, they seek to ensure that key elements of care are

Table 1 Key Terms

Term	Definition	Example	Goal
Clinical practice guideline	A guideline developed to aid practitioner and patient pursuit of the most appropriate health care responses to specific clinical circumstances	ACC/AHA guidelines for evaluation and management of chronic heart failure (2)	Defining optimal care.
Care plan	A clinical practice guideline detailing the usual sequence of decisions and nature and duration of services for a defined episode of care	Care plan for outpatient evaluation and management of heart failure	Reduce errors of underuse; improve the reliability of care.
Critical pathway	The core set of decisions and services described in an appropriate sequence and schedule most likely to effect an efficient, coordinated program of treatment	Description of the critical features of the care experience essential to most efficiently manage the usual patient admitted to hospital with congestive heart failure	Reduce errors of underuse and overuse; improve efficiency as well as reliability of care
Disease-management program	Systems aimed at following patients with a chronic condition over time to ensure that they receive interventions supported by clinical research	Multidisciplinary team to follow patients with heart failure on outpatient basis (3)	Reduce errors of over-use, under-use, and mis-use; improve overall coordination of care

Source: Adapted from Ref. 1.

reliably delivered, e.g., assessment of left ventricular function during the hospitalization. However, critical pathways often differ from care plans by attempting to improve efficiency. They introduce the element of *timing* of key actions, with the goal of avoiding unnecessary prolongations of hospital stay or of reducing the chances of readmission [5]. In addition, critical pathways try to focus attention on a small number of *essential* steps that are most likely to affect the effectiveness and efficiency of care. Thus, a care plan may be a detailed summary of all routine interventions, whereas a true critical pathway might be distilled down to a few lines on a 3×5 card.

"Disease-management programs" go one step further by trying to improve overall coordination of the care of patients with heart failure. Most (but not all) heart failure disease-management programs use nonphysicians who have frequent contact with patients to check on their clinical status and ensure that key interventions are being delivered [6]. These nonphysicians use protocols so that they do not necessarily have to check with physicians before recommending changes in medication regimens and arranging key tests. Some disease-management programs use computer programs and home monitoring devices to reduce or even eliminate the need for nonphysician clinicians to be in contact with patients.

HEART FAILURE PRACTICE GUIDELINE CONTENT

Many organizations develop practice guidelines in cardiovascular medicine, including individual hospitals and groups of providers. Among the most respected and widely cited guidelines are those developed by the joint task force of the American College of Cardiology and American Heart Association. The authors of these guidelines include leading authorities in their respective fields, and the guidelines themselves are updated regularly and made available on the Internet (www.americanheart.org).

ACC/AHA guidelines all use a common format, in which indications for various interventions are placed in one of three classes:

Class I: Conditions for which there is evidence and/or general agreement that a given procedure/therapy is useful and effective.

Class II: Conditions for which there is conflicting evidence and/or a divergence of opinion about the usefulness/efficacy of performing the procedure/therapy.

Class IIa: Weight of evidence/opinion is in favor of usefulness/efficacy.

Class IIb: Usefulness/efficacy is less well established by evidence/opinion.

Class III: Conditions for which there is evidence and/or general agreement that a procedure/therapy is not useful/effective and in some cases may be harmful.

More recent ACC/AHA guidelines also assess the level of evidence that supports the recommendations. Level A means that the data were derived from multiple randomized clinical trials; level B means the data were derived from a single randomized trial or nonrandomized studies; and level C means that the consensus opinion of experts was the primary source of the recommendation.

Evaluation of Patients

A major innovation of the most recent ACC/AHA guidelines is the introduction of a new system of classification of patients that emphasizes the evolution and risks of progression of heart failure (Fig. 2). Stage A patients are at high risk of developing heart failure due to conditions such as systemic hypertension, coronary artery disease, or diabetes mellitus,

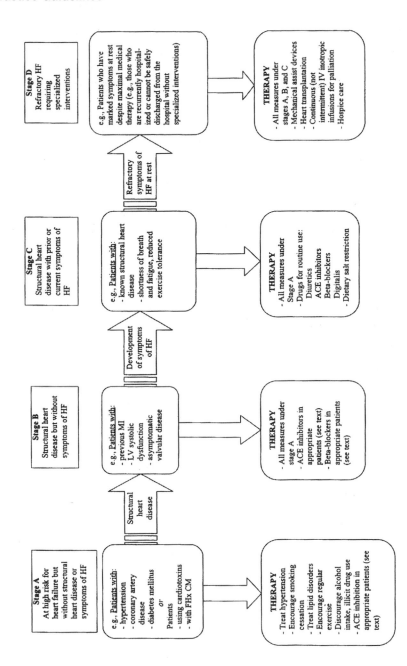

Figure 2 ACC/AHA Guidelines for treatment according to stages in the evolution of heart failure. FHx CM indicates family history of cardiomyopathy; MI, myocardial infarction; LV, left ventricular; and IV, intravenous. (From Ref. 3.)

but have no identified structural or functional cardiac abnormalities and have never shown signs or symptoms of HF. Stage B patients have developed structural heart disease that is strongly associated with heart failure, but have never shown signs or symptoms of this condition. Stage C patients have current or prior symptoms of heart failure associated with underlying structural heart disease. Stage D patients have advanced structural heart disease and marked symptoms of heart failure at rest.

This new classification system is most important for highlighting patients in stages A and B, who are at increased risk for heart failure but have not yet met criteria for diagnosis of this condition. By including these patients in the guidelines, the ACC/AHA task force emphasizes the importance of preventing heart failure, and the evidence supporting interventions to improve prognosis for patients who are at risk for this syndrome. Thus, the guidelines have effectively increased their scope , and now address issues such as use of ACE inhibitors for patients who have survived acute myocardial infarction.

The traditional New York Heart Association classification system has not been replaced, and continues to be used to stratify patients with known heart failure, i.e., those patients within stages C and D. The authors of the ACC/AHA guidelines recognized that functional classification systems are subjective, and that treatment paradigms are not strongly influenced by these clinical assessments. The new staging system is expected to have a more direct relationship to specific treatment strategies.

In the initial evaluation of patients with potential or known heart failure, the ACC/AHA guidelines note the importance of a complete history and physical examination, with particular emphasis on the value of assessment of patients' functional status (Table 2). The class I indications also include recommendations for baseline laboratory testing, including noninvasive assessment of left ventricular function. Cardiac catheterization is routinely recommended for patients with angina who would be candidates for revascularization, reflecting evidence for survival benefit for patients who undergo coronary artery bypass graft surgery for three vessel coronary disease and left ventricular dysfunction.

These guidelines offer some support for coronary angiography (class IIa indications) for patients with heart failure and suspected (but not definite) coronary artery disease. They do not routinely recommend maximal exercise testing with respiratory gas exchange,

Table 2   ACC/AHA Class I Recommendations for Evaluation of Patients with Heart Failure

Recommendation	Level of Evidence
1. Thorough history and physical examination to identify cardiac and noncardiac disorders that might lead to the development of HF or accelerate the progression of HF.	C
2. Initial and ongoing assessment of a patient's ability to perform routine and desired activities of daily living.	C
3. Initial and ongoing assessment of volume status.	C
4. Initial measurement of complete blood count, urinalysis, serum electrolytes (including calcium and magnesium), blood urea nitrogen, serum creatinine, blood glucose, liver function tests, and thyroid-stimulating hormone.	C
5. Serial monitoring of serum electrolytes and renal function.	C
6. Initial 12-lead electrocardiogram and chest radiograph.	C
7. Initial 2-dimensional echocardiography with Doppler or radionuclide ventriculography to assess left ventricular systolic function.	C
8. Cardiac catheterization with coronary arteriography in patients with angina who are candidates for revascularization.	B

but do support this assessment (class IIa) when it is uncertain whether heart failure is the cause of patients' exercise limitation or when patients are candidates for advanced treatments, such as heart transplantation.

The ACC/AHA task force discouraged routine use of several tests (class IIb or III indications), including endomyocardial biopsy, measurement of respiratory gas exchange to guide prescription of an appropriate exercise program, or routine Holter monitoring or signal-averaged electrocardiography.

Therapy

The broad themes of treatment recommended by the ACC/AHA guidelines are summarized in Figure 2. As risk for heart failure and its complications increase, the focus of the recommendations broadens from prevention to treatment with therapies proven to improve survival and/or symptomatic status. As severity of illness increases, preventive recommendations are not dropped; treatment recommendations are added. The level of evidence to support the recommended therapeutic interventions for patients increases as the severity of illness of patients increases (Tables 3 through 6). The availability of evidence to support these recommendations reflects the large number of randomized trials performed for treatment of advanced heart failure in the last two decades.

The preventive strategies for patients with stages A and B heart failure are not solely the focus of cardiovascular specialists. These strategies are also the responsibilities of primary-care physicians and other clinical personnel caring for these patients, and the patients themselves. The strategies include treatment of risk factors for progression of left ventricular dysfunction through medications and modifications of life style. This broadened approach to ''disease management'' is becoming increasingly widespread, as health care organizations recognize that they cannot mitigate the impact of heart failure through excellent care of patients with severe disease alone. Efforts must be made to decrease the incidence of the condition as well.

For patients with a high risk for developing left ventricular dysfunction (stage A), the guidelines emphasize preventive interventions such as control of blood pressure, lipid disorders, and life-style patterns that may contribute to development of cardiomyopathy or ischemic heart disease (Table 3). A low threshold is advocated for recommending

Table 3 ACC/AHA Class I Recommendations for Patients at High Risk of Developing Heart Failure (Stage A)

Recommendation	Level of Evidence
1. Control of systolic and diastolic hypertension in accordance with recommended guidelines.	A
2. Treatment of lipid disorders, in accordance with recommended guidelines.	B
3. Avoidance of patient behaviors that may increase the risk of HF (e.g., smoking, alcohol consumption, and illicit drug use).	C
4. ACE inhibition in patients with a history of atherosclerotic vascular disease, diabetes mellitus, or hypertension and associated cardiovascular risk factors.	B
5. Control of ventricular rate in patients with supraventricular tachyarrhythmias.	B
6. Treatment of thyroid disorders.	C
7. Periodic evaluation for signs and symptoms of HF.	C

Table 4   ACC/AHA Class I Recommendations for Patients with Asymptomatic Left Ventricular Systolic Dysfunction (Stage B)

Recommendation	Level of Evidence
1. ACE inhibition in patients with a recent or remote history of myocardial infarction regardless of ejection fraction.	A
2. ACE inhibition in patients with a reduced ejection fraction, whether or not they have experienced a myocardial infarction.	B
3. Beta-blockade in patients with a recent myocardial infarction regardless of ejection fraction.	A
4. Beta-blockade in patients with a reduced ejection fraction, whether or not they have experienced a myocardial infarction.	B
5. Valve replacement or repair for patients with hemodynamically significant valvular stenosis or regurgitation.	B
6. Regular evaluation for signs and symptoms of HF.	C
7. Measures listed as Class I recommendations for patients in stage A. (See Table 3)	

Table 5   ACC/AHA Class I Recommendations for Treatment of Symptomatic Left Ventricular Systolic Dysfunction (Stage C)

Recommendation	Level of Evidence
1. Diuretics in patients who have evidence of fluid retention.	A
2. ACE inhibition in all patients, unless contraindicated.	A
3. Beta-adrenergic blockade in all stable patients, unless contraindicated. Patients should have no or minimal evidence of fluid retention and should not have required treatment recently with an intravenous positive inotropic agent.	A
4. Digitalis for the treatment of symptoms of HF, unless contraindicated.	A
5. Withdrawal of drugs known to adversely affect the clinical status of patients (e.g., nonsteroidal antiinflammatory drugs, most antiarrhythmic drugs, and most calcium channel blocking drugs).	B
6. Measures listed as Class I recommendations for patients in stages A and B.	

Table 6   ACC/AHA Class I Recommendations for Patients with Refractory End-Stage Heart Failure (Stage D)

Recommendation	Level of Evidence
1. Meticulous identification and control of fluid retention.	B
2. Referral for cardiac transplantation in eligible patients.	B
3. Referral to an HF program with expertise in the management of refractory heart failure.	A
4. Measures listed as class I recommendations for patients in stages A, B, and C.	

angiotensin-converting enzyme (ACE) inhibitors. The guidelines do not recommend routine use of nutritional supplements to prevent development of structural heart disease, or routine testing of left ventricular function for patients without signs or symptoms of heart failure or structural heart disease.

For patients with asymptomatic left ventricular dysfunction (stage B), the guidelines provide strong support for use of ACE inhibition in all patients with reduced ejection fractions and in all patients with histories of myocardial infarction. Similar support is offered for use of beta blockade (Table 4). The guidelines recommend consideration of valve replacement or repair for patients with hemodynamically significant valve abnormalities that may lead to permanent left ventricular dysfunction. They do not support use of long-term vasodilator therapy for patients with severe aortic regurgitation (class IIb). The ACC/AHA guidelines also discourage use of digoxin for asymptomatic patients who are in sinus rhythm (class III indication).

For patients with symptomatic left ventricular dysfunction (stage C), the ACC/AHA guidelines provide strong support for use of ACE inhibition and beta-adrenergic blockade in the absence of contraindications (Table 5). Diuretics are recommended for patients with fluid retention, and digitalis is endorsed for patients with symptoms of heart failure. The guidelines also support careful review of patients' other medications, and withdrawal of drugs known to adversely affect patients' clinical status, such as nonsteroidal antiinflammatory drugs.

The ACC/AHA task force thought there was encouraging evidence for use of spironolactone (class IIa indication) for patients with recent or current class IV symptoms, preserved renal function, and a normal potassium concentration. These guidelines also provided support for consideration of angiotensin-receptor blockade (ARB) in patients who are being treated with digitalis, diuretics, and a beta-blocker and who cannot be given an ACE inhibitor because of cough or angioedema. The Valsartan Heart Failure Trial, which showed adverse effects from addition of this angiotensin-receptor blocker to patients already receiving an ACE inhibitor and a beta-blocker in a post-hoc analysis, was published during the same month as these guidelines [7], and is not directly reflected in the recommendations; however, the findings of this trial do not directly change any of the guidelines. Subsequent trials have not demonstrated an adverse effect of combination therapy with an ACE-inhibitor beta-blockade and ARB on outcome.

The guidelines directly discourage routine use of nutritional supplements, such as coenzyme Q10, carnitine, taurine, and antioxidants, or hormonal therapies, such as growth hormone for heart failure, calling them class III indications. They also did not find evidence to support use of intermittent infusions of positive inotropic drugs or calcium channel blocking drugs.

For patients with refractory end-stage heart failure (stage D), the guidelines support referral of patients to a heart failure program with expertise in management of patients with refractory disease (Table 6). They do not support partial left ventriculectomy or routine use of infusions of positive inotropic agents.

Patients Without Left Ventricular Dysfunction

Although as many as 40% of patients with heart failure do not have left ventricular systolic dysfunction, the absence of clinical trials defining the efficacy of therapeutic interventions compromises the ability of guidelines to address this patient population. Studies of the use of beta-blockers, ACE inhibitors, other vasodilators, calcium blockers, and diuretics have generally been small, and not designed to demonstrate impact on mortality. These medications are nevertheless often used for patients with heart failure without systolic dysfunction because of the presence of comorbid conditions, such as hypertension and diabetes.

In the absence of controlled clinical trials, the guidelines endorse principles of treatment aimed at mitigating factors expected to exert important effects on left ventricular relaxation, including blood pressure, heart rate, blood volume, and myocardial ischemia, The guidelines strongly support control of systolic and diastolic hypertension for patients with heart failure and preserved left ventricular systolic function; and also recommend control of ventricular rate in patients with atrial fibrillation and use of diuretics to control pulmonary congestion. The ACC/AHA task force found only weak evidence to support use of beta-adrenergic blocking agents, ACE inhibitors, angiotensin-receptor blockers, or calcium antagonists in patients with controlled hypertension to minimize symptoms of heart failure (class IIb indications).

Other Special Populations

The ACC/AHA guidelines make a variety of recommendations that remind clinicians to provide evidence-based care for other conditions in patients with heart failure (Table 7). They emphasize the importance of good control of hypertension and use of nitrates and beta-blockers in conjunction with diuretics for patients with angina and heart failure. Anticoagulants are recommended for patients with atrial fibrillation, but not for heart failure without atrial fibrillation. Coronary revascularization is recommended for patients with both heart failure and angina, but not for patients with heart failure and coronary disease who do *not* have angina (class IIb indication).

End of Life Care

The importance of beginning end-of-life planning before patients become too ill to participate in decisions is also noted in these guidelines (Table 7). The guidelines recommend initiation of education of the patient and family regarding the expected course of illness, final treatment options, and end-of-life planning before the patient becomes too ill to participate in decisions. Discussions regarding treatment preferences should address likely scenarios, such as cardiac arrest, catastrophic events, such as a severe cerebrovascular accident, and marked exacerbations of heart failure. The guidelines recommend making a clear distinction between short-term interventions aimed at achieving a rapid recovery vs. prolonged life support without reasonable expectation of return to good functional capacity.

The guidelines note that hospice services have been extended to heart failure patients relatively recently in most regions, and they support the hospice concept for this population. Hospice care is aimed at relieving symptoms, and the guidelines support compassionate care that is directed at symptoms, such as breathlessness, even if it may in some cases actually shorten survival. The guidelines oppose use of a cardioverter-defibrillator in patients with class IV symptoms of heart failure who are not expected to improve.

Exercise

Although much of the focus of the ACC/AHA and other guidelines tends to be on use of medications, nonpharmacologic interventions are an important part of care of patients with heart failure. The American Heart Association released a Scientific Statement in 2003 [8] that summarizes research on risks and benefits of exercise training for patients with heart failure, and concludes that exercise training appears effective for improving exercise capacity and quality of life. The Scientific Statement specifically urges insurers to support exercise training programs for heart failure as described in these guidelines.

Table 7 ACC/AHA Class I Recommendations for Special Populations, Patients with Diastolic Dysfunction, and End-of-Life Care

Population or Concomitant Condition	Recommendation	Level of Evidence
Hypertension	1. Control of systolic and diastolic hypertension in patients with heart failure in accordance with recommended guidelines.	A
Angina	1. Nitrates and beta-blockers (in conjunction with diuretics) for the treatment of angina in patients with heart failure.	B
	2. Coronary revascularization in patients who have both HF and angina.	A
Atrial fibrillation	1. Anticoagulants in patients with HF who have paroxysmal or chronic atrial fibrillation or a previous thromboembolic event.	A
	2. Control of the ventricular response in patients with HF and atrial fibrillation with a beta-blocker (or amiodarone, if the beta-blocker is contraindicated or not tolerated).	A
Ventricular arrhythmia	1. Implantable cardioverter-defibrillator (alone or in combination with amiodarone) in patients with heart failure who have a history of sudden death, ventricular fibrillation, or hemodynamically destabilizing ventricular tachycardia.	A
Preserved left ventricular function	1. Control of systolic and diastolic hypertension, in accordance with published guidelines.	A
	2. Control of ventricular rate in patients with atrial fibrillation.	C
	3. Diuretics to control pulmonary congestion and peripheral edema.	C
End-of-life care	1. Ongoing patient and family education regarding prognosis for function and survival.	C
	2. Patient and family education about options for formulating and implementing advance directives.	C
	3. Continuity of medical care between inpatient and outpatient settings.	C
	4. Components of hospice care that are appropriate to the relief of suffering.	C

The recommendations describe a standard approach to assessment of patients' functional capacity, including lower targets for intensity of exercise in very debilitated patients or those who are not accustomed to aerobic activity (e.g., 60% or 65% of peak oxygen consumption, vs. the more frequently used range of 70% to 80%). Duration of exercise should include an adequate warm-up period, such as 10 to 15 minutes. The most frequently recommended exercise duration is 20 to 30 minutes, followed by a cool-down period. Most studies have used 3 to 5 times per week as the optimal training frequency.

The AHA statement recommends that exercise be performed in a setting with direct monitoring and supervision, including telemetry monitoring, especially during the initial training session. These recommendations echo those of the American Association for Cardiovascular and Pulmonary Rehabilitation [9]. Home training can follow a period of initial supervision, but continued monitoring of patients with exercise-induced arrhythmias and more advanced forms of heart failure is considered "prudent." Although the duration of exercise training is not well studied, the Scientific Statement recommends that patients with heart failure remain active either in a formal exercise program or one at home indefinitely.

The Scientific Statement notes the lack of definitive data on the safety and efficacy of resistive training, but supports use of resistive training to strengthen individual muscle groups using small free weights (1, 2, or 5 lb), elastic bands, or repetitive isolated muscle training. This recommendation is based upon research indicating functional benefits in small numbers of patients, but the Scientific Statement explicitly notes need for studies in larger trials.

The Scientific Statement encourages candidates for heart transplantation to participate in exercise training with both aerobic training and resistive exercise before and after transplantation, and even while using left ventricular assist devices. These recommendations echo those of the Agency for Health Care Policy and Research Guidelines on Cardiac Rehabilitation [10].

Drugs and Devices Under Investigation

The guidelines explicitly note that there are numerous drug and device interventions for heart failure that are under active investigation, but data were not sufficiently conclusive at the time the guidelines were written to allow development of consensus on their roles. These interventions, including pharmacologic innovations such as vasopeptidase inhibitors, cytokine antagonists, endothelin antagonists, synchronized biventricular pacing, external counterpulsation, and techniques for respiratory support, such as nocturnal oxygen and continuous positive airway pressure. Before any of these interventions can achieve a class I indication reflecting strong support from the ACC/AHA guidelines, definitive clinical trials must be performed. Since the guidelines were written, studies have been published on some of these interventions, particularly synchronized biventricular pacing. For this reason, modifications of ACC/AHA and other guidelines are planned every few years.

GUIDELINE IMPLEMENTATION

The achievement of consensus on what should be done in the care of any patient population is only one step in the process of improvement of care. The next challenge is to develop systems that make these interventions occur with reliability. The limited impact of information alone was demonstrated in one trial in which simple dissemination of guidelines followed by written and verbal reminders failed to change treatment of heart failure in an intensive care unit setting [11]. Consensus has emerged that implementation of guidelines requires a multidimensional approach, including education and coordination of efforts among physicians, other clinical personnel, and patients themselves [3].

The organization of such efforts is usually led by physicians because of their special leadership role in health care, but success does not always come easily. Physicians are trained to meet the acute needs of individual patients before them; when faced with the responsibility for improving the care over time of populations of patients with heart failure and other chronic conditions, physician leaders are often forced to recognize that they may not have the tools and expertise to succeed. The American College of Cardiology and other organizations are attempting to develop and disseminate tools that use continuous quality improvement (CQI) [12]. CQI uses principles adapted from industrial manufacturers to improve quality through repetitive cycles of process and outcomes measurement, implementation of interventions to improve care, followed by remeasurement to assess the impact of interventions [13].

The simplest application of CQI is the use of critical pathways for hospitalized patients. These pathways are standardized protocols that define key steps in the care of common syndromes. Whether critical pathways actually improve efficiency and quality is unclear, as some data suggest that improvement associated with them may result simply from focusing physicians' and nurses' attention on the patient population, not from the protocols themselves [14]. Thus, the most important step in pathway implementation may be multidisciplinary team development, not the pathway itself.

Team-based care has proved especially beneficial in the care of patients with heart failure. Multidisciplinary teams that combine physicians, nurses, and other personnel in following patients with heart failure over time have been shown to improve patient survival and quality of life, while reducing costs of care [6]. Many hospitals and other organizations report success in reducing hospitalizations through their heart failure disease-management programs, but more rigorous assessments suggest that outcomes vary according to the program design. A systematic review pooled publish data from a total of 11 trials involving 2067 patients with heart failure, and found that disease-management programs were cost saving in seven of the eight trials that reported cost data and also improved prescribing practices [15]. Programs that used multidisciplinary teams and specialized follow-up led to a substantial reduction in the risk of hospitalization (RR = 0.77, 95% CI 0.68 to 0.86, N = 1366). In contrast, trials using telephone contact with improved coordination of primary care services failed to find any benefit (RR = 1.15, 95% CI 0.96 to 1.37, N = 646). Thus, the model used by many payer "carve out" companies seems less guaranteed of success than the model used by health-care provider organizations. Examples of the impact of key trials of multidisciplinary heart failure programs are summarized in Table 8 [6,16–24].

Table 8 Major Randomized Trials of Multidisciplinary Heart Failure Management

Author/Year	No. of patients	Findings
Rich, et al., 1993 (17)	98	Nurse-directed multidisciplinary team reduced admissions 27% over 90-day follow-up period for patients ≥70 years with mean NYHA class 2 heart failure
Schneider, et al., 1993 (18)	54	Nurse-directed medication discharge planning reduced readmissions by 73% over 1 month of follow-up
Kostis, et al., 1994 (19)	20	Exercise, cognitive therapy, and stress management led to improvement in exercise tolerance and quality of life, and enhanced weight loss over 12-week period
Rich, et al., 1995 (6)	282	Nurse-directed multidisciplinary team led to 44% fewer admissions and lower costs with improved quality of life for patients with average age of 79 years during 90-day follow-up period; benefits persisted up to 1 year.
Stewart, et al., 1998 (20)	97	Home-based nurse-pharmacist team led to 42% fewer admissions and lower hospital costs for patients with mean age of 75 years over 6-month follow-up period.
Serxner, et al., 1998 (21)	109	Educational mailings and compliance aids led to 52% fewer admissions and improved health status for patients with mean age of 71 years over 6-month follow-up period.

Source: Adapted from Ref. 16.

Table 9 ACC/AHA Recommendations for Implementation of Heart Failure Practice Guidelines

Strength of Recommendation	Recommendation
Strongest (class I)	1. Multifactorial interventions that attack different barriers to behavioral change. *(Level of Evidence: A)* 2. Multidisciplinary disease-management programs for patients at high risk for hospital admission or clinical deterioration. *(Level of Evidence: B)* 3. Academic detailing or educational outreach visits. *(Level of Evidence: A)*
Encouraging (class IIa)	1. Chart audit and feedback of results. *(Level of Evidence: A)* 2. Reminder systems. *(Level of Evidence: A)* 3. Local opinion leaders. *(Level of Evidence: A)*
Modest (class IIb)	Multidisciplinary disease-management programs for patients at low risk for hospital admission or clinical deterioration. *(Level of Evidence: B)*
Weak (class III)	1. Dissemination of guidelines without more intensive behavioral change efforts. *(Level of Evidence: A)* 2. Basic provider education alone. *(Level of Evidence: A)*

Source: From Ref. 3.

The ACC/AHA guidelines [3] also make recommendations supporting the use of multidisciplinary disease-management programs for patients at high risk for hospital admission or clinical deterioration, as well as multifactorial educational efforts for patients and physicians (Table 9). These recommendations reflect pessimism for the impact of educational effort alone, and the greater impact expected from multidisciplinary interventions aimed at higher-risk patients.

An AHA Scientific Statement on Team Management of Patients with Heart Failure provides a detailed description for the elements required for successful heart failure programs [25]. These recommendations encourage a structured patient assessment, including evaluation of psychosocial issues that can influence patient compliance with the management plan and their overall quality of life. Nonphysician personnel are particularly important in this approach for education and counseling of patients, and follow-up to ensure that patients are following recommendations and are clinically stable. Other key components of management include increased access to health-care professionals for problems by telephone or ''walk-in'' appointment, early attention to signs and symptoms of fluid overload, and attention to behavioral strategies to increase compliance.

MEASUREMENT OF QUALITY FOR THE PURPOSE OF IMPROVEMENT

A final element needed for programs to reliably improve care for patients with heart failure is a ''feedback'' system whereby quality is measured and improved. This issue was the focus of an ACC/AHA scientific forum, which included a specific discussion of quality measurement for heart failure [26]. This report emphasized that guidelines are not the same as performance measures. Performance measures ''are explicit standards of care against which actual clinical care is judged,'' whereas guidelines ''are written to suggest diagnostic or therapeutic interventions for most patients in most circumstances.'' The implication is that guidelines represent recommendations, and performance measures suggest rules from which deviation should occur only after careful consideration and documentation of the rationale.

The ACC/AHA working group endorsed four specific *structural* (i.e., descriptive of systems) measures for consideration as quality measures:

1. Clinicians should have clear, evidence-based facility guidelines for care of patients with heart failure. The guidelines may take the form of either pathways or recommendations, but the facility should have a document that describes or endorses best practices and aligns them with existing medical evidence.
2. Clinicians should have a mechanism to systematically monitor patient care and outcomes, with domains of care that align with the guideline recommendations endorsed by the clinicians. This information should be reviewed by clinical staff at least annually.
3. The clinicians and care facility staff must have an organizational structure to move patients to the appropriate level of care.
4. Clinicians and care facilities should have specific programs to address end-of-life needs.

Four *process* measures (i.e., describing specific functions) were endorsed by the working group:

1. Documentation of left ventricular function.
2. Use of ACE inhibitors for patients with heart failure, left ventricular systolic dysfunction and no contraindications.
3. Use of digoxin for patients hospitalized with heart failure and left ventricular systolic dysfunction.
4. Use of beta-blockers for patients with NYHA class II and III heart failure, left ventricular systolic dysfunction, and no contraindications.

Note that these recommendations were published in 2000, and may be altered by recent and future clinical trials.

The working group did not believe that performance measures based upon actual patient outcomes (e.g., mortality, hospitalization) should be used to inform consumer choice because of difficulty in risk adjustment and lack of standards for sample size. Nevertheless, the working group believed that outcome measures should be collected by clinicians and used for internal quality improvement activities.

The use of such performance measures can no longer be considered optional by cardiovascular physicians and others involved in the care of patients with heart failure. Measurement of these and other dimensions of quality of care are now being used to assess all hospitals as part of the JCAHO accreditation process, and data are expected to be made public by the middle of this decade. To reduce the costs of the mandatory collection of these data, hospitals are developing systems to integrate their measurement into the routine processes of care (e.g., special data collection tools used as part of discharge planning). For business purposes as well as the pursuit of better care, hospitals must invest in systems for improvement of their performance, or else confront the possibility that they will appear to be providers of inferior care compared to their competitors.

CONCLUSION

Much of the progress in the care of patients with heart failure has resulted from research on new pharmacologic and device-based strategies for treatment of patients with this condition. However, comparable if not greater impact has resulted from the interventions aimed at improving the speed and reliability with which evidence-based management strategies are used. These interventions include the development of consensus-based guidelines and the use of CQI tactics (e.g., multidisciplinary disease-management teams). The development of guidelines and measures of quality, followed by the measurement and improvement of performance are essential parts of the advancement of care of patients with heart failure and other cardiovascular diseases.

REFERENCES

1. Califf RM, Peterson ED, Gibbons RJ, Garson A Jr, Brindus RG, Beller GA, Smith SC Jr. Integrating quality into the cycle of therapeutic development. J Am Coll Cardiol 2002; 40: 1895–1901.
2. Ritchie JL, Forrester JS, Fye WB JS. (conference co-chairs). 28th Bethesda Conference Practice Guidelines and the Quality of Care. J Am Coll Cardiol 1997; 29:1125–1179.
3. Hunt SA, Baker DW, Gildstein S, et al. ACC/AHA guidelines for the evaluation and management of chronic heart failure in the adult: executive summary: a report of the American College of Cardiology/American Heart Association Task Force on Practice Guidelines (Committee to Revise the 1995 Guidelines for the Evaluation and Management of Heart Failure). J Am Coll Cardiol 2001; 38:2101–2113.
4. Giugliano RP, Camargo CA, Lloyd-Jones DM, et al. Elderly patients receive less aggressive medical and invasive management of unstable angina: potential impact of practice guidelines. Arch Intern Med 1998; 158:1113–1120.
5. Polanczyk CA, Newton C, Dec GW, Di Salvo TG. Quality of care and hospital readmission in congestive heart failure: an explicit review process. J Card Fail 2001; 7:299–301.
6. Rich MW, Beckham V, Wittenberg C, Leven CL, Freedland KE, Carney RM. A multidisciplinary intervention to prevent the readmission of elderly patients with congestive heart failure. N Engl J Med 1995; 333:1190–1195.
7. Cohn JN, Tognoni G. for the Valsartan Heart Failure Trial Investigators. A randomized trial of the angiotensin-receptor blocker valsartan in chronic heart failure. N Engl J Med 2001; 345:1667–1675.
8. Pina IL, Apstein CS, Balady GJ, et al. Exercise and heart failure. A statement from the American Heart Association Committee on Exercise, Rehabilitation, and Prevention. Circulation 2003; 107:1210–1225.
9. American Association of Cardiovascular and Pulmonary Rehabilitation. Guidelines for Cardiac Rehabilitation and Secondary Prevention Programs. Champaign. IL: Human Kinetics Publishers:1999.
10. U.S. Department of Health and Human Services. Agency for Health Care Policy and Research. Clinical Practice Guideline No. 17: Cardiac Rehabilitation, Agency for Health Care Policy and Research, Washington, DC, Human Kinetics Publishers, October 1995 AHCPR Publication No. 96-0672.
11. Weingarten S, Riedinger M, Conner L, Johnson B, Ellrodt AG. Reducing lengths of stay in the coronary care unit with a practice guideline for patients with congestive heart failure: insights from a controlled clinical trial. Med Care 1994; 32:1232–1243.
12. Mehta RH, Montoye CK, Gallogly M, et al. Improving quality of care for acute myocardial infarction: the Guidelines Applied in Practice (GAP) Initiative. JAMA 2002; 287:1269–1276.
13. Berwick DM. Continuous improvement as an ideal in health care. N Engl J Med 1989; 320: 53–56.
14. Pearson SD, Kleefield SF, Roukop JR, Cook EF, Lee TH. Critical pathways intervention to reduce length of hospital stay. Am J Med 2001; 110:175–180.
15. McAlister FA, Lawson FME, Koon KT, Armstrong PW. A systematic review of randomized trials of disease management programs in heat failure. Am J Med 2001; 110:378–384.
16. Rich MW. Heart failure disease management: a critical review. J Cardiac Fail 1999; 5:64–75.

17. Rich MW, Vinson JM, Sperry JC, et al. Prevention of readmission in elderly patients with congestive heart failure: results of a prospective, randomized pilot study. J Gen Intern Med 1993; 8:585–590.
18. Schneider JK, Nornberger S, Booker J, Davis A, Kralicek R. A medication discharge planning program: measuring the effect on readmissions. Clin Nurs Res 1993; 2:41–53.
19. Kostis JB, Rosen RC, Cosgrove NM, Shindler DM, Wilson AC. Nonpharmacologic therapy improves functional and emotional status in congestive heart failure. Chest 1994; 106: 996–1001.
20. Stewart S, Pearson S, Horowitz JD. Effects of a home-based intervention among patients with congestive heart failure discharged from acute hospital care. Arch Intern Med 1998; 158: 1067–1072.
21. Serxner S, Miyaji M, Jeffortds J. Congestive heart failure disease management study: a patient education intervention. Congest Heart Fail 1998; 4:23–28.
22. Stewart S, Horowitz JD. Home-based intervention in congestive heart failure. Long-term implications on readmission and survival. Circulation 2002; 105:2861–6.
23. Frumhulz NM, Amatruda J, Smith GL, Mattera JA, Roumani SA, Radford MJ, Crombie P, Vaccarino V. Randomized trial of education and support intervention to prevent readmission of patients with heart failure. J Am Cell Cardiol 2002; 39:83–9.
24. Phillips CO, Wright SM, Kern DE, Singa RM, Shepperd S, Raubin HR. Comprehensive discharge pregnancy with post-discharge support for older patients with congestive heart failure. JAMA 2004; 291:1358–67.
25. Grady KL, Dracup K, Kennedy G, et al. Team management of patients with heart failure: a statement for healthcare professionals from the Cardiovascular Nursing Council of the American Heart Association. Circulation 2000; 102:2443–2456.
26. Quality of Care and Outcomes Research in CVD and Stroke Working Groups. Measuring and improving quality of care. A report from the American Heart Association/American College of Cardiology First Scientific Forum on Assessment of Healthcare Quality in Cardiovascular Disease and Stroke. Circulation 2000; 101:1483–1493.

22

Coronary Revascularization, Mitral Valve Repair, Left Ventricular Remodeling, Procedures and Devices

Patrick M. McCarthy
Departments of Cardiovascular and Thoracic Surgery,
Northwestern University Medical Center,
Chicago, Illinois, USA

Katherine J. Hoercher and Richard Lee
George M. and Linda H. Kaufman Center for Heart Failure,
Cleveland Clinic Foundation
Cleveland, Ohio, USA

INTRODUCTION

The significant increase in the prevalence, morbidity, and mortality from heart failure has resulted in a profound health crisis in the United States [1]. The impact of heart failure is observed not only in the loss of both quantity and quality of life, but also on the enormous financial burden it has placed on an already strained health care system. The practice of cardiovascular surgery has also been radically impacted as a consequence of the heart failure epidemic, as evidenced by the increased application of nontransplant surgical therapies, thereby creating a new subspecialty within the field.

Surgical therapies for patients with heart failure are not an entirely new concept, as interventions on this population have been performed for decades, albeit with a high perioperative morbidity and mortality as observed in the 1970s and 1980s. These unacceptable early outcomes served to limit the role of surgery to cases of failed medical management, and historically, many of these patients were referred for cardiac transplantation. Although still very successful for end-stage heart failure, the field of transplantation will continue to be plagued by a finite number of organ donors (Chapter 23). Perhaps even more alarming, as recently reported by Sheehy and colleagues, is that even in a ''perfect world'' where all potential organ donors became actual donors, the supply of cardiac donors would not meet the growing demand [2]. As the number of patients suffering from heart failure continues to escalate, it is imperative to avoid or delay the need for cardiac transplantation whenever possible.

Surgery for heart failure is rapidly evolving. We are observing increased referrals for ''conventional'' surgery; fortunately, many aspects have evolved to improve survival, and as a result, surgical outcomes for patients with even the most advanced heart failure have made tremendous improvements.

Contemporary surgical management of heart failure addresses the geometry of the failing left ventricle, which is one that has progressed from a normal elliptical ventricular shape to that of a dilated, spherical muscle or pathologically "remodeled" ventricle. The emergence of devices and procedures to arrest or reverse remodeling and, thus, improve cardiac function are at the forefront of surgical heart failure management.

Insights into the pathophysiological process of heart failure have also yielded major advances in pharmacological therapy and have helped us design specific evidence-based treatment paradigms that have clearly improved outcomes in these patients. Hence, a key ingredient to the success of any heart failure surgery is the combination of state-of-the-art pharmacologic therapy, thereby creating a true synergy. A coordinated team of clinicians with both medical and surgical expertise provides these patients with the best chance for a meaningful future.

This chapter will review the current and evolving surgical strategies and devices to treat both ischemic and nonischemic heart failure with a focus on coronary artery bypass grafting (CABG), mitral valve repair, and left ventricular reconstruction.

CORONARY BYPASS SURGERY

Ischemic cardiomyopathy (ICM) is the most common cause of congestive heart failure (CHF) and although estimates vary, it may be the direct cause of CHF in 40% to 70% of cases [3,4]. Clinical manifestations of ICM include congestive heart failure, angina, arrhythmias, and sudden death.

Historically, the outcome of ischemic cardiomyopathy with medical therapy is overall poor. However, it should be noted, that there are no current published randomized trials comparing surgery with advanced pharmacologic and nonoperative therapies.

Earlier observational studies comparing medical vs. surgical therapy demonstrate that patients with ICM have a 1-year survival rate of 50% to 90% and a 5-year survival rate of 4% to 47% [5–11]. From the Coronary Artery Surgery Study (CASS) registry, patients who did not have surgery had a 21% 12-year survival [12]. The Veteran's Affairs (VA) Cooperative Study also clearly demonstrated a survival benefit for patients with impaired LV function (LVEF < 40%) who underwent bypass surgery compared with initial medical management [13]. These findings have led to a broader application of coronary revascularization to include patients with severely diseased ventricles.

The major benefit of revascularization is functional improvement of myocardium, with secondary effects of retarding ventricular remodeling and reducing substrate for malignant ventricular arrhythmias. In determining appropriate candidates for revascularization, patient evaluation and selection have a critical role for patients with ICM. As with patients with normal ventricular function, evaluation includes assessment of symptoms (especially angina), functional status, age, and major medical comorbidities (especially pulmonary, renal, cerebrovascular, and peripheral vascular disease). Coronary angiography identifies the extent of disease and quality of the distal vessels. Attention is also directed to assessment of global and regional ventricular function and myocardial viability.

As our experience with coronary artery bypass grafting has grown, revascularization has become an integral component of the surgical treatment for heart failure. However, prior to an attempt at intervention, an understanding of where the patient lies on the ischemia-infarction continuum must be made [14–16]. Revascularization of tissue that will never contribute to ventricular function will not benefit a patient.

Myocardial tissue with compromised blood flow may be ischemic, stunned, hibernating, or infarcted. Ischemia is defined by adequate blood flow and intact function at rest but with impaired flow reserve and rapidly reversible functional impairment with exercise. These patients will quickly benefit from revascularization. Stunned myocardial tissue is ischemic myocardium with prolonged post ischemic dysfunction. These patients should improve over time after revascularization. Hibernating myocardium is tissue with impaired resting blood flow and function, without response to exercise. This tissue may contribute to myocardial function with increased blood flow. Infarcted tissue is no longer myocardium [14–16]. All of these states frequently coexist in patients with ICM (their relative proportions varying among different patients), and have tremendous importance for predicting improvement after CABG.

Several imaging techniques are available to prospectively evaluate the relative proportions of recruitable myocardium. There is no individual "gold standard," rather, the modalities are somewhat complementary and include radionuclide, echocardiographic and magnetic resonance imaging techniques.

Nuclear medicine techniques include single photon emission computed tomography (SPECT) (using thallium-201), and positron emission tomography (PET) (using rubidium-82 or ^{13}N-ammonia metabolic F-18 deoxyglucose [FDG] or carbon-11 acetate tracers).

Thallium uptake by the myocardium is related to blood flow and cellular integrity, and, hence, is predictive of viability. In a SPECT injection/delayed redistribution exam, thallium is injected at rest. Images are obtained early and after 4 hours of redistribution [15,17]. Delayed imaging up to 24 hours may uncover additional viable areas. This implies that "fixed" defects on routine thallium-201 rest-redistribution imaging may actually represent hibernating rather than irreversibly damaged myocardium. The SPECT examination predicts functional improvement after CABG in 62% of asynergic, viable segments but only in 23% of nonviable segments [15].

Stress-redistribution thallium imaging is another technique used to assess myocardial viability [18,19]. However, up to 50% of regions with fixed irreversible perfusion defects exhibit some degree of metabolic activity using other more sensitive viability measures. Reinjection of thallium after 24-hour interval may improve the negative predictive value [20]. However, the identification of viable regions by rest-redistribution thallium imaging is still less than ideal. Positive and negative predictive accuracy range from 45% to 79% and 62% to 80%, respectively [15,17,18].

The PET scan may better assess myocardial viability [21,22]. A region of myocardium showing high FDG uptake relative to myocardial blood flow (perfusion/metabolic mismatch) represents ischemic, stunned, or hibernating myocardium. Myocardial scar is identified by an area with decreased perfusion at rest that corresponds to decreased metabolism (perfusion/metabolic match). The number of viable segments predicts improvement after revascularization. The average positive and negative predictive accuracy of PET for predicting improved function after revascularization are 82% and 83%, respectively, with an overall predictive accuracy of 82% [23].

Dobutamine stress echocardiography (DSE) also helps to differentiate between stunned and hibernating myocardium [24]. Segmental wall motion is monitored during dobutamine administration from a low to a high dose. A uniphase response (segmental wall augmentation that continues from low to high dobutamine doses) is suggestive of myocardial stunning. However, a biphasic response (augmentation at low doses followed by a reduction in function at higher doses) is indicative of ischemia and hibernation. DSE has been useful in the preoperative prediction of viable myocardium [25]. DSE has been found to have an overall accuracy of 86%, a specificity of 91% and a sensitivity of 68%. When compared to ^{201}TL injection/delayed redistribution imaging, the accuracy of the nuclear imaging and DSE techniques appear to be similar [26]. (Table 1)

Cardiac magnetic resonance imaging (MRI) is a relatively new tool to assess myocardial viability. It has three important roles: assessment of tissue perfusion, evaluation of myocardial contractile reserve, and characterization of myocardial cellular membrane function. In patients with ventricular dysfunction, MRI exams accompanied by the intravenous

Table 1 Sensitivity and Specificity of NonInvasive Techniques to Predict Functional Recovery Following Coronary Revascularization in Patients with Left Ventricular Dysfunction Due to Coronary Artery Disease

Technique	No. of Patients	% (95% CI)	
		Sensitivity[a]	Specificity[b]
Technitium[99m] sestamibi imaging	207	83 (78–87)	69 (63–74)
Dobutamine echocardiography	448	84 (82–86)	81 (79–84)
Thallium[201] stress-redistribution imaging	209	86 (83–89)	47 (43–51)
Thallium[201] rest-redistribution imaging	145	90 (87–93)	54 (49–60)
[18F]fluorodeoxyglucose PET	327	88 (84–91)	73 (69–74)

CI, confidence intervals; PET, positron-emission tomography.

[a] Sensitivity is defined as the number of viable segments of myocardium divided by the number with recovery of function.

[b] Specificity is defined as the number of nonviable segments divided by the number without recovery of function postoperatively. Values are weighted means. There is no significant difference in sensitivity among methods.
Source: From Ref. 26a.

infusion of low-dose dobutamine may help identify additional viable areas [27]. Dobutamine MRI is a specific (81%) but insensitive (50%) predictor of myocardial functional recovery following revascularization [28]. However, MRI may be particularly useful in patients for whom physiological stress is impractical [29].

Cine MRI with gadolinium-based contrast agent evaluates the transmural extent of myocardial viability. Gadolinium-based contrast agents are biologically inert and diffuse into the interstitial space, where their exit is delayed in zones of irreversible myocardial injury (hence, ''hyperenchancement''). Hyperenhancement of dysfunctional myocardial segments is indicative of nonviability. Improvement in regional contractility after revascularization is inversely related to the extent of hyperenhancement before revascularization (30). (Fig. 1) In their study of 50 patients, contractility improved after CABG in 78% of regions without hyperenhancement but in only 2% of segments with severe hyperenhancement [30]. A larger percentage of the left ventricle that is both dysfunctional and not hyperenhanced before revascularization predicts a greater the improvement in the global mean wall-motion score and ejection fraction after revascularization. Cine MRI studies are also useful to identify areas of scar that may be amenable to surgical ventricular reconstruction.

At the Cleveland Clinic, MRI (when feasible) and PET are the methods of choice. Newer MRI protocols assess the extent and distribution of scar and segmental perfusion/ function relations, as well as associated aneurysm, LV thrombus, and mitral regurgitation. After complete evaluation, we will tend to offer surgery to patients who have compensated heart failure.

Surgical techniques for CABG in ischemic cardiomyopathy are similar to that for patients with normal LV function. However, intraoperative myocardial protection, complete revascularization, and optimal conduit selection become even more critical.

The outcome after CABG in the setting of severe LV dysfunction has improved significantly over time. This may be in part due to advances in intraoperative myocardial protection, increasing surgeon experience, and more consistent postoperative care strategies. Also, in the earlier randomized surgical trials, the internal thoracic arteries were not commonly utilized and we now know that these grafts have superior early and late patency rates vs. vein grafts [31]. The modern era of coronary artery bypass also has the advantage

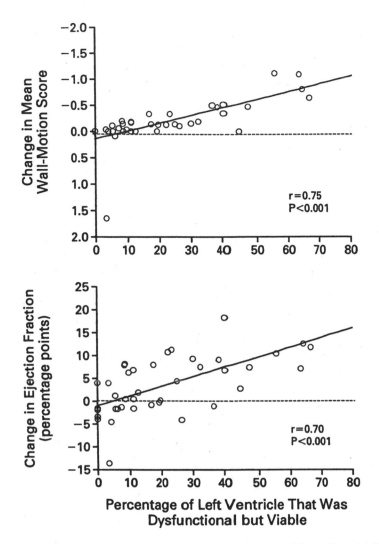

Figure 1 Relationship between the percentage of the left ventricle that was dysfunctional but assessed as viable (n = 41) before revascularization and the changes in mean wall-motion score and ejection fraction after coronary revascularization. Decreases in wall-motion scores indicate improvements in myocardial contractility. The mean left ventricular ejection fraction was 43 ± 13% before and 47 ± 12% after surgery. (From Ref. 30.)

of the availability of platelet inhibitors, which have been shown to improve vein graft patency rates and HMG coenzyme A inhibitors or ''statins,'' which decrease the angiographic progression of atherosclerosis in bypass grafts [32–34].

Middleborough and colleagues reported their experience in 125 consecutive patients who underwent coronary revascularization and had a preoperative left ventricular ejection fraction less than 20% [34a]. Although preoperative viability studies were not routinely performed, more than 90% of patients had either active angina pectoris (79%) or critical coronary anatomy (13%). The 5-year actuarial survival was 72%. Multivariate analysis indicated older age, NYHA class IV symptoms, and poorly visualized distal vessels as adverse predictors of outcome. Further justification for surgical revascularization can be

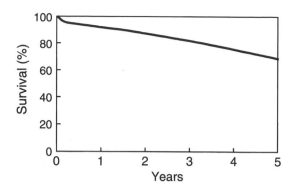

Figure 2 Survival of 788 patients who underwent coronary revascularization at the Cleveland Clinic who had severe left ventricular dysfunction and underwent primary coronary artery bypass grafting between 1997 and 2001.

demonstrated by the authors' own experience. The Cleveland Clinic recently studied a contemporaneous cohort of 788 patients with severe LV dysfunction ($\leq$ 35%) who had undergone primary CABG between 1997 and 2001. Hospital mortality was 2.4%. Survival was 92%, 82%, and 69% at 1, 3, and 5 years, respectively; freedom from admission for heart failure was 95%, 89%, and 82 % at the same time points (mean follow-up 2.4 $\pm$ 1.8 years). (Fig. 2)

Although LV dysfunction remains a marker of increased morbidity and mortality after CABG, its impact as a predictor of poor postoperative outcomes has decreased [35–37]. Other factors, such as urgent surgery, worse preoperative functional status (NYHA class III or IV), reoperative CABG, and extent of CAD (coronery artery disease), have become more important. In the CABG Patch trial [38], patients with preoperative heart failure had 2 times greater perioperative mortality compared to those without. Significantly, symptomatic heart failure was a more important predictor of mortality than preoperative ejection fraction [39]. The impact of CHF on outcome after CABG was also noted in the SHOCK trial [40]. Other factors, such as LV end systolic volume index are also independent predictors of poor 5-year survival after CABG [41].

In the current era, coronary bypass surgery remains an important treatment for ischemic cardiomyopathy with compensated CHF. CABG has acceptably low mortality and morbidity over previous studies when performed by an experienced surgical team applying the latest techniques in appropriately selected candidates. The STITCH trial is now prospectively evaluating the benefits of coronary revascularization vs. optimized medical therapy for patients with multivessel coronary artery disease and impaired left ventricular function.

VALVULAR DISEASE IN HEART FAILURE

Valvular disease alone may contribute to heart failure or may be the effect of heart failure due to other disease etiologies. In either case, once present, it continues to adversely effect patient survival and may benefit from surgical correction.

Mitral Regurgitation

Severe mitral regurgitation (MR) is a frequent complication of both ischemic and nonischemic cardiomyopathy with the culprit again being adverse left ventricle remodeling.

Left ventricular enlargement results in papillary muscle displacement and the decreased coaptation of the mitral valve leaflets, which creates a central jet of mitral regurgitation. This process results in greater left ventricular volume overload, increasing ventricular dilatation and dysfunction, and worsening mitral regurgitation.

The issues regarding the appropriate management of patients with MR and advanced left ventricular dysfunction remain controversial. Mitral valve surgery in these patients has long thought to be associated with a prohibitive operative mortality due, in part, to earlier reports identifying severe left ventricular dysfunction as highly significant for adverse outcomes. However, these observations were largely based on the use of traditional mitral valve replacement with disruption of the subvalvular apparatus [42–44]. Mitral valve repair and replacement with chordal preservation techniques can now be successfully applied in patients with severe LV dysfunction, and there is now an increasing body of evidence demonstrating low operative mortality, good long-term survival, and freedom from readmissions for heart failure [45,46]. Today, the symptomatic patient with mitral regurgitation and severe left ventricular dysfunction should be considered for surgery; in most instances, mitral valve *repair* has become the surgery of choice [44a]. The authors' mitral valve repair strategy utilizes an undersized flexible annuloplasty ring. If the annulus is very dilated and there is little tethering, a 26 mmm or 28 mm ring is used and, conversely, if the annulus is small and/or there is much tethering then a 24 mm is used.

At the Cleveland Clinic between 1990 and 1998, 44 patients with severe mitral regurgitation and a LV ejection fraction less than 35% underwent isolated mitral repair (n = 35) or replacement (n = 9). All patients had been hospitalized one to six times for management of heart failure (mean 2.3 ± 1.5) and had NYHA class III or IV symptoms despite optimal pharmacologic therapy. The 1-, 2-, and 5-year survival rates were 89%, 86%, and 67%, respectively. Freedom from readmission for heart failure averaged 88%, 82%, and 72% during the same follow-up [47]. (Fig. 3) Favorable results have also been reported from Badwar and Bolling in 125 patients with refractory 4 + mitral regurgitation and NYHA class III–IV heart failure. In this series, there was one operative death with 1- and 2-year actuarial survival rates of 80% and 70% [48]. Overall, mitral valve surgery in patients with severe left ventricular function offers improvement of symptoms of heart failure and reasonable intermediate-term (2–3 year) survival; in many instances, it may provide an alternative to transplantation.

Successes in mitral valve surgery in the setting of severe LV dysfunction have increased attention on patients with aortic valve disease and severe LV dysfunction. Clini-

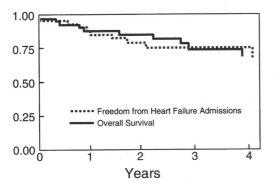

Figure 3 Survival and freedom from heart failure hospital admission after mitral valve repair for a cohort of patients who underwent surgery at Cleveland Clinic.

cians must commonly make a judgment about the wisdom of operative intervention in patients with poor left ventricular function in two types of aortic valve disease: (a) presumed severe aortic stenosis but a low gradient, and (b) severe aortic insufficiency with left ventricular dilatation.

Aortic Stenosis

The increased afterload with aortic stenosis contributes to a host of symptoms such as angina, dyspnea, syncope and sudden death [49]. The guidelines for the management of adult patients with symptomatic aortic valve disease are generally clear, but for patients with the high risk combination of severe LV dysfunction, low cardiac output, and low transvalvular gradient, survival after surgery has generally been poor [50]. Recent ACC/ AHA (American College of Cardiology/American Heart Association) guidelines for managing valvular heart disease recommend hemodynamic evaluation of low-flow, low-gradient aortic stenosis using dobutamine echocardiography to distinguish patients with fixed anatomic aortic stenosis from those with flow-related (''relative'') aortic stenosis and advanced left ventricular dysfunction [42]. Nishimura and colleagues have utilized a dobutamine challenge in the catheterization laboratory to assess ventricular contractile reserve in patients with low-gradient aortic stenosis and LVEF less than 40%. Among patients in whom contractile reserve was identified (stroke volume increase greater than 20%), operative mortality was 7% compared with more than 60% for those who did not respond to dobutamine stimulation [50a].

Outcomes from the Cleveland Clinic were reviewed for three groups of patients with aortic stenosis treated between 1990 and 1998 [51]. Group I included 68 patients who had AVR (aortic valve replacement) with aortic valve area (AVA) of 0.75 cm^2 or less, LV ejection fraction (LVEF) of 35% or less, and mean gradient of 30 mm Hg or less. Group II included 297 patients who had AVR with AVA of 0.75 cm^2 or less, LVEF of 50% or less, and mean gradient of 35 mm Hg or less. Finally, Group III included 89 patients who did not receive AVR but had an AVA of 0.75 cm^2 or less, LVEF of 35% or less, and mean gradient of 30 mm Hg or less.

The perioperative mortality between the surgical group with severe LV dysfunction (group I) and group II were similar (5.9% vs. 4%). The 1-and 4-year survival were also acceptable for both groups (82% and 75% for group I; 92% and 82% for group II, P = 0.03). These results demonstrate that in the modern era, patients with severe LV dysfunction and a low transvalvular gradient can undergo aortic valve replacement, albeit at a slightly higher risk than patients with better ventricular function. Certainly when one examines the dismal outcome in the patients who did not undergo aortic valve replacement, this strategy should be pursued whenever feasible. (Fig. 4)

Aortic Insufficiency

Historically, the natural history of patients with severe aortic regurgitation (AR) and ventricular dysfunction managed medically is dismal [52]. Currently, the indications for operative intervention include: (a) functional NYHA class III or IV symptoms with preserved LV function, (b) class II symptoms with progressive LV dilatation or angina, (c) asymptomatic patients with mild-to-moderate LV dysfunction, and (d) those who are undergoing coronary artery bypass or other operations who have moderate-to-severe aortic insufficiency [42]. In the presence of severe LV dysfunction these guidelines are less clear. For patients with chronic AR with severe LV dysfunction, previous outcomes from earlier eras have been poor [53]. Symptomatic patients with advanced LV dysfunction (ejection fraction <25%,

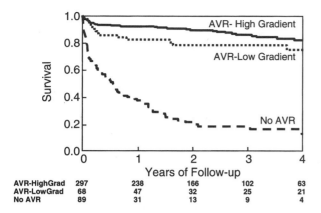

AVR-HighGrad	297	238	166	102	63
AVR-LowGrad	68	47	32	25	21
No AVR	89	31	13	9	4

Figure 4 Comparison of survival at Cleveland Clinic in patients with aortic valve stenosis after aortic valve replacement (for high and low gradients) and medical management.

and/or end-systolic dimension greater than 60 mm) may have developed irreversible myocardial changes that will not be improved by correction of the regurgitation [49]. Unfortunately, a minority of patients may not present until they develop advanced heart failure.

At the Cleveland Clinic, we recently reviewed our experience with valve surgery for AR with severe LV dysfunction to determine survival and to further investigate whether the impact of LV dysfunction as a predictor of outcome after AVR had changed over time. From 1972 through 1999, 724 patients had isolated aortic valve surgery for chronic AR. Of this group, 88 patients had LVEF of 30% or less with the remaining 636 patients having an LVEF greater than 30%. Survival after propensity matching and adjustment at 5, 10, 15, 20 and 25 years in patients with severe left ventricular dysfunction was 68%, 46%, 41%, 18%, and 9% vs. the nonsevere LV dysfunction group which was 82%, 62%, 41%, 27%, and 18% ($P = 0.04$). Importantly, hospital mortality in the propensity matched patients reduced in both groups over time ($P = 0.0008$) and long-term survival in 1985 and later was similar between the two groups ($P = 0.96$) (Fig. 5). Based on this analysis, it is evident that improvements in technique, medical and surgical management, and prostheses type have had a positive impact on the long-term outcome.

In the age of implantable left ventricular assist devices, these operations should be carried out in centers that have LVAD capability as a "safety net" in case of the rare

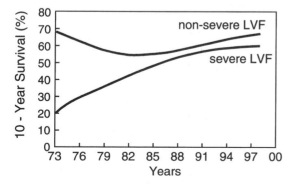

Figure 5 Survival following aortic valve surgery in patients with severe left ventricular dysfunction has improved over time and demonstrates similar long-term mortality since 1985.

early failure. Today, with improved myocardial protection, better perioperative use of inotropic and vasodilator agents, and more advanced valve prostheses with low gradients, aortic valve replacement can safely be performed for aortic insufficiency, even in patients with severe LV dysfunction.

LEFT VENTRICULAR RECONSTRUCTION FOR ISCHEMIC CARDIOMYOPATHY

Ventricular reconstruction is the active surgical attempt to restore the shape of the pathologically remodeled ventricle to one that is physiologically superior to the shape created in diseased states. In patients with ischemic cardiomyopathy, anterior myocardial infarction is a common initiating event, which leads to loss of function of the anterior wall as well as parts of the interventricular septum [54]. This initial insult initiates progressive LV remodeling leading to the clinical manifestations of heart failure. Although the definitions are not universally standardized, dyskinetic segments are aneurysmal transmural scars, whereas akinetic segments should be viewed as noncontributing segments of myocardium. The purpose of LV reconstruction (either alone or in conjunction with the correction of other cardiac disease) is to remove the diseased segment from the remaining functional segments of the left ventricle in an effort to improve cardiac function. At the Cleveland Clinic we frequently resect dyskinetic segments, and may resect discrete near-transmural akinetic scars. We do not resect akinetic areas that have no scar.

The concept of surgical LV reconstruction has existed since the first reported LV aneurysmectomy in 1958 by Denton Cooley in describing his technique of open resection and simple closure on cardiopulmonary bypass [55]. This technique would become the standard of the profession for the next 30 years.

Although the technique remained unchanged, our understanding of left ventricular aneurysm pathology and its role in heart failure continued to evolve. The long-term survival in patients who were managed medically was disappointing. In 1953, Brushke reported a 5-year survival rate of 12% in patients with left ventricular aneurysms who were medically managed [56]. One year later, Shlichter reported the same 5-year survival of 12%, with the leading cause of death as heart failure [57]. This led to a more aggressive surgical approach by pioneers like Rene Favaloro. In 1968, he reported a series of 130 patients who underwent resection for left ventricular aneurysm with a hospital mortality of 13% [58]. Follow-up was obtained in 80 patients. There were 12 hospital deaths and 19 late deaths. However, notably, in the 49 long-term survivors, 41 were free of heart failure symptoms.

The surgical resection of left ventricular aneurysms slowly became applied, however, the results were not always predictable, and as a result prompted an alteration of the traditional surgical technique. In 1985, Jatene and Dor described their procedure, which excluded the dysfunctional segment from the ventricular septum, as well as the free ventricular wall [59,60]. As a result, Jatene reduced his hospital mortality from 11.6% to 4.3%, and his late mortality from 12.6% to 3.5%. Dor applied his technique to areas of akinesia as well as dyskinesia. Although operative mortality was 12% in patients with large areas of akinesia, it was 0% in patients with small akinetic wall motion abnormalities [61]. In the subgroup of survivors with large akinetic areas, ejection fraction increased from 25% to 41%. Although other reports suggested an inferior outcome after reconstruction of akinetic segments as compared with dyskinetic segments, these surgeons used the traditional methods of aneurysm resection and linear closure [62,63]. A multiinstitutional trial of Surgical Anterior Ventricular Endocardial Restoration (SAVER) evaluated the efficacy and safety of this technique in 439 patients following anterior myocardial infarction [63a]. Concomitant procedures included coronary artery bypass grafting (89%), mitral valve repair (27%), and mitral valve replacement (4%). Postprocedure ejection fraction increased from 29% ± 10% to 39% ± 12%. Actuarial survival at 18 months was 89%.

Why has surgical LV reconstruction come into the forefront of the management of heart failure? The research of the 1990s has shown the dramatic impact ventricular size and shape have on the morbidity and mortality in heart failure. Lee followed 382 patients with NYHA class III and IV heart failure referred for evaluation of cardiac transplantation [64]. In patients with massively dilated left ventricles greater than 4cm/m^2, 2-year survival was 49%. In contrast, patients with left ventricles less than 4 cm/m^2 had a 75% 2-year survival.

Ventricular dilatation also affects survival after acute myocardial infarction. As part of the GUSTO (Global Utilization of Streptokinase and t-PA for Occluded Arteries) trial, Migrino evaluated end-systolic volume at 90 to 180 minutes into reperfusion during acute myocardial infarction [65]. Patients with an end-systolic volume index greater than 40mL/m^2 had a higher probability of mortality at 1 month and 1 year. In the SAVE (Survival and Ventricular Enlargement) trial, left ventricular size was a strong, independent risk factor for mortality after 2 years [66].

Even after coronary artery bypass surgery, patients with large ventricles have a worse prognosis. Yamaguchi identified left ventricular end-systolic volume index greater than 100 ml/m^2 as an independent risk factor for the development of heart failure in ischemic cardiomyopathy [67]. These reports have helped cardiac surgeons focus on the importance of reconstruction of the left ventricle in ischemic cardiomyopathy.

There are presently four variations of left ventricular reconstruction used to exclude the septum. These include a linear closure by Jatente, a modified linear closure by Mickleborough, a circular closure with a patch by Dor, and a double cerclage closure without a patch by McCarthy. (Fig. 6) All of these techniques involve an incision into the diseased anterior wall, an exclusion of the entire diseased segment, and a reduction in ventricular cavity size. In the majority of patients, reconstruction is done in the LAD (left anterior descending) distribution on the anterior portion of the left ventricle. However, reconstruction has also been performed on the posterior wall after circumflex or right coronary artery occlusion. Most of these patients undergo concomitant coronary artery bypass grafting. Many also undergo mitral valve repair. Indications for the operation include patients with ischemic cardiomyopathy with worsening LV dysfunction, heart failure, angina pectoris, thromboembolism, or recurrent ventricular tachycardia. In other patients severe coronary artery disease or mitral valve disease are the primary indication for surgical intervention and the LV scar is reconstructed as a secondary procedure.

At the Cleveland Clinic, LV reconstruction was performed in patients with a discrete left anterior descending scar, frequently with preoperative imaging consisting of magnetic resonance imaging scan and/or three-dimensional echocardiography. Most patients had compensated heart failure or other indications for surgery, such as severe coronary artery disease or mitral regurgitation. Currently, our technique of LV reconstruction is a double cerclage circular closure without the use of a patch on the beating heart. One hundred and two consecutive patients with this technique were reported with a 1% hospital mortality [68]. A patch is utilized only in rare patients with a calcified aneurysm in whom the purse-string sutures may not create a neck, or in patients with a small LV cavity to avoid creating too small a cavity with a low stroke volume. Since January 1997, 224 patients (80% male, mean age 62 ±10 years) underwent LV reconstruction, 69% for dyskinetic and 31% for akinetic regions, as part of comprehensive surgical management of ischemic cardiomyopathy. Before surgery, 66% were in NYHA class III or IV. The mean preoperative ejection

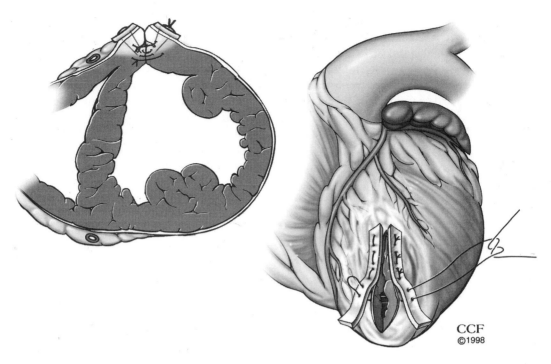

Figure 6 This technique completely excludes the nonfunctional left ventricular segment with a Fontan stitch, but closes the ventricle in a manner that does not require any prosthetic material.

fraction was 26 ± 8.5% and QRS duration was 121.8 ± 31.6 milliseconds. Concomitant procedures included coronary artery bypass grafting in 85% and mitral valve repair in 43%.

Overall survival at 30 days, 1, 2 and 3 years was 98%, 92%, 90% and 86%, respectively. Freedom from readmission for heart failure at 1, 2 and 3 years was 80%, 70% and 61%. Readmission was more common in older patients and those with a longer QRS duration, higher preoperative pulmonary artery diastolic pressures, elevated postoperative pulmonary artery systolic pressures and longer cardiopulmonary bypass times. Freedom from adverse events (transplant listing, return to NYHA IV, left ventricular assist device insertion, or death) at 1, 2 and 3 years was 89%, 85% and 83%. Preoperative ventricular dysrhythmia was a powerful predictor of worse outcomes. Both adverse events (p = 0.002) and readmission (p = 0.02) were significantly higher in patients with a longer QRS duration. The presence of a preoperative implantable cardioverter defibrillator (ICD) was also associated with early mortality (p = 0.001). On the other hand, preoperative NYHA class, LV ejection fraction, preoperative ventricular volumes, prior cardiac surgery, and need for mitral valve repair were not risk factors for worse outcomes, after accounting for the influence of conduction disturbances.

Advances in imaging technology should permit better prediction of those patients who will benefit from reconstruction and those who would benefit from revascularization and valvular correction alone. In addition, the distinction between akinetic and dyskinetic segments must be more clearly defined. Although there are several different methods of defining segment function, a simple, reproducible method has not yet been established.

Lastly, the effect of location of the aneurysm, the effect of a patch, and the indications for postoperative arrhythmia treatment needs to be more completely understood.

ALTERNATIVE DEVICE THERAPIES

The previous sections have outlined direct surgical reconstruction of coronary arteries, valves, or left ventricle. Lessons learned from the detrimental effects of LV remodeling have resulted in the development of new devices to inhibit this process and alter the disease course of heart failure. Two of these devices have been developed to either prevent myocyte overstretch and provide passive LV constraint (Acorn CorCap®) or reshape the LV without removal of functioning myocardium (Myocor Myosplint®).

The first example of such a device is the Acorn CorCap®, a mesh-like polyester jacket that is surgically placed around the ventricles of the heart to provide diastolic support. (Fig. 7) The concept of passive diastolic constraint is not new. The Acorn CorCap® was developed following the experience with dynamic cardiomyoplasty, which demonstrated the benefit of the girdling effect of the latissimus dorsi preventing further LV dilation [69,70]. Constructed from a compliant woven mesh, it is designed to provide both flexibility and strength. The design of the mesh permits bidirectional compliance of the fabric, which allows it to conform easily to the heart, hence allowing the heart to return to a more normal ellipsoidal shape. CorCap® placement is often performed with concomitant valve repair or coronary artery bypass.

Preclinical studies with CorCap® have been reported from two different heart failure models. In a canine heart failure model, Saavedra has shown that the long-term use of CorCap® results in lowered end-diastolic and end-systolic volumes by 19% and 22%, respectively, and shifted the end systolic pressure volume relation to the left, compatible

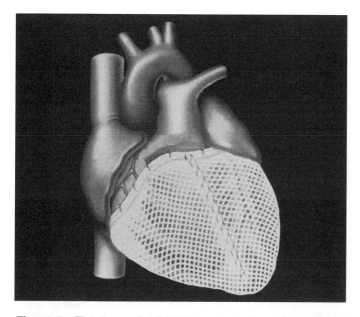

Figure 7 The Acorn CorCap® is a mesh-like polyester jacket that is surgically wrapped around a dilated left ventricle, often in conjunction with another cardiac procedure. Results of the randomized trial utilizing the device will soon be released.

with reverse remodeling [71]. No change in density or affinity of the β-receptors was observed. Further, the systolic response to dobutamine stimulation was markedly improved, and diastolic compliance was unaffected. Chaudrey demonstrated an improvement in LV diastolic function and chamber sphericity, decreased wall stress, and no evidence of functional mitral regurgitation [72]. Power, using an ovine heart failure model, reported similar findings of improved cardiac function, as evidenced by increased ejection fraction and LV fractional shortening [73].

Based on the preclinical results, clinical trials were initiated to establish safety and potential efficacy of CorCap® therapy in heart failure patients. Konertz and colleagues examined the safety and efficacy of the CorCap® in a series of 27 patients suffering from cardiomyopathy with a mean NYHA of 2.6 ± 0.1. Of these, 16 received concomitant cardiac surgery, principally mitral valve repair or replacement, and the remaining 11 patients received CorCap® only. In the device-only group, 5 of the 11 patients experienced adverse events, including two deaths during an average follow-up of 12.2 ± 1.1 months, but none of the events were device related. Follow-up at 3 and 6 months reflected a significant improvement from pretreatment in EF (21% to 28% and 33%) and NYHA functional class (2.5 to 1.6 and 1.7), as well as a significant decrease in LVEDD (74 mm to 68 mm and 65 mm), and LVESD (65 mm to 62 mm and 57 mm) [74].

Raman and associates reported similar findings in a cohort of five patients undergoing CorCap® with concomitant CABG. Mid-term outcomes at 12-months follow-up demonstrated a significant decrease in LVEDD and LVESD, with an improvement in LVEF and NYHA functional class (75).

From these early safety/feasibility studies it appears the CorCap® may be useful in preventing further cardiac dilation and may improve symptoms of heart failure without device related morbidity or mortality. A randomized, prospective clinical trial of the Acorn CorCap® is currently under way in Europe, Australia, and North America to confirm these early observations. Enrollment will be completed in June of 2004 with study results available at that time.

Myocor Myosplint®

Developed from the lessons learned with partial left ventriculectomy (Batista procedure), the Myocor Myosplint® was designed to change the geometry of the LV, thereby decreasing wall stress and improving hemodynamics. The implant consists of two epicardial pads and a transventricular tension member. The two pads are located on the surface of the heart with the load bearing tension member passing through the ventricle connecting the pads and drawing the ventricular walls toward one another. (Fig. 8) Typically, three Myosplints are placed on the beating heart from the lateral LV through the posterior intraventricular septum. The splints are then tightened to create a bilobular shape.

The Myosplint® was initially studied in the canine heart failure model to assess outcomes at 1 month following application. In this trial, heart failure was induced in 15 dogs over a period of 27 days. Of these, seven animals underwent sham surgery and eight animals received the Myosplint® device. By 3-D echocardiographic calculations, LVEF significantly increased from 19% at baseline to 36% acutely and remained at 39% at 1 month after Myosplint® implant. Also, LVEDV and LVESV significantly decreased and were sustained at 1 month. End-systolic wall stress significantly decreased by 39% acutely, and by 31% at 1 month. Also, EDWS (end diastolic wall stress) was significantly reduced by 30% acutely and by 41% at 1 month [76].

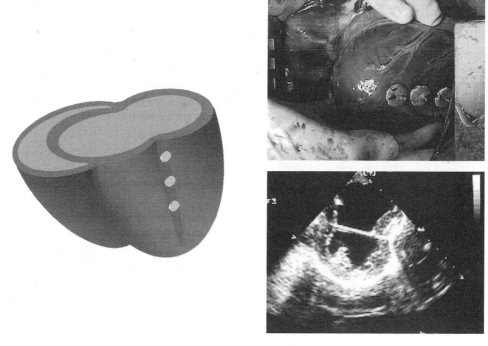

Figure 8   The Myosplint implants transventricular tension members to alter the geometry of the LV into a bilobular shape. This reduces the tension on each of the individual ventricular segments and may promote reverse remodeling.

Chronic human studies were first performed in seven patients with dilated cardiomyopathy and NYHA class III–IV symptoms [77]. LVEDD in this group ranged from 72 to 102 mm; mitral valve regurgitation was mild in three patients and moderate in four cases. Four patients underwent concomitant mitral valve repair at the time of Myosplint® implant. At 3 month follow-up, one patient experienced worsening heart failure attributed to unrepaired, significant mitral regurgitation. The remaining six patients had improvement in symptoms of heart failure with two of the patients being removed from the transplant waiting list. This early experience demonstrated that Myosplint® implantation can be safely performed without significant adverse affects, however, these investigators noted that mitral valve repair should be done in any patient undergoing the procedure with significant mitral valve incompetence.

Early results from the newest devices suggest that surgical therapies to halt and/or reverse LV remodeling are feasible and may play a significant role when applied earlier in the natural history of patients with cardiomyopathy before the development of decompensated CHF.

SUMMARY

Heart transplantation and ventricular assist devices are options for only a small percentage of people afflicted with advanced heart failure and as a result, thousands of people will die from this disease, and even more will have limited lives. The surgical options for heart failure are a part of a larger paradigm shift in management. Viable and effective surgical options and devices clearly exist and are applicable to a large portion of patients with heart failure. However, patient selection is paramount, as any intervention must improve cardiac function in order to improve the duration and quality of life in this high-risk group. In addition, this strategy should only be employed at a center that is prepared to offer all the resources that may be needed in the most challenging patients. Even more importantly, long-term medical management must be individually tailored to give these patients their best chance for a meaningful life.

REFERENCES

1. Levy D, Kenchaiah S, Larson MG, et al. Long term trends in the incidence and survival with heart failure. N Engl J Med 2002; 347:1397–1402.
2. Sheehy E, Conrad SL, Brigham LE, et al. Estimating the number of potential donors in the United States. N Engl J Med 2003; 349(7):667–674.
3. McMurray JJ, Stewart S. Epidemiology, etiology, and prognosis of heart failure. Heart 2000; 83(5):596–602.
4. Sutton GC. Epidemiological aspects of heart failure. Am Heart J 1990; 120:1538–1540.
5. Faulkner SL, Stoney WS, Alford WC, et al. Ischemic cardiomyopathy: medical versus surgical treatment. J Thorac Cardiovasc Surg 1977; 74(1):77–82.
6. Franciosa JA, Wilen M, Ziesche S, Cohn J. Survival in men with severe chronic left ventricular failure due to either coronary heart disease or idiopathic dilated cardiomyopathy. Am J Cardiol 1983; 51:831–8–16.
7. Harris PJ, Lee KL, Harrell FE, Behar VS, Rosati RA. Outcome in medically treated coronary artery disease. Ischemic events: nonfatal infarction and death. Circulation 1980; 62:718–726.
8. Manley JC, King JF, Zeft HJ, Johnson WD. The ''bad'' left ventricle. Results of coronary surgery and effect on late survival. J Thorac Cardiovasc Surg 1976; 72:841–847.
9. Vlietstra RE, Assad-Morell JL, Frye RL, et al. Survival predictors in coronary artery disease: medical and surgical comparisons. Mayo Clinic Proc 1977; 52:85–90.
10. Yatteau RF, Peter RH, Behar VS, Bartel AG, Rosati RA, Kong Y. Ischemic cardiomyopathy: the myopathy of coronary artery disease, natural history, and results of medical versus surgical treatment. Am J Cardiol 1974; 34:520–525.
11. Zubiate P, Kay JH, Dunne EF. Myocardial revascularization for patients with ejection fraction of 0.2 or less: 12 years' results. West J Med 1984; 140:745–749.
12. Emond M, Mock MB, Davis KB, et al. Long-term survival of medically treated patients in the Coronary Artery Surgery Study (CASS) Registry. Circulation 1994; 90:2645–2657.
13. The VA Cooperative Study Group. Eighteen-year follow-up in the Veterans Affairs Cooperative Study of Coronary Artery Bypass Surgery for Stable Angina. Circulation 1992; 86:121–130.
12a. Myers WO, Blackstone EM, Davis K, Foster E, Kiaser GG. CASS Registry. Long-Term Surgical Survival. J Am Coll Cardiol 1999; 33:488–98.
13. The VA Cooperative Study Group. Eighteen-year follow-up in the Veterans Affairs Cooperative Study of Coronary Artery Bypass Surgery for Stable Angina. Circulation 1992; 86:121–130.
14. Saraste A, Pulkki K, Kallajoki M, Henricksen K, Parvinen M, Voipio-Pulkki L. Apoptosis in human acute myocardial infarction. Circulation 1997; 95:320–323.
15. Ragosta M, Beller GA, Watson DD, Kaul S, Gimple LW. Quantitative planar rest-redistribution ^{201}TL imaging in detection of myocardial viability and prediction of improvement in left ventricular function after coronary bypass surgery in patients with severely depressed left ventricular function. Circulation 1993; 87:1630–1641.
16. Haas F, Haehnel C, Picker W, et al. Preoperative positron emission tomographic viability assessment and perioperative and postoperative risk in patients with advanced ischemic heart disease. J Am Coll Cardiol 1997; 30:1693–1700.
17. Mori T, Minamiji K, Kurogane H, et al. Rest-reinjected thallium-201 imaging for assessing viability of severe asynergic regions. J Nucl Med 1991; 32:1718–1724.

18. Dilszian V, Rocco TP, Freedman NMT, et al. Enhanced detection of ischemic but viable myocardium by the reinjection of thallium after stress-redistribution imaging. N Engl J Med 1990; 323:141–146.

19. Kiat H, Berman DS, Maddahi J, et al. Late reversibility of tomographic myocardial thallium-201 defects: an accurate marker of myocardial viability. J Am Coll Cardiol 1988; 12: 1456–1463.

20. Ohtani H, Tamaki N, Yonekura Y. Value of thallium-201 reinjection after delayed SPECT imaging for predicting reversible ischemia after coronary bypass grafting. Am J Cardiol 1990; 66:194–199.

21. Tillish J, Brunken R, Marshal R, et al. Reversibility of cardiac wall motion abnormalities predicted by positron tomography. N Engl J Med 1986; 314:884–888.

22. Gould KL, Yoshida K, Hess MJ, et al. Myocardial metabolism of fluorodeoxyglucose compared to cell membrane integrity for the potassium analogue Rubidium-82 for assessing infarct size in man by PET. J Nucl Med 1991; 32:1–9.

23. Beanlands RSB, Ruddy TD, de Temp RA, Iwanochho RM, Coate SG, Freeman M, Nahmius C, Hendry P, Burns RJ, Lamy A, Michleborogle L, Kostuh W, Fallen E, Nichol G and the PARR Investigator. Positron emission tomography and recovery following revasculazation (PARR-1): the importance of scar and re-development of a predicament for the degree of recovery of left ventricular function. J Am Coll Cardiol 2002; 40:1735–43.

24. LaCanna G, Alfieri O, Giubbini M, Ferrari R, Visioli O. Echocardiography during infusion of dobutamine for identification of reversible dysfunction in patients with coronary artery disease. J Am Coll Cardiol 1994; 23:617–626.

25. Vanverschelde JL, Gerber BL, AM DH, et al. Preoperative selection of patients with severely impaired left ventricular function for coronary revascularization. Role of low-dose dobutamine echocardiography and exercise-redistribution-reinjection thallium SPECT. Circulation 1995; 92(Suppl):II37–II44.

26. Vanverschelde JL, D'Hondt AM, Marwick T, Gerber BL, Wijns W, Melin JA. Head to head comparison of exercise–redistribution-reinjection thallium SPECT and low-dose dobutamine echocardiography for prediction of the reversibility chronic left ventricular ischemic dysfunction. J Am Coll Cardiol 1996; 28:432–442.

26a. Wijns W, Vatner SF, Camici PG. Mcberngting myocardium 1998; 339:176–181.

27. Baer FM, Theissen P, Schneider CA, et al. Dobutamine magnetic resonance imaging predicts contractile recovery of chronically dysfunction myocardium after successful revascularization. J Am Coll Cardiol 1998; 31:1040–1048.

28. Gunning MG, Anagnostopulos C, Knight CJ, et al. Comparison of [201]TL, ^{99}Tc-fetrofosmin, and dobutamine magnetic resonance imaging for identifying hibernating myocardium. Circulation 1998; 98(18):1869–1874.

29. Pasquet AA, White RD, Zuchowski RD, Marwick TH. A one-stop shop for delineation of viable myocardium? Comparison of function and perfusion assessment by resting MRI with dobutamine echocardiography. Circulation 1998; 98(17):I-514.

30. Kim RJ, Wu E, Rafael A, et al. The use of contrast-enhanced magnetic resonance imaging to identify reversible myocardial dysfunction. New Engl J Med 2000; 343(20):1445–1453.

31. Leavitt BJ, O'Connor GT, Olmstead EM, Martin JR, Mahoney CT, Durey LI, Hernandez F, Lahey SJ for the Northern New England, Cardiovascular Disease Study Group. Use of the internal mammary artery graft and in-hospital mortality and adverse outcomes associated with coronary artery bypass surgery. Circulation 2001; 103:507–12.

31a. Klein C, Nekolla SG, Bengel FM, Momose M, Sumner A, Haas F, Schnackenberg B, Delius W, Mydra M, Wolfram D, Schwalger M. Assessment of myocardial viability with contrast-enhanced magnetic resonance imaging. Comparison with position emission tomography. Circulation 2002; 105:162–67.

32. Gavaghan TP, Gebski V, Baron DW. Immediate postoperative aspirin improves vein graft patency early and late after coronary artery bypass graft surgery. A placebo-controlled, randomized study. Circulation 1991; 83:1526–1533.

33. Flaker GC, Warnica JW, Sacks FM, et al. Pravastatin prevents clinical events in revascularized patients with average cholesterol concentrations: Cholesterol and Recurrent Events (CARE) Investigators. J Am Coll Cardiol 1999; 34:106–112.

34. The Post-Coronary Artery Bypass Graft Trial Investigators. The effect of aggressive lowering of low-density lipoprotein cholesterol levels and low-dose anticoagulation on obstructive changes in saphenous-vein-coronary-artery bypass grafts. N Engl J Med 1997; 336:153–162.

34a. Mickleborough L, Carson S, Tamariz M, Iranov J. Results of revascularization with severe left ventricular dysfunction. J Thorac Cardiovasc Surg 2000; 119:550–557.

35. Cosgrove DM, Loop FD, Lytle BW, et al. Primary myocardial revascularization trends in surgical mortality. J Thorac Cardiovasc Surg 1984; 88:673–684.

36. Estafanous FG, Loop FD, Higgins TL, et al. Increased risk and decreased morbidity of coronary artery grafting between 1986 and 1994. Ann Thorac Surg 1998; 65:383–389.

37. Yau TM, Fedak PW, Weisel RD, Teng C, Ivanov J. Predictors of operative risk for coronary bypass operations in patients with left ventricular dysfunction. J Thorac Cardiovasc Surg 1999; 118(6):1006–1013.

38. Argenziano M, Spotnitz HM, Whang W, Bigger JT, Parides M, Rose EA. Risk stratification for coronary bypass surgery in patients with left ventricular dysfunction: analysis of the coronary artery bypass grafting patch trial database. Circulation 1999; 100(19 Suppl): II119–II124.

39. Olshansky B, Telfer EA, Curtis AB, Bigger JT. Predictive value of preoperative left ventricular ejection fraction and functional class for mortality and morbidity after high-risk coronary artery bypass grafting. Am J Cardiol 2000; 85(12):1489–1491.

40. Hochman JS, Sleeper LA, Webb JG, et al. Early revascularization in acute myocardial infarction complicated by cardiogenic shock. New Engl J Med 1999; 341:625–634.

41. Yamaguchi A, Ino T, Adachi H, et al. Left ventricular volume verdicts postoperative course in patients with ischemic cardiomyopathy. Ann Thorac Surg 1998; 65:434–8.

42. Bonow RO, Carabello B, deLeon AC, et al. ACC/AHA practice guidelines for the management of patients with valvular heart disease. Circulation 1998; 98:1949–1984.

43. Lee SJ, Bay KS. Mortality risk factors associated with mitral valve replacement: a survival analysis of 10 year follow-up data. Can J Cardiol 1991; 7:11–18.

44. Tribouilloy CM, Enriquez-Sarano M, Schaff HV, et al. Impact of preoperative symptoms on survival after surgical correction of organic mitral regurgitation: rationale for optimizing surgical indications. Circulation 1999; 99(3):400–405.

45. David TE, Uden DE, Strauss HD. The importance of the mitral apparatus in left ventricular function after correction of mitral regurgitation. Circulation 1983; 68(Suppl II):I176–I182.

46. Lillehei CW, Levy MJ, Bonnabeau RC. Mitral valve replacement with preservation of papillary muscles and chordae tendinea. Circulation 1996; 94:2117–2123.

47. Bishay ES, McCarthy PM, Cosgrove DM, et al. Mitral valve surgery in patients with severe left ventricular dysfunction. Eur J Cardiothorac Surg 2000; 17(3):213–221.

48. Badhwar V, Bowling S. Mitral valve surgery in the patient with left ventricular dysfunction. Semin Thorac Cardiovasc Surg 2002; 14:133–136.

49. Pathophysiology of Aortic Valve Disease in cardiac surgery in the adult. Edmunds LH, Ed: McGraw Hill, 1997:835–858.

50. Connolly HM, Oh JK, Schaff HV, et al. Severe aortic stenosis with low transvalvular gradient and severe left ventricular dysfunction: result of aortic valve replacement in 52 patients. Circulation 2000; 101(16):1940–1946.

50a. Nishimura RA, Grantham JA, Connolly HM, et al. Low-output, low-gradient aortic stenosis in patients with depressed left ventricular systolic function: the clinical utility of dobutamine challenge in the catheterization laboratory. Circulation 2002; 106:809–813.

51. Pereira JJ, Lauer MS, Bashir M, Afridi I, Blackstone EH, Stewart WJ, McCarthy PM, Thomas JD, Asher CR. Survival after aortic valve replacement for severe aortic stenosis with low transvalvular gradients and severe left ventricular dysfunction. J Am Coll Cardiol 2002; 39(8): 1356–1363.

52. Aronow WS, Ahn C, Kronzon I, Nanna M. Prognosis of patients with heart failure and unoperated severe aortic valvular regurgitation and relation to ejection fraction. Am J Cardiol 1994; 74:286–288.

53. Bonow RO, Nikas D, Elefteriades JA. Valve replacement for the regurgitant lesions of the aortic or mitral valve in advanced left ventricular dysfunction. Card Clin 1995; 13:73–83.

54. Buckberg GD. Commonality of ischemic and dilated cardiomyopathy: laplace and ventricular restoration. J Cardiac Surg 1999; 14:53–59.

55. Cooley DA, Collins HA, Morris GC, Chapman DW. Ventricular aneurysm after myocardial infarction. Surgical excision with the use of temporary cardiopulmonary bypass. JAMA 1958; 167:557.

56. Bruschke AVG, Proudfit WF, Sones FM. Progress study of 590 consecutive non-surgical cases of coronary disease followed 5 to 9 years. II Ventriculographic and other correlations. Circulation 1973; 47(6):1154–1163.

57. Schlichter J, Hellerstein HK, Katz LN. Aneurysm of the heart: a correlative study of 102 proved cases. Medicine 1954; 33:43.

58. Favaloro RG, Effler DB, Groves LK, Wescott RN, Suarez E, Lozada J. Ventricular aneurysm-clinical experience. Ann Thorac Surg 1968; 6(3):227–245.

59. Jatene AD. Left ventricular aneurysmectomy: resection or reconstruction. J Thorac Cardiovasc Surg 1985; 89:321–331.

60. Dor V, Kreitmann P, Jourdan J, et al. Interest of physiological closure (circumferential plasty on contractile areas) of left ventricle after resection and endocardectomy for aneurysm or akinetic zone. Comparasion with classical technique about a series of 209 left ventricular resections [abstr]. J Thorac Cardiovasc Surg 1985; 26:73.

61. Dor V. Reconstructive left ventricular surgery for post-ischemic akinetic dilatation. Semin Thorac Cardiovasc Surg 1997; 9:139–145.

62. Mangschau A. Akinetic versus dyskinetic left ventricular aneurysms diagnosed by gated scintigraphy: difference in surgical outcome. Ann Thorac Surg 1989; 4795:746–751.

63. Couper GS, Bunton RW, Birjiniuk V, DiSesa VJ, Fallon MP, Collins JJ, Cohn LH. Relative risks of left ventricular aneurysmectomy in patients with akinetic scars versus true dyskinetic aneurysms. Circulation 1990; 82(5Suppl: IV):248–256.

63a. Athanasuleas C, Stanley AWH, Buckberg GD, et al. Surgical anterior ventricular endocardial restoration (SAVER) in the dilated remodeled ventricle after anterior myocardial infarction. J Am Coll Cardiol 2001; 37:1199–1209.

64. Lee TH, Hamilton MA, Stevenson LW, Moriguchi JD, Fonarow GC, Child JS, Laks H, Walden JA. Impact of left ventricular cavity size on survival in advanced heart failure. Am J Cardiol 1993; 72(9):672–676.

65. Migrino RQ, Young JB, Ellis SG, White HD, Lundergan CF, Miller DP, Granger CB, Ross AM, Califf RM, Topol EJ. End-systolic volume index at 90 to 180 minutes into reperfusion therapy for acute myocardial infarction is a strong predictor of early and late mortality. Circulation 1997; 96:116–121.

66. Sutton MSJ, Pfeffer MA, Moye L, Plappert T, Rouleau JL, Lamas G, Rouleau J, Parker JO, Arnold MO, Sussex B, Braunwald E. Cardiovascular death and left ventricular remodeling two years after myocardial infarction. Circulation 1997; 96:3294.

67. Yamaguchi A, Ino T, Adachi H, Murata S, Kamio H, Okada M, Tsuboi J. Left ventricular volume predicts postoperative course in patients with ischemic cardiomyopathy. Ann Thorac Surg 1998; 65:434–438.

68. Caldeira C, McCarthy PM. A simple method of left ventricular reconstruction without patch for ischemic cardiomyopathy. Ann Thorac Surg 2001; 72:2148–2149.

69. Chachques JC, Grandjean PA, Schwartz K, et al. Effects of latissimus dorsi dynamic cardiomyoplasty on ventricular function. Circulation 1988; 78:203–216.

70. Capouya ER, Gerber RS, Drinkwater DC et al. Girdling effect of nonstimulated cardiomyoplasty on left ventricular function. Ann Thorac Surg 1993; 56:867–870.

71. Saavedra FW, Tunn R, Mishima T, et al. Reverse remodeling and enhanced adrenergic reserve from a passive external ventricular support in experimental dilated heart failure. Circulation 2000; 102(supp II):501.

72. Chaudry PA, Mishima T, Sharov VG, et al. Passive epicardial containment prevents ventricular remodeling in heart failure. Ann Thorac Surg 2000; 70:1275–1280.

73. Power J, Raman J, Byrne M. Passive ventricular constraint is a trigger for a significant degree of reverse remodeling in an experimental model of degenerative heart failure and dilated cardiomyopathy. Circulation 2000; 102(supp I):II-501.

74. Konertz WF, Shapland JE, Hotz H, et al. Passive containment and reverse remodeling by a novel textile cardiac support device. Circulation 2001; 104(suppl I):I-270–I-275.

75. Raman JS, Hata M, Storere JM, et al. The mid-term results of ventricular containment (Acorn Wrap) for end stage ischemic cardiomyopathy. Ann Thorac Surg 2001; 5:278–281.

76. McCarthy PM, Takagaki M, Ochiai Y, Young JB, Tabata T, Shiota T, Qin JX, Thomas JD, Mortier TJ, Schroeder RF, Schweich CJ, Fukamachi K. Device-based change in left ventricular shape: a new concept for the treatment of dilated cardiomyopathy. J Thorac Cardiovasc Surg 2001; 122(3):482–490.

77. Schenk S, Reichenspurner H, Boehm DH, et al. Myosplint implant and shape-change procedure: intra-and peri-operative safety and feasibility. J Heart Lung Transplant 2002; 21(6):680–686.

23

Long Term Mechanical Circulatory Support and Cardiac Transplantation

Peter C. Kouretas, Susan Moffatt-Bruce, and Robert C. Robbins
Department of Cardiothoracic Surgery, Stanford University
Stanford, California, USA

SYNOPSIS

Congestive heart failure remains a clinical syndrome characterized by a vicious cycle leading to progressive circulatory failure and end-organ dysfunction in an ever-increasing number of patients. The long-term goal in the treatment of these victims of heart failure is the improvement of their quality of life. We have outlined the current cardiac replacement strategies for individuals who have failed current medical therapies and are otherwise appropriate candidates for further therapeutic interventions. These cardiac replacement strategies include mechanical circulatory support devices, which are implemented both as a bridge to transplantation as well as permanent or destination therapy. The concept of bridging end-stage heart failure patients to recovery with mechanical circulatory systems is also addressed. Finally, the current state of cardiac transplantation including patient selection, operative techniques, postoperative management, immunosuppression strategies, and the most current results of cardiac transplantation is reviewed.

INTRODUCTION

The earliest application of mechanical circulatory support was used for acute cardiovascular collapse, specifically postcardiotomy failure. During the past decade, the application of ventricular assist devices (VADs) for longer-term support has become possible. Ventricular assist devices are now routinely used as bridges to transplantation as well as for permanent circulatory support or destination therapy. The role of VADs as bridges to myocardial recovery has also recently been the topic of extensive clinical and experimental investigation. Although cardiac transplantation is the therapeutic option of choice for end-stage heart failure, there are several limitations to this approach for the management of an ever-increasing number of individuals. The supply of donor hearts will never fully meet the demands of transplant candidates whose disease has reached its final stage. Furthermore, donor heart availability is completely unpredictable, rendering individuals on the waiting list vulnerable in the setting of acute deterioration. Given the ever-increasing time on the waiting list, bridging individuals to transplantation using mechanical circulatory support (MCS) systems has become the therapeutic option of choice in the setting of acute deterioration not responsive to medical management. This chapter will focus on MCS as a long-term support strategy to transplantation, recovery, and permanent support. In addition, we will review the current status of cardiac transplantation, which continues to remain the accepted treatment for end-stage heart failure.

MECHANICAL CIRCULATORY SUPPORT

Background

The possibility of supporting the circulation for an extended period of time became feasible with the implementation of cardiopulmonary bypass (CPB) in 1953 [1]. The use of cardiopulmonary bypass for postcardiotomy recovery of cardiac function [2] inspired the rapid development of other assist devices for longer-term support of the circulation. The first successful use of an mechanical assist device for temporary left heart assistance was implanted by Dr. Michael E. DeBakey at Baylor College of Medicine in 1963 [3]. This intrathoracic device was a pulsatile, air-driven, ventricular assist device that supported a patient for 4 days after an aortic valve operation. A subsequent version of this DeBakey blood pump was implanted extracorporeally between the left atrium and the axillary artery in 1966 [4]. This marked the first successful implementation of a mechanical assist device bridging a patient to myocardial recovery after postcardiotomy failure. In addition to an implantable left ventricular assist system (LVAS), which partially supported the circulation, a total artificial heart was also employed, in 1969, to support the circulation of a patient who could not be weaned from CPB after resection of a left ventricular aneurysm [5]. Application of this TAH (total artificial heart), developed by Liotta and the Baylor-Rice team, represents the first application of a VAD as a bridge to cardiac transplantation. The success of these pioneering surgeons resulted in directives at the national level, supported by the National Heart, Lung, and Blood Institute, aimed at producing MCS systems for long-term use as well as for permanent cardiac replacement. As a result of extensive animal and in vitro testing, the safety and efficacy of these MCS systems were tested, evaluated, and ultimately applied in the clinical setting. These MCS systems now serve as bridges to transplantation in terminally ill patients who cannot wait until a suitable donor heart is available.

Patient Selection

Identification of appropriate candidates for MCS is of paramount importance given that universal criteria do not exist. In addition, the timing of device implantation is also critical for optimum outcomes. Potential MCS recipients are usually transplant candidates, but this criterion is being redefined given the recent results from the Randomized Evaluation of Mechanical Assistance for the Treatment of Congestive Heart Failure (REMATCH) trial [6]. The patient considered for MCS support should fulfill the general criteria for transplant recipient selection and be a suitable candidate for cardiac transplantation. The MCS recipient should have adequate psychosocial support for a potentially prolonged period of mechanical support.

Typically, MCS systems are used to support the circulation of patients who are in NYHA class IV heart failure despite aggressive medical therapy and who are at imminent risk of death before a donor heart becomes available. These patients with end-stage heart disease should not have any irreversible end-organ failure. The tendency should be to implant the assist device before significant clinical deterioration is present. In a recent review of the Novacor European Registry, preimplant clinical parameters were analyzed in an effort to determine the impact on postimplant survival [7]. Multivariate analysis revealed that the following preimplant conditions were independent risk factors for survival after LVAS placement: respiratory failure associated with septicemia, right heart failure, age greater than 65 years, acute postcardiotomy, and acute infarction. The 1-year survival after LVAS implantation, including posttransplant, significantly dropped from 60% to 24% with the presence of one risk factor. Temporary end-organ dysfunction, however, has been demonstrated to recover after device placement. Therefore, dysfunction of one or more organs is not necessarily a contraindication to placement of a device [8,9].

The hemodynamic criteria for circulatory failure that is refractory to maximal medical management include a cardiac index of less than $2.0 \, L/min/m^2$, a systolic blood pressure less than 80 mmHg, and pulmonary capillary wedge pressure of greater than 20 mmHg despite adequate preload, inotropic therapy or intraaortic balloon counterpulsation [10]. These criteria simply serve as a guide but the downward trend in hemodynamics as well as an escalation in pharmacologic support may be more important in deciding the timing of device placement.

Mechanical Circulatory Support Systems

The MCS systems currently used as intermediate to long-term bridges to transplantation include: the Novacor LVAS (World Heart Corporation, Ottawa, Canada), the HeartMate LVAS (Thoratec Laboratories, Pleasanton, CA), the CardioWest total artificial heart (CardioWest Technologies Inc., Tucson, AZ), and the Thoratec VAD (Thoratec Laboratories, Pleasanton, CA). The HeartMate and Novacor LVAS are fully implantable, intracorporeal systems that mechanically bypass the left ventricle without removal of the native heart. These systems do not provide support for the right ventricle. The Thoratec VAD is a paracorporeal system that provides either univentricular or biventricular support. The implantable CardioWest TAH replaces the entire native heart and, thus, offers biventricular support. These systems have unique advantages and disadvantages depending on the patient profile and the type of circulatory support required. All of these systems, however, have been demonstrated to provide circulatory support for extended periods of time. The benefits and complications of each of these systems coupled with specific patient considerations need to be evaluated when deciding upon the type and timing of each device.

The four devices listed above represent MCS systems that are not completely implantable and provide pulsatile flow. Advances in technology have resulted in the introduction of new MCS devices that are designed to provide circulatory support with fewer complications. These advances include new-generation blood pumps that are smaller, more durable and in some instances, completely implantable. The LionHeart LVAD 2000 (Arrow International, Reading, PA) is a totally implantable pulsatile LVAS currently being tested in human trials. The power supply to the LVAS is achieved through a transcutaneous energy transmission system (TETS) and a compliance chamber to compensate for air displacement (Fig. 1). Alternatives to pulsatile systems are axial flow devices that provide continuous, nonpulsatile flow. There are numerous axial flow pumps that are undergoing experimental investigation in human trials: the Jarvik 2000 Heart (Jarvik Heart Inc, New York, NY, Figure 2), MicroMed DeBakey VAD (MicroMed Technology Inc, Houston, TX), and the HeartMate II (Thoratec Laboratories Inc, Pleasanton, CA). These nonpulsatile axial pumps are smaller, potentially more durable, and have reduced energy requirements (Fig. 3). The results of ongoing trials will help elucidate the role that these pumps will assume in the management of patients with end-stage heart failure.

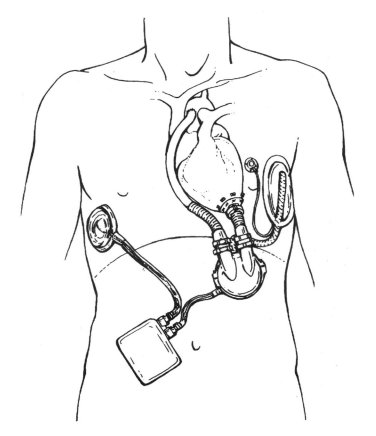

Figure 1   The LionHeart LVS-2000, a completely implantable left ventricular assist device with a transcutaneous energy transmission system.

Novacor Left Ventricular Assist System

The Novacor LVAS was originally designed as a totally implantable system intended for destination therapy. An interim system consisting of a portable, partially implantable, electrically powered device with a percutaneous power lead/vent has functioned well primarily as a bridge to transplantation since 1984 [11]. The Novacor N100PC LVAS consists of a seamless, smooth-surfaced polyurethane sac bonded to dual, symmetrically opposed pusher plates and to a lightweight fiberglass/epoxy housing that incorporates the valve fittings [12]. The inflow and outflow conduits are 25 mm in diameter and contain custom porcine bioprostheses with sinuses behind each of the valve leaflets. The inflow conduits and outflow grafts that connect the pump between the left ventricular apex and ascending aorta were fabricated from low-porosity, woven, crimped polyester (Cooley; Meadox Medical, Oakland, NJ). Since 1998, a gelatin-sealed, knitted polyester graft with integral wall reinforcement has been used for the inflow conduit (Sulzer Vascutek Ltd, Renfrewshire, Scotland) [13].

The system controller is located extracorporeally and is connected to the implanted energy converter via a percutaneous lead, which also provides a pump vent. The wearable control system provides electrical energy to a pulsed-solenoid energy converter, which is coupled to the pusher plates through a flat spring mechanism. This actuator design allows efficient, reliable transformation of electrical to mechanical energy with an overall effi-

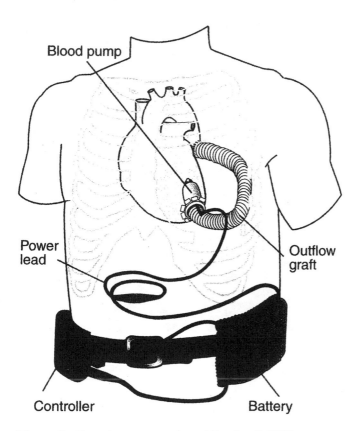

Figure 2 Percutaneous version of the Jarvik 2000.

ciency of 65%. Transducers within the pump send signals to the external control unit to regulate the pumping rate. The system can be operated in either fixed-rate, synchronous, or fill-to-empty mode.

The Novacor LVAS was converted from a console-based system into a portable, wearable system in 1993. The wearable system incorporates a compact controller and rechargeable power packs that are worn on the patient's belt [14]. (Fig. 4) The wearable system has optimized out-of-hospital use, with more than 60% of the worldwide recipients spending greater than 80% of their support time outside of the hospital [15]. The wearable system has significantly improved patient mobility, discharge to home, and aggressive rehabilitation while waiting for transplantation.

The operative technique for implantation of the Novacor pump is via a midline incision from the sternal notch to the umbilicus. The pump pocket is placed in a preperitoneal space anterior to the posterior rectus sheath between the left costal margin and the iliac crest [12]. A smaller pocket is created in the right rectus sheath for lateral placement of the outflow conduit to avoid kinking. The percutaneous vent tube is tunneled in a subcutaneous manner from the pump pocket and exits between the right costal margin and the iliac crest. After institution of normothermic cardiopulmonary bypass, the outflow conduit is anastomosed to the proximal right lateral aspect of the partially clamped ascending aorta. This anastomosis may be performed off cardiopulmonary bypass in selected patients who can tolerate the increased left ventricular afterload. The inflow cannulae are placed through a ventriculotomy at the left ventricular apex. Alternatively, the anastomoses

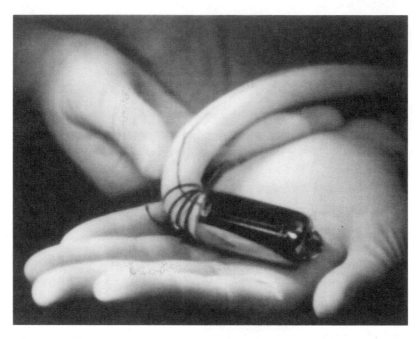

Figure 3 The Jarvik 2000 axial flow pump is constructed of titanium and has a 16-mm Hemashield outflow graft. The pump weighs 90 g and is 2.5 cm in diameter.

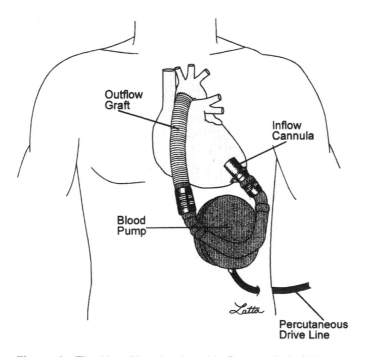

Figure 4 The HeartMate Implantable Pneumatic Left Ventricular Assist System.

may be performed in an antegrade manner, with the inflow conduit placed first. After appropriate de-airing of the pump and conduits via a needle-vent in the outflow graft, the pump is started at a slow fixed-rate mode. After the patient is separated from cardiopulmonary bypass, the operating mode is switched to fill-to-empty.

HeartMate Left Ventricular Assist System

The HeartMate LVAS is an implantable, pulsatile blood pump that is available in a pneumatically driven version (implantable pneumatic or IP-LVAS) (Fig. 5) or electrically powered version (vented electric or VE-LVAS) (Fig. 6) [16,17]. The same blood pump is employed in both versions but differs in the method of actuation. In the IP-LVAS device, the console delivers a pulse of air that displaces the polyurethane diaphragm, compressing the blood chamber within the rigid titanium housing and causing the ejection of blood. The VE-LVAS, available since 1991, contains an electric motor that actuates the same pusher-plate mechanism as in the IP version. The low-speed torque electric motor is positioned below the diaphragm and drives a pair of nested helical cams. Two lines, contained in a single conduit in the most recent VE-LAS version, are tunneled percutaneously and exit through the skin and connect to the external control system. One line contains the electric cable, whereas the second line serves as an external vent and also permits pneumatic actuation in the event of an emergency. The inflow and outflow conduits each contain a 25 mm porcine valve for unidirectional blood flow.

Surgical implantation also requires placement on cardiopulmonary bypass and the anastomotic techniques to the ascending aorta and LV apex are similar to those used for the Novacor device. The pump is placed beneath the left hemidiaphragm either in a

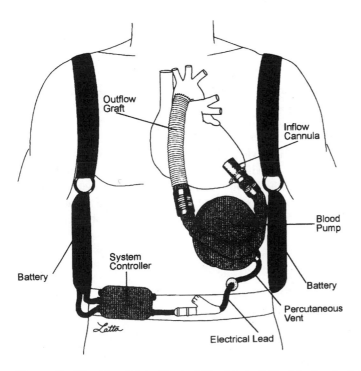

Figure 5   The HeartMate Vented Electric Left Ventricular Assist System.

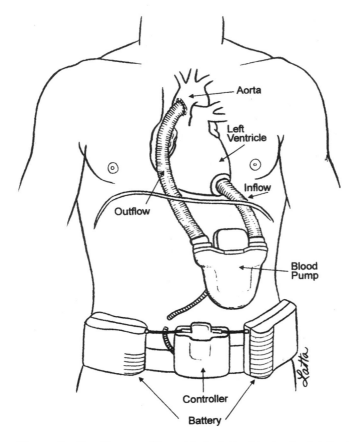

Figure 6 The Novacor Wearable Left Ventricular Assist System.

preperitoneal pocket [18] or within the peritoneal cavity [19]. Both pumps can generate a maximum stroke volume of 85 ml and a maximum pump output of 11 L/min. The pumps can be operated in fixed rate or an automatic mode. The automatic mode is more physiological, maximizes flow by ejecting only after the blood pump is at least 90% filled, and is thus, responsive to circulatory demand.

The most unique property of the HeartMate LVAS is the textured, blood-contacting surface that lines the blood pump. The blood-contacting portion of the titanium housing incorporates titanium microspheres and the flexible diaphragm is covered with integrally textured polyurethane. These textured surfaces promote the formation of a pseudointimal layer [20]. As a result of this unique feature, systemic anticoagulation with heparin and warfarin are avoided. Anticoagulation with aspirin or antiplatelet agents is used with low thromboembolic risks [21].

Thoratec Ventricular Assist System

The Thoratec VAS is a pneumatically powered, paracorporeal device that can provide univentricular or biventricular support (Fig. 7) [22]. The Thoratec VAS device consists of four main components: a drive console, inflow cannulae, outflow cannulae, and a pump. The pump contains a seamless polyurethane blood sac within a rigid polycarbonate housing. The pump connects to a dual drive console, which sends both positive and nega-

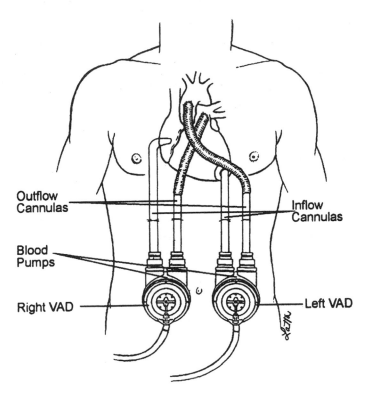

Outflow Cannulas

Inflow Cannulas

Blood Pumps

Right VAD

Left VAD

Figure 7 The Thoratec Ventricular Assist System in the biventricular support configuration.

tive pressurized air to fill and empty the pump. Bjork-Shiley tilting-disc mechanical valves in the inflow and outflow conduits ensure unidirectional blood flow through the device. The Thoratec VAS can operate in three different modes: volume, fixed-rate, and external-synchronous mode. The volume mode, or fill-to-empty mode of operation allows the pump to change speed as determined by the amount of filling. In the fixed-rate mode, the pump rate is set by the operator and functions independently of the patient's heart rate. The external-synchronous mode triggers the pump to empty based on the patient's R-wave on the electrocardiogram. The preferred mode of operation is the volume mode because it maximizes support of the cardiac output. The other two modes of operation are used for de-airing after implantation, weaning prior to explantation, or when a pump rate of 80 beats/min cannot be achieved. In order to provide adequate blood ejection, the operator must adjust the systolic driveline pressure to 200 mmHg, an ejection time of 300 milliseconds, and diastolic vacuum pressure is adjusted to optimize filling. The pump has a maximum stroke volume of 65 ml and a maximum flow of 6.5 L/min. When biventricular support is needed, right pump flow should be lower than left pump flow in order to prevent pulmonary congestion and injury.

The Thoratec VAS is typically implanted through a median sternotomy with the use of cardiopulmonary bypass. An alternative technique includes placement via a left thoracotomy without the use of CPB [23]. For left-ventricular assistance, the inflow conduit is placed either in the left ventricular apex or the left atrium. Left ventricular apical cannulation provides the best filling of the device and is the preferred site of insertion for bridge-to-transplant patients. The outflow conduit, a 12-mm preclotted woven Dacron graft, is anastomosed to the ascending aorta using a side-biting clamp. For right-ventricular assistance, the inflow cannula is placed either in the right ventricle or right atrium and the outflow cannula is anastomosed to the main pulmonary artery. The cannulae are exteriorized below each respective costal margin and connected to the pump or pumps. The pumps rest on the anterior surface of the abdomen in a paracorporeal position. Systemic anticoagulation with heparin and warfarin are implemented during the support period.

CardioWest Total Artificial Heart

The CardioWest TAH, formerly called the Jarvik-7 or Symbion TAH, is a pneumatically actuated, pulsatile biventricular pump that is implanted in the orthotopic position. The pump consists of two ventricles that are connected to the respective native atria and great vessels (Fig. 8). Pulses of air delivered from the drive console compress a smooth, flexible polyurethane diaphragm within the ventricular blood chambers, causing ejection of blood. Two Medtronic-Hall mechanical valves provide unidirectional blood flow. The maximal stroke volume of this pump is 70 ml with an output between 6 and 8 L/min [24].

Implantation of the CardioWest TAH is through a median sternotomy and requires excision of both ventricles with retention of both atrial cuffs. The device is then anastomosed to both atria and great vessels. The pneumatic drivelines from each ventricle are externalized percutaneously and attached to the drive console. Patients may be ambulatory by using battery power and air tanks that permit a few hours away from the drive console. Anticoagulation typically requires a regimen with heparin, warfarin, and dipyridamole to prevent thrombus formation.

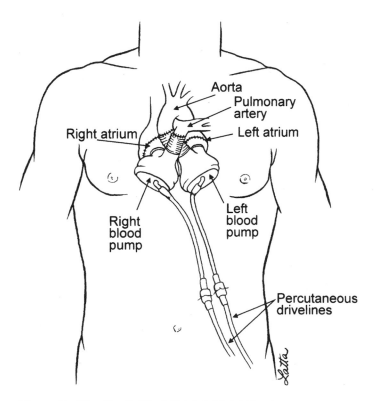

Figure 8   The CardioWest Total Artificial Heart.

The CardioWest TAH is currently undergoing Food and Drug Administration (FDA) approval in the United States. This device, however, is already approved as a bridge to transplantation in other countries. A significantly smaller, portable drive console is currently being developed for out-of-hospital use.

Summary of Mechanical Circulatory Support Systems

The most commonly used LVAS for long-term mechanical support and FDA-approved as bridges-to-transplantation include the Novacor, HeartMate and Thoratec. The Novacor and HeartMate are both implantable and provide left ventricular support alone. The Thoratec is a paracorporeal device and provides left and right ventricular support, as needed. One of the main differences between the HeartMate and the other devices is the blood-contacting surfaces used and the type of anti-coagulation required. The HeartMate uses textured blood-contacting surfaces allowing the formation of a "pseudointimal" lining and, therefore, does not require any systemic anticoagulation. All other devices require systemic anticoagulation with heparin and warfarin. The CardioWest TAH, in addition to the Thoratec, provides biventricular support. The main differences between these two pumps, however, is that the CardioWest TAH only provides biventricular support, whereas the Thoratec VAS can be used for left, right and biventricular support. Furthermore, the CardioWest TAH requires removal of the native heart and is placed in an orthotopic position. The CardioWest TAH remains in clinical trials under an investigational device exemption begun in 1993 and a multicenter trial has been undertaken [25]. Table 1 summarizes the four long-term circulatory support systems previously discussed.

Complications with Mechanical Circulatory Support

In addition to advancements in technology, better patient selection, and improved perioperative management, the incidence of morbidity and mortality after LVAS implementation has significantly declined. The most frequent complications include bleeding, infection, thromboembolism, neurologic dysfunction, organ failure, right heart failure, hemolysis, and technical problems. The most prevalent acute complication in the immediate postoperative period remains bleeding. Bleeding is a consequence of coagulopathy often secondary

Table 1 Summary of the Long-Term Circulatory Support Systems

Device	FDA Approval	Indication	Position	Anti-Coagulation
Novacor	1985–Bridge to Transplant	LV alone	Intracorporeal	Systemic
HeartMate (IP)	1986–Bridge to Transplant	LV alone	Intracorporeal	NONE
HeartMate (VE)	1991–Bridge to Transplant 2002–Destination	LV alone	Intracorporeal	NONE
Thoratec	1996–Bridge to Transplant 1999–Bridge to Recovery	LV alone or RV alone or Biventricular	Paracorporeal	Systemic
CardioWest	No FDA approval	Biventricular only	Intracorporeal	Systemic

to hepatic insufficiency, fibrinolysis, and platelet consumption secondary to cardiopulmonary bypass, as well as the extensive surgical dissection required for implantation. The incidence of bleeding requiring reexploration ranges from 21% to 48% [26,27]. The introduction of the serine protease inhibitor aprotinin in LVAS recipients has significantly decreased the incidence of bleeding, blood product requirement, and perioperative mortality [28].

Infection is another very common complication during mechanical support. The incidence of infection ranges from 40% to 49% [29,30]. Recipients of MCS implants are susceptible to both nosocomial and device-related infections, with the most common site being the drive-line [31,32]. Antimicrobial drive-lines as well as modification of the implant techniques may significantly decreases the incidence of device-related infections [32,33]. A longer drive-line tunnel may provide greater protection from ascending infection than shorter subcutaneous tunneled tracts. In addition, covering the upper surface of the implantable pump with a patch of knitted graft material has significantly decreased the incidence of pocket infections [32]. LVAD infection is associated with significantly decreased survival when compared to patients without infectious complications who survived to transplantation [34]. Infection, however, does not preclude successful bridging to transplantation, which remains an effective treatment option [35].

Another important long-term complication of mechanical support devices is thromboembolism. The reported incidence ranges from 4% with HeartMate [36] to 12% with the Novacor device [15]. The HeartMate's textured surface promotes formation of an adherent pseudointimal cellular lining, which is presumably more biocompatible than the blood contacting surfaces of other devices [20]. This freedom from thrombogenicity translates into the lower thromboembolic rates observed despite the absence of systemic anticoagulation [21]. Modifications to the Novacor inflow conduit design have markedly diminished the thromboembolic rate from 31% to 12% [13,15], which is similar to the thromboembolic rate of 10% observed in the REMATCH trial [6]. The original inflow conduit was a woven, unsupported, and crimped polyester graft. The new Vascutek inflow conduit is a knitted, gelatin-sealed, integrally supported polyester graft resulting in substantially improved neointimal morphology and significantly reduced embolic rates [15].

Right heart failure after LVAD support has a poor prognosis and is largely unpredictable. The need for perioperative RVAD support after LVAD insertion ranges from 9% to 11% [37,38]. In a recent retrospective study, the best predictors of severe right ventricular failure after implantable LVAD insertion by multivariable logistic regression analysis were preoperative circulatory support, female gender, and nonischemic etiology [37]. Interestingly, pulmonary hypertension with elevated pulmonary artery pressures and pulmonary vascular resistance were not risk factors for RV failure, which suggests that RV contractility was not strong enough to generate an increase in pressure [37].

Management of right heart failure after LVAD placement remains a continual challenge that is best treated by avoidance and institution of aggressive preventive measures [39]. Some of these maneuvers include management of pulmonary hypertension with the selective endothelial vasodilator, inhaled nitric oxide [40]; pharmacologic measures to decrease right ventricular afterload and enhance contractility; and ventilatory adjustments made to prevent respiratory acidosis and enhance pulmonary compliance. Furthermore, some of the preventive measures employed are aimed at diminishing the deleterious effects of the amplified inflammatory cascade, which contributes to right-sided circulatory failure. These strategies include use of the serine protease inhibitor aprotinin both to prevent fibrinolysis and inhibit the kallikrein system [28]; leukocyte depletion strategies while on cardiopulmonary bypass; and modified ultrafiltration both intraoperatively and postoperatively. Despite these maneuvers, patients with severe right heart failure, intractable ventricular arrhythmias, and circulatory failure secondary to insufficient filling of the LVAD, require placement of a Thoratec RVAD.

One major limitation after implantation of mechanical circulatory support systems is the post-VAD immunologic sensitization and its subsequent implications on allograft function and survival. Reports indicate that after LVAD implantation, antibodies to major histocompatibility (HLA) class I or II antigens develop in approximately 60% of patients [41]. The mechanism of immunologic sensitization after mechanical circulatory support, as evidenced by elevated titers of panel reactive antibody (PRA) greater than 10, is not entirely clear [42]. Several potential risk factors for sensitization include blood product administration, specifically platelet transfusion during the post-operative period after LVAD placement [43]. Furthermore, the LVAD surface itself has been demonstrated to activate the immune system. The textured surface of the HeartMate initiates a proinflammatory cascade with subsequent upregulation of cytokines as well as adhesion molecules [44]. In addition, CD4 T-cell levels accompanying LVAD implantation are significantly reduced [45] and demonstrate a heightened susceptibility to apoptosis [46]. This selective activation of the immune system on the LVAD surface results in enhanced immunosensitization with the attendant adverse sequelae of rejection, opportunistic infection, and decreased survival.

The most important preventive measure to reduce allosensitization is avoidance of blood product administration after LVAD implantation. Other effective interventions employed to depress the surface-activated immune response include plasmapheresis, intravenous immunoglobulin, and simply aspirin [46,47]. A recent study demonstrated that intravenous immunoglobulin, in conjunction with cyclophosphamide, reduced serum anti-HLA alloreactivity and shortened the duration to transplantation in highly sensitized LVAD recipients [47]. The development of novel biomaterials and pharmacologic interventions aimed at modulating the immune response to LVAD implantation remains a critical step for improved long-term outcomes.

Clinical Results of MCS as Bridges to Transplant

Survival to Transplantation

Extensive clinical experience has been obtained over the last decade with mechanical circulatory systems used as bridges to transplantation. Once believed to be a risk factor for poor survival after transplantation, ventricular assist devices have convincingly been demonstrated to improve posttransplant survival [48,49]. Clinical studies have shown that implantable LVAD therapy is safe, provides effective hemodynamic support with a low incidence of adverse events, and improves survival in transplant candidates [48]. In a multicenter trial of the HeartMate IP LVAS in patients awaiting transplantation, Frazier reported a significant increase in survival to transplantation for patients treated with an LVAD when compared to control patients (71% of device patients *vs.* 36% of control patients) [36]. Furthermore, posttransplant survival after 1 year was also significantly greater in the device group when compared with the control group (90% vs. 67%, p < 0.03) [36]. In another multicenter evaluation of the HeartMate VE LVAS in patients awaiting heart transplantation, survival to transplantation was once again significantly improved with LVAD therapy when compared with a similarly matched cohort of controls treated medically (67% vs. 33%, p < 0.0001) [48]. All patients in both groups had to meet specific selection criteria, which required approval for transplantation as well as reliance on current intravenous inotropic therapy.

The multicenter bridge-to-transplant series in the United States using the Novacor LVAS also demonstrated improved survival to transplantation when compared with controls without LVAS support (77% vs. 37%, p < 0.0001) [50]. The European experience with the Novacor LVAS is similar with an overall survival of 64% with 33% of patients being discharged to home after LVAS placement [30]. The median implant time was 115 days with no device or system failures. Since the introduction of the wearable system in 1993, both the duration of support and number of patients discharged to home have progressively increased. In the overall experience of patients receiving MCS as a bridge to transplantation, more than 60% have actually received a transplant. More than 85% of those individuals transplanted have survived to be discharged from the hospital [30,51,52].

The most common cause of death in patients with long-term MCS not surviving to transplantation is usually multiorgan failure. In an attempt to elucidate upon predictors of survival to transplantation, a multiinstitutional study of patients bridged to transplantation with the HeartMate VE LAS and Thoratec VAD were reviewed [27,53]. Risk factors for decreased survival to transplantation after HeartMate VE LVAS included increased age, prior heart surgery, elevated creatinine, and total bilirubin [48]. In a multiinstitutional study of patient's bridged to transplantation with a Thoratec VAD, elevated blood urea nitrogen levels was the only sensitive predictor of survival to transplantation [53]. Elevations in serum creatinine and total bilirubin were also associated with decreased survival to transplantation.

Survival and Outcomes After Transplantation

In addition to improved survival *to* transplantation after mechanical circulatory support, there is now growing evidence demonstrating improved outcomes *after* transplantation in LVAS recipients when compared with patients managed on inotropic support [54,55]. Clinical outcomes posttransplantation, including renal failure and right heart failure, were significantly increased in patients on inotropic support *vs.* LVAS recipients [54]. Six-month survival, however, was not significantly different between the two groups. Aaronson and colleagues have recently demonstrated improved posttransplant survival (95% vs. 65%, p < 0.007) and overall survival (77% vs. 44%, p < 0.01) at 3 years in patients receiving an implantable LVAD (HeartMate VE LVAS) when compared with patients on inotropic support [55]. Bridging to transplantation with an implantable LVAD, therefore, improves utilization of donor hearts [55]. In the multicenter clinical evaluation of the HeartMate VE LVAS, Frazier and associates also demonstrated a significant improvement in posttransplant survival after 1 year in LVAD patients bridged to transplant when compared with controls managed medically (84% vs. 63%, p < 0.01) [48].

Recovery, Rehabilitation, and Quality of Life

Given that transplant recipients are waiting longer periods of time, the duration of support while on MCS has progressively increased. In 1998, half of the Novacor LVAS recipients were supported for greater than 6 months, and the median waiting time in HeartMate VE LVAS group was 105 days. Furthermore, a significant number of implantable LVAS recipients are being discharged to home. The potential for recovery and rehabilitation both in-hospital and ultimately at home has translated into improved clinical and survival outcomes. With mechanical circulatory support, device recipients have recovery of end organ function, improvement in New York Heart Association functional class, and advanced physical rehabilitation. Patients on MCS who experience this accelerated functional rehabilitation are enrolled in hospital release programs [48]. In a recent study, outpatients spent a mean of 326 days at home, which corresponded to 72% of their time on support [56]. There was no increased mortality and the number of readmissions per patient per year was only 2.8. Hospital discharge has enabled individuals to return to near-normal lifestyles with resumption of physical activities and a return to employment. Significant improvement in exercise capacity also occurs with chronic LVAD therapy [57]. Interestingly, the exercise capacity of device patients is better than that of transplant candidates [58]. These benefits clearly translate into an enhanced quality of life while these individuals are being bridged to transplantation.

Cost of LVAD Support

The economics of devices used for mechanical circulatory support remains an important focus of concern significantly impacting the patient, provider, and society as a whole. Based on the experience with "bridge-to-transplantation" patients, the average first-year cost of LVAD implantation is estimated to be $222,460 including professional fees, and $192,154 excluding professional fees [59]. The latter figure is comparable to average first-year costs for cardiac transplantation, which was $176,605 without professional fees. With the introduction of safe and efficient outpatient programs, increasing numbers of LVAD recipients are being discharged to home sooner. In a recent report by the Columbia group, 49% of their patients who received a wearable HeartMate VE-LVAS were discharged to home, spending an average of 103 days of outpatient support [60]. All patients were either successfully transplanted or explanted with no outpatient deaths. The estimated average cost to bridge a patient to transplantation or explanation after discharge to home was $13,200 compared with the cost of inpatient therapy of $165,200. Efficient and timely implantation of mechanical support systems in addition to enrollment in outpatient programs will allow for more cost-effective management as well as improved quality of life for the patient.

Long-Term MCS as a Transplant Alternative

Permanent LVAS

The FDA has recently approved the use of the HeartMate VE LVAS for permanent use or destination therapy for patients with severe end-stage heart failure. This approval was based on the recent findings from the REMATCH trial. The efficacy and safety of the HeartMate VE LVAS as a long-term myocardial replacement therapy was investigated in a prospective, randomized multicenter trial comparing LVAD therapy with optimal medical management [6]. Patients with NYHA class IV heart failure, who were not eligible for heart transplantation, were randomly assigned to receive an LVAD (68 patients) or medical treatment (61 patients). The trial demonstrated a significant improvement in survival in patients who received the LVAD with a 48% reduction in the risk of death from any cause [6]. The Kaplan-Meier estimates of survival at 1 year were 52% in the device group and 25% in the medical-therapy group (p = 0.002), and at 2 years were 23% and 8% (p = 0.09), respectively (Fig. 9). Furthermore, the quality of life was significantly improved at 1 year in the device group. The frequency of serious adverse events in the device group, however, was significantly higher than in the medical group and included neurologic dysfunction, bleeding, infection, and malfunction of the device. The leading cause of death in the device group was sepsis, accounting for 25% of the mortalities. Mechanical failure of the LVAD, including inflow-valve failure, erosion, and kinking of the outflow graft, was the second most frequent cause of death in the device group, resulting in 10% of the mortalities.

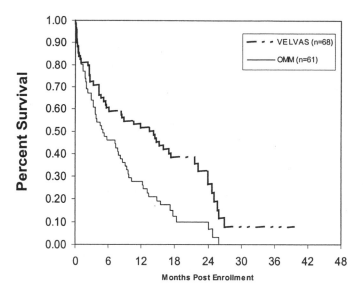

Figure 9 Kaplan Meier actuarial patient survival for patients enrolled in the REMATCH trial. (From Ref. 6.)

The promise of establishing permanent mechanical support as a therapeutic option is very encouraging given the enormous population of patients with severe end-stage heart disease who could potentially benefit from this strategy. The future challenge will be to minimize the adverse events by application of new technology, such as fully implantable devices, which would decrease the infection risk and device malfunction. The ultimate goal is to improve device durability so the long-term capabilities of MCS will translate into comparable survival and may serve as an alternative to heart transplantation.

Bridge to Recovery

A second possible approach to the application of long-term MCS as an alternative to heart transplantation is as a bridge to myocardial recovery. In addition to the dramatic clinical improvement with LVAD therapy, numerous studies have documented the improvement in the structure and function of the native myocardium with chronic unloading [61,62]. Left ventricular unloading with MCS induces an increase in wall thickness, decreased wall stress with a reduction in myocyte damage based on histological examination [61]. Prolonged unloading also improved native ventricular function with improved left-ventricular end-diastolic dimension, ejection fraction, and cardiac index [62]. Further studies have also demonstrated dramatic changes in the myocardial ultrastructure after LVAD implantation with regression of fibrosis and hypertrophy as well as decreased myocyte apoptosis and necrosis [63–65]. Potential mechanisms to explain this myocardial healing include decreased expression of the cytokine tumor necrosis factor-α, downregulation of matrix metalloproteinases, reduction in collagen damage as well decreased activation of nuclear factor-κB in the failing heart after LVAD support [66–68]. Furthermore, unloading of the ventricle with MCS reverses the downregulation of β-adrenergic receptors and restores myocardial responsiveness to inotropic stimulation [69]. Myocardial contractile strength is also improved with long-term MCS by upregulating genes encoding for proteins involved in calcium cycling resulting in reversal of contractile dysfunction [70].

Given the significant beneficial effects of long-term MCS on myocardial structure and function, the concept of bridging to myocardial recovery in select patients is becoming a reality [71,72]. The population most likely to benefit from bridging to recovery is patients with idiopathic dilated cardiomyopathy (IDC). In a recent report by Hetzer and colleagues, they report on the midterm follow-up of patients, all with IDC, who underwent removal of their LVAS [73]. Thirty-five percent of their patients with IDC (23 of 65) underwent elective explantation of the LVAD after mean assist duration of 5 months. Removal of the LVAS was performed when cardiac function was restored as determined by echocardiographic measurement of left ventricular ejection fraction and left ventricular internal diameter in diastole. Fifty-seven percent (13 of 23) have experienced a lasting recovery with a mean follow-up of 23 months. Lasting cardiac recovery after explantation was related to patients with a shorter history of heart failure and a more rapid recovery during the unloading period [73]. In contrast to this report, Mancini and co-workers report that only 8% of their patient population with IDC were explant candidates based on exercise testing [74].

Weaning from cardiac assist devices appears to be feasible in a very select group of patients. Identifying reliable predictors of myocardial remodeling, application of the appropriate modalities to predict the timing and efficacy of explantation, and assessing the degree and durability of recovery are critical questions that need to be further evaluated. Further elucidation of the cellular and molecular changes that occur in the myocardium after mechanical unloading will allow implementation of additional therapeutic strategies aimed at complete myocardial recovery.

CARDIAC TRANSPLANTATION

Historical Overview

Cardiac transplantation has evolved over a century with Alexis Carrel and Charles Guthrie performing the first heterotopic heart transplant in a dog in 1905 [75]. Twenty years later Frank Mayo described a "biological incompatibility between donor and recipient" that become known as transplant rejection [76]. In 1967, Christian Barnard performed the first human heart transplant [77] and 3 days later, the first American heart transplant was performed in a 17-day-old baby using hypothermic circulatory arrest [78]. In 1968, Norman Shumway at Stanford performed the fourth human heart transplant, which initiated a clinical program that has been instrumental in developing heart transplantation as it is known today [78]. Due to the enthusiasm surrounding these initial procedures, 102 transplants were performed in 1968. However, disappointing results reduced this number by half in 1969, and a moratorium on heart transplantation was imposed. Shumway and his colleagues eventually lead the way for the reemergence of cardiac transplantation in the late 1970s. The introduction of the transvenous endomyocardial biopsy technique for monitoring rejection by Philip Caves and Margaret Billingham [79] and the use of cyclosporine facilitated successful cardiac transplantation in the early 1980s, with more than 100 heart transplants performed in 1981 [80]. The International Society for Heart and Lung Transplantation (ISHLT) now consists of a registry compiling data from more than 223 centers in 18 countries worldwide representing more than 61,000 heart transplant recipients [81].

Cardiac Transplant Recipient

Indications for transplantation

The benefits of transplantation are obvious; what is less obvious is which patient is a transplant candidate and when should that patient be transplanted. The survival benefit of cardiac transplantation compared with conventional heart failure treatment has never been tested in a prospective, randomized trial. The early experience at Stanford included 109 patients with a 1- and 2-year survival of 52% and 43%, respectively [82]. Of the 40 patients selected for transplantation for which donors did not become available, 38 died in less than 6 months. With these data, the Stanford group concluded that cardiac transplantation prolonged survival and returned patients to active lives [82]. More recently UNOS (United Network of Organ Sharing) data has demonstrated that patients at greatest risk from dying of heart failure have a survival benefit after cardiac transplantation [83]. It has not been established however if cardiac transplantation prolongs life or improves quality of life for patients at low risk of dying.

The major diagnoses leading to heart transplantation as reported by the ISHLT are idiopathic dilated cardiomyopathy (44%) and ischemic cardiomyopathy (41%) (Fig. 10) [81]. The known causes of dilated cardiomyopathy include infectious (viral), inflammatory, toxic, metabolic and familial etiologies. Infrequent indications for transplantation include intractable angina, refractory malignant ventricular arrhythmias, cardiac tumors and cardiac failure secondary to valvular or congenital heart disease.

Cardiac transplantation is for patients with end-stage heart disease that have failed or cannot tolerate medical or surgical therapy. Recipients typically have NYHA class III or IV symptoms despite optimal medical therapy and their prognosis for 1-year survival without transplantation is less than 50%. Measurement of oxygen consumption (VO_2) during maximal exercise is an objective and reproducible means to risk stratify patients with heart failure. Patients with a peak VO_2 greater than 14 ml/kg/min have a 1-year survival of approximately 94%, allowing transplantation to be safely deferred [84–86]. Left ventricular ejection fraction is also measured to assess timing of transplantation but this has greater limitations. Those with ejection fractions less than 20% are typically deemed appropriate for transplantation, but ejection fraction does not predict functional capacity whereby very dyskinetic hearts can remain well compensated for long periods. Therefore, ejection fraction less than 20%, reduced maximal VO_2 (<14 ml/kg/min) as well as reduced serum sodium (<135 mEq/dL), high pulmonary capillary wedge pressure (>25 mmHg) and elevated plasma norepinephrine (>600 pg/ml) have all been proposed as objective guidelines that indicate poor survival for patients if left untransplanted [84–87]. The Thoracic Organ Transplantation Committee of UNOS have proposed guidelines for placing patients on the waiting list as outlined in Table 2 [88]. Conversely,

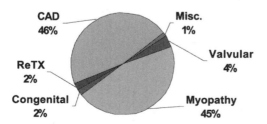

Figure 10 Diagnosis in adult heart transplant recipients as reported to the registry of the ISHLT.

Table 2 Guidelines for Placing Patients on the Waiting List for Cardiac Transplantation

Heart Failure

Cardiogenic shock or low-output state with reversible end-organ dysfunction requiring mechanical support

Low-output state or refractory heart failure requiring continuous inotropic support

Advanced heart failure signs and symptoms (New York Heart Association class III and IV) with objective documentation of marked functional limitation

Recurrent or rapidly progressive heart failure symptoms unresponsive to maximized vasodilators and diuretics

Refractory Angina Pectoris

Severe ischemic symptoms consistently limiting day-to-day activity and not amenable to conventional revascularization, with objective evidence for angina pectoris and extensive myocardial ischemia after optimization of medical therapy

Recurrent unstable myocardial ischemic syndromes requiring multiple hospitalizations unable to undergo conventional revascularization

Life-threatening Refractory Ventricular Arrhythmia

Recurrent symptomatic life-threatening ventricular arrhythmias that cannot be controlled by all appropriate conventional medical and surgical modalities

Prolonged periods of documented electromechanical disassociation following AICD conversion of ventricular tachycardia or ventricular fibrillation to normal sinus rhythm

Cardiac Tumor

Tumor confined to the myocardium

patients that should not be immediately transplanted are those with peak VO_2 greater than 14 ml/kg/min without other indications, those with left ventricular ejection fraction <20% alone, those with a history of NYHA class III or IV symptoms alone, or ventricular arrhythmias only [88,89]. In patients with advanced left ventricular dysfunction (EF < 30%) and a prior myocardial infarction, prophylactic implantation of a defibrillator improves survival and should be considered as a recommended therapy [90]. Patients should be continuously reevaluated by the transplant team so that the potential for improved quality of life is not lost.

Cardiac Transplant Recipient Selection

The evaluation of a potential cardiac transplant recipient is performed by a multidisciplinary team of transplant surgeons, cardiologists, psychologists, and social workers. Eligibility criteria need to be strictly followed in order to ensure an equitable, objective, and medically justified allocation of a very limited donor pool. The traditional eligibility criteria include age less than 65 years, absence of major noncardiac comorbidities, compliance with medical therapy, and psychosocial stability. Contraindications to cardiac transplantation are not easily categorized and many of the traditional contraindications listed in Table 3 have changed.

Age is the most controversial criteria for transplantation whereby many studies have indicated that older age is a risk factor in cardiac transplantation [91–93]. In particular, patients older than 55 years with a pretransplant diagnosis of ischemic cardiomyopathy have been reported to be at a particularly high risk for death with a 5-year survival rate of 56% as compared with 78% for younger patients [92]. In contrast, both Stanford and the Cleveland Clinic, using careful selection criteria, have not found age to adversely impact survival and have reported 5-year survival rates as high as 80% for both young

Table 3 Traditional Contraindications to Heart
Transplantation

Age >65 years
Systemic illness with a poor prognosis
Myocardial infiltrative and inflammatory disease
Irreversible pulmonary arterial hypertension
Irreversible pulmonary parenchymal disease
Acute pulmonary parenchymal disease
Severe peripheral and/or cerebrovascular disease
Irreversible renal dysfunction
Irreversible hepatic dysfunction
Active peptic ulcer disease
Active diverticular disease
Insulin-dependent diabetes with end-organ damage
Active infection
Psychosocial instability
Severe obesity
Severe osteoporosis

and old recipients [91,93]. In addition, some have found a decreased incidence of rejection events in older transplant recipients [94]. Emphasis on physiological rather than chronological age must, therefore, be considered during the selection process.

Pulmonary vascular hypertension has been identified as an independent predictor of mortality. Earlier ISHLT data indicated that increased PVR correlated with mortality after cardiac transplantation [95]. More recently, it has been reported that accurate testing of pharmacologic reversibility of pulmonary hypertension has permitted a significant decrease in postoperative morbidity and mortality [96–98]. In pediatric heart transplantation, pulmonary hypertension leading to donor right ventricular dysfunction remains a major risk factor associated with poor outcomes [99–101]. Fortunately, experience with pulmonary vasodilators in children demonstrating pharmacologic reduction in pulmonary vascular resistance is increasing and favorable results have been reported [99,100].

Other than cardiac disease, transplant recipients should in general be free of other end-organ dysfunction. A systemic illness with a poor prognosis and severe lung disease are definite exclusion criteria. Although irreversible renal and liver dysfunction alone exclude a patient from transplantation, many transplant centers will now evaluate patients for a combined heart-kidney or heart-liver transplant.

Diabetes mellitus causes many concerns relative to transplantation, including wound healing, hyperglycemia, and steroid use, compounded renal insufficiency and neural toxicity due to immunosuppressive drugs. Controversy exists as to whether survival of patients with and without diabetes is comparable [102,103]. Concurrent use of insulin is reported to have no effect on survival, and the rates of infection and acute rejection do not appear to differ from those recipients without diabetes [103]. Currently, most programs would be cautious transplanting diabetic patients with end organ damage until more long-term outcomes become available.

Very few data are available for patients with HIV, hepatitis B and C disease. HIV remains a contraindication to transplantation but hepatitis is controversial. In a recent study concerning hepatitis B, it was found that new onset of clinical liver disease was common posttransplantation in antigen-positive patients with the majority of deaths due to hepatitis B infection [104]. In contrast, hepatitis C does not seem to carry such significant

Table 4   Modified Recipient Contraindications to
Heart Transplantation

Absolute Contraindications

Severe irreversible pulmonary hypertension (> 6 Wood units)
Active systemic infection
Active systemic disease with poor prognosis
Active gastrointestinal bleeding

Probable Contraindications

Irreversible renal and/or hepatic dysfunction
Hepatitis B positive serology
HIV positive serology
Active alcohol or drug abuse
Recent pulmonary infarction
Peripheral vascular or cerebrovascular disease
Psychosocial instability and lack of compliance

Potential Contraindications

Hepatitis C positive serology
Chronic obstructive pulmonary disease
Renal insufficiency
Hepatic insufficiency
Peptic ulcer disease
Diverticular bowel disease
Active or recent malignancy
Diabetes mellitus
Excessive obesity

implications posttransplantation although significant long-term experience is lacking
[105]. With advanced medical therapy and clinical experience evolving, contraindications
to cardiac transplantation should be considered as absolute, probable and potential contraindications as outlined in Table 4.

Donor selection

Absolute donor criteria typically include ABO compatibility, age less than 55 years, and
absence of prolonged cardiac arrest, hypotension or thoracic trauma, underlying structural
cardiac disease, sepsis, extracranial malignancy or positive HIV serology. Size mismatch
between donor and recipient should ideally be less than 25%. Echocardiographic evaluation
is used for evaluating ventricular function and intracardiac pathology. Coronary artery
angiography is indicated in men older than 45 and women older than 50 years and for
donors with significant risk factors for coronary artery disease. The ultimate determination
of suitability is made after direct visualization of the heart.

  The number of donor hearts available continues to limit cardiac transplantation.
Recently, a consensus conference report was published to provide recommendations to
improve the evaluation and successful utilization of potential cardiac donors and Table 5
outlines these recommendations [106]. Transplant programs have subsequently expanded
their donor criteria to age greater than 55 years, hepatitis B and C positive serology,
reduced ventricular function and inotropic support being only relative contraindications

Table 5 Recommendations to Improve Donor Evaluation and Utilization

Age > 55 years can be used selectively
A normal sized 70 kg heart is suitable for most recipients
Hepatitis C positive and hepatitis B virus (core IgM negative) may be used in high-risk recipients
Left ventricular hypertrophy less than 13 mm does not preclude transplantation
Valvular abnormalities should be assessed as repairable after explanting the heart
Coronary angiograms may not be necessary in every patient over 45 years if low risk
Elevated cardiac enzymes without evidence of cardiac dysfunction does not preclude donation

to donation [107,108]. A system of donor and recipient risk matching has therefore evolved [109]. "Alternative recipients" are high-risk recipients, with probable or potential contraindications to transplantation that are deemed suitable to receive marginal donor hearts. Marginal donors may have coronary artery disease, high-risk behavior, hepatitis seropositivity, decreased left ventricular fraction, high inotropic requirement, left ventricular hypertrophy or be over 55 years.

Medical management of the donor is complicated by the physiological phenomenon of brain death and the need to coordinate procurement of multiple organs. Poor resuscitation and management results in poorly functioning allografts. Hypothermia is the most important component of organ preservation and is considered essential to the procurement procedure. At the time of organ procurement, a bolus of ice-cold cardioplegia solution is administered proximal to the aortic cross clamp. Rapid topical cooling of the heart is achieved with cold saline poured into the pericardial well. The heart is explanted quickly and placed into sterile bowel bags, filled with cold saline inside an airtight container. This technique allows for "safe" ischemic period of 4 to 6 hours. With these time constraints, careful consideration of the timing of the explant must be made by the donor surgeon. Sufficient time is required for the recipient surgeon to prepare the recipient particularly in the case of a redo sternotomy, which requires up to 90 minutes lead time before returning with the donor heart.

Operative Techniques

Drs. Lower and Shumway described the key technical aspects of successful orthotopic cardiac transplantation in 1960 and now more than 40 years later it mirrors the technique of choice [110]. Both the donor and the recipient hearts are removed by transecting the atria at the midatrial level, leaving the pulmonary venous connections to the left atrium intact in the posterior wall and transecting the aorta and pulmonary valves just above their respective valves.

In recent years, there has been a move to alter the surgical technique to leave the donor atria intact and make the anastomosis at the level of the superior vena cava and the inferior vena cava, which is referred to as the bicaval anastomotic technique. (Fig. 10) This change in technique was instigated in an attempt to preserve as much donor atrium as possible so to decrease the requirement for pacemaker placement due to donor sinus node dysfunction, lessen atrioventricular valve regurgitation and also facilitate endomyocardial biopsies [111,112].

The transplant operation begins with line placement and patient preparation. After performing a median sternotomy, cannulation of the recipients' aorta and vena cavae is performed, as with any standard cardiac surgery procedure. Variations particular to transplantation include snaring of both vena cavae and insertion of the aortic cannulae

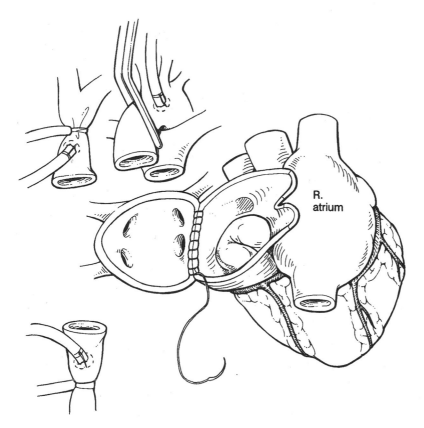

Figure 11 Bicaval technique in adult heart transplant recipient. After the left atrial anastomoses, the superior and inferior vena cavae are anastomosed in an end-to-end manner followed by the aortic and pulmonary anastomoses.

high on the recipient aorta. The recipient heart is excised only after the donor heart is visualized and deemed appropriate for transplantation.

The left atrial anastomosis is performed first, followed by the superior and inferior vena cava anastomosed to the right atrium (Fig. 11). The heart is continuously bathed in ice-cold saline during the implantation and a cold line is placed in the left ventricle for endomyocardial cooling. The pulmonary artery anastomosis is then performed with the cross-clamp on, followed by the aortic anastomosis. With the completion of the pulmonary artery anastomosis, the tapes around the vena cavae are released, allowing blood to flow into the lungs and, with concomitant ventilation, to displace air from the left side of the heart. Carbon dioxide is also continuously pumped into the field to reduce air in the heart. In general, 3.0 or 4.0 polypropylene sutures are used in a running fashion for all of the vascular anastomoses. Before the aortic anastomosis is completed, agitation of the left atrium and ventricle is performed to further dislodge air from the heart. A leukocyte filtering process is completed just prior to the removal of the cross clamp. The patient is placed in steep Trendelenburg position, and a needle vent site is created in the ascending aorta before releasing the aortic cross clamp [113].

Post Operative Care

The care required postoperatively differs little from that of patients who undergo cardiac revascularization or valvular surgery. Hemodynamic monitoring including a Swan-Ganz catheter and radial arterial line serve to facilitate care when pulmonary artery pressures and cardiac indices are needed to treat more complex transplant recipients. Routinely, however, central venous and arterial blood pressure monitoring suffices. Ventilatory support is weaned as tolerated and the average patient can be extubated within 4 to 6 hours postoperatively. Early cardiac failure accounts for up to 25% of perioperative deaths of transplant recipients, the causes of which include pulmonary hypertension and subsequent right heart failure, ischemic graft injury during preservation and acute rejection [108]. Poor cardiac function may also be due to cardiac tamponade.

Atrial pacing or atrioventricular sequential pacing may be necessary in the early postoperative period when AV block is usually temporary, resolving in 24 hours or less. Dopamine infusion may also be used in an attempt to improve renal blood flow as well

Table 6 Clinically Used Immunosuppressive Agents

Agent	Mechanism of Action	Toxicities
Induction Immunosuppression		
Antilymphocyte/Antithymocyte Immunoglobulin	Deplete activated lymphocytes Deplete activated thymocytes	Antibody response Allergic reaction
OKT3	Sequestration of $CD3^+$ T cells	Cytokine release syndrome Antibody response
Interleukin-2 Receptor Blocker	Inhibits T cell activation	None known
Maintenance Immunosuppression		
Glucocorticoids	Anti-inflammatory	Cushingoid habitus Glucose intolerance Osteoporosis Cataracts Hypertension Hyperlipidemia Poor wound healing
Cyclosporine	Calcineurin inhibitor Inhibits T cell proliferation	Nephrotoxicity Neurotoxicity Hypertension Gingival hyperplasia Hyperlipidemia
Tacrolimus	Calcineurin inhibitor Inhibits T cell proliferation	Nephrotoxicity Neurotoxicity Hypertension Gingival hyperplasia Diabetes Alopecia
Azathioprine	Purine analogue Inhibits de novo and salvage purine synthesis pathways	Marrow toxicity Hepatotoxicity Hepatotoxicity
Mycophenolate Mofetil	Inhibits inosine monophosphate dehydrogenase: inhibits de novo purine synthesis	Gastrointestinal disturbance
Rapamycin	Inhibits T cell activation? unknown mechanism	Hyperlipidemia Myelosuppression

as reduce the nephrotoxic effective of immunosuppressive therapy used early postoperative period. The use of preoperative angiotensin inhibitors combined with prolonged cardiopulmonary bypass times may result in substantial decreases in systemic vascular resistance and norepinephrine or vasopressin infusions are used to improve resistance.

Elevated pulmonary artery vascular resistance following heart transplantation is usually best approached with an aggressive preventative plan. The use of nitric oxide from the time of weaning from cardiopulmonary bypass can alleviate the strain on the right heart and permit it time to accommodate. Phosphodiesterase inhibitors with or without epinephrine and prostaglandin E_1 may also improve pulmonary vascular resistance and decrease the work of the right heart immediately postoperatively. A right ventricular assist device should be considered if right heart failure persists despite aggressive medical management [114].

Immunosuppression

Successful cardiac transplantation is dependent on effective immunosuppression since allograft rejection is the major cause of morbidity and mortality. Currently available immunosuppressive agents, their mode of action and side effects are outlined in Table 6. Presently, induction therapy followed by maintenance immunosuppression with corticosteroids, cyclosporine, and rapamycin is used at Stanford (Table 7). Figure 12 demonstrates the various agents employed for induction immunosuppression as reported to the registry of the ISHLT [81]. Figure 13 portrays the maintenance immunosuppressive protocols in place at the 1- and 5-year follow-up reports [81].

The introduction of cyclosporine, a T cell inhibitor, revolutionized solid organ transplantation [80]. Cyclosporine is administered in its oral formulation 2 to 3 days after transplantation when renal function has stabilized. The whole blood cyclosporine level target is 325 ng/ml for 1 to 6 weeks, 275 ng/ml for 6 weeks to 3 months, 225 ng/ml for 3 to 6 months and 200 ng/ml thereafter. Despite its substantial benefits, cyclosporine is associated with substantial side effects, including renal dysfunction, neurotoxicity and hypertension.

If cyclosporine is not tolerated, tacrolimus is substituted. Tacrolimus' use in heart transplantation began in the 1990s as a rescue agent [115,116]. Tacrolimus is also associated with renal and neurotoxicity, although perhaps to a lesser degree. Seizures and cerebral changes associated with cyclosporine can be ameliorated with the use of tacrolimus [117,118]. Multicenter, comparative trials of tacrolimus and cyclosporine in Europe and the United States have found that recipient survival is similar but tacrolimus is associated

Table 7 Stanford Immunosuppressive Regimen for Cardiac Transplantation

Induction Immunosuppression	
Methylprednisolone	500 mg IV coming off bypass
Daclizumab	1 mg/kg coming off bypass (q2weeks for a total of 5 weeks)
Maintenance Immunosuppression	
Sirolimus	2 mg per day 4 hours after Cyclosporine dose
Corticosteroids	Methylprednisolone 125 mg IV q8h for 3 doses post op
	Prednisone 1.0 mg/kg divided b.i.d. Days 1–14
	Prednisone Days 14+ taper to off as tolerated
Cyclosporine	25 mg p.o. b.i.d. postoperative day 1

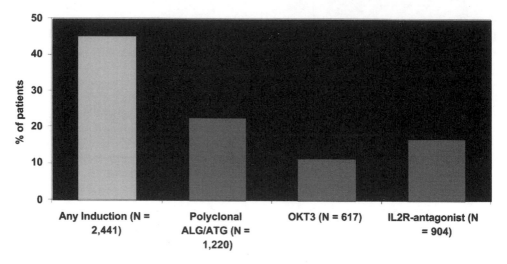

Figure 12 Induction immunosuppression agents in adult heart transplant recipients reported between January 2000 and June 2002.

with a reduced number of rejection episodes and decreased need for treatment of hypertension and hyperlipidemia [118–121].

Sirolimus is a macrolide antibiotic that is structurally similar to tacrolimus but has a yet undefined mechanism of action. The significant potential for renal and neurotoxicity associated with cyclosporine and tacrolimus have been attributed to their calcineurin blockade and are, therefore, potentially avoidable with the use of sirolimus [122,123]. In addition, sirolimus has been shown to prevent allograft coronary artery disease in animal models [124]. Recently, Stanford has introduced sirolimus into the standard cardiac trans-

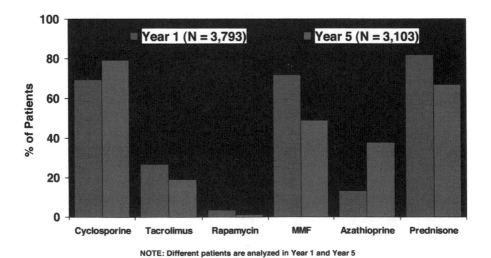

NOTE: Different patients are analyzed in Year 1 and Year 5

Figure 13 Maintenance immunosuppressive combinations at 1 and 5 years posttransplantation reported between January 2000 and June 2002. MMF, mycophenolate mofetil; AZA, azathioprine.

plant maintenance immunosuppressive regimen with target blood levels of 10 to 13 ng/ml.

Perhaps the most controversial aspect of immunosuppression in heart transplantation is the role of induction therapy [125–130]. Induction therapy is the use of perioperative therapy to potentially induce donor specific tolerance. The agents used include antithymocyte globulin, antilymphocyte globulin, OKT3, daclizumab, and basiliximab, IL-2 receptor antagonists (Fig. 11). The proponents of induction therapy argue that tolerance is achievable given the correct conditions; opponents of induction therapy argue that an increased potential for infectious and neoplastic complications secondary to severe immunosuppression is not warranted [125,126].

Clinical experience comparing outcomes with and without induction therapy has revealed that survival is the same but suggests that the incidence of rejection is reduced with induction therapy [127,128]. Interleukin 2 receptor inhibitors, such as daclizumab and basiliximab, act by arresting the proliferation of alloreactive T cells and have been shown effective in reducing rejection in renal transplantation [129]. Limited experience in heart transplantation has revealed that daclizumab induction therapy safely reduces the frequency and severity of acute allograft rejection without any notable side effects [130]. It has since been introduced into the immunosuppressive regimen at Stanford. (Table 7)

Complications of Cardiac Transplantation

Rejection: Acute and Chronic

Rejection exists in three forms: hyperacute, acute, and chronic. Hyperacute rejection is an antibody-mediated response that occurs when preexisting antibodies bind to donor ABO and HLA antigens upon graft revascularization. Gross inspection of the graft reveals a mottled or dark red, flaccid allograft, and histologically has global interstitial hemorrhage and edema without lymphocyte infiltrate. This form of rejection is most likely in a highly sensitized recipient and typically requires biventricular support or retransplantation and is often catastrophic [131].

Acute rejection is a T-cell mediated response. In a nonsensitized host, it is rare to see acute rejection before day 5 posttransplant with the incidence being highest in the first 3 months. At Stanford, endomyocardial biopsies are taken weekly starting at week 2 for 4 weeks, every other week for 2 months, monthly for 3 months and then every other month until the first anniversary of the transplant. Biopsies are performed yearly thereafter or when clinically indicated and are graded according to the International Society of Heart and Lung Transplantation (ISHLT) standardized criteria [132,133]. In the absence of allograft dysfunction, grades 1A and 1B are not normally treated, whereas grades 2 and above are treated with corticosteroids and augmented immunosuppressive regimens as outlined in Table 8.

Chronic rejection has proven to be the most difficult form of rejection to understand, prevent, and treat and remains the major cause of late morbidity and mortality. Chronic rejection is usually seen many years after transplantation but can also occur in an accelerated fashion. The pathology of chronic rejection is likely a humoral process resulting in fibrosis with loss of normal organ architecture and accelerated arteriosclerosis referred to as cardiac allograft vasculopathy. Many factors have been implicated in the pathogenesis of chronic rejection including organ preservation, minor and major histocompatibility mismatches, induction immunosuppression, race, gender, cytomegalovirus infection, and immunosuppressive regimens [134,135].

Table 8 Acute Cardiac Transplant Rejection

Acute Cellular Grade 2 or Greater

Methylprednisolone 1000 mg IV q.d. × 3 days
Prednisone 0.6 mg/kg tapering to 0.2 mg/kg over 3 weeks

Cellular Recurrent Grade 2 or Greater

Methylprednisolone 500–1000 mg IV q.d. × 3 days
Prednisone 0.6 mg/kg with 3 week taper
RATG or OKT3
Change Cyclosporine to Tacrolimus

Cellular, Intractable

Total lymphoid irradiation 800 cGy total dose twice weekly
(Mantel and inverted Y distribution)

Infection

In the early postoperative period (<1 month) infections are attributed to continuation of a presurgical infection, transmission by the donor allograft, and reactivation of viruses, most notably herpes simplex virus and human herpes virus 6. Absent during this period, despite immunosuppression, are opportunistic infections. Between 1 and 6 months after transplantation, cytomegalovirus (CMV) and Epstein Barr virus (EBV) infection become problematic. All endemic fungi can cause infection at this time and protection against *Aspergillus* and *Pneumocystis carinii* are critical. Six months posttransplant, patients are at risk for diseases similar to those in nonimmunocompromised hosts.

In an effort to reduce the incidence of infectious complications, antimicrobial prophylaxis regimens are followed. These regimens include ganciclovir, trimethoprim/sulfamethoxazole and aerosolized Amphotericin B therapy. Table 9 outlines the current antimicrobial prophylaxis for Stanford heart transplant recipients.

Post transplant malignancy

Allograft function depends on maintaining an immunosuppressive state, which leaves transplant recipients with a three- to four-fold increased risk of developing neoplasms [136–138]. Apart from skin malignancies, common malignancies seen in the general population are not increased in transplant recipients; instead, rare tumors, including posttransplant lymphoproliferative disorders (PTLD) and various sarcomas, are seen. The Epstein–Barr virus has been associated with PTLD, which is abnormal monoclonal B cell proliferation, is frequently extranodal and has a predilection for brain and allograft involvement [136]. Therapy includes reduction of immunosuppression, local therapy, chemotherapy, antiviral therapy and the use of monoclonal antibodies to CD20 [138,139].

The incidence of nonmelanoma skin cancers after transplantation outweighs the incidence of PTLD [140]. Transplant recipients tend to have a greater tendency towards squamous cell carcinoma as compared with basal cell carcinoma, which is opposite to the general population. Most therapy follows standard dermatologic approaches according to the histology and the clinical stage of the disease.

Results of Cardiac Transplantation

The survival benefit of cardiac transplantation compared with medical treatment of heart failure has never been tested in a prospective randomized trial. As noted earlier, the early

Table 9 Antimicrobial Prophylaxis Regimen Post Cardiac Transplantation

	Cytomegalovirus Prophylaxis	
	Donor CMV Negative	Donor CMV Positive
Recipient CMV Negative	No treatment	DHPG Prophylaxis 34 days/ Cytovene/ Cytogam
Recipient CMV Positive	DHPG Prophylaxis 24 days	DHPG Prophylaxis 24 days
DHPG (Ganciclovir IV)		
24 Day Regimen:	5 mg/kg IV b.i.d. for 14 days 6 mg/kg IV q.d. for 10 days	
34 Day Regimen:	5 mg/kg IV b.i.d. for 14 days 6 mg/kg IV b.i.d. for 20 days	
Cytovene (Ganciclovir PO)		
1000 mg PO TID for 6 weeks		
Cytogam (IgG Gamma Globulin)		
Within 72 hours posttransplant:	150 mg/kg	
Weeks 2, 4, 6, 8 posttransplant:	100 mg/kg	
Weeks 12 and 16 posttransplant:	50 mg/kg	
Pneumocystis Carinii Pneumonia Prophylaxis		
Bactrim SS 1 tablet q.d. for life		
If Bactrim allergic: Pentamidine 300 mg nebulized Q month		
Aspergillus Prophylaxis		
Amphotericin B aerosolized:20 mg b.i.d. while hospitalized		

Stanford experience provided evidence for improved survival posttransplant [82]. The 24th American College of Cardiology Bethesda Conference on Cardiac Transplantation recommended heart transplantation as the gold standard of treatment of patients with refractory advanced heart failure [141].

The Stanford experience has since been reexamined with 1-, 5- and 10-year survival rates of 85%, 68% and 46%, respectively, likely as a result of three decades of clinical experience [142]. The UNOS and ISHLT database have reported 1-, 5- and 10-year survival rates of 83%, 70% and 50% respectively [81]. Heart transplant actuarial survival curves and calculations as reported to the registry of the ISHLT are shown in Figures 14 [81]. Similar results have been reported by transplant groups worldwide [143–145]. The incidence of rejection and death from infection and allograft coronary artery disease have decreased over time likely due to improvements in immunosuppression and treatment of infection.

When comparing U.S. cardiac transplantation with European transplantation, it has been found that U.S. recipients were more likely to be on ventricular assist devices or inotropes preoperatively compared with European recipients. Also, living donor (domino) transplants, which are virtually nonexistent in the United States, make up 7% of UK transplants [144]. The long-term outcomes of retransplanted recipients are comparable with that of recipients undergoing their first transplant in some series, but inferior to initial transplant in other series, especially in patients with cardiac allograft vasculopathy [146].

Risk factors for poor outcomes after cardiac transplantation have been investigated by many groups [49,147]. The ISHLT Registry analysis has reported the need for extracorporeal membrane oxygenation and mechanical ventilation as the top risk factors for poor

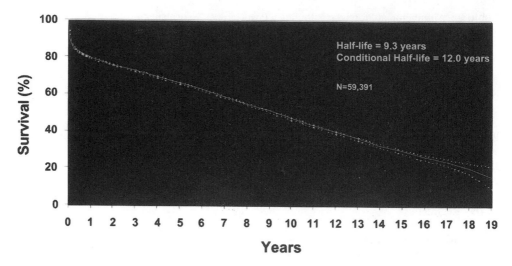

Figure 14 Actuarial survival for adult heart transplants performed between January 1982 and June 2001. Conditional half-life is the time to 50% survival for those recipients surviving the first year posttransplantation.

outcomes [81]. Adults with congenital heart disease, a previous transplant, ventricular assist device, diagnosis of ischemic cardiomyopathy, and male recipient of a female donor heart have all been reported to affect 1-year mortality. Table 10 demonstrates the risk factors for mortality within 1 year for adult heart transplants as reported to the registry for the ISHLT [81].

The cause of death amongst cardiac transplant recipients varies according to the posttransplant time period [81]. The largest single cause of death during the first 30 days is due to primary failure and acute rejection during the ensuing 11 months (Fig. 15). From 1 to 3 years posttransplant, infection, rejection, malignancy, and allograft coronary artery vasculopathy are equally responsible for recipient death. After year 3, malignancy and allograft coronary artery vasculopathy are the most common causes of death after adult heart transplantation (Fig. 15) [81].

Table 10 Risk Factors for 1-Year Mortality following Heart Transplantation (1996–2001) in Descending Order of Magnitude

Variable	Odds Ratio	95% Confidence Interval	P-value
ECMO	3.00	1.32–6.85	0.009
Ventilator	2.94	2.23–3.86	<.0001
Diagnosis: CHD	2.34	1.66–3.31	<.0001
IABP	1.53	1.21–1.94	0.0005
Previous Transplant	1.50	1.10–2.06	0.01
VAD	1.45	1.25–1.69	<.0001
Male recipient/female donor	1.18	1.05–1.33	0.005

CHD: congenital heart disease; ECMO: extracorporeal membrane oxygenator support; IABP: intra-aortic balloon pump; VAD: ventricular assist device
Source: Ref. 96.

ADULT HEART TRANSPLANT RECIPIENTS:
Cause of Death (Deaths: January 1992 - June 2002)

CAUSE OF DEATH	0-30 Days (N = 2,454)		31 Days - 1 Year (N = 2,155)		>1 Year - 3 Years (N = 1,642)		>3 Years - 5 Years (N = 1,391)		>5 Years (N = 3,454)	
CAV	44	(1.8%)	108	(5.0%)	243	(14.8%)	251	(18.0%)	588	(17.0%)
ACUTE REJECTION	157	(6.4%)	264	(12.3%)	156	(9.5%)	60	(4.3%)	39	(1.1%)
LYMPHOMA	1	(0.0%)	44	(2.0%)	78	(4.8%)	79	(5.7%)	181	(5.2%)
MALIGNANCY, OTHER	2	(0.1%)	49	(2.3%)	171	(10.4%)	269	(19.3%)	661	(19.1%)
CMV	3	(0.1%)	27	(1.3%)	14	(0.9%)	3	(0.2%)	4	(0.1%)
INFECTION, NON-CMV	348	(14.2%)	745	(34.6%)	216	(13.2%)	138	(9.9%)	333	(9.6%)
PRIMARY FAILURE	602	(24.5%)	183	(8.5%)	118	(7.2%)	67	(4.8%)	191	(5.5%)
GRAFT FAILURE	403	(16.4%)	226	(10.5%)	282	(17.2%)	201	(14.5%)	466	(13.5%)
TECHNICAL	183	(7.5%)	24	(1.1%)	15	(0.9%)	17	(1.2%)	36	(1.0%)
OTHER	83	(3.4%)	103	(4.8%)	114	(6.9%)	97	(7.0%)	205	(5.9%)
MULTIPLE ORGAN FAILURE	342	(13.9%)	204	(9.5%)	80	(4.9%)	73	(5.2%)	270	(7.8%)
RENAL FAILURE	14	(0.6%)	16	(0.7%)	27	(1.6%)	44	(3.2%)	203	(5.9%)
PULMONARY	109	(4.4%)	71	(3.3%)	72	(4.4%)	51	(3.7%)	128	(3.7%)
CEREBROVASCULAR	163	(6.6%)	91	(4.2%)	56	(3.4%)	41	(2.9%)	149	(4.3%)

Figure 15 Risk factors for mortality in adult heart transplant recipients performed between January 1992 and June 2002.

Future of Transplantation

Xenotransplantation, as the future of heart transplantation, has been thwarted by multiple challenges, including ethical, infectious, physiological and immunologic obstacles [148]. The physiologic and immunologic obstacles were approached first, and limited success has been realized [149,150]. At present the pig appears to be the most realistic source of organs but further research is required [148–150]. The concern for zoonotic infections and social acceptance of xenotransplantation will be future obstacles to overcome.

Cell transplantation is one of the newest treatment modalities proposed to improve patients with cardiac failure (Chapter 25) [151]. Experimental data have shown that the implantation of contractile cells into fibrous postinfarction scar allows the myocardium to regain functionality. Autologous skeletal myoblasts have been tested but other cell types can be considered including bone marrow and hematopoietic stem cells [152]. Recent reports describe a novel contractile bioartificial tissue that can be engineered in vitro that holds promise for use in reconstructive heart surgery [153].

SUMMARY

Cardiac transplantation is definitive therapy for end-stage heart failure. Absolute numbers of transplants performed is limited by donor supply; ways in which to expand donor criteria are being actively sought. Immunosuppression is required for all transplant recipients but is associated with toxicity and infectious and neoplastic complications. Ongoing research on how to improve immunosuppressive drugs and regimens will potentially reduce the associated morbidity. Chronic rejection continues to be the limiting factor in long-term outcomes. Currently the half-life of a transplant recipient is approximately 10 years with the longest living transplant recipient having survived 25 years posttransplant [81]. Clearly, the realm of cardiac transplantation has yet to be perfected, but tremendous strides have been made over 30 years of experience.

REFERENCES

1. Gibbon JH. Application of a mechanical heart and lung apparatus to cardiac surgery. Minn. Med 1954; 37:171–185.
2. Spencer FC, Eiseman B, Trinkle JK, Rodd NP. Assisted circulation for cardiac failure following intracardiac surgery with cardiorespiratory bypass. J Thorac Cardiovasc Surg 1965; 49: 56–73.
3. Hall CP, Liotta D, Henly WS, Crawford ES, DeBakey ME. Development of artificial intrathoracic circulatory pumps. Am J Surg 1964; 108:685–692.
4. DeBakey ME. Left ventricular bypass pump for cardiac assistance. Clinical experience. Am J Cardiol 1971; 27:3–11.
5. Cooley DA, Liotta D, Hallman GL, Bloodwell RD, Leachman RD, Milam JD. Orthotopic cardiac prosthesis for two-staged cardiac replacement. Am J Cardiol 1969; 24:723–730.
6. Rose EA, Gelijns AC, Moskowitz AJ, Heitjan DF, Stevenson LW, Dembitsky W, Long JW, Ascheim DD, Tierney AR, Levitan RG, Watson JT, Meier P, Ronan NS, Shapiro PA, Lazar RM, Miller LW, Gupta L, Frazier OH, Desvigne-Nickens P, Oz MC, Poirier VL. Long-term mechanical left ventricular assistance for end-stage heart failure. N Engl J Med 2001; 345: 1435–1443.
7. Deng MC, Loebe M, El Banayosy A, Gronda E, Jansen PG, Vigano M, Wieselthaler GM, Reichart B, Vitali E, Pavie A, Mesana T, Loisance DY, Wheeldon DR, Portner PM. Mechanical circulatory support for advanced heart failure: effect of patient selection on outcome. Circulation 2001; 103:231–237.
8. Khot UN, Mishra M, Yamani MH, Smedira NG, Paganini E, Yeager M, Buda T, McCarthy PM, Young JB, Starling RC. Severe renal dysfunction complicating cardiogenic shock is not a contraindication to mechanical support as a bridge to cardiac transplantation. J Am Coll Cardiol 2003; 41:381–385.
9. Farrar DJ, Hill JD. Recovery of major organ function in patients awaiting heart transplantation with Thoratec ventricular assist devices. Thoratec Ventricular Assist Device Principal Investigators. J Heart Lung Transplant 1994; 13:1125–1132.
10. Delgado DH, Rao V, Ross HJ, Verma S, Smedira NG. Mechanical circulatory assistance: state of art. Circulation 2002; 106:2046–2050.
11. Portner PM, Oyer PE, McGregor CGA. First human use of an electrically powered implantable ventricular assist system. Artif Organs 1985; 9:36.
12. Robbins RC, Oyer PE. Bridge to transplant with the Novacor left ventricular assist system. Ann Thorac Surg 1999; 68:695–697.
13. Robbins RC, Kown MH, Portner PM, Oyer PE. The totally implantable Novacor left ventricular assist system. Ann Thorac Surg 2001; 71:S162–S165.
14. Miller PJ, Billich TJ, LaForge DH, Lee J, Naegeli A, Ramasamy N, Jassawalla JS, Portner PM. Initial clinical experience with a wearable controller for the Novacor left ventricular assist system. ASAIO J 1994; 40:M465–M470.
15. Portner PM, Jansen PG, Oyer PE, Wheeldon DR, Ramasamy N. Improved outcomes with an implantable left ventricular assist system: a multicenter study. Ann Thorac Surg 2001; 71:205–209.
16. Frazier OH, Rose EA, Macmanus Q, Burton NA, Lefrak EA, Poirier VL, Dasse KA. Multicenter clinical evaluation of the HeartMate 1000 IP left ventricular assist device. Ann Thorac Surg 1992; 53:1080–1090.
17. Frazier OH. Chronic left ventricular support with a vented electric assist device. Ann Thorac Surg 1993; 55:273–275.

18. McCarthy PM, Wang N, Vargo R. Preperitoneal insertion of the HeartMate 1000 IP implantable left ventricular assist device. Ann Thorac Surg 1994; 57:634–637.
19. Radovancevic B, Frazier OH, Duncan JM. Implantation technique for the HeartMate left ventricular assist device. J Card Surg 1992; 7:203–207.
20. Rose EA, Levin HR, Oz MC, Frazier OH, Macmanus Q, Burton NA, Lefrak EA. Artificial circulatory support with textured interior surfaces. A counterintuitive approach to minimizing thromboembolism. Circulation 1994; 90:II87–II91.
21. Slater JP, Rose EA, Levin HR, Frazier OH, Roberts JK, Weinberg AD, Oz MC. Low thromboembolic risk without anticoagulation using advanced-design left ventricular assist devices. Ann Thorac Surg 1996; 62:1321–1327.
22. Farrar DJ, Hill JD. Univentricular and biventricular Thoratec VAD support as a bridge to transplantation. Ann Thorac Surg 1993; 55:276–282.
23. Pasic M, Bergs P, Hennig E, Loebe M, Weng Y, Hetzer R. Simplified technique for implantation of a left ventricular assist system after previous cardiac operations. Ann Thorac Surg 1999; 67:562–564.
24. Arabia FA, Smith RG, Rose DS, Arzouman DA, Sethi GK, Copeland JG. Success rates of long-term circulatory assist devices used currently for bridge to heart transplantation. ASAIO J 1996; 42:M542–M546.
25. Copeland JG, Arabia FA, Banchy ME, Sethi GK, Foy B, Long J, Kormos RL, Smith RG. The CardioWest total artificial heart bridge to transplantation: 1993 to 1996 national trial. Ann Thorac Surg 1998; 66:1662–1669.
26. McCarthy PM, Smedira NO, Vargo RL, Goormastic M, Hobbs RE, Starling RC, Young JB. One hundred patients with the HeartMate left ventricular assist device: evolving concepts and technology. J Thorac Cardiovasc Surg 1998; 115:904–912.
27. Frazier OH, Rose EA, Oz MC, Dembitsky WP, McCarthy PM, Radovancevic B, Poirier VL, Dasse KA. Multicenter clinical evaluation of the HeartMate; vented electric left ventricular assist system in patients awaiting heart transplantation. J Heart Lung Transplant 2001; 20:201–202.
28. Goldstein DJ, Seldomridge JA, Chen JM, Catanese KA, DeRosa CM, Weinberg AD, Smith CR, Rose EA, Levin HR, Oz MC. Use of aprotinin in LVAD recipients reduces blood loss, blood use, and perioperative mortality. Ann Thorac Surg 1995; 59:1063–1067.
29. Holman WL, Skinner JL, Waites KB, Benza RL, McGiffin DC, Kirklin JK. Infection during circulatory support with ventricular assist devices. Ann Thorac Surg 1999; 68:711–716.
30. El Banayosy A, Deng M, Loisance DY, Vetter H, Gronda E, Loebe M, Vigano M. The European experience of Novacor left ventricular assist (LVAS) therapy as a bridge to transplant: a retrospective multi-centre study. Eur J Cardiothorac Surg 1999; 15:835–841.
31. Gordon SM, Schmitt SK, Jacobs M, Smedira NM, Goormastic M, Banbury MK, Yeager M, Serkey J, Hoercher K, McCarthy PM. Nosocomial bloodstream infections in patients with implantable left ventricular assist devices. Ann Thorac Surg 2001; 72:725–730.
32. Arusoglu L, Koerfer R, Tenderich G, Alexander WA, El Banayosy A. A novel method to reduce device-related infections in patients supported with the HeartMate device. Ann Thorac Surg 1999; 68:1875–1877.
33. Choi L, Choudhri AF, Pillarisetty VG, Sampath LA, Caraos L, Brunnert SR, Oz MC, Modak SM. Development of an infection-resistant LVAD driveline: a novel approach to the prevention of device-related infections. J Heart Lung Transplant 1999; 18:1103–1110.
34. Herrmann M, Weyand M, Greshake B, von Eiff C, Proctor RA, Scheld HH, Peters G. Left ventricular assist device infection is associated with increased mortality but is not a contraindication to transplantation. Circulation 1997; 95:814–817.
35. Prendergast TW, Todd BA, Beyer AJ, Furukawa S, Eisen HJ, Addonizio VP, Browne BJ, Jeevanandam V. Management of left ventricular assist device infection with heart transplantation. Ann Thorac Surg 1997; 64:142–147.
36. Frazier OH, Rose EA, McCarthy P, Burton NA, Tector A, Levin H, Kayne HL, Poirier VL, Dasse KA. Improved mortality and rehabilitation of transplant candidates treated with a long-term implantable left ventricular assist system. Ann Surg 1995; 222:327–336.

37. Ochiai Y, McCarthy PM, Smedira NG, Banbury MK, Navia JL, Feng J, Hsu AP, Yeager ML, Buda T, Hoercher KJ, Howard MW, Takagaki M, Doi K, Fukamachi K. Predictors of severe right ventricular failure after implantable left ventricular assist device insertion: analysis of 245 patients. Circulation 2002; 106:I198–I202.

38. Fukamachi K, McCarthy PM, Smedira NG, Vargo RL, Starling RC, Young JB. Preoperative risk factors for right ventricular failure after implantable left ventricular assist device insertion. Ann Thorac Surg 1999; 68:2181–2184.

39. Van MC. Right heart failure: best treated by avoidance. Ann Thorac Surg 2001; 71: S220–S222.

40. Wagner F, Dandel M, Gunther G, Loebe M, Schulze-Neick I, Laucke U, Kuhly R, Weng Y, Hetzer R. Nitric oxide inhalation in the treatment of right ventricular dysfunction following left ventricular assist device implantation. Circulation 1997; 96:II-6.

41. Itescu S, Tung TC, Burke EM, Weinberg A, Moazami N, Artrip JH, Suciu-Foca N, Rose EA, Oz MC, Michler RE. Preformed IgG antibodies against major histocompatibility complex class II antigens are major risk factors for high-grade cellular rejection in recipients of heart transplantation. Circulation 1998; 98:786–793.

42. Tsau PH, Arabia FA, Toporoff B, Paramesh V, Sethi GK, Copeland JG. Positive panel reactive antibody titers in patients bridged to transplantation with a mechanical assist device: risk factors and treatment. ASAIO J 1998; 44:M634–M637.

43. Moazami N, Itescu S, Williams MR, Argenziano M, Weinberg A, Oz MC. Platelet transfusions are associated with the development of anti-major histocompatibility complex class I antibodies in patients with left ventricular assist support. J Heart Lung Transplant 1998; 17:876–880.

44. Spanier TB, Chen JM, Oz MC, Stern DM, Rose EA, Schmidt AM. Time-dependent cellular population of textured-surface left ventricular assist devices contributes to the development of a biphasic systemic procoagulant response. J Thorac Cardiovasc Surg 1999; 118:404–413.

45. Ankersmit HJ, Edwards NM, Schuster M, John R, Kocher A, Rose EA, Oz M, Itescu S. Quantitative changes in T-cell populations after left ventricular assist device implantation: relationship to T-cell apoptosis and soluble CD95. Circulation 1999; 100:II211–II215.

46. Ankersmit HJ, Tugulea S, Spanier T, Weinberg AD, Artrip JH, Burke EM, Flannery M, Mancini D, Rose EA, Edwards NM, Oz MC, Itescu S. Activation-induced T-cell death and immune dysfunction after implantation of left-ventricular assist device. Lancet 1999; 354: 550–555.

47. John R, Lietz K, Burke E, Ankersmit J, Mancini D, Suciu-Foca N, Edwards N, Rose E, Oz M, Itescu S. Intravenous immunoglobulin reduces anti-HLA alloreactivity and shortens waiting time to cardiac transplantation in highly sensitized left ventricular assist device recipients. Circulation 1999; 100:II229–II235.

48. Frazier OH, Rose EA, Oz MC, Dembitsky W, McCarthy P, Radovancevic B, Poirier VL, Dasse KA. Multicenter clinical evaluation of the HeartMate vented electric left ventricular assist system in patients awaiting heart transplantation. J Thorac Cardiovasc Surg 2001; 122: 1186–1195.

49. John R, Rajasinghe H, Chen JM, Weinberg AD, Sinha P, Itescu S, Lietz K, Mancini D, Oz MC, Smith CR, Rose EA, Edwards NM. Impact of current management practices on early and late death in more than 500 consecutive cardiac transplant recipients. Ann Surg 2000; 232:302–311.

50. Kormos RL, Ramasamy N, Sit S, Griffith BP. Bridge to transplant experience with the Novacor left ventricular assist system: results of a multicenter US study. J Heart Lung Transplant 1999; 18:143–Abstract.

51. Farrar DJ, Hill JD, Pennington DG, McBride LR, Holman WL, Kormos RL, Esmore D, Gray LA, Seifert PE, Schoettle GP, Moore CH, Hendry PJ, Bhayana JN. Preoperative and postoperative comparison of patients with univentricular and biventricular support with the Thoratec ventricular assist device as a bridge to cardiac transplantation. J Thorac Cardiovasc Surg 1997; 113:202–209.

52. Poirier VL. Worldwide experience with the TCI HeartMate system: issues and future perspective. Thorac Cardiovasc Surg 1999; 47(suppl 2):316–320.

53. Farrar DJ. Preoperative predictors of survival in patients with Thoratec ventricular assist devices as a bridge to heart transplantation. Thoratec Ventricular Assist Device Principal Investigators. J Heart Lung Transplant 1994; 13:93–100.
54. Bank AJ, Mir SH, Nguyen DQ, Bolman RM, Shumway SJ, Miller LW, Kaiser DR, Ormaza SM, Park SJ. Effects of left ventricular assist devices on outcomes in patients undergoing heart transplantation. Ann Thorac Surg 2000; 69:1369–1374.
55. Aaronson KD, Eppinger MJ, Dyke DB, Wright S, Pagani FD. Left ventricular assist device therapy improves utilization of donor hearts. J Am Coll Cardiol 2002; 39:1247–1254.
56. Drews TN, Loebe M, Jurmann MJ, Weng Y, Wendelmuth C, Hetzer R. Outpatients on mechanical circulatory support. Ann Thorac Surg 2003; 75:780–785.
57. Foray A, Williams D, Reemtsma K, Oz M, Mancini D. Assessment of submaximal exercise capacity in patients with left ventricular assist devices. Circulation 1996; 94:II222–II226.
58. Mancini D, Goldsmith R, Levin H, Beniaminovitz A, Rose E, Catanese K, Flannery M, Oz M. Comparison of exercise performance in patients with chronic severe heart failure versus left ventricular assist devices. Circulation 1998; 98:1178–1183.
59. Moskowitz AJ, Rose EA, Gelijns AC. The cost of long-term LVAD implantation. Ann Thorac Surg 2001; 71:S195–S198.
60. Morales DL, Catanese KA, Helman DN, Williams MR, Weinberg A, Goldstein DJ, Rose EA, Oz MC. Six-year experience of caring for forty-four patients with a left ventricular assist device at home: safe, economical, necessary. J Thorac Cardiovasc Surg 2000; 119:251–259.
61. Nakatani S, McCarthy PM, Kottke-Marchant K, Harasaki H, James KB, Savage RM, Thomas JD. Left ventricular echocardiographic and histologic changes: impact of chronic unloading by an implantable ventricular assist device. J Am Coll Cardiol 1996; 27:894–901.
62. Frazier OH, Benedict CR, Radovancevic B, Bick RJ, Capek P, Springer WE, Macris MP, Delgado R, Buja LM. Improved left ventricular function after chronic left ventricular unloading. Ann Thorac Surg 1996; 62:675–681.
63. Bruckner BA, Stetson SJ, Perez-Verdia A, Youker KA, Radovancevic B, Connelly JH, Koerner MM, Entman ME, Frazier OH, Noon GP, Torre-Amione G. Regression of fibrosis and hypertrophy in failing myocardium following mechanical circulatory support. J Heart Lung Transplant 2001; 20:457–464.
64. Bartling B, Milting H, Schumann H, Darmer D, Arusoglu L, Koerner MM, El Banayosy A, Koerfer R, Holtz J, Zerkowski HR. Myocardial gene expression of regulators of myocyte apoptosis and myocyte calcium homeostasis during hemodynamic unloading by ventricular assist devices in patients with end-stage heart failure. Circulation 1999; 100:II216–II223.
65. McCarthy PM, Nakatani S, Vargo R, Kottke-Marchant K, Harasaki H, James KB, Savage RM, Thomas JD. Structural and left ventricular histologic changes after implantable LVAD insertion. Ann Thorac Surg 1995; 59:609–613.
66. Torre-Amione G, Stetson SJ, Youker KA, Durand JB, Radovancevic B, Delgado RM, Frazier OH, Entman ML, Noon GP. Decreased expression of tumor necrosis factor-alpha in failing human myocardium after mechanical circulatory support: a potential mechanism for cardiac recovery. Circulation 1999; 100:1189–1193.
67. Li YY, Feng Y, McTiernan CF, Pei W, Moravec CS, Wang P, Rosenblum W, Kormos RL, Feldman AM. Downregulation of matrix metalloproteinases and reduction in collagen damage in the failing human heart after support with left ventricular assist devices. Circulation 2001; 104:1147–1152.
68. Grabellus F, Levkau B, Sokoll A, Welp H, Schmid C, Deng MC, Takeda A, Breithardt G, Baba HA. Reversible activation of nuclear factor-kappa B in human end-stage heart failure after left ventricular mechanical support. Cardiovasc Res 2002; 53:124–130.
69. Ogletree-Hughes ML, Stull LB, Sweet WE, Smedira NG, McCarthy PM, Moravec CS. Mechanical unloading restores beta-adrenergic responsiveness and reverses receptor downregulation in the failing human heart. Circulation 2001; 104:881–886.
70. Heerdt PM, Holmes JW, Cai B, Barbone A, Madigan JD, Reiken S, Lee DL, Oz MC, Marks AR, Burkhoff D. Chronic unloading by left ventricular assist device reverses contractile dysfunction and alters gene expression in end-stage heart failure. Circulation 2000; 102:2713–2719.

71. Hetzer R, Muller JH, Weng Y, Meyer R, Dandel M. Bridging-to-recovery. Ann Thorac Surg 2001; 71:S109–S113.

72. Muller J, Wallukat G, Weng YG, Dandel M, Spiegelsberger S, Semrau S, Brandes K, Theodoridis V, Loebe M, Meyer R, Hetzer R. Weaning from mechanical cardiac support in patients with idiopathic dilated cardiomyopathy. Circulation 1997; 96:542–549.

73. Hetzer R, Muller JH, Weng YG, Loebe M, Wallukat G. Midterm follow-up of patients who underwent removal of a left ventricular assist device after cardiac recovery from end-stage dilated cardiomyopathy. J Thorac Cardiovasc Surg 2000; 120:843–853.

74. Mancini DM, Beniaminovitz A, Levin H, Catanese K, Flannery M, DiTullio M, Savin S, Cordisco ME, Rose E, Oz M. Low incidence of myocardial recovery after left ventricular assist device implantation in patients with chronic heart failure. Circulation 1998; 98:2383–2389.

75. Carrel A, Guthrie CC. The transplantation of veins and organs. Am Med 1905; 10:1101–1102.

76. Mann FC, Priestly JT, Markowitz J, Yater WM. Transplantation of the intact mammalian heart. Arch Surg 1993; 26:219–224.

77. Barnard CN. The operation. A human cardiac transplant: an interim report of a successful operation performed at Groote Schuur Hospital, Cape Town. S Afr Med J 1967; 41: 1271–1274.

78. Reitz BA. History of heart and heart-lung transplantation. In: Baumgartner WA, Reitz BA, Kasper EK, Theodore J, Eds. Heart and Lung Transplantation., WB Saunders Company. 2002:3–14.

79. Caves PK, Stinson EB, Billingham M, Shumway NE. Percutaneous transvenous endomyocardial biopsy in human heart recipients. Experience with a new technique. Ann Thorac Surg 1973; 16:325–336.

80. Oyer PE. Heart transplantation in the cyclosporine era. Ann Thorac Surg 1988; 46:489–490.

81. Taylor DO, Edwards LB, Mohacsi PJ, Boucek MM, Trulock EP, Keck BM, Hertz MI. The registry of the international society for heart and lung transplantation: twentieth official adult heart transplant report-2003. J Heart Lung Transplant 2003; 22:616–624.

82. Hunt SA, Rider AK, Stinson EB, Griepp RB, Schroeder JS, Harrison DC, Shumway NE. Does cardiac transplantation prolong life and improve its quality? An updated report. Circulation 1976; 54:III56–III60.

83. Deng MC, Smits JM, Young JB. Proposition: the benefit of cardiac transplantation in stable outpatients with heart failure should be tested in a randomized trial. J Heart Lung Transplant 2003; 22:113–117.

84. Aaronson KD, Schwartz JS, Chen TM, Wong KL, Goin JE, Mancini DM. Development and prospective validation of a clinical index to predict survival in ambulatory patients referred for cardiac transplant evaluation. Circulation 1997; 95:2660–2667.

85. Mancini DM, Eisen H, Kussmaul W, Mull R, Edmunds LH, Wilson JR. Value of peak exercise oxygen consumption for optimal timing of cardiac transplantation in ambulatory patients with heart failure. Circulation 1991; 83:778–786.

86. Cimato TR, Jessup M. Recipient selection in cardiac transplantation: contraindications and risk factors for mortality. J Heart Lung Transplant 2002; 21:1161–1173.

87. Argenziano M, Rose EA. Cardiac transplantation: current concepts and future directions. In: Balady GJ, Pina IL, Eds. Exercise and Heart Failure. Armonk, NY: Futura Publishing Company, 1997:171–184.

88. Koerner MM, Durand JB, Lafuente JA, Noon GP, Torre-Amione G. Cardiac transplantation: the final therapeutic option for the treatment of heart failure. Curr Opin Cardiol 2000; 15: 178–182.

89. Deng MC, Smits JM, Packer M. Selecting patients for heart transplantation: which patients are too well for transplant?. Curr Opin Cardiol 2002; 17:137–144.

90. Moss AJ, Zareba W, Hall WJ, Klein H, Wilber DJ, Cannom DS, Daubert JP, Higgins SL, Brown MW, Andrews ML. Prophylactic implantation of a defibrillator in patients with myocardial infarction and reduced ejection fraction. N Engl J Med 2002; 346:877–883.

91. Rickenbacher PR, Lewis NP, Valantine HA, Luikart H, Stinson EB, Hunt SA. Heart transplantation in patients over 54 years of age. Mortality, morbidity and quality of life. Eur Heart J 1997; 18:870–878.

92. Borkon AM, Muehlebach GF, Jones PG, Bresnahan DR, Genton RE, Gorton ME, Long ND, Magalski A, Porter CB, Reed WA, Rowe SK. An analysis of the effect of age on survival after heart transplant. J Heart Lung Transplant 1999; 18:668–674.

93. Mccarthy JF, McCarthy PM, Massad MG, Cook DJ, Smedira NG, Kasirajan V, Goormastic M, Hoercher K, Young JB. Risk factors for death after heart transplantation: does a single-center experience correlate with multicenter registries?. Ann Thorac Surg 1998; 65: 1574–1578.

94. Baron O, Trochu JN, Treilhaud M, Al Habash O, Remadi JP, Petit T, Duveau D, Despins P, Michaud JL. Cardiac transplantation in patients over 60 years of age. Transplant Proc 1999; 31:75–78.

95. Hosenpud JD, Bennett LE, Keck BM, Boucek MM, Novick RJ. The Registry of the International Society for Heart and Lung Transplantation: seventeenth official report-2000. J Heart Lung Transplant 2000; 19:909–931.

96. Hertz MI, Taylor DO, Trulock EP, Boucek MM, Mohacsi PJ, Edwards LB, Keck BM. The registry of the international society for heart and lung transplantation: nineteenth official report-2002. J Heart Lung Transplant 2002; 21:950–970.

97. Chen JM, Levin HR, Michler RE, Prusmack CJ, Rose EA, Aaronson KD. Reevaluating the significance of pulmonary hypertension before cardiac transplantation: determination of optimal thresholds and quantification of the effect of reversibility on perioperative mortality. J Thorac Cardiovasc Surg 1997; 114:627–634.

98. Espinoza C, Manito N, Roca J, Castells E, Mauri J, Ribas M, Claret G. Reversibility of pulmonary hypertension in patients evaluated for orthotopic heart transplantation: importance in the postoperative morbidity and mortality. Transplant Proc 1999; 31:2503–2504.

99. Zales VR, Pahl E, Backer CL, Crawford S, Mavroudis C, Benson DW. Pharmacologic reduction of pretransplantation pulmonary vascular resistance predicts outcome after pediatric heart transplantation. J Heart Lung Transplant 1993; 12:965–972.

100. Bando K, Konishi H, Komatsu K, Fricker FJ, del Nido PJ, Francalancia NA, Hardesty RL, Griffith BP, Armitage JM. Improved survival following pediatric cardiac transplantation in high-risk patients. Circulation 1993; 88:II218–II223.

101. Addonizio LJ, Hsu DT, Fuzesi L, Smith CR, Rose EA. Optimal timing of pediatric heart transplantation. Circulation 1989; 80:III84–III89.

102. Mancini D, Beniaminovitz A, Edwards N, Chen J, Maybaum S. Survival of diabetic patients following cardiac transplant. J Heart Lung Transplant 2001; 20:168.

103. Czerny M, Sahin V, Zuckermann A, Zimpfer D, Kilo J, Baumer H, Wolner E, Grimm M. Diabetes affects long-term survival after heart transplantation. J Heart Lung Transplant 2001; 20:245.

104. Hosenpud JD, Pamidi SR, Fiol BS, Cinquegrani MP, Keck BM. Outcomes in patients who are hepatitis B surface antigen-positive before transplantation: an analysis and study using the joint ISHLT/UNOS thoracic registry. J Heart Lung Transplant 2000; 19:781–785.

105. Castella M, Tenderich G, Koerner MM, Arusoglu L, El Banayosy A, Schulz U, Schulze B, Schulte-Eistrup S, Wolff C, Minami K, Koerfer R. Outcome of heart transplantation in patients previously infected with hepatitis C virus. J Heart Lung Transplant 2001; 20:595–598.

106. Zaroff JG, Rosengard BR, Armstrong WF, Babcock WD, D'Alessandro A, Dec GW, Edwards NM, Higgins RS, Jeevanandum V, Kauffman M, Kirklin JK, Large SR, Marelli D, Peterson TS, Ring WS, Robbins RC, Russell SD, Taylor DO, Van Bakel A, Wallwork J, Young JB. Consensus conference report: maximizing use of organs recovered from the cadaver donor: cardiac recommendations, March 28–29, 2001, Crystal City, Va. Circulation 2002; 106: 836–841.

107. Chen JM, Sinha P, Rajasinghe HA, Suratwala SJ, McCue JD, McCarty MJ, Caliste X, Hauff HM, John R, Edwards NM. Do donor characteristics really matter? Short- and long-term impact of donor characteristics on recipient survival, 1995- 1999. J Heart Lung Transplant 2002; 21:608–610.

108. Potapov EV, Loebe M, Hubler M, Musci M, Hummel M, Weng Y, Hetzer R. Medium-term results of heart transplantation using donors over 63 years of age. Transplantation 1999; 68: 1834–1838.

109. Laks H, Marelli D, Fonarow GC, Hamilton MA, Ardehali A, Moriguchi JD, Bresson J, Gjertson D, Kobashigawa JA. Use of two recipient lists for adults requiring heart transplantation. J Thorac Cardiovasc Surg 2003; 125:49–59.

110. Lower RR, Shumway NE. Studies on the orthotopic homotransplantation of the canine heart. Surg Forum 1960; 11:18.

111. Aziz T, Burgess M, Khafagy R, Wynn HA, Campbell C, Rahman A, Deiraniya A, Yonan N. Bicaval and standard techniques in orthotopic heart transplantation: medium-term experience in cardiac performance and survival. J Thorac Cardiovasc Surg 1999; 118:115–122.

112. Beniaminovitz A, Savoia MT, Oz M, Galantowicz M, Di Tullio MR, Homma S, Mancini D. Improved atrial function in bicaval versus standard orthotopic techniques in cardiac transplantation. Am J Cardiol 1997; 80:1631–1635.

113. Baumgartner WA. Operative techniques used in heart transplantation. In: Baumgartner WA, Reitz BA, Kasper EK, Theodore J, Eds. Heart and Lung Transplantation. Philadelphia: WB Saunders Company, 2002:180–199.

114. Fleischer KJ, Baumgartner WA. Heart Transplantation. In: Cardiac Surgery in the Adult. Edmunds LH, Ed. Philadelphia: McGraw-Hill Companies, 1997:1409–1449.

115. Yamani MH, Starling RC, Pelegrin D, Platt L, Majercik M, Hobbs RE, McCarthy P, Young JB. Efficacy of tacrolimus in patients with steroid-resistant cardiac allograft cellular rejection. J Heart Lung Transplant 2000; 19:337–342.

116. De Bonis M, Reynolds L, Barros J, Madden BP. Tacrolimus as a rescue immunosuppressant after heart transplantation. Eur J Cardiothorac Surg 2001; 19:690–695.

117. Klein IH, Abrahams A, van Ede T, Hene RJ, Koomans HA, Ligtenberg G. Different effects of tacrolimus and cyclosporine on renal hemodynamics and blood pressure in healthy subjects. Transplantation 2002; 73:732–736.

118. Taylor DO, Barr ML, Meiser BM, Pham SM, Mentzer RM, Gass AL. Suggested guidelines for the use of tacrolimus in cardiac transplant recipients. J Heart Lung Transplant 2001; 20: 734–738.

119. Meiser BM, Uberfuhr P, Fuchs A, Schmidt D, Pfeiffer M, Paulus D, Schulze C, Wildhirt S, Scheidt WV, Angermann C, Klauss V, Martin S, Reichenspurner H, Kreuzer E, Reichart B. Single-center randomized trial comparing tacrolimus (FK506) and cyclosporine in the prevention of acute myocardial rejection. J Heart Lung Transplant 1998; 17:782–788.

120. Taylor DO, Barr ML, Radovancevic B, Renlund DG, Mentzer RMJr, Smart FW, Tolman DE, Frazier OH, Young JB, VanVeldhuisen P. A randomized, multicenter comparison of tacrolimus and cyclosporine immunosuppressive regimens in cardiac transplantation: decreased hyperlipidemia and hypertension with tacrolimus. J Heart Lung Transplant 1999; 18: 336–345.

121. Baran DA, Galin I, Sandler D, Segura L, Cheng J, Courtney MC, Correa R, Chan M, Fallon JT, Spielvogel D, Lansman SL, Gass AL. Tacrolimus in cardiac transplantation: efficacy and safety of a novel dosing protocol. Transplantation 2002; 74:1136–1141.

122. Snell GI, Levvey BJ, Chin W, Kotsimbos AT, Whitford H, Williams TJ, Richardson M. Rescue therapy: a role for sirolimus in lung and heart transplant recipients. Transplant Proc 2001; 33:1084–1085.

123. Snell GI, Levvey BJ, Chin W, Kotsimbos T, Whitford H, Waters KN, Richardson M, Williams TJ. Sirolimus allows renal recovery in lung and heart transplant recipients with chronic renal impairment. J Heart Lung Transplant 2002; 21:540–546.

124. Dambrin C, Klupp J, Birsan T, Luna J, Suzuki T, Lam T, Stahr P, Hausen B, Christians U, Fitzgerald P, Berry G, Morris R. Sirolimus (rapamycin) monotherapy prevents graft vascular disease in nonhuman primate recipients of orthotopic aortic allografts. Circulation 2003; 107: 2369–2374.

125. van Gelder T, Balk AH, Jonkman FA, Zietse R, Zondervan P, Hesse CJ, Vaessen LM, Mochtar B, Weimar W. A randomized trial comparing safety and efficacy of OKT3 and a monoclonal anti-interleukin-2 receptor antibody (BT563) in the prevention of acute rejection after heart transplantation. Transplantation 1996; 62:51–55.

126. Swinnen LJ, Costanzo-Nordin MR, Fisher SG, O'Sullivan EJ, Johnson MR, Heroux AL, Dizikes GJ, Pifarre R, Fisher RI. Increased incidence of lymphoproliferative disorder after

immunosuppression with the monoclonal antibody OKT3 in cardiac-transplant recipients. N Engl J Med 1990; 323:1723–1728.

127. Copeland JG, Icenogle TB, Williams RJ, Rosado LJ, Butman SM, Vasu MA, Sethi GK, McDonald AN, Klees E, Rhenman MJ. Rabbit antithymocyte globulin. A 10-year experience in cardiac transplantation. J Thorac Cardiovasc Surg 1990; 99:852–860.

128. Carrier M, White M, Perrault LP, Pelletier GB, Pellerin M, Robitaille D, Pelletier LC. A 10-year experience with intravenous thymoglobuline in induction of immunosuppression following heart transplantation. J Heart Lung Transplant 1999; 18:1218–1223.

129. Vincenti F, Kirkman R, Light S, Bumgardner G, Pescovitz M, Halloran P, Neylan J, Wilkinson A, Ekberg H, Gaston R, Backman L, Burdick J. Interleukin-2-receptor blockade with daclizumab to prevent acute rejection in renal transplantation. Daclizumab Triple Therapy Study Group. N Engl J Med 1998; 338:161–165.

130. Beniaminovitz A, Itescu S, Lietz K, Donovan M, Burke EM, Groff BD, Edwards N, Mancini DM. Prevention of rejection in cardiac transplantation by blockade of the interleukin-2 receptor with a monoclonal antibody. N Engl J Med 2000; 342:613–619.

131. Weil R, Clarke DR, Iwaki Y, Porter KA, Koep LJ, Paton BC, Terasaki PI, Starzl TE. Hyperacute rejection of a transplanted human heart. Transplantation 1981; 32:71–72.

132. Billingham ME, Cary NR, Hammond ME, Kemnitz J, Marboe C, McCallister HA, Snovar DC, Winters GL, Zerbe A. A working formulation for the standardization of nomenclature in the diagnosis of heart and lung rejection: Heart Rejection Study Group. The International Society for Heart Transplantation. J Heart Transplant 1990; 9:587–593.

133. Winters GL, Marboe CC, Billingham ME. The International Society for Heart and Lung Transplantation grading system for heart transplant biopsy specimens: clarification and commentary. J Heart Lung Transplant 1998; 17:754–760.

134. Young JB. Perspectives on cardiac allograft vasculopathy. Curr Atheroscler Rep 2000; 2:259–271.

135. Valantine HA, Luikart H, Doyle R, Theodore J, Hunt S, Oyer P, Robbins R, Berry G, Reitz B. Impact of cytomegalovirus hyperimmune globulin on outcome after cardiothoracic transplantation: a comparative study of combined prophylaxis with CMV hyperimmune globulin plus ganciclovir versus ganciclovir alone. Transplantation 2001; 72:1647–1652.

136. Penn I. Post-transplant malignancy: the role of immunosuppression. Drug Safety 2000; 23:101–113.

137. Hunt SA. Malignancy in organ transplantation: heart. Transplant Proc 2002; 34:1874–1876.

138. Tenderich G, Deyerling W, Schulz U, Heller R, Hornik L, Schulze B, Jahanyar J, Koerfer R. Malignant neoplastic disorders following long-term immunosuppression after orthotopic heart transplantation. Transplant Proc 2001; 33:3653–3655.

139. Zilz ND, Olson LJ, McGregor CG. Treatment of post-transplant lymphoproliferative disorder with monoclonal CD20 antibody (rituximab) after heart transplantation. J Heart Lung Transplant 2001; 20:770–772.

140. Fortina AB, Caforio AL, Piaserico S, Alaibac M, Tona F, Feltrin G, Livi U, Peserico A. Skin cancer in heart transplant recipients: frequency and risk factor analysis. J Heart Lung Transplant 2000; 19:249–255.

141. Hunt SA. 24th Bethesda Conference: cardiac transplantation. J Am Coll Cardiol 1993; 22:1–64.

142. Robbins RC, Barlow CW, Oyer PE, Hunt SA, Miller JL, Reitz BA, Stinson EB, Shumway NE. Thirty years of cardiac transplantation at Stanford university. J Thorac Cardiovasc Surg 1999; 117:939–951.

143. Marelli D, Laks H, Kobashigawa JA, Bresson J, Ardehali A, Esmailian F, Plunkett MD, Kubak B. Seventeen-year experience with 1,083 heart transplants at a single institution. Ann. Thorac. Surg 2002; 74:1558–1566.

144. Anyanwu AC, Rogers CA, Murday AJ. Variations in cardiac transplantation: comparisons between the United Kingdom and the United States. J Heart Lung Transplant 1999; 18:297–303.

145. Smits JM, De Meester J, Deng MC, Scheld HH, Hummel M, Schoendube F, Haverich A, Vanhaecke J, van Houwelingen HC. Mortality rates after heart transplantation: how to compare center-specific outcome data?. Transplantation 2003; 75:90–96.

146. John R, Chen JM, Weinberg A, Oz MC, Mancini D, Itescu S, Galantowicz ME, Smith CR, Rose EA, Edwards NM. Long-term survival after cardiac retransplantation: a twenty-year single-center experience. J Thorac Cardiovasc Surg 1999; 117:543–555.

147. John R, Rajasinghe HA, Itescu S, Suratwalla S, Lietz K, Weinberg AD, Kocher A, Mancini DM, Drusin RE, Oz MC, Smith CR, Rose EA, Edwards NM. Factors affecting long-term survival (>10 years) after cardiac transplantation in the cyclosporine era. J Am Coll Cardiol 2001; 37:189–194.

148. Dorling A, Riesbeck K, Warrens A, Lechler R. Clinical xenotransplantation of solid organs. Lancet 1997; 349:867–871.

149. Lawson JH, Platt JL. Molecular barriers to xenotransplantation. Transplantation 1996; 62: 303–310.

150. Lambrigts D, Sachs DH, Cooper DK. Discordant organ xenotransplantation in primates: world experience and current status. Transplantation 1998; 66:547–561.

151. Li RK, Jia ZQ, Weisel RD, Mickle DA, Zhang J, Mohabeer MK, Rao V, Ivanov J. Cardiomyocyte transplantation improves heart function. Ann Thorac Surg 1996; 62:654–660.

152. Menasche P. Cell transplantation for the treatment of heart failure. Semin Thorac Cardiovasc Surg 2002; 14:157–166.

153. Kofidis T, Akhyari P, Wachsmann B, Boublik J, Mueller-Stahl K, Leyh R, Fischer S, Haverich A. A novel bioartificial myocardial tissue and its prospective use in cardiac surgery. Eur J Cardiothorac Surg 2002; 22:238–243.

24

Targeted Gene Transfer in Heart Failure

Roger J. Hajjar and Anthony Rosenzweig
The Program in Cardiovascular Gene Therapy, Cardiovascular Research Center and Cardiology Division, Massachusetts General Hospital, Harvard Medical School Boston, Massachusetts, USA

SUMMARY

Heart failure is a major cause of morbidity and mortality in the Western World, and as the population ages, the disease burden will continue to increase. Even though current treatments for heart failure have made significant progress in prolonging the survival of patients with heart failure, complete correction of ventricular function is still elusive in the treatment of heart failure. With the advent of novel intracellular targets involving cell contractility and survival, and increasingly efficient gene transfer methodologies, gene-based therapies are emerging as promising therapeutic strategies in patients afflicted with heart failure. Both viral and nonviral vector systems have been developed and continue to undergo improvements for gene delivery in the heart. Major advances in transcript analysis will ensure that many molecular targets will be available in the near future for targeting. In this chapter, we will provide an overview of gene delivery systems and vectors along with a number of targets that have had promising results in animal models of heart failure.

INTRODUCTION

Congestive heart failure (CHF) represents an enormous clinical problem demanding effective therapeutic approaches. Despite advances in approaches to its treatment, including novel pharmacologic management, myocardial revascularization, mechanical assist, and transplantation, CHF remains a leading cause of death in the United States and Europe [1,2]. Even though new treatments for congestive heart failure have had a significant impact on mortality and the course of the disease, they do not reverse or cure the underlying pathological state of the heart. The cells and microcirculation that make up the failing heart contribute to the contractile dysfunction are shown in Figure 1. The contributions of the microcirculation and fibroblasts to the phenotype of the failing heart are beyond the scope of this review [3,4]. Within the failing heart, there are many types of cardiomyocytes, including ones that have undergone either apoptosis or necrosis, diseased cardiomyocytes that are characterized by contractile dysfunction, and nondiseased cardiomyocytes that are exposed to neurohormonal stimulation and are at risk of becoming dysfunctional or

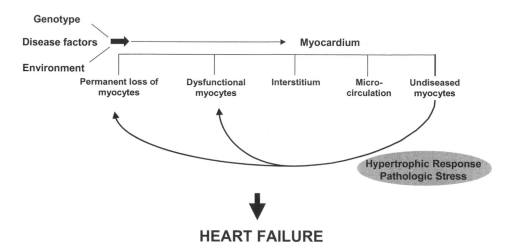

Figure 1 Cardiomyocytes, fibroblasts and microcirculation that make up the failing heart contribute to the contractile dysfunction observed in systolic heart failure. Within the failing heart, there are many types of cardiomyocytes, including ones that have undergone either apoptosis or necrosis, diseased cardiomyocytes that are characterized by contractile dysfunction, and nondiseased cardiomyocytes that are exposed to neurohormonal stimulation and are at risk of becoming dysfunctional or undergoing necrosis and apoptosis.

undergoing necrosis and apoptosis [5]. We have focused on using gene transfer to restore the diseased cardiomyocytes in order to improve contractile function and survival in failing cardiac myocytes [5]. Targets for gene transfer include membrane channels, intracellular transporters involved in calcium homeostasis, and other intracellular pathways involved in cell survival. The myopathic heart has a number of abnormalities that have been characterized at the cellular level, including changes at the level of the sarcolemma, sarcoplasmic reticulum, myofilaments, and mitochondria, all of which contribute to depressed contractile function and reserve. Identifying the mechanisms by which these changes contribute to the observed pathology is frequently confounded by simultaneous alterations in multiple signaling pathways in the complex milieu of the failing or myopathic heart. For this reason, gene transfer has the potential to alter our approach to understanding these different mechanisms in heart failure in two distinct, yet related, ways. First, the ability to genetically reprogram the heart in relevant in vitro and in vivo models of cardiovascular disease allows us to test the role of the specific restored molecular pathways in disease pathogenesis. In this way, mechanistic hypotheses can be tested and potential targets for therapeutic intervention can be identified. Gene transfer allows us to rapidly translate the latest developments in molecular and cell biology into clinically relevant models. Once validated, a potential target can be approached with the full spectrum of therapeutic options, including traditional pharmaceuticals, targeted synthesis of small molecule agonists or antagonists, biological agents (cells, antibodies, genetic material), or gene-based therapy. Undoubtedly, lessons gleaned from gene transfer experiments about local modulation of cardiac genetic programs will better guide attempts to transform early investigations into established therapy.

VECTORS FOR CARDIAC GENE DELIVERY

Vectors available for gene transfer have recently improved significantly [6,7]. A growing number of vectors are available for experimental and clinical gene transfer experiments

Table 1 Vector Systems for Gene Transfer

	Duration of Expression	Advantages	Disadvantages
Naked DNA	4–7 days	No viral proteins	Low efficiency, low level transgene expression that is transient
Adenovirus	7–28 days	High titer, high efficiency and level of transgene expression	Transient expression, immune/inflammatory response of host
Adeno-Associated Virus	Onset of expression at 4 weeks; long-term expression (? lifelong)	Long-term expression Evokes minimal immune response in host	Large-scale production remains difficult Limited insert size Integration can cause insertional mutagenesis and/or adverse activation of neighboring genes
Lentivirus (pseudo-typed virus)	Longterm (? lifelong)	Long term expression High efficiency	Large-scale production remains difficult Integration can cause insertional mutagenesis and/or adverse activation of neighboring genes Potential biosafety concerns because of relationship to HIV strains
Herpes virus/Amplicor	10–20 days	Large transgenes	Complex construction

[8] as shown in Table 1. Moreover, many of these systems are not applicable to cardiac gene transfer, which requires in vivo gene transfer (in contrast to *ex vivo* transduction of cells) to cells that are generally not replicating. For these reasons, discussion will focus on the systems most relevant to cardiac gene transfer.

Plasmid DNA

Plasmid DNA is often referred to as "naked DNA" to indicate the absence of a more elaborate packaging system. Over the past decade, multiple investigators have demonstrated the ability of the heart to take up and express genes directly injected as plasmids. A major advantage of this approach is that it avoids many of the biosafety concerns associated with viral vectors. However, in general the *level* of transgene expression and the *efficiency* of gene transfer (per cent of target cells expressing the transgene) are substantially lower with unmodified plasmid DNA than with more elaborate chemical or biological packaging systems. Whether the expression level and efficiency are adequate to achieve the experimental or clinical goals will depend on the particular application. For example, expression of secreted angiogenesis factors after muscle injection of plasmid DNA, despite relatively low levels of focal transgene expression, has demonstrated significant biological effects in animals models [9–11] and appears promising clinically. However, efforts to more directly target cardiac dysfunction have generally focused on gene transfer approaches that achieve more effective transgene expression, such as the viral vectors considered in the following text.

Adenoviruses

Recombinant adenoviral vectors offer several significant advantages for cardiac gene transfer. The viruses can be prepared at extremely high titer, infect nonreplicating cells, and confer high-efficiency and high-level transduction of cardiomyocytes in vivo after direct injection or perfusion approaches [12]. The major disadvantages to adenoviral gene transfer have been its transience and the immune response it evokes. In animal models, adenoviral gene transfer to adult myocardium in vivo has generally been found to mediate high-level expression for approximately 1 week [12–15]. Importantly, the immune response evoked does not appear to require transgene expression in professional antigen-presenting cells [16]. It does appear feasible to mitigate the inflammatory response and prolong transgene expression through a variety of other strategies. For example, further attenuation of adenoviral gene expression either through incorporation of specific mutations in additional early adenoviral genes, as in so-called "second generation" vectors [17] or recombinase-mediated deletion of virtually all the viral genes, as in "gutless" vectors [18], have both been reported to attenuate the host immune response and prolong transgene expression. Conversely, retention of some specific adenoviral genes involved in minimizing the inflammatory response are ordinarily deleted to make room for the transgene, may also help. For example, Wen and colleagues found that inclusion of the adenoviral E3 region in gene transfer vectors reduced vascular inflammation and neointima formation after arterial gene transfer in vivo [19]. However, little information is currently available about the long-term effects of such modified vectors in the cardiovascular system and large-scale, clinical-grade production of some of these vector designs remains problematic.

Adeno-Associated Viruses

Recombinant adeno-associated viruses (rAAV) are derived from nonpathogenic parvoviruses, evoke essentially no cellular immune response, and produce transgene expression lasting months in most systems [20–22]. They appear promising for sustained cardiac gene transfer [6,22,23]. In comparison with adenoviral gene transfer, cardiac injection of rAAV produces less initial but more sustained transgene expression [6,22,23]. rAAV vectors appear particularly promising for sustained expression of secreted gene products. Whether the expression level and efficiency produced by rAAV will also be sufficient to modulate overall cardiac function, as has been achieved with adenoviral vectors [24], remains to be seen. Although systems for initial generation and purification of rAAV have improved, large scale production for clinical applications remains challenging.

Lentiviruses

Lentiviruses are derived from a family of retroviruses that includes human immunodeficiency virus, and feline immunodeficiency virus. These viruses are have enveloped capsids and a plus-stranded RNA genome. As with other retroviruses, the RNA genome is converted to DNA by reverse transcriptase after infection and is then stably integrated into the host genome. However, unlike retroviruses that only infect dividing cells, lentiviruses can infect both dividing and nondividing cells. Lentiviruses have specific tropisms that restrict their targets. However, by pseudotyping the viral envelope with the envelope from vesicular stomatitis virus, lentiviruses have a much broader range. Importantly, lentiviral vectors have the ability, in contrast to standard retroviral vectors, to transduce both dividing and nonreplicating cells, critically important for cardiac gene transfer. As with other retroviruses, however, lentiviruses usually integrate into the host chromosomes, promoting stable transgene expression but potentially also inducing adverse effects through insertional mutagenesis or transactivation of neighboring genes [25,26]. Success with lentiviral gene transfer was first reported for HeLa cells and fibroblasts in vitro, as well as neurons in vivo [27,28]. Subsequently, lentiviral gene transfer has been reported in a wide variety of cell types, including cardiomyocytes [29–32].

Herpes Virus/Amplicons

Herpes Simplex 1 has a number of characteristics that make it a valuable gene delivery vector in vivo. There are two types of HSV-1 based vectors: (a) those produced by inserting the exogenous genes into a backbone virus genome, and (b) HSV amplicon virions, which are produced by inserting the exogenous gene into an amplicon plasmid that is subsequently replicated and then packaged into virion particles. HSV-1 can infect a wide variety of cells both dividing and nondividing but has strong tropism towards nerve cells. It has a very large genome size and can accommodate very large transgenes (>35 kb). In cardiovascular gene transfer, ryanodine receptors and titin (both very large proteins) have been successfully encoded in herpes viruses [33].

Concerns and Limitations

The biological advantages and limitations of the viral vectors have been detailed in the previous text and in Table 1. These vectors have also been used clinically with variable success. Through these early clinical experiences, a concerning number of complications have occurred. The most widely publicized case was that of Jesse Gelsinger. Gelsinger was a 17-year-old patient with partial ornithine transcarbamylase (OTC) deficiency, an X-linked defect of the urea cycle in which nitrogen metabolism is affected leading to a spectrum of neurological symptoms including seizures and mental retardation [34]. Therapy for the condition relies on alternative substrate administration, but mortality rates with the disease are high. Following the administration of an adenovirus carrying OTC, Gelsinger developed acute respiratory distress syndrome (ARDS) and died 2 days later of multiple organ failure. Measurements of inflammatory cytokines suggested that the vector had caused systemic inflammatory response syndrome and suggested that activation of the complement cascade may have played an important role [35,36]. This case illustrated that the immune response mounted against the viral vectors not only limits the efficiency of such vectors but can have catastrophic consequences.

Cardiac gene delivery

A number of mechanical approaches have been used to transduce myocardium using adenoviral vectors. Techniques used have included intracoronary catheter delivery, direct injection into the myocardium, intraventricular delivery with retroinfusion of the coronary vein, and injection of adenovirus into the pericardial sac [14,37–40]. Most of these approaches lead to focal transduction of the myocardium, with viral expression in only specified regional areas of the heart. This may not be adequate in heart failure where effective therapy may requires generalized transduction of the heart. More recently, a new technique for cardiac gene delivery has been developed in rodents that involves injecting adenovirus into the aortic root just above the aortic valve, while the aorta and pulmonary artery are transiently cross-clamped [37]. This technique achieved relatively homogeneous and diffuse transduction of the myocardium, and has also been shown to produce transgene-specific physiological effects on ventricular function in vivo. More recently, the cross-clamping technique was extended to hamsters where cooling the animals allowed prolonged cross-clamping (~5 minutes) and better efficiency of gene transfer [41]. Further animal studies have established that in vivo adenoviral gene transfer can not only achieve transgene expression in the myocardium but also modulate intrinsic functional properties of the intact heart. These studies have also been extended to larger animals and have involved retrograde perfusion through the coronary sinus and cardiopulmonary bypass with viral perfusion to the heart. These latter approaches may be more amenable to translation into the clinical arena.

CALCIUM HANDLING IN HEART FAILURE

The myopathic heart exhibits abnormalities in both the systolic and diastolic phase. Changes in diastolic function often appear earlier than systolic dysfunction. In fact, compensated hypertrophy phenotypically demonstrates impaired relaxation parameters in the presence of normal or increased systolic function [42]. Abnormalities in calcium handling were noted more than 15 years ago when calcium transients recorded with the calcium indicator aequorin from trabeculae from myopathic human hearts removed at the time of cardiac transplantation revealed a significantly prolonged calcium transient with an elevated end-diastolic intracellular calcium [43]. These defects were subsequently found in single isolated cardiomyocytes loaded with the fluorescent indicator Fura-2 from myopathic hearts [44]. The calcium transients were characterized as having elevated diastolic calcium levels, a decreased systolic Ca^{2+}, and prolonged relaxation phase. Studies both in muscle strips and isolated cardiomyocytes found that systolic calcium concentration were decreased in the failing state, while diastolic calcium concentration were elevated [44]. These differences were accentuated at higher stimulation rates.

The slow relaxation and abnormal force-frequency relationship observed in isolated muscles as well as in isolated myocytes from failing hearts, suggest a deficiency in calcium reuptake by the sarcoplasmic reticulum (SR). Calcium transport into the SR occurs via the SR calcium ATPase calcium pump (SERCA2a). Failing hearts have been characterized by defects in SR function. Specifically, "relaxation abnormalities" correlated with deficient SR Ca^{2+} uptake have been associated with a decreased expression level of SR Ca^{2+}-ATPase and reduction in SR Ca^{2+}-ATPase activity [45–49]. A number of investigators have shown that the levels of SERCA2a message and protein to be consistently decreased in heart failure [45–51] in relation to phospholamban. Associated with a decrease in mRNA, there is a decrease in SR Ca^{2+}-ATPase activity and SR Ca^{2+} uptake from SR vesicles and membranes isolated from failing human heart as shown in Figure 2. Indeed, in experiments where the SR vesicles were isolated from human hearts, vesicles from failing human hearts had decreased rates of Ca^{2+} uptake when compared with normal hearts. Furthermore, the SR Ca^{2+} ATPase activity is inversely related to diastolic calcium (Fig. 2) [45–51]. In failing hearts diastolic calcium is elevated and ATPase activity low relative to normal hearts.

Calcium is removed from the cytosol by the sarcolemmal Na^+/Ca^{2+} exchanger, which has high capacity but low affinity and is the major calcium extrusion mechanism of the cardiac myocyte [52]. This system returns calcium concentrations to diastolic levels (~100–300 nM) and may, therefore, contribute significantly to myocardial relaxation.

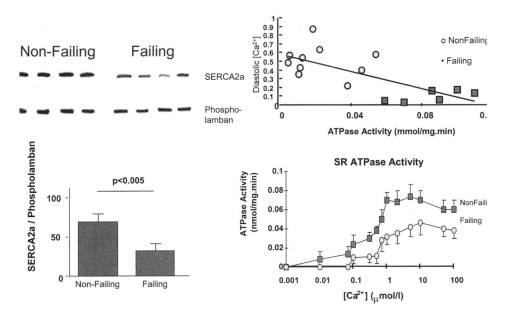

Figure 2 Failing hearts are characterized by reduced SERCA2a protein levels as shown in the *upper left panel*. Relative to phospholamban, SERCA2a levels are substantially decreased as shown in the *bottom left panel*. The decrease in SERCA2a activity is inversely related to diastolic calcium as shown in the *upper right panel*. Throughout a large range of calcium concentration, SERCA2a activity is decreased in failing hearts as shown in *lower right panel*.

Most studies indicate that mRNA and protein levels of the Na^+/Ca^{2+} exchanger are increased in human myopathic hearts, but not in all preparations [52–55]. Likewise, studies find the functional capacity of the Na^+/Ca^{2+} exchanger to transport calcium is increased. The consequence of an increased activity of the Na^+/Ca^{2+} exchanger in failing hearts may be to compensate for the reduction in SR Ca^{2+}-ATPase activity. Increased activity of the Na^+/Ca^{2+} exchanger should aid in myocardial relaxation, albeit at the cost of reduced calcium release from the SR during systole. This would be particularly evident at higher rates of stimulation and, thus, lead to a blunted frequency response as is commonly seen in myopathic human myocardium.

The Na^+/Ca^{2+} exchanger can operate to bring calcium into the cell or extrude calcium out from the cell [52–56]. There is an increase in sensitivity to compounds that produce positive inotropic effects through raised intracellular Na^+, either by inhibiting the Na/K-ATPase or by opening Na^+ channels, in muscle strips from failing human hearts. It has been suggested that the relaxation abnormalities produced by the loss of SERCA2a activity could be, at least partially, compensated for by an increase in the activity of the Na^+/Ca^{2+} exchanger [52–58].

GENE TRANSFER OF CALCIUM HANDLING PROTEINS

Gene transfer provides a unique opportunity to manipulate the expression of essential proteins and alter the expression of specific downstream signaling pathways implicated in the pathogenesis of heart failure. Contractile dysfunction of the myocardium results from abnormalities in many subcellular mechanisms. Specifically, three major areas of calcium handling have been targeted: the calcium handling proteins involved in excitation-contraction coupling, potassium channels and their role in arrhythmia genesis, and abnormalities in neurohormonal receptors–specifically the beta-adrenoceptor signaling pathways as shown in Figure 3.

Adenoviral gene transfer has been instrumental in elucidating the molecular basis of these abnormalities, and has also shown that many of these changes seen in excitation-contraction coupling can be halted and even reversed in failing myocardium. Gene transfer of SERCA2a, for example, has been shown to lead to an increase in SR Ca^{2+} ATPase activity, an increase in the amount of Ca^{2+} released, a faster relaxation phase, and a decrease in diastolic calcium [13,59,60]. Conversely, using gene transfer to increase phospholamban relative to SERCA 2a in isolated myocytes, simulates abnormalities of calcium handling seen in failing ventricular myocardium [12,61]. These include prolongation of the relaxation phase of the calcium transient, a decrease in Ca^{2+} release, and increase in resting Ca. Furthermore, overexpressing SERCA2a can largely rescue the phenotype created by increasing the phospholamban/SERCA2a ratio. More recently, restoration of SERCA2a in failing human cardiomyocytes was shown to restore the contractile function of these failing human cells to normal as shown in Figure 4 [59]. This study validated the premise that targeting SERCA2a by gene transfer may offer a new therapeutic modality in patients with heart failure.

SERCA2a
Phospholamban
Kv4.3
Na/Ca Exchanger
Phosphatases

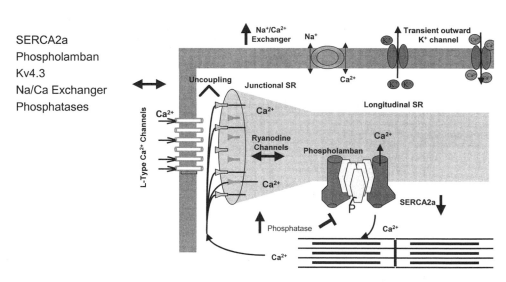

Figure 3 Excitation-contraction coupling in heart failure and molecular targets amenable to gene therapy. Excitation of the cardiac cell induces the entry of a small amount of calcium, which in turn causes the release of a larger amount of calcium from the sarcoplasmic reticulum, which in turn activates the myofilaments and eventually produces force. During relaxation, most of the calcium is taken up by SERCA2a back into the SR and a smaller amount of the calcium is extruded outside the cell by the Na/Ca exchanger. SERCA2a is under the endogenous control of phospholamban, a protein that when unphosphorylated inhibits SERCA2a and when phosphorylated the inhibition is removed. The action potential duration is also determined by the transient outward current, which is dependent on he expression of the potassium channel (Kv4.3). In heart failure, there is a downregulation of SERCA2a, an increase in Na^+/Ca^{++} exchanges and a decrease in Kv4.3, which constitute targets for molecular repair.

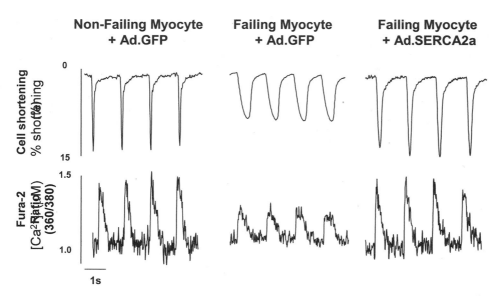

Figure 4 Effect of adenoviral gene transfer of SERCA2a (Ad.SERCA2a) in failing cardiac myocytes loaded with the fluorescent calcium indicator, Fura-2. In failing cardiac myocytes (infected with the adenovirus carrying the reporter gene green fluorescent protein, GFP), contraction amplitude is decreased and prolonged compared to nonfailing cardiac myocytes. Gene transfer of SERCA2a in the failing cardiac myocytes restores contraction to normal levels. (From Ref. 59.)

We recently investigated whether increasing SERCA2a expression can improve ventricular function in a rat model of pressure-overload hypertrophy and failure. After 19 to 23 weeks of banding, during the transition from compensated hypertrophy to heart failure, overexpression of SERCA2a restored both SERCA2a expression and ATPase activity to nonfailing levels. Furthermore, rats infected with Ad.SERCA2a had significant improvement in left ventricular systolic pressure (LVSP), +dP/dt, -dP/dt, and rate of isovolumic relaxation normalizing them back to levels comparable to sham-operated rats [62]. Load independent parameters of contractility also improved. More recently, transfer of SER-CA2a in a rat model of heart failure was shown to effectively decrease mortality [13]. In fact, survival was increased significantly in animals receiving gene transfer compared with those who did not (63% vs. 9%) as shown in Figure 5. Furthermore, cardiac metabolism measured by the ratio of creatine phosphate to ATP was also restored to normal. The restoration of the energetics was surprising because enhanced contractility is associated with increased energy demand. The fact that gene transfer of SERCA2a was not associated with a compromise in energetics means that a beneficial remodeling occurred within the cardiac cell restoring the metabolic machinery. The decrease in diastolic calcium seen with restoration of SERCA 2a levels to normal has also been postulated to reduce proapoptotic and prohypertrophic signaling (as sustained elevations of intracellular calcium lead to activation of serine-threonine phosphatases, including calcineurin, inducing hypertrophy and cell death).

β-ADRENERGIC SIGNALING

The β-adrenergic signaling pathway provides an important target for intervention in heart failure. β-adrenergic signaling defects including downregulation of myocardial adrenergic

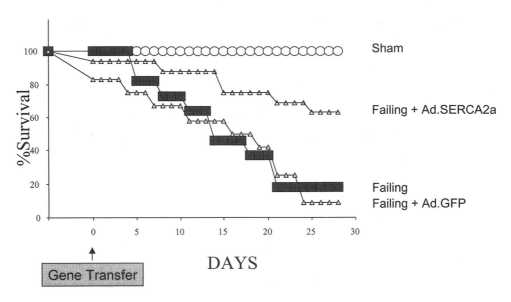

Figure 5 Survival curves in failing rats compared with failing rats who have received SER-CA2a gene transfer. Note the improved survival compared with failing rats who either had no gene transfer or received the reporter gene GFP (Ad.GFP). (From Ref. 13.)

receptors, β-AR uncoupling, and an upregulation of the β-AR kinase (β24ARK1) are central features of human and animal heart failure. In isolated ventricular myocytes from a model of heart failure in the rabbit, adenoviral gene transfer of the human β2-AR or an inhibitor of β ARK1 led to the restoration of β-AR signaling and an increase in cytosolic cAMP levels [63]. More recently overexpression of an inhibitor of β ARK1 by gene transfer of a truncated and dysfunctional βARK1 (β ARKct) rescued function in a model of left ventricular dysfunction in the rabbit [64]. These studies along with the finding that overexpression of β ARKct prevents the development of cardiomyopathy in a murine model of heart failure emphasize importance of β-adrenergic signaling defects in the pathogenesis of heart failure and raises the possibility that targeting this system may restore function in failing cardiomyocytes [65,66]. However, stimulation of the β-adrenergic system induces an increase in intracellular cAMP which, when sustained, can be cardiotoxic and arrhythmogenic. In fact overexpression of the β_1 receptor induces fibrosis, severe left ventricular dysfunction and arrhythmias [67]. It is possible that this mechanism may underlie the clinical observation that inotropic interventions that increase cellular cAMP increase mortality in chronic heart failure. In fact, a recent study found that in mice overexpressing β_2-adrenergic receptors development of heart failure was exacerbated when these mice were subjected to aortic stenosis. Moreover, the transgenic mice had more severe left ventricular dysfunction and higher incidence of premature deaths. Interestingly, intracoronary injection of a recombinant adenovirus encoding adenylyl cyclase provided enduring increases in cardiac function in normal pigs even though adenylyl cyclase modulates cAMP [68]. Nevertheless, the critical role of the β-adrenergic pathway suggests further investigation of this pathway as a target for intervention despite the cautionary clinical and experimental experience of direct β-agonism. As shown in Figure 6, a summary of the effects of overexpressing SERCA2a by gene transfer on cAMP, intracellular calcium, arrhythmias, survival, and energetics while at the same time enhancing contractility point toward an overall beneficial effect of this mode of inotropy over conventional inotropic agents.

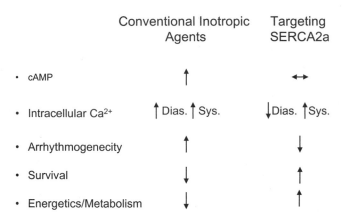

Figure 6 Differences in conventional treatment for heart failure vs. targeting specifically SERCA2a on survival, cAMP, calcium handling, energetics, and arrhythmogenic potential.

SURVIVAL SIGNALING

Cardiomyocyte programmed cell death or has been identified in a wide variety of human cardiac disorders including myocardial infarction, congestive heart failure, dilated cardiomyopathy, and arrhythmogenic right ventricular dysplasia [69–72]. However, although apoptosis has been documented in many settings, quantitation of the number of apoptotic cells in human heart disease has varied widely and the role of this process in the pathophysiology of disease remains controversial [70,71]. However, multiple studies suggest that apoptosis and the caspase proteases central to this process play a role in the pathogenesis of cardiac disease. Transgenic cardiac expression of a ligand-activatable procaspase-8 is causes dilated cardiomyopathy [73] that can be prevented by administration of a broadspectrum caspase inhibitor [74]. In addition, mice with a cardiac-specific deletion of the gp130 cytokine receptor develop massive myocyte apoptosis and cardiomyopathy in response to pressure overload [75]. These important studies suggest apoptosis can induce cardiomyopathy in genetic murine models that either lack endogenous protective signaling mechanisms (gp130 knock-out) or in which caspases are activated. However, the therapeutic potential of antiapoptotic interventions in more common cardiac diseases remains incompletely delineated. Pharmacologic caspase inhibition reduces both DNA fragmentation and infarct size after transient ischemia [76,77]. Such studies encourage consideration of apoptosis as a therapeutic target. However, clinically meaningful rescue of cardiomyocytes obviously requires not only inhibition of apoptosis, but also prevention of other mechanisms of cell death as well as restoration of function (as previously discussed). As presented in the following text, evidence suggests that specific signaling pathways can mediate favorable effects on cardiomyocyte survival and function, and thus hold promise as the basis for therapeutic intervention.

In many systems, activation of PI 3-kinase and its downstream serine-threonine kinase effector, Akt (or Protein Kinase B), provide potent prosurvival signals likely working through multiple downstream effectors. In cardiomyocytes, IGF-I activates PI 3-kinase and Akt, and activation of PI 3-kinase appears necessary for the antiapoptotic effects of IGF-I in cardiomyocytes [78]. Adenoviral gene transfer of constitutively active mutants of both PI 3-kinase and Akt reduce cardiomyocyte apoptosis in vitro and gene transfer of constitutively active Akt to the heart in vivo substantially reduces cardiomyocyte apoptosis as well as infarct size after transient ischemia [79]. Importantly, Akt activation also substantially improves regional and overall cardiac function [79]. This remarkable degree of functional rescue appears related to the ability of Akt activation to not only block myocyte apoptosis, but also to preserve excitation-contraction coupling in surviving cells [79]. Moreover, inhibition of Akt activity with a dominant negative construct accelerates hypoxia-induced cardiomyocyte dysfunction, suggesting the signaling via endogenous Akt is playing a protective role as well [79]. The clinical implication of these observations are that the benefits of Akt activation (or similar interventions) may be even greater than one would predict based simply on the number of apoptotic cardiomyocytes. It is possible that apoptotic signaling contributes to overall cardiac dysfunction both through direct *loss* of cardiomyocytes and *dysfunction* of surviving cardiomyocytes and thus may be a particularly attractive target for therapeutic intervention.

The studies previously mentioned suggest an important role for Akt in myocyte survival and function. However, the practical implications of this finding may be limited by the cell autonomous nature of the protective effect. Effective therapy through gene transfer of such a gene product would require transduction of a large number of cardiomyocytes. As noted, several approaches to these appear promising and may be extrapolated into clinical application. However, an alternative approach to modulating cardiomyocyte survival would be to express a secreted ligand that activates these signaling pathways locally. One example of such a ligand would be IGF-I. However, prior clinical studies have suggested that elevated systemic IGF-I levels may be linked to an increased risk of cancer, as well as hypotension and hypoglycemia after acute administration [80–84]. Interestingly, gene transfer of IGF-I protects cardiomyocytes from hypoxia-induced apoptosis in both an autocrine and paracrine manner [85]. Moreover, in vivo gene transfer of IGF-I significantly reduces infarct size after transient ischemia *without* increasing serum levels of IGF-I. Thus, ultimately, local expression of a secreted prosurvival ligand may have strategic advantages over either systemic peptide delivery or expression of downstream effectors.

FUTURE DIRECTIONS

Substantial progress has been made in vector technology, cardiac gene delivery, and our understanding of heart failure pathogenesis. These advances make consideration of gene therapy for heart failure a reasonable consideration at this time. Multiple targets are undergoing consideration. Currently, strategies that enhance sarcoplasmic calcium transport are supported by substantial evidence in both cardiomyocytes derived from patients with heart failure and in animal models and in vivo animal studies. Initial studies evaluating other novel targets appear promising but have not been as fully evaluated. In ongoing efforts to target cardiac dysfunction, gene transfer provides an important tool to improve our understanding of the relative contribution of specific pathways. In this way, specific therapeutic targets can be validated for intervention whether pharmacologic or genetic. However, formidable challenges remain to translating the results of these basic studies into clinical gene therapy for heart failure. Further development of concepts established in rodent models will be required in large animal models with clinical grade vectors and delivery systems to evaluate both efficacy and safety of these approaches. Nevertheless, both the practical advances in vector and delivery systems, as well as a growing insight into the molecular pathogenesis of heart failure provide reason for cautious optimism.

REFERENCES

1. Levy D, Garrison RJ, Savage DD, Kannel WB, Castelli WP. Prognostic implications of echocardiographically determined left ventricular mass in the Framingham Heart Study. N Engl J Med 1990; 322:1561–1566.

2. Cowie MR, Wood DA, Coats AJ, Thompson SG, Poole-Wilson PA, Suresh V, Sutton GC. Incidence and aetiology of heart failure; a population-based study. Eur Heart J 1999; 20: 421–428.

3. Gavin JB, Maxwell L, Edgar SG. Microvascular involvement in cardiac pathology. J Mol Cell Cardiol 1998; 30:2531–2540.

4. Swynghedauw B. Molecular mechanisms of myocardial remodeling. Physiol Rev 1999; 79: 215–262.

5. Hajjar RJ, del Monte F, Matsui T, Rosenzweig A. Prospects for gene therapy for heart failure. Circ Res 2000; 86:616–621.

6. Gao GP, Wilson JM, Wivel NA. Production of recombinant adeno-associated virus. Adv Virus Res 2000; 55:529–543.

7. Cemazar M, Sersa G, Wilson J, Tozer GM, Hart SL, Grosel A, Dachs GU. Effective gene transfer to solid tumors using different nonviral gene delivery techniques: electroporation, liposomes, and integrin-targeted vector. Cancer Gene Ther 2002; 9:399–406.

8. Rosenzweig A, EdVectors for Gene Therapy. New York: John Wiley & Sons 2001.

9. Isner JM. Myocardial gene therapy. Nature 2002; 415:234–239.

10. Marban E. Cardiac channelopathies. Nature 2002; 415:213–218.

11. Towbin JA, Bowles NE. The failing heart. Nature 2002; 415:227–233.

12. Hajjar RJ, Schmidt U, Matsui T, Guerrero JL, Lee KH, Gwathmey JK, Dec GW, Semigran MJ, Rosenzweig A. Modulation of ventricular function through gene transfer in vivo. Proc Natl Acad Sci USA 1998; 95:5251–5256.

13. del Monte F, William E, Lebeche D, Schmidt U, Rosenzweig A, Gwathmey JK, Lewandowski DE, Hajjar RJ. Improvement in survival and cardiac metabolism following gene transfer of SERCA2a in a rat model of heart failure. Circulation 2001; 104:1424–1429.

14. del Monte F, Butler K, Boecker W, Gwathmey JK, Hajjar RJ. Novel technique of aortic banding followed by gene transfer during hypertrophy and heart failure. Physiol Genomics 2002; 9:49–56.

15. del Monte F, Harding SE, Dec GW, Gwathmey JK, Hajjar RJ. Targeting phospholamban by gene transfer in human heart failure. Circulation 2002; 105:904–907.

16. Prasad SA, Norbury CC, Chen W, Bennink JR, Yewdell JW. Cutting edge: recombinant adenoviruses induce CD8 T cell responses to an inserted protein whose expression is limited to nonimmune cells. J Immunol 2001; 166:4809–4812.

17. Engelhardt JF, Ye X, Doranz B, Wilson JM. Ablation of E2A in recombinant adenoviruses improves transgene persistence and decreases inflammatory response in mouse liver. Proc Natl Acad Sci USA 1994; 91:6196–6200.

18. Kochanek S, Clemens PR, Mitani K, Chen HH, Chan S, Caskey CT. A new adenoviral vector: replacement of all viral coding sequences with 28 kb of DNA independently expressing both full-length dystrophin and beta-galactosidase. Proc Natl Acad Sci USA 1996; 93:5731–5736.

19. Wen S, Driscoll RM, Schneider DB, Dichek DA. Inclusion of the E3 region in an adenoviral vector decreases inflammation and neointima formation after arterial gene transfer. Arterioscler Thromb Vasc Biol 2001; 21:1777–1782.

20. Ng P, Parks RJ, Cummings DT, Evelegh CM, Sankar U, Graham FL. A high-efficiency Cre/loxP-based system for construction of adenoviral vectors. Hum Gene Ther 1999; 10: 2667–2672.

21. Cordier L, Gao GP, Hack AA, McNally EM, Wilson JM, Chirmule N, Sweeney HL. Muscle-specific promoters may be necessary for adeno-associated virus- mediated gene transfer in the treatment of muscular dystrophies. Hum Gene Ther 2001; 12:205–215.

22. Ng P, Evelegh C, Cummings D, Graham FL. Cre levels limit packaging signal excision efficiency in the Cre/loxP helper-dependent adenoviral vector system. J Virol 2002; 76:4181–4189.

23. Gao G, Qu G, Burnham MS, Huang J, Chirmule N, Joshi B, Yu QC, Marsh JA, Conceicao CM, Wilson JM. Purification of recombinant adeno-associated virus vectors by column chromatography and its performance in vivo. Hum Gene Ther 2000; 11:2079–2091.

24. Svensson EC, Marshall DJ, Woodard K, Lin H, Jiang F, Chu L, Leiden JM. Efficient and stable transduction of cardiomyocytes after intramyocardial injection or intracoronary perfusion with recombinant adeno-associated virus vectors. Circulation 1999; 99:201–205.

25. Check E. Second cancer case halts gene-therapy trials. Nature 2003; 421:305.
26. Hacein-Bey-Abina S, von Kalle C, Schmidt M, Le Deist F, Wulffraat N, McIntyre E, Radford I, Villeval JL, Fraser CC, Cavazzana-Calvo M, Fischer A. A serious adverse event after successful gene therapy for X-linked severe combined immunodeficiency. N Engl J Med 2003; 348:255–256.
27. Naldini L, Blomer U, Gallay P, Ory D, Mulligan R, Gage FH, Verma IM, Trono D. In vivo gene delivery and stable transduction of nondividing cells by a lentiviral vector. Science 1996; 272:263–267.
28. Naldini L, Blomer U, Gage FH, Trono D, Verma IM. Efficient transfer, integration, and sustained long-term expression of the transgene in adult rat brains injected with a lentiviral vector. Proc Natl Acad Sci U S A 1996; 93:11382–11388.
29. Sakoda T, Kasahara N, Hamamori Y, Kedes L. A high-titer lentiviral production system mediates efficient transduction of differentiated cells including beating cardiac myocytes. J Mol Cell Cardiol 1999; 31:2037–2047.
30. Peng KW, Pham L, Ye H, Zufferey R, Trono D, Cosset FL, Russell SJ. Organ distribution of gene expression after intravenous infusion of targeted and untargeted lentiviral vectors. Gene Ther 2001; 8:1456–1463.
31. MacKenzie TC, Kobinger GP, Kootstra NA, Radu A, Sena-Esteves M, Bouchard S, Wilson JM, Verma IM, Flake AW. Efficient transduction of liver and muscle after in utero injection of lentiviral vectors with different pseudotypes. Mol Ther 2002; 6:349–358.
32. Zhao J, Pettigrew GJ, Thomas J, Vandenberg JI, Delriviere L, Bolton EM, Carmichael A, Martin JL, Marber MS, Lever AM. Lentiviral vectors for delivery of genes into neonatal and adult ventricular cardiac myocytes in vitro and in vivo. Basic Res Cardiol 2002; 97:348–358.
33. Goins WF, Krisky DM, Wolfe DP, Fink DJ, Glorioso JC. Development of replication-defective herpes simplex virus vectors. Methods Mol Med 2002; 69:481–507.
34. Hollon T. Researchers and regulators reflect on first gene therapy death. Nat Med 2000; 6:6.
35. Bostanci A. Gene therapy. Blood test flags agent in death of Penn subject. Science 2002; 295:604–605.
36. Marshall E. Gene therapy death prompts review of adenovirus vector. Science 1999; 286:2244–2245.
37. Hajjar RJ, Schmidt U, Matsui T, Guerrero JL, Lee KH, Gwathmey JK, Dec GW, Semigran MJ, Rosenzweig A. Modulation of ventricular function through gene transfer in vivo. Proc Natl Acad Sci USA 1998; 95:5251–5256.
38. Donahue JK, Kikkawa K, Thomas AD, Marban E, Lawrence JH. Acceleration of widespread adenoviral gene transfer to intact rabbit hearts by coronary perfusion with low calcium and serotonin. Gene Ther 1998; 5:630–634.
39. Fromes Y, Salmon A, Wang X, Collin H, Rouche A, Hagege A, Schwartz K, Fiszman MY. Gene delivery to the myocardium by intrapericardial injection. Gene Ther 1999; 6:683–688.
40. Guzman RJ, Lemarchand P, Crystal RG, Epstein SE, Finkel T. Efficient gene transfer into myocardium by direct injection of adenovirus vectors. Circ Res 1993; 73:1202–1207.
41. Ikeda Y, Gu Y, Iwanaga Y, Hoshijima M, Oh SS, Giordano FJ, Chen J, Nigro V, Peterson KL, Chien KR, Ross J. Restoration of deficient membrane proteins in the cardiomyopathic hamster by in vivo cardiac gene transfer. Circulation 2002; 105:502–508.
42. Gwathmey JK, Morgan JP. Altered calcium handling in experimental pressure-overload hypertrophy in the ferret. Circ Res 1985; 57:836–843.
43. Gwathmey JK, Copelas L, MacKinnon R, Schoen FJ, Feldman MD, Grossman W, Morgan JP. Abnormal intracellular calcium handling in myocardium from patients with end-stage heart failure. Circ Res 1987; 61:70–76.
44. Beuckelmann DJ, Nabauer M, Erdmann E. Intracellular calcium handling in isolated ventricular myocytes from patients with terminal heart failure [see comments]. Circulation 1992; 85:1046–1055.
45. Hasenfuss G, Reinecke H, Studer R, Meyer M, Pieske B, Holtz J, Holubarsch C, Posival H, Just H, Drexler H. Relation between myocardial function and expression of sarcoplasmic

reticulum Ca(2 +)-ATPase in failing and nonfailing human myocardium. Circ Res 1994; 75: 434–442.

46. Hasenfuss G, Reinecke H, Studer R, Pieske B, Meyer M, Drexler H, Just H. Calcium cycling proteins and force-frequency relationship in heart failure. Basic Res Cardiol 1996; 91(suppl 2):17–22.

47. Hasenfuss G. Calcium pump overexpression and myocardial function. Implications for gene therapy of myocardial failure. Circ Res 1998; 83:966–968.

48. Schmidt U, Hajjar RJ, Helm PA, Kim CS, Doye AA, Gwathmey JK. Contribution of abnormal sarcoplasmic reticulum ATPase activity to systolic and diastolic dysfunction in human heart failure. J Mol Cell Cardiol 1998; 30:1929–1937.

49. Schmidt U, Hajjar RJ, Kim CS, Lebeche D, Doye AA, Gwathmey JK. Human heart failure: cAMP stimulation of SR Ca(2 +)-ATPase activity and phosphorylation level of phospholamban. Am J Physiol 1999; 277:H474–H480.

50. Meyer M, Dillmann WH. Sarcoplasmic reticulum Ca(2 +)-ATPase overexpression by adenovirus mediated gene transfer and in transgenic mice. Cardiovasc Res 1998; 37:360–366.

51. Schwinger RH, Bohm M, Schmidt U, Karczewski P, Bavendiek U, Flesch M, Krause EG, Erdmann E. Unchanged protein levels of SERCA II and phospholamban but reduced Ca2 + uptake and Ca(2 +)-ATPase activity of cardiac sarcoplasmic reticulum from dilated cardiomyopathy patients compared with patients with nonfailing hearts. Circulation 1995; 92: 3220–3228.

52. Bers DM. Cardiac Na/Ca exchange function in rabbit, mouse and man: what's the difference?. J Mol Cell Cardiol 2002; 34:369–373.

53. Hasenfuss G, Schillinger W, Lehnart SE, Preuss M, Pieske B, Maier LS, Prestle J, Minami K, Just H. Relationship between Na + -Ca2 + -exchanger protein levels and diastolic function of failing human myocardium. Circulation 1999; 99:641–648.

54. Pogwizd SM, Qi M, Yuan W, Samarel AM, Bers DM. Upregulation of Na(+)/Ca(2 +) exchanger expression and function in an arrhythmogenic rabbit model of heart failure. Circ Res 1999; 85:1009–1019.

55. Pogwizd SM, Schlotthauer K, Li L, Yuan W, Bers DM. Arrhythmogenesis and contractile dysfunction in heart failure: roles of sodium-calcium exchange, inward rectifier potassium current, and residual beta-adrenergic responsiveness. Circ Res 2001; 88:1159–1167.

56. Studer R, Reinecke H, Bilger J, Eschenhagen T, Bohm M, Hasenfuss G, Just H, Holtz J, Drexler H. Gene expression of the cardiac Na(+)-Ca2 + exchanger in end-stage human heart failure. Circ Res 1994; 75:443–453.

57. Brittsan AG, Carr AN, Schmidt AG, Kranias EG. Maximal inhibition of SERCA2 Ca(2 +) affinity by phospholamban in transgenic hearts overexpressing a non-phosphorylatable form of phospholamban. J Biol Chem 2000; 275:12129–12135.

58. Carr AN, Schmidt AG, Suzuki Y, del Monte F, Sato Y, Lanner C, Breeden K, Jing SL, Allen PB, Greengard P, Yatani A, Hoit BD, Grupp IL, Hajjar RJ, DePaoli-Roach AA, Kranias EG. Type 1 phosphatase, a negative regulator of cardiac function. Mol Cell Biol 2002; 22: 4124–4135.

59. del Monte F, Harding SE, Schmidt U, Matsui T, Kang ZB, Dec GW, Gwathmey JK, Rosenzweig A, Hajjar RJ. Restoration of contractile function in isolated cardiomyocytes from failing human hearts by gene transfer of SERCA2a. Circulation 1999; 100:2308–2311.

60. Hajjar RJ, Kang JX, Gwathmey JK, Rosenzweig A. Physiological effects of adenoviral gene transfer of sarcoplasmic reticulum calcium ATPase in isolated rat myocytes. Circulation 1997; 95:423–429.

61. Hajjar RJ, Schmidt U, Kang JX, Matsui T, Rosenzweig A. Adenoviral gene transfer of phospholamban in isolated rat cardiomyocytes rescue efects by concomitant gene transfer of sarcoplasmic reticulum Ca2 + ATPase. Circ Res 1997; 81:145–153.

62. Miyamoto MI, del Monte F, Schmidt U, DiSalvo TS, Kang ZB, Matsui T, Guerrero JL, Gwathmey JK, Rosenzweig A, Hajjar RJ. Adenoviral gene transfer of SERCA2a improves left-ventricular function in aortic-banded rats in transition to heart failure. Proc Natl Acad Sci USA 2000; 97:793–798.

63. Maurice JP, Hata JA, Shah AS, White DC, McDonald PH, Dolber PC, Wilson KH, Lefkowitz RJ, Glower DD, Koch WJ. Enhancement of cardiac function after adenoviral-mediated in vivo intracoronary beta2-adrenergic receptor gene delivery. J Clin Invest 1999; 104:21–29.

64. Tevaearai HT, Eckhart AD, Shotwell KF, Wilson K, Koch WJ. Ventricular dysfunction after cardioplegic arrest is improved after myocardial gene transfer of a beta-adrenergic receptor kinase inhibitor. Circulation 2001; 104:2069–2074.

65. Rockman HA, Chien KR, Choi DJ, Iaccarino G, Hunter JJ, Ross J, Lefkowitz RJ, Koch WJ. Expression of a beta-adrenergic receptor kinase 1 inhibitor prevents the development of myocardial failure in gene-targeted mice. Proc Natl Acad Sci USA 1998; 95:7000–7005.

66. Shah AS, White DC, Tai O, Hata JA, Wilson KH, Pippen A, Kypson AP, Glower DD, Lefkowitz RJ, Koch WJ. Adenovirus-mediated genetic manipulation of the myocardial beta- adrenergic signaling system in transplanted hearts. J Thorac Cardiovasc Surg 2000; 120:581–588.

67. Engelhardt S, Hein L, Wiesmann F, Lohse MJ. Progressive hypertrophy and heart failure in beta1-adrenergic receptor transgenic mice. Proc Natl Acad Sci USA 1999; 96:7059–7064.

68. Lai NC, Roth DM, Gao MH, Fine S, Head BP, Zhu J, McKirnan MD, Kwong C, Dalton N, Urasawa K, Roth DA, Hammond HK. Intracoronary delivery of adenovirus encoding adenylyl cyclase VI increases left ventricular function and cAMP-generating capacity. Circulation 2000; 102:2396–2401.

69. Saraste A, Pulkki K, Kallajoki M, Henriksen K, Parvinen M, Voipio-Pulkki LM. Apoptosis in human acute myocardial infarction. Circulation 1997; 95:320–323.

70. Narula J, Haider N, Virmani R, DiSalvo TG, Kolodgie DF, Hajjar RJ, Schmidt U, Semigran MJ, Dec GW, Khaw BA. Apoptosis in myocytes in end-stage heart failure. N Engl J Med 1996; 335:1182–1189.

71. Olivetti G, Abbi R, Quaini F, Kajstura J, Cheng W, Nitahara JA, Quaini E, Di LC, Beltrami CA, Krajewski S, Reed JC, Anversa P. Apoptosis in the failing human heart. N Engl J Med 1997; 336:1131–1141.

72. Mallat Z, Tedgui A, Fontaliran F, Frank R, Durigon M, Fontaine G. Evidence of apoptosis in arrhythmogenic right ventricular dysplasia. N Engl J Med 1996; 335:1190–1196.

73. Wencker D, Nguyen N, Khine CC, Chandra M, Garantziotis S, Ng K, Factor SM, Shirani J, Kitsis RN. Myocyte apoptosis is sufficient to cause dilated cardiomyopathy. Circulation 1999; 100:I-83.

74. Wencker D, Chandra M, Armstrong RC, Garantziotis S, Factor SM, Shirani J, Kitsis RN. Rescue of dilated cardiomyopathy by caspase inhibition in FKBP-caspase-8 transgenic mice. Circulation 2000; 102:28 I-28.

75. Hirota H, Chen J, Betz UA, Rajewsky K, Gu Y, Ross J, Muller W, Chien KR. Loss of a gp130 cardiac muscle cell survival pathway is a critical event in the onset of heart failure during biomechanical stress. Cell 1999; 97:189–198.

76. Yaoita H, Ogawa K, Maehara K, Maruyama Y. Attenuation of ischemia/reperfusion injury in rats by a caspase inhibitor. Circulation 1998; 97:276–281.

77. Holly TA, Drincic A, Byun Y, Nakamura S, Harris K, Klocke FJ, Cryns VL. Caspase inhibition reduces myocyte cell death induced by myocardial ischemia and reperfusion in vivo. J Mol Cell Cardiol 1999; 31:1709–1715.

78. Matsui T, Li L, del Monte F, Fukui Y, Franke T, Hajjar R, Rosenzweig A. Adenoviral gene transfer of activated PI 3-kinase and Akt inhibits apoptosis of hypoxic cardiomyocytes in vitro. Circulation 1999; 100:2373–2379.

79. Matsui T, Tao J, del Monte F, Lee K-H, Li L, Picard M, Force TL, Franke TF, Hajjar RJ, Rosenzweig A. Akt activation preserves cardiac function and prevents injury after transient cardiac ischemia in vivo. Circulation 2001; 104:330–335.

80. Donath MY, Jenni R, Brunner HP, Anrig M, Kohli S, Glatz Y, Froesch ER. Cardiovascular and metabolic effects of insulin-like growth factor I at rest and during exercise in humans. J Clin Endocrinol Metab 1996; 81:4089–4094.

81. Jones JI, Clemmons DR. Insulin-like growth factors and their binding proteins: biological actions. Endocr Rev 1995; 16:3–34.

82. Hankinson SE, Willett WC, Colditz GA, Hunter DJ, Michaud DS, Deroo B, Rosner B, Speizer FE, Pollak M. Circulating concentrations of insulin-like growth factor-I and risk of breast cancer. Lancet 1998; 351:1393–1396.

83. Chan JM, Stampfer MJ, Giovannucci E, Gann PH, Ma J, Wilkinson P, Hennekens CH, Pollak M. Plasma insulin-like growth factor-I and prostate cancer risk: a prospective study. Science 1998; 279:563–566.

84. Rosen CJ, Pollak M. Circulating IGF-I: new perspectives for a new century. Trends Endocrinol Metab 1999; 10:136–141.

85. Chao W, Matsui T, Novikov M, Tao J, Li L, Liu H, Ahn YK, Rosenzweig A. Strategic advantages of IGF-I expression for cardioprotection. J Gen Medicine 2003; 5:277–286.

25
Cellular Transplantation

Philippe Menasché
*Department of Cardiovascular Surgery & INSERM U-633 Hôpital Européen Georges Pompidou
Paris, France*

INTRODUCTION

Over the past decade, cellular transplantation has progressively emerged as a potential new means of repairing infarcted myocardium, particularly in patients who have already exhausted the currently available medical, interventional, and surgical treatment options. The underlying concept is that replacement of irreversibly damaged muscle by new contractile cells should restore functionality in these necrotic areas and subsequently contribute to improvement of global heart function. Because the regenerative capacity of the adult mammalian heart [1,2] is by far too limited to compensate for the loss of cardiac cells resulting from a large infarct, and although attempts at converting the infarcted myocardium into contractile tissue by direct injection of viral vectors encoding the muscle-specific *Myo-D* master gene have been rather disappointing [3], the most clinically relevant approach is considered to be the direct transplantation of exogenously supplied cells. After extensive laboratory work, early clinical trials of surgical autologous skeletal myoblast transplantation was initiated in June, 2000 in heart failure patients [4], and rapidly followed by catheter-based intracoronary delivery of bone marrow–derived stem cells in the setting of acute myocardial infarction [5,6]. These phase I studies have primarily established the feasibility and safety of this novel approach and efficacy remains to be validated by prospective trials, which are under way or in preparation. In parallel, a large amount of experimental work is still mandatory to address some basic issues, particularly those pertaining to the choice of the optimal cell type, the technique most appropriate for intramyocardial cell transfer, and the adjunctive strategies required for optimizing postengraftment cell survival. The chapter will concentrate on these issues before highlighting the major lessons gained from the preliminary clinical trials.

TYPE OF CELLS TO BE CONSIDERED FOR INTRAMYOCARDIAL TRANSPLANTATION

The ''ideal'' cell for transplantation has to meet several stringent criteria: it should be easy to collect and expand, relatively tolerant to ischemia so as to survive in a poorly vascularized scar tissue, and establish connexions with host cardiomyocytes

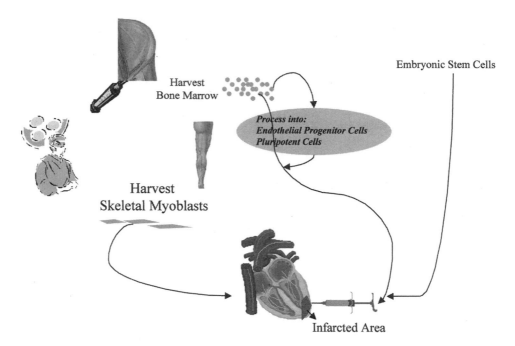

Figure 1   Different sources for stem cells used in cardiac cell transplantation.

allowing its effective and synchronous contribution to heartbeats. Unfortunately, none of the various cell lineages that have been considered so far matches all these require-ments [6a]. (See Fig. 1)

Fetal Cardiomyocytes

Initial studies with fetal and neonatal cardiomyocytes have been pivotal to establish the "proof-of-concept" in that they have showed, in rodent models of coronary artery ligation or cryoinjury-induced myocardial infarction, that these cells successfully engrafted, were coupled with host cardiomyocytes through connexin 43–supported gap junctions, im-proved left ventricular function [7–9] and maintained their cardioprotective effects up to 6 months after transplantation [10]. Additional evidence that transplanted cells could functionally integrate within the host tissue has been brought by the findings that fetal cells harvested from the sino-atrial area exerted a pacemaker activity following their trans-plantation in recipient animals whose conduction system had been irreversibly damaged [11]. However, in a clinical perspective, the transplantation of fetal or neonatal cardiac cells raises significant issues related to ethics, availability, and immunogenicity. In an attempt to overcome these problems, it has been proposed to use xenogenic neonatal cardiomyocytes along with the combined blockade of the CD28/B7 and CD40 costimula-tory pathways, but in spite of encouraging experimental results suggesting the ability of this immunosuppressive regimen to enhance graft survival [12], the clinical relevance of xenogenic Adult cell transplantation remains questionable, and there is currently a good agreement that emphasis should be put on autologous cells. In this context, both skeletal myoblasts and bone marrow–derived cells are particularly attractive "natural" candidates.

Skeletal Myoblasts

Satellite cells can be considered as stem cells for the muscle in that they normally lie in a quiescent state under the basal membrane of skeletal muscular fibers but, following tissue injury, they are rapidly recruited, proliferate (taking the name of myoblasts) and fuse, thereby effecting repair and regeneration of the damaged fibers. In the perspective of clinical applications, these cells feature several attractive characteristics including their autologous origin, a high potential for in vitro expansion, a commitment to their myogenic lineage, which virtually eliminates the oncogenic risk, and a high resistance to ischemia, which is a major advantage given the relatively avascular nature of the postinfarct scars in which they are intended to be implanted. Importantly, our clinical experience shows that neither recovery nor expansion or functionality (i.e., the capacity to generate myofibers) of satellite cells are impeded by advanced age or heart failure. Consequently, we are not convinced that the use of *Myo-D*-transfected fibroblasts as an alternative source of myogenic cells [13] has a true clinical relevance.

Experimental studies have consistently shown that the injected myoblasts differentiated into typical multinucleated cross-striated myotubes, which occupy areas of postinfarction fibrosis [14], but without any evidence for *transdifferentiation* into cardiac cells [15], the only manifestation of a milieu-induced phenotypic change being the emergence of a composite population of fibers that coexpress fast, skeletal muscle-type and slow myosin isoforms [14]. Consequently, and in contrast to fetal cardiomyocytes, engrafted skeletal myotubes do not communicate (at least directly) with host cardiac cells as the expression of the major proteins responsible for mechanical and electrical coupling in the heart (N-cadherin and connexin-43, respectively), although detectable in cultured skeletal myoblasts, is downregulated following intramyocardial grafting [16]. Likewise, our electrophysiological studies show that the membrane properties of engrafted myotubes retain typical skeletal muscle patterns with, for example, action potential durations almost ten times shorter than those of host cardiomyocytes [17].

These observations functionally translate into an improvement in left ventricular function, which has been demonstrated in small and large animal models of myocardial infarction [14,18–21]. The direct contribution of engrafted skeletal myoblasts to the amelioration of the functional outcome is strongly suggested by tissue Doppler imaging studies showing an improvement in the transmyocardial velocity gradients across the infarcted area that has been transplanted [14] and is consistent with the previous finding that function only improves in hearts where implanted cells are detectable [19]. These benefits are sustained over time, as shown by our 1-year echocardiographic values of ejection fraction that were found unchanged from those measured at the 2-month posttransplant time point [22], an effect possibly due to the increased proportion of slow-type myosin expressed by engrafted muscle fibers and the related resistance to fatigue. Importantly, we [23] and others [24] have found that the functional improvement yielded by skeletal myoblast transplantation was tightly dependent on the number of injected cells. Although one study [25] has raised the possibility of cell overgrowth leading to distorsion of the ventricular contours, in clinical practice, the concern would rather be opposite, i.e., that the high rate of early cell death (see following text) reduces graft size to the point that its functional efficacy is not as great as it could be. This relationship between the number of injected cells and the functional outcome should be clarified by the dose-ranging protocol of our ongoing phase II trial.

The mechanism(s) by which myoblast transplantation improves function of the failing heart still remain elusive and different hypotheses can be considered. First, the elastic properties of implanted cells could act as a scaffold that thickens the ventricular wall, which would result in reduced wall stress and limitation of infarct expansion. In our clinical study, however, myoblast transplantation, performed an average of 6 years after the infarct, did not alter end-diastolic volumes. It is, therefore, likely that although early postinfarct cell transplantation may *prevent* ventricular dilatation, it cannot *reverse* remodeling once it is completed. Second, a direct contribution to contractility is suggested by the experimental observations that myoblast transplantation improves *systolic* indices of regional and global left ventricular function, as assessed by pressure-volume loops [22] and tissue Doppler imaging [14], respectively. Furthermore, the pathological findings made in human hearts [26,27] that engrafted myotubes retain typical cross-striations provide an indirect argument for their persisting functionality (nonfunctioning skeletal muscle cells usually feature a disorganized pattern). On the other hand, the lack of connexin – 43 expression on myotubes raises the question of how they could synchronously contract with host cardiomyocytes. In keeping with this observation, our electrophysiological studies [17] have failed to detect coupling between donor and recipient cells but have also shown that, in response to a depolarizing current, grafted myotubes elicited action potentials followed by active contractions. It is, thus, conceivable that in areas where grafted and recipient cells are in close physical contact, myotubes could be excited by direct transmembrane currents (i.e., currents that are not channelled through the classic gap junctions pathway) fired by the neighbouring cardiomyocytes (the so-called field effect).

The finding that grafted myotubes retain both their excitable and contractile properties provides evidence for their viability which, in turn, leads to a third hypothesis by which these cells would increase inotropism of the recipient heart through paracrine effects, i.e., the release of cytokines and/or growth factors acting as signals for resident cardiac stem cells [28] and, therefore, promoting recruitment of new contractile elements. Indeed, the involvement of humoral mediators would be consistent with the results of our sheep experiments showing a reduced collagen density in infarcted areas repopulated by engrafted myoblasts [14] and, therefore, suggesting some effect of these cells on the extracellular matrix. Likewise, the beneficial effects reported after engraftment of Langerhans islets in diabetic patients and fetal cerebral tissue in those suffering from Parkinson's disease are likely related to the secretion of insulin and dopamine by the transplanted cells, respectively. The identification of the mediator(s) released by skeletal myoblasts that could trigger an endogenous myocardial regeneration from the quiescent pool of cardiac resident cells remains to be done, but it is noteworthy that recent data from our laboratory have shown that insulin growth factor-1, a growth factor whose cardioprotective effects have been largely documented [29,30], was produced by myoblasts and myotubes across a wide variety of species, including human beings.

Bone Marrow–Derived Cells

Transplantation of bone marrow cells is raising a growing interest because these cells share with myoblasts the possibility of being used as autografts but also have the presumably additional advantage of a transdifferentiation potential allowing them to convert into cardiac and/or endothelial cells. Indeed, the question is not so much whether bone marrow – derived cells can change their phenotype — there is accumulating experimental evidence that they can. The key issues are to determine whether they incur a transdifferentiation into true cardiomyocytes and, if yes, which populations are responsible for this switch and whether the magnitude of these phenotypic changes can reasonably account for an improvement in function.

Several studies have now reported that bone marrow – derived cells could change their phenotype either in vitro under the influence of specific culture conditions or in vivo in response to cues present in the target organ in which they are implanted. These results, however, have to be analyzed carefully because definite proof of transdifferentiation requires the combination of two strict criteria: accurate lineage determination bringing unequivocal evidence that the transdifferentiated cells really originate from the graft; and phenotypic characterization of these cells relying preferentially on tissue-specific gene markers. Indeed, many reports on the cardiac transdifferentiation of bone-marrow cells have failed to meet these criteria. Assuming, however, that bone- marrow cells feature a plasticity that enables them to change their phenotype, the first basic question is to identify the populations responsible for this conversion. From this standpoint, the bone-marrow cell pool can be broadly divided into two major categories: hematopoietic progenitors and stromal (or mesenchymal) cells.

Hematopoietic progenitors have been reported to "regenerate" the myocardium in rodent models of myocardial infarction where cell transplantation (either intravenous or intramyocardial) was almost consistently done very early (i.e., within a few hours) after the ischemic insult. These results raise two major questions. The first is to identify the progenitor population most appropriate for effecting this regeneration. Thus, Kocher and associates [31] have shown that intravenous injection of human $CD34^+$ cells into athymic nude rats 48 hours after myocardial infarction resulted in angiogenesis, decreased apoptosis in the periinfact region and improved function. Other studies have proposed to use $CD133^+$ progenitors, which are precursors to both endothelial and hematopoietic lineages and are, thus, credited for an angiogenic potential [32]. To further add to the confusion, most $CD133^+$ cells are also positive for the $CD34^+$ antigen, but recent data suggest that the $CD34^-$ fraction of the $CD34^+$ pool would be more effective for engraftment [33]. Importantly, all these subpopulations are present in very small percentages in the circulating blood (2%–3% for the $CD34^+$, about 1% for the $CD133^+$ cells), which expectedly translates into a low rate of engraftment. Thus, in a mouse model of coronary occlusion-reperfusion intravenously injected with hematopoietic stem cells, only 3.3% of the endothelial cells and 0.02% of the cardiomyocytes of the recipient heart were derived from donor cells [34]; likewise, injection of green fluorescence-labeled $CD34^+$ cells into ischemic rat limbs was found to result in minimal incorporation of these cells into capillaries [35]. These data lead to the second question which pertains to the means of scaling-up this small number of progenitors to potentiate their functional benefits. This remains a technical challenge. One option is to try to expand these cells in vitro, but this approach is fraught with the risk that they loose their pluripotentiality. Alternatively, it has been proposed to use a cytokine-based in vivo mobilization. Although this technique has been successful for regenerating infarcted mouse myocardium by Lin-$ckit^{POS}$ cells [36], its application in primates has failed to yield any benefit and concerns have even been expressed about the safety of administering granulocyte colony-stimulating factor in the early phase of myocardial infarction.

A second strategy then consists of using bone marrow mesenchymal cells. In both rat [37] and swine [38] infarction models, these cells have been shown to differentiate into cardiac and blood vessel cells, which correlated with improved regional perfusion and wall motion, greater scar thickness, and augmented global heart function. However, the cardiomyogenic transdifferentiation of these cells is also plagued with clinically relevant issues. Thus, one means of inducing their phenotypic conversion is to culture them in the presence of 5-azacytidine, a DNA demethylating agent expected to raise safety concerns. Using a process that did not involve exposure to 5-azacytidine, Shake and coworkers [39] recently reported that in a swine model of occlusion-reperfusion, intramyo-cardially injected autologous mesenchymal cells only expressed *myogenic* markers, none of which were *cardio*specific, which correlated with an attenuation of regional systolic dysfunction, too limited, however, for affecting ultimate infarct size. Another means of driving mesenchymal cells towards a cardiomyogenic lineage consists of bringing them in direct contact with host cardiomyocytes, which can be achieved through cocultures [40] or coimplantations [41]. Indeed, this concept of a direct cell-to-cell contact for inducing transdifferentiation is quite consistent with what has been previously shown about the cardiomyogenic conversion of endothelial cells [42], and it is strengthened by a recent study showing that human endothelial progenitor cells can also turn to functionally effec-tive cardiomyocytes provided that they are cocultured with rat cardiac cells [43]. However, in the perspective of clinical applications, neither of the two previously mentioned ap-proaches (5-azacytidine pretreatment or cocultures/coimplantations with native xenogenic cardiomyocytes) is likely to be easy to implement. Data are also lacking regarding the quantitative importance of this transdifferentiation phenomenon but a recent study reported a percentage not higher than 1% to 2% after cocultures of human mesenchymal cells with neonatal rat cardiomyocytes [44]. In this setting, a great deal of interest has been raised by the identification of a select subpopulation of multipotent adult pluripotent cells (MAPCs) [45] isolated from the bone-marrow stroma. Whether these cells can be success-fully used for repairing human infarcted myocardium still remains speculative as they are difficult to grow (it takes several weeks) and identify (their phenotypic characterization is only made "by default," i.e., based on a negative staining for the most common surface markers), and their conversion into true cardiomyocytes has not yet been established conclusively.

These uncertainties regarding the choice of the optimal subpopulation for myocardial repair has led several groups to advocate the use of total, unfractionated bone marrow with the premise that, in addition to its simplicity (cells are easily collected from peripheral blood or bone marrow and reinjected immediately or after a few days of cultivation), this technique should have the advantage of fully exploiting the regenerative potential of the mixed cell lineages that comprise the bone marrow through a combined supply of an-giogenic growth factors and their receptors [5,35,46–48]. However, keeping in mind that nobody would give a drug without knowing its exact composition, it can be equally worri-some to inject a poorly characterized cell therapy product. Forthcoming clinical trials should hopefully help define whether this concern is merely academic or not.

From the presented considerations, two major conclusions can be drawn. First, the regenerating effects of bone marrow transplantation are probably maximal when cells are injected early after the infarction, i.e., at a stage where they can find, in a freshly ischemic tissue, the appropriate cues for transdifferentiation. Conversely, it is likely that, at the later stage of the fibrous scar, these signals are lost, except, maybe, in the border zones, which is probably insufficient for yielding a meaningful improvement in function (at worst, injection of bone marrow in the core of the infarcted area could convey a transdifferentia-tion of grafted cells into fibroblasts). In support of this concept, we [49] and others [50] have shown that injection of total unfractionated bone marrow into chronically infarcted myocardium failed to improve function and subsequent transplantation of human CD133[+] progenitors into nude rats equally failed to be more effective than skeletal myoblasts [50a]. Attempts at repopulating nonischemic doxorubicin-injured hearts with mononuclear or sca-1[+] progenitor cells have also been unsuccessful [51]. The second conclusion is that although the conversion of bone marrow cells into cardiomyocytes, as well as the quantita-tive magnitude of this event, are still debatable, there is more compelling evidence for the angiogenic potential of these cells. Interestingly, recent studies [46,47,52] suggest that, in keeping with the paracrine hypothesis mentioned about skeletal myoblasts, this cell-induced angiogenesis is more related to the release of growth factors than to the anatomic incorporation of the grafted cells into foci of neovascularization. Put together, these observations fit a paradigm where bone marrow cell transplantation would be electively targeted at increasing *angiogenesis* in *ischemic* patients, whereas skeletal myoblasts would be indicated for augmentation of *function* in those suffering from *heart failure*.

Embryonic Stem Cells

Embryonic cells are conceptually attractive because their totipotency should make it possible to prepare cardiomyocyte cell lines in vitro before injecting them into myocardial scars. These cells can be derived from fertilized oocytes that are no longer targeted for childbearing; alternatively, they could be obtained after nuclear transfer into enucleated recipient oocytes (therapeutic cloning), which would avoid immune reactions because the grafted cells then recapitulate the whole genetic program of the future recipient. However, apart from the major ethical and regulatory issues raised by this approach, and which are far beyond the scope of this review, the clinical applicability of embryonic cells for cell replacement therapy is plagued by major technical challenges [53] including the purification of specific cell lineages (i.e., ventricular, atrial, or pacemaker cells), in vitro demonstration that the differentiated cells effect normal physiological functions, in vivo confirmation of the efficacy of transplantation in animal models of myocardial infarction, and avoidance of cell-related tumor development (teratoma). In the pivotal study of Kehat and colleagues [54], in which human undifferentiated embryonic stem cells were grown from a single-cell clone, only 8.1% of the embryoid bodies generated from these cells spontaneously contracted and stained positively for cardiac-specific markers, thereby indicating that the first objective of purity, which is fundamental for abrogating the oncogenic potential of residual undifferentiated cells, is still far from being achieved.

METHODS OF CELL DELIVERY

Surgical Approach

This technique entails multiple punctures, a few millimeters apart, in the core and around the borders of the scar, care being taken to inject cells parallel to the epicardium to avoid their inadvertent delivery into the left ventricular cavity (for this purpose, we have designed a 27 gauge prebent needle). Another technical issue is to minimize cell leakage through the needle holes. To address this question, we have found useful to first create subepicardial pockets into which cells are dropped and then to wait for a few seconds before withdrawing the needle to limit the backflow of cells along the needle tracts.

Catheter-Based Approach

In an attempt to reduce the invasiveness of cell transfer, catheter-based techniques have been rapidly developed [54a]. They basically rely on three routes: endoventricular, intracoronary, and transvenous, guidance of cell delivery being achieved with electromagnetic mapping, coronary angiography, and endovascular ultrasounds, respectively. In our experience, the latter technique has been found particularly user-friendly and we are currently testing its potential benefits in a sheep model of myocardial infarction. However, although these percutaneous approaches have been expeditiously applied in patients, they have actually undergone limited preclinical testing. Thus, the extent of intramyocardial cell trapping following endoventricular injections has not been fully investigated, nor is the ability of intracoronarily injected bone marrow cells to gain access to myocardial tissue, even if their transendothelial migration is thought to be enhanced by high-pressure infusion and angioplasty balloon inflation to prevent backflow [5]. Indeed, *viability* of cells following passage through the catheters has usually been assessed but their *functionality* (i.e., ability of skeletal myoblasts and bone-marrow cells to differentiate into myotubes and cardiac/vascular cells, respectively), which is an equally important end point, as well as their long-term survival have often been underlooked. For example, in a recent study [55], follow-up of myoblasts injected through an endoventricular catheter was limited to 10 days. Likewise, there are also limited data regarding the functional efficacy of these techniques and we only found one experimental study [52] in which the effects of transendocardially injected bone marrow cells were extensively investigated. Clearly, there is still much work to be done in this area, particularly for comparing the results of percutaneous cell delivery with that of the surgical approach, which remains the benchmark against which alternate modes of cell transplantation should be tested. This remark does not only apply to percutaneous approaches but also to biografts made of bioresorbable cell-seeded scaffolds, which could represent an effective means of repairing wall defects in adult and pediatric open-heart operations.

The Problem of Cell Death

Regardless of the route of delivery, cell death remains a major problem of cell transplantation common to all cell lineages. Thus, up to 90% of transplanted cardiomyocytes have been shown to die within the first 24 hours [56]; we have made quantitatively similar observations with myoblasts and in the study of Toma and associates [57], the 4-day survival rate of human mesenchymal cells injected into *normal* (noninfarcted) mice only averaged 0.44%. The mechanisms of this high death rate are multiple and include particularly physical strain during injections, ischemia due to the poor vascularity of the target scar, and apoptosis. As it is uncertain whether multiplication of surviving cells can catch up to this initially high attrition rate, the development of cell survival-enhancing strategies appears critical for optimizing the functional benefits of the procedure. Two of them are of potentially great clinical relevance. The first consists of enhancing angiogenesis to limit the ischemic component of cell death, an approach based on the observation that the survival of cardiomyocytes grafted into highly vascularized granulation tissue is two-fold greater than that observed after grafting into acutely necrotic myocardium [56]. In practice, increased angiogenesis can be achieved by pretransplantation transfection of cells with genes encoding vascular growth factors [58], direct coinjection of these factors [59] or concomitant revascularization of cell-transplanted segments (an approach which appears sound but only be confirmed when efficacy is demonstrated by ongoing randomized trials committed to avoiding bypass surgery in these segments to avoid confounding factors in the interpretation of outcome measures). The second strategy aimed at increasing the survival rate of transplanted cells relies on limitation of apoptosis, which can be successfully achieved by heat shocking cells just prior to their implantation [56]. Finally, it is also likely that even though an immune response is unlikely to occur in the case of autologous transplantation, the inflammatory state created by needle punctures can contribute to cell damage. This mechanism is expected to be still greater if it superimposes upon the inflammation that occurs during the early phase of infarction. Conversely, late injections may equally reduce the effectiveness of the procedure if they are performed once the remodeling process has been completed. These observations suggest that there is probably an optimal time window for cell transplantation following myocardial infarction and that bracketing this time frame is another means of optimizing the benefits of the procedure.

ANALYSIS OF EARLY CLINICAL DATA

Skeletal myoblasts

On June 15, 2000, we performed the first human transplantation of autologous skeletal myoblasts [4]. The operation was uneventful, the cardiac condition markedly improved, including the scarred segment which had been grafted, and the patient died 18 months later from a stroke. At autopsy, myotubes were identified in scar tissue and found to express in roughly similar proportions fast, slow, and composite (fast and slow) myosin isoforms [26]. This operation was the first of a series of 10 [61], designed to assess the feasibility and safety of the procedure and included patients meeting the following three criteria: severe left ventricular dysfunction (ejection fraction ≤ 0.35); history of myocardial infarct with a residual discrete, echocardiographically akinetic (after dobutamine challenge) and metabolically nonviable scar (as assessed by fluorodeoxyglucose positron emission tomography); and indication for concomitant coronary artery bypass grafting in remote (i.e., different from the transplanted area), ischemic myocardium. Since then, two other series have been reported, one [62] in Poland (10 patients) and the other [63] in the United States (16 patients). Similar to the protocol of our phase I trial, all these patients underwent cell transplantation during a conventional coronary artery bypass operation, except for five of the American study who underwent placement of a left ventricular assist device at the time of cell transplantation with the objective of assessing the fate of the engrafted cells at the time of subsequent transplantation [27]. Finally, catheter-based endoventricular or transvenous myoblast transplantations have also been performed in Europe as part of both physican-driven and industry-sponsored trials and, based on the presentation made by P. Serruys at the TCT meeting in October, 2002, totalled 13 patients before the study was stopped because of serious adverse events (it has then been reinitiated after protocol changes).

The protocol of the surgical procedure that we originally designed (and which has remained unchanged over time) is fairly straightforward and involves three steps: a biopsy of the *vastus lateralis* retrieved from the thigh under local anesthesia; a 2- to 3-week period of cell expansion and the reimplantation of the final cell yield concentrated in a small volume (5–6 mL) in and around the postinfarct scar while remote ischemic areas are revascularized by bypass grafts.

Overall, these phase I trials have now established the feasibility of the procedure, i.e., the possibility of growing hundreds million of cells (an average of 871×10^6 cells were injected in our study, of which 86% were identified as myogenic by specific antibodies and 90% were viable at the time of the final collection), in compliance with Good Medical Practice standards and within a clinically relevant time frame (2–3 weeks). The operation, by itself, has also turned out to be safe, without specific procedure-related complications, while companion experiments have documented the persisting functionality of myoblasts harvested from heart failure patients (i.e., their ability to differentiate in vitro into myotubes when allowed to grow to confluence) as well as their lack of oncogenic potential (when injected into immunodeficient mice). The only adverse event ascribed to cell transplantation is sustained ventricular tachycardia, which has occurred in some patients (and presumably caused two deaths in the catheter-based trial). These arrhythmias have been documented within the first postoperative weeks, with a seemingly low rate of late recurrences, as demonstrated by interrogation of the automatic internal cardioverter-defibrillator (AICD) implanted in these cases. The mechanism of these arrhythmias is being investigated and although the involvement of inflammatory reactions (triggered by needle punctures and cell injections) would fit their early posttransplantation timing of onset, we rather favor the hypothesis that differences in action potential duration between engrafted myotubes and native cardiomyocytes [17] provide a substrate for microreentry circuits. This hypothesis could account for the efficacy of amiodarone [61,62] to blunt these arrhythmias since one of the mechanisms of action of this drug is to reduce repolarization dispersion [64]. The arrhythmogenic potential of engrafted myotubes might be further enhanced by their capacity to generate depolarizing rebounds from which bursts of action potentials can be fired and interfere with those of host cardiomyocytes in areas where the two cell populations are not insulated by scar tissue but close enough (which is not unlikely given the patchy pattern of human infarcts) to allow electrotonic currents to be operative. Regardless of the mechanism, and even if data derived from phase I studies do not conclusively establish a causal relationship between cell transplantation and arrhythmias, in particular in a patient population particularly susceptible to this complication, it has been considered safe by most investigators to include implantation of AICDs in the protocol of phase II studies. In addition to providing protection against the potential proarrhythmic risk of cell grafting, the device may offer long-term survival benefits in this high-risk subset of heart failure patients [65] while its interrogation should yield useful information about the true incidence of these arrhythmias by comparison with control placebo-injected groups.

The small number of patients operated on so far, the lack of control groups, and the confounding effect of concomitant revascularization clearly preclude any definite conclusion pertaining to the efficacy of the procedure. It is, encouraging, however, that in our series [61] approximately 60% of the cell-implanted scar areas demonstrated a new postoperative systolic thickening that did not deteriorate over the 1- to 2.5-year follow-up, whereas at most 10% of segments meeting their inclusion criteria (lack of contractile reserve and of metabolic viability) would have been expected to improve following bypass surgery alone. Efficacy data are more difficult to interpret in the US dose-escalating adjunct-to-bypass trial, in that the number of injected cells peaked at the relatively low value of 300 million [63]. The same caveat applies to the series of Siminiak et al. [62]. Put together, however, these data are encouraging enough to warrant further confirmation by randomized phase II trials designed and powered so as to demonstrate efficacy, if any. It is in this context that we started in November 2002 a multicenter dose-ranging study (the Myoblast Autograft Grafting in Ischemic Cardiomyopathy [MAGIC] trial) planned to include 300 patients with severe postinfarction left ventricular dysfunction (ejection fraction $\leq 35\%$), a residual akinetic scar not amenable to revascularization, and an indication of bypass in remote ischemic areas. These patients will be randomized into three groups (a placebo group receiving injections of culture medium and two transplanted cohorts differing by the number of injected cells) and the echocardiographic centralized and blinded assessment at 6 months of contractile changes in cell-grafted nonrevascularized myocardial segments (primary end point) should hopefully allow meaningful conclusions about the efficacy of the procedure.

Bone Marrow-Derived Cells

The number of clinical studies of bone-marrow cell transplantation is growing tremendously, with some of them being reported in peer-reviewed journals while others are limited to isolated and anectodal cases agressively announced through Internet-mediated press releases. So far, surgical approaches have entailed intramyocardial implantation of bone marrow mononuclear cells [66] or CD133$^+$ progenitors [67] at the time of concomitant coronary artery bypass grafting whereas catheter-based approaches have consisted of intracoronary injections of mononuclear cells coupled with balloon angioplasty and stenting in patients with acute myocardial infarction [5,6] or endoventricular stand-alone injections in ischemic patients targeted for increased angiogenesis [68]. Overall, these phase I studies should be credited for documenting the feasibility of the procedure, the apparent lack of adverse events, and the similarity of results with both blood-derived and bone marrow–derived cells [6]. The claims for efficacy, based on improved perfusion and function, are more questionable in the absence of control randomized groups of patients, particularly if one keeps in mind the powerful placebo effect seen in end-stage ischemic heart disease—a remark equally relevant to the previously mentioned trials of skeletal myoblast transplantation. Hopefully, a forthcoming phase II trial involving intracoronary injections of bone marrow (fresh or briefly cultivated) or placebo solution in patients with acute myocardial infarction should allow more objective assessment of the expected benefits of this modality of cell therapy.

The recent observation [47] that the majority of endothelial progenitor cells are derived from the monocyte/macrophage pathway [47] also makes it clinically relevant to know whether injection of these cells, alone or as part of the mononuclear cell mix, carries a specific risk related to the recognized role of macrophages in atherosclerotic plaque instability and rupture.

In conclusion, cellular transplantation appears as a promising means of ''rejuvenating'' infarcted myocardium through the engraftment of cells that may positively affect heart function by various mechanisms involving elastic, contractile, and paracrine effects. Although still scarce, laboratory investigations also suggest that the regenerating capacity of the transplanted cells could also be relevant to nonischemic cardiomyopathies [69,70], thereby contributing to expanding the potential for cell replacement therapy. As mentioned in this review, several basic issues remain to be addressed to better characterize the optimal cell type, define the most effective mode and timing of cell delivery, optimize graft survival and understand the mechanism(s) of action of the donor cells. In parallel, the initial encouraging efficacy data collected in a still limited number of patients need to be validated by large prospective randomized trials complying with the stringent methodologic rules commonly applied to drug trials. Only such an approach will conclusively establish whether the hopes currently raised by cellular transplantation are met, to what extent the cell-related regeneration process affects patient function and clinical outcome and, consequently, the place this novel strategy may occupy within the armamentarium of techniques designed to treat heart failure.

ADDENDUM

Since the time of this writing, three important clinical studies have been published. One entailed surgical implantation of skeletal myoblasts (71) and reported improved functional outcomes without adverse events but interpretation of the data is confounded by the fact that the cell-transplanted segments were also concomitantly revascularized. Two other studies have looked at the effects of bone marrow-derived mononuclear (72) or mesenchymal stem cells (73) injected directly into the coronary arteries shortly after myocardial infarction. The strength of these two trials is that they have been randomized although only the latter included a placebo-controlled group. Both have reported improvement in function and perfusion, thereby supporting the concept that these cell types may be beneficial in acutely infarcted patients undergoing concomitant revascularization of the culprit vessel. Their conclusions, however, still require validation by additional, larger-scale placebo-controlled, double-blind randomized trials.

REFERENCES

1. Kajstura J, Leri A, Finato N, Di Loreto C, Beltrami CA. Myocyte proliferation in end stage cardiac failure in humans. Proc Natl Acad Sci USA 1998; 95:8801–8805.

2. Beltrami AP, Urbanek K, Kajstura J, Yan SM, Finato N, Bussani R, Nadal-Ginard B, Silvestri F, Leri A, Beltrami CA, Anversa P. Evidence that human cardiac myocytes divide after myocardial infarction. N Engl J Med 2001; 344:1750–1757.

3. Leor J, Prentice H, Sartorelli V, Quinones MJ, Patterson M, Kedes LK, Kloner RA. Gene transfer and cell transplant: an experimental approach to repair a 'broken heart'. Cardiovasc Res 1997; 35:431–441.

4. Menasché P, Hagège AA, Scorsin M, Pouzet B, Desnos M, Duboc D, Schwartz K, Vilquin JT, Marolleau JP. Clinical myoblast transplantation for heart failure. Lancet 2001; 367:279–280.

5. Strauer BE, Brehm M, Zeus T, Kostering M, Hernandez A, Sorg RV, Kogler G, Wernet P. Repair of infarcted myocardium by autologous intracoronary mononuclear bone marrow cell transplantation in humans. Circulation 2002; 106:1913–1918.

6. Assmus B, Schachinger V, Teupe C, Britten M, Lehmann R, Dobert N, Grunwald F, Aicher A, Urbich C, Martin H, Hoelzer D, Dimmeler S, Zeiher AM. Transplantation of progenitor cells and regeneration enhancement in acute myocardial infarction (TOPCARE-AMI). Circulation 2002:3009–3017.

6a. Struver BE, Kornowski R. Stem cell therapy in perspective. Circulation 2003; 107:929–934.

7. Leor J, Patterson M, Quinones MJ, Kedes LH, Kloner RA. Transplantation of fetal myocardial tissue into the infarcted myocardium of rat. Circulation 1996; 94(suppl II):II-332–II-336.

8. Scorsin M, Hagege AA, Marotte F, Mirochnik N, Copin H, Barnoux M, Sabri A, Samuel JL, Rappaport L, Menasche P. Does transplantation of cardiomyocytes improve function of infarcted myocardium. Circulation 1997; 96(suppl II):II-188–II-193.

9. Li RK, Jia ZQ, Weisel RD, Mickle DA, Zhang J, Mohabeer MK, Rao V, Ivanov J. Cardiomyocyte transplantation improves heart function. Ann Thorac Surg 1996; 62:654–661.

10. Muller-Ehmsen J, Peterson KL, Kedes L, Whittaker P, Dow JS, Long TI, Laird PW, Kloner RA. Long term survival of transplanted neonatal rat cardiomyocytes after myocardial infarction and effect on cardiac function. Circulation 2002; 105:1720–1726.

11. Ruhparwar A, Tebbenjohanns J, Niehaus M, Mengel M, Irtel T, Kofidis T, Pichlmaier AM, Haverich A. Transplanted fetal cardiomyocytes as cardiac pacemaker. Eur J Cardiothoracic Surg 2002; 21:853–857.

12. Li TS, Hamano K, Kajiwara K, Nishida M, Zempo N, Esato K. Prolonged survival of xenograft fetal cardiomyocytes by adenovirus-mediated CTLA4-Ig expression. Transplantation 2001; 72:1983–1985.

13. Etzion S, Barbash IM, Feinberg MF, Zarin P, Miller L, Guetta E, Holbova R, Kloner RA, Kedes LH, Leor J. Cellular cardiomyoplasty of cardiac fibroblasts by adenoviral delivery of *MyoD* ex vivo: an unlimited source of cells for myocardial repair. Circulation 2002; 106(suppl I):I-125–I-130.

14. Ghostine S, Carrion C, Guarita Souza LC, Richard P, Bruneval P, Vilquin JT, Pouzet B, Schwartz K, Menasché P, Hagège AA. Long-term efficacy of myoblast transplantation on regional structure and function after myocardial infarction. Circulation 2002; 106(suppl I): I-131–I-136.

15. Reinecke H, Poppa V, Murry CE. Skeletal muscle stem cells do not transdifferentiate into cardiomyocytes after cardiac grafting. J Mol Cell Cardiol 2002; 34:241–249.

16. Reinecke H, MacDonald GH, Hauschka SD, Murry CE. Electromechanical coupling between skeletal and cardiac muscle: implications for infarct repair. J Cell Biol 2000; 149:731–740.

17. Léobon B, Garcin I, Menasché P, Vilquin JT, Audinat E, Charpak S. Myoblasts transplanted into rat infarcted myocardium are functionally isolated from their host. Proc Natl Acad Sci USA. 2003; 100:7808–7811.

18. Kao RL, Chin TK, Ganote CE, Hossler FE, Li C, Browder W. Satellite cell transplantation to repair injured myocardium. CVR 2000; 1:31–42.

19. Taylor DA, Atkins BZ, Hungspreugs P, Jones TR, Reedy MC, Hutcheson KA, Glower DD, Kraus WE. Regenerating functional myocardium: improved performance after skeletal myoblast transplantation. Nat Medi 1998; 4:929–933.

20. Rajnoch C, Chachques JC, Berrebi A, Bruneval P, Benoit MO, Carpentier A. Cellular therapy reverses myocardial dysfunction. J Thorac Cardiovasc Surg 2001; 121:871–878.

21. Jain M, DerSimonian H, Brenner DA, Ngoy S, Teller P, Edge AS, Zawadzka A, Wetzel K, Sawyer DB, Colucci WS, Apstein CS, Liao R. Cell therapy attenuates deleterious ventricular remodeling and improves cardiac performance after myocardial infarction. Circulation 2001; 103:1920–1927.

22. Al Attar N, Carrion C, Ghostine S, Garcin I, Vilquin JT, Hagège AA, Menasché P. Long-term (1 year) functional and histological results of autologous skeletal muscle cells transplantation in rat. Cardiovasc Res 2003; 58:142–148.

23. Pouzet B, Vilquin JT, Hagege AA, Scorsin M, Messas E, Fiszman M, Schwartz K, Menasché P. Factors affecting functional outcome after autologous skeletal myoblast transplantation. Ann Thorac Surg 2001; 71:844–851.

24. Tambara K, Sakakibara Y, Sakaguchi G, Premaratne GU, Lin X, Nishimura K, Komeda M. Transplanted skeletal myoblasts can fully replace the infarcted myocardium when they survive in the host in large numbers. [abstr]. Circulation 2002; 106(suppl II):II-549.

25. Reinecke H, Murry CE. Transmural replacement of myocardium after skeletal myoblast grafting into the heart: too much of a good thing?. Cardiovasc Pathol 2000; 9:337–344.

26. Hagège AA, Carrion C, Menasché P, Vilquin JT, Duboc D, Marolleau JP, Desnos M, Bruneval P. Autologous skeletal myoblast grafting in ischemic cardiomyopathy. Clinical validation of long-term cell viability and differentiation. Lancet 2003; 361:491–492.

27. Pagani F, DerSimonian R, Zawadska A, Wetzel K, Edge ASB, Jacoby DB, Dinsmore JH, Wright S, Aretz TH, Eisen HJ, Aaronson KD. Autologous skeletal myoblasts transplanted to ischemia damaged myocardium in humans. J Am Coll Cardiol 2003; 41:879–888.

28. Anversa P, Nadal-Ginard B. Myocyte renewal and ventricular remodelling. Nature 2002; 415:240–243.

29. Wang PH. Roads to survival. Insulin-like growth factor-1 signaling pathways in cardiac muscle. Circ Res 2001; 88:552–554.

30. Welch S, Plank D, Witt S, Glascock B, Schaefer E, Chimenti S, Andreoli AM, Limana F, Leri A, Kajstura J, Anversa P, Sussman MA. Cardiac-specific IGF-1 expression attenuates dilated cardiomyopathy in tropomodulin-expressing transgenic mice. Circ Res 2002; 90: 641–648.

31. Kocher AA, Schuster MD, Szabolcs MJ, Takuma S, Burkhoff D, Wang J, Homma S, Edwards NM, Itescu S. Neovascularization of ischemic myocardium by human bone-marrow-derived angioblasts prevents cardiomyocyte apoptosis, reduces remodeling and improves cardiac function. Nat Med 2001; 4:430–436.

32. Quirici N, Soligo D, Caneva L, Servida F, Bossolasco P, Deliliers GL. Differentiation and expansion of endothelial cells from human bone marrow CD133⁺ cells. Br J Haematol 2001; 115:186–194.

33. Kuci S, Wessels JT, Buehring HJ, Schilbach K, Schumm M, Seitz G, Loeffler J, Bader P, Sclegel PG, Niethammer D, Handgretinger R. Idetification of a novel class of human adherent CD34- stem cells that give rise to SCID-repopulating cells. Blood 2003; 10:869–876.

34. Jackson KA, Majka SM, Wang H, Pocius J, Hartley CJ, Majesky MW, Entman ML, Michael LH, Hirschi KK, Goodell MA. Regeneration of ischemic cardiac muscle and vascular endothelium by adult stem cells. J Clin Invest 2001; 107:1395–1402.

35. Iba O, Matsubara H, Nozawa Y, Fujiyama S, Amano K, Mori Y, Kojima H, Iwasaka T. Angiogenesis by implantation of peripheral blood mononuclear cells and platelets into ischemic limbs. Circulation 2002; 106:2019–2025.

36. Orlic D, Kajstura J, Chimenti S, Limana F, Jakoniuk I, Quaini F, Nadal-Ginard B, Bodine DM, Leri A, Anversa P. Mobilized bone marrow cells repair the infarcted heart, improving function and survival. Proc Natl Acad Sci USA 2001; 98:10344–10349.

37. Tomita S, Li RK, Weisel RD. Autologous transplantation of bone marrow cells improves damaged heart function. Circulation 1999; 100(suppl II):II-247–II-256.

38. Tomita S, Mickle DA, Weisel RD, Jia ZQ, Tumiati LC, Allidina Y, Liu P, Li RK. Improved heart function with myogenesis and angiogenesis after autologous porcine bone marrow stromal cell transplantation. J Thorac Cardiovasc Surg 2002; 123:1132–1140.

39. Shake JG, Gruber PJ, Baumgartner WA, Senechal G, Meyers J, Redmond JM, Pittenger MF, Martin BJ. Mesenchymal stem cell implantation in a swine myocardial infarct model: engraftment and functional effects. Ann Thorac Surg 2002; 73:1919–1926.

40. Rangappa S, Entwistle JWC, Wechsler AS. Cardiomyocytes can induce human mesenchymal cells to express cardiac phenotype and genotype [asbtr]. Circulation 2002; 106(suppl II):II-235.

41. Min JY, Sullivan MF, Yang Y, Zhang JP, Converso KL, Morgan JP, Xiao XF. Significant improvement of heart function by cotransplantationof human mesenchymal stem cells and fetal cardiomyocytes in postinfarcted pigs. Ann Thorac Surg 2002; 74:1568–1575.

42. Condorelli G, Borello U, De Angelis L, Latronico M, Sirabella D, Coletta M, Galli R, Balconi G, Follenzi A, Frati G, Cusella de Angelis MG, Gioglio L, Amuchastegui S, Adorini D, Nalini L, Vescovi A, Dejana E, Cossu G. Cardiomyocyte induce endothelial cells to transdifferentiate into cardiac muscle: implications for myocardium regeneration. Proc Natl Acad Sci USA 2001; 98:10733–10738.

43. Badorff C, Brandes RP, Popp R, Rupp S, Urbich C, Aicher A, Fleming I, Busse R, Zeiher AM, Dimmeler S. Transdifferentiation of blood-derived human adult endothelial progenitor cells into functionally active cardiomyocytes. Circulation 2003; 107:1024–1032.

44. Kahill KS, Pittenger MF, Byrne BJ. Differentiation of human mesenchymal stem cells to cardiomyocytes by co-culture [abstr]. Circulation 2002; 106(suppl II):II-198.

45. Jiang Y, Jahagirdar BN, Reinhardt RL, Schwartz RE, Keene CD, Ortiz-Gonzalez XR, Reyes M, Lenvik T, Lund T, Blackstad M, Du J, Aldrich S, Lisberg A, Low WC, Largaespada DA, Verfaillie CM. Pluripotency of mesenchymal stem cells derived from adult marrow. Nature 2002; 418:41–49.

46. Kamihata H, Matsubara H, Nishiue T, Fujiyama S, Tsutsumi Y, Ozono R, Masaki H, Mori Y, Iba O, Tateishi E, Kosaki A, Shintani S, Murohara T, Imaizumi T, Iwasaka T. Implantation of bone marrow mononuclear cells into ischemic myocardium enhances collateral perfusion and regional function via side-supply of angioblasts, angiogenic ligands, and cytokines. Circulation 2001; 104:1046–1052.

47. Rehman J, Li J, Orschell CM, March KL. Peripheral blood "endothelial progenitor cells" are derived from monocytes/macrophages and secrete angiogenic growth factors. Circulation 2003; 107:1164–1169.

48. Tateishi-Yuyama E, Matsubara H, Murohara T, Ikeda U, Shintani S, Masaki H, Amano K, Kishimoto Y, Yoshimoto K, Akashi H, Shimada K, Iwasaka T, Imaizumi T. Therapeutic Angiogenesis using Cell Transplantation (TACT) Study Investigators. Therapeutic angiogenesis for patients with limb ischaemia by autologous transplantation of bone-marrow cells: a pilot study and a randomised controlled trial. Lancet 2002; 360:427–435.

49. Bel A, Messas E, Agbulut O, Richard P, Samuel JL, Bruneval P, Hagege AA, Menasche P. Transplantation of autologous fresh bone marrow into infarcted myocardium. Circulation 2003; 108(suppl II):II-247–252.

50. Hamano K, Li TS, Kobayashi T, Hirata K, Yano M, Kohno M, Matsuzaki M. Therapeutic angiogenesis induced by local autologous bone marrow cell implantation. Ann Thorac Surg 2002; 73:1210–1215.

50a. Agbulut O, Vandervelde S, Al Attar N, Larghero J, Ghostine S, Léobon B, Robidel E, Borsani P, Le Lor'ch M, Bissery A, Chomienne C, Bruneval P, Marolleau JP, Vilquin JT, Hagège A, Sameul JL, Menasché PH. Comparison of human skeletal myoblasts and bone marrow-derived CD133+ progenitors for repair of infarted myocardium. J Am Coll Cardiol 2004; 44:458-463.

51. Agbulut O, Menot ML, Li Z, Marotte F, Paulin D, Hagège A, Chomienne C, Rappaport L, Samuel JL, Menasché P. Temporal patterns of bone marrow cell differentiation following transplantation in nonischemic cardiomyopathy. Cardiovasc Res 2003; 58:451–459.

52. Fuchs S, Baffour R, Zhou YF, Shou M, Pierre A, Tio FO, Weissman NJ, Leon M, Epstein SE, Kornowski R. Transendocardial delivery of autologous bone marrow enhances collateral perfusion and regional function in pigs with chronic experimental myocardial ischemia. J Am Coll Cardiol 2001; 37:1726–1732.

53. Odorico JS, Kaufman DS, Thomson JA. Multilineage differentiation from human embryonic stem cell lines. Stem Cells 2001; 19:193–204.

54. Kehat I, Kenyagin-Karsenti D, Snir M, Segev H, Amit M, Gepstein A, Livne E, Binah O, Itskovitz-Eldor J, Gepstein L. Human embryonic stem cells can differentiate into myocytes with structural and functional properties of cardiomyocytes. J Clin Invest 2001; 108:407–414.

54a. Thompson CA, Nasseri BA, Makower J, Houser S, McGarry M, Lamson T, Pumerantseva I, Chang JY, Gold HZ, Vacanti JP, Oesterle SN. Percutaneous transvenous cellular cardiomyoplasty. A novel nonsurgical approach for myocardial cell transplantation. J Am Coll Cardiol 2003; 41:1964–1971.

55. Dib N, Diethrich EB, Campbell A, Goodwin N, Robinson B, Gilbert J, Hobohm DW, Taylor DA. Endoventricular transplantation of allogenic skeletal myoblasts in a porcine model of myocardial infarction. J Endovasc Ther 2002; 9:313–319.

56. Zhang M, Methot D, Poppa V, Fujio Y, Walsh K, Murry CE. Cardiomyocyte grafting for cardiac repair: graft cell death and anti-death strategies. J Mol Cell Cardiol 2001; 33:907–921.

57. Toma C, Pittenger MF, Cahill KS, Byrne JB, Kessler PD. Human mesenchymal stem cells differentiate to a cardiomyocyte phenotype in the adult murine heart. Circulation 2002; 105: 93–98.

58. Suzuki K, Murtuza B, Smolenski RT, Sammut IA, Suzuki N, Kaneda Y, Yacoub MH. Cell transplantation for the treatment of acute myocardial infarction using vascular endothelial growth factor-expressing skeletal myoblasts. Circulation 2001; 104(suppl I):207–I-212.

59. Sakakibara Y, Nishimura K, Tambara K, Yamamoto M, Lu F, Tabata Y, Komeda M. Prevascularization with gelatin microspheres containing basic fibroblast growth factor enhances the benefits of cardiomyocyte transplantation. J Thorac Cardiovasc Surg 2002; 124:50–56.

60. Suzuki K, Smolenski RT, Jayakumar J, Murtuza B, Brand NJ, Yacoub MH. Heat shock treatment enhances graft cell survival in skeletal myoblast transplantation to the heart. Circulation 2000; 102(suppl III):III-216–III-221.

61. Menasché P, Hagège AA, Vilquin JT, Desnos M, Abergel E, Pouzet B, Bel A, Sarateanu S, Scorsin M, Schwartz K, Bruneval P, Benbunan M, Marolleau JP, Duboc D. Autologous skeletal myoblast transplantation for severe postinfarction left ventricular dysfunction. J Am Coll Cardiol 2003; 41:1078–1083.

62. Siminiak T, Kalawski R, Fiszer D, Jerzykowska O, Rozwadowska N, Rzeniczak J, Kurpisz M. Transplantation of autologous skeletal myoblasts in the treatment of patients with postinfarction heart failure. Early results of phase I clinical trial [abstr]. Circulation 2002; 106(suppl II):II-626.

63. Dib N, McCarthy P, Dinsmore J, Yeager M, Pagani FD, Wright S, McLellan WR, Fonarow G, Eisen HJ, Furukawa S, Michler RE, Buchele D, Ghazoul M, Diethrich EB. Safety and feasibility of autologous myoblast transplantation in patients with ischemic cardiomyopathy: interim analysis from the United States experience [abstr]. Circulation 2002; 106(suppl II): II-463.

64. Drouin E, Lande G, Charpentier F. Amiodarone reduces transmural heterogeneity of repolarization in the human heart. J Am Coll Cardiol 1998; 32:1063–1067.

65. Moss AJ, Zareba W, Hall WJ, Klein H, Wilber DJ, Cannon DS, Daubert JP, Higgins SL, Brown MW, Andrews ML. The Multicenter Automatic Defibrillator Implantation Trial II Investigators. Prophylactic implantation of a defibrillator in patients with myocardial infarction and reduced ejection fraction. New Engl J Med 2002; 346:877–883.

66. Hamano H, Nishida M, Hirata K, Mikamo A, Li TS, Harada M, Miura T, Matsusaki M, Esato K. Local implantation of autologous bone marrow cells for therapeutic angiogenesis

in patients with ichemic heart disease. Clinical trial and preliminary results. Jpn Circ J 2001; 65:845–847.

67. Stamm C, Westphal B, Kleine HD, Petzsch M, Kittner C, Klinge H, Schümichen C, Nienaber CA, Freund M, Steinhoff G. Autologous bone-marrow stem-cell transplantation for myocardial regeneration. Lancet 2003; 361:45–46.

68. Tse HF, Kwong YM, Chan JKF, Lo G, Ho CL, Lau CP. Angiogenesis in ischaemic myocardium by intramyocardial autologous bone marrow mononuclear cell implantation. Lancet 2003; 361:47–49.

69. Yoo KJ, Li RK, Weisel RD, Mickle DA, Jia ZQ, Kim EJ, Tomita S, Yau TM. Heart cell transplantation improves heart function in dilated cardiomyopathic hamsters. Circulation 2000; 102(suppl III):III-204–III-209.

70. Scorsin M, Hagege AA, Dolizy I, Marotte F, Mirochnik N, Copin H, Barnoux M, le Bert M, Samuel JL, Rappaport L, Menasche P. Can cellular transplantation improve function in doxorubicin-induced heart failure?. Circulation 1998; 98(suppl II):II-151–II-156.

71. Herreros J, Prosper F, Perez A, Gavira JJ, Garcia-Velloso MJ, Barba J, Sanchez PL, Canizo C, Rabago G, Marti-Climent JM, Hernandez M, Lopez-Holgado N, Gonzalez-Santos JM, Martin-Luengo C, Alegria E. Autologous intramyocardial injection of cultured skeletal muscle-derived stem cells in patients with non-acute myocardial infarction. Eur Heart J 2003; 24:2012–2020.

72. Wollert KC, Meyer GP, Lotz J, Ringes-Lichtenberg S, Lippolt P, Breidenbach C, Fichtner S, Korte T, Hornig B, Messinger D, Arseniev L, Hertenstein B, Ganser A, Drexler H. Intracoronary autologous bone-marrow cell transfer after myocardial infarction: the BOOST randomised controlled clinical trial. Lancet 2004; 364:141–148.

73. Chen SL, Fang WW, Ye F, Liu YH, Qian J, Shan SJ, Zhang JJ, Chunhua RZ, Liao LM, Lin S, Sun JP. Effect on left ventricular function of intracoronary transplantation of autologous bone marrow mesenchymal stem cell in patients with acute myocardial infarction. Am J Cardiol 2004; 94:92–95.

Index